Sang-Do Lee
Editor

COPD

Heterogeneity and Personalized Treatment

Springer

Editor
Sang-Do Lee
Department of Pulmonary and Critical Care Medicine
Asan Medical Center University
of Ulsan College of Medicine
Seoul
South Korea

ISBN 978-3-662-47177-7 ISBN 978-3-662-47178-4 (eBook)
DOI 10.1007/978-3-662-47178-4

Library of Congress Control Number: 2017947875

Printed on acid-free paper

This Springer imprint is published by Springer Nature
The registered company is Springer-Verlag GmbH Germany
The registered company address is: Heidelberger Platz 3, 14197 Berlin, Germany

COPD

Preface

Chronic obstructive pulmonary disease (COPD) is a leading cause of morbidity and mortality worldwide. Over the last few decades, the study of COPD has become one of the most rapidly developing fields in medicine. The recent years have provided clinicians and researchers with major advances in the understanding of underlying mechanisms in COPD. In the past decades, COPD was classified solely on the basis of the degree of airflow limitation. Nowadays, COPD is regarded as a heterogeneous disease, with multiple etiological factors, clinical phenotypes, and comorbidities. One of the main reasons for poor understanding and poor treatment is the heterogeneity of COPD. The strategy for the management of COPD is moving toward a more personalized approach compared with the historical approach. Dissecting the heterogeneity would lead to a better understanding and effective personalized treatment of COPD.

Airway Vista, also known as Chronic Obstructive Airway Diseases Symposium, has been hosted by the Obstructive Lung Disease Research Foundation in South Korea since 2008. This academic event is designed to offer respiratory health professionals new horizons in their understanding of COPD and asthma. The scientific program of the symposium includes the most significant advances in the researches of chronic airway diseases, COPD, asthma, and pulmonary functional imaging. We have held Airway Vista successfully every year, featuring more than 50 world-renowned speakers respectively. This year (2017) has marked the 10th anniversary of Airway Vista. To celebrate the achievements of this 10-year-old symposium, we decided to publish a textbook by gathering the contents of previous symposium programs. We have tried to provide readers with an overview of COPD, the current understanding of its pathobiology, and a contemporary approach to diagnosis and treatment. With this goal in mind, a group of experts took the task of developing this publication, focusing on essential issues that all providers should be aware of.

The first chapter of this book covers overviews of COPD which include the current definition, epidemiology, risk factors, and pathogenesis of COPD. The second chapter is comprised of diagnosis and assessment given to COPD patients. In Chap. 3, COPD heterogeneity was described in a clinical phenotype as well as radiological and genetic aspects. Various pharmacological and nonpharmacological management strategies are reviewed based on evidence in the fourth chapter. The final chapter outlines a future perspective on COPD.

This book presents state-of-the-art knowledge on issues related to heterogeneity, such as phenotypes (clinical, physiological, radiological, etc.), genotypes, tools to be used for dissecting heterogeneity (CT/MRI/Scan, Biomarkers etc.), and tailored treatment strategies in each subgroup of patients. Especially, radiologic imaging is a new promising tool for this issue and will be presented in detail with numerous figures. A further key feature is presentation about the current and future treatment strategies for tailored medicine including bronchoscopic lung volume reduction, pulmonary hypertension, and comorbidity management. This textbook will become a great asset in clinical practice and research to all who are involved or interested in COPD.

I would like to acknowledge the work done by the members of the Korean Obstructive Lung Disease (KOLD) Cohort Study who contributed to the preparation of this book. We are especially grateful to all contributing authors from abroad: Norbert Voelkel, Edwin Silverman, Meilan Han, Paul Jones, Rubin Tuder, and Nurdan Kokturk. Finally we wish to thank our families for their patience and consistent support during our academic lives.

I hope that all readers will find these chapters as helpful and insightful as we have.

Seoul, South Korea Sang-Do Lee

Contents

Part I

Overview

Definition and Epidemiology of COPD

1

Young Sam Kim

Definition of COPD

Chronic Obstructive Pulmonary Disease (COPD) is a common disease and prevalence is increasing worldwide. It is characterized by persistent airway obstruction that is partially reversible but it is considered preventable and treatable disease now. Airflow limitation is associated with chronic and abnormal inflammatory response in the airways and the lung to noxious stimuli [1]. Airway obstruction is defined by a reduction of expiratory airflow. Generally, forced expiratory volume in 1 s/forced volume capacity (FEV_1/FVC) ratio of less than 70% after bronchodilator has been used to identify COPD patient. The use of lower limit of normal (LLN) values has been proposed to define airflow limitation by spirometry, but current Global initiative for chronic Obstructive Lung Disease (GOLD) and American Thoracic Society/European Respiratory Society guidelines continue to recommend the fixed ratio criteria instead of an LLN for the diagnosis of COPD [1]. Patients with COPD have shown a great deal of heterogeneity and can be classified according to their clinical and radiologic parameters, biomarkers, lung function impairment and prognosis [2]. Traditionally, COPD has been classified as chronic bronchitis (CB) and emphysema. CB is defined as the presence of a chronic productive cough for 3 months in each of two consecutive years. Emphysema is defined as the destruction of alveolar walls and permanent enlargement of the airspaces distal to the terminal bronchioles. Current GOLD guidelines do not include the use of these terms in the definition of COPD. Asthma and COPD represent different disease entity with different pathogeneses and risk factors. Sometimes clinical manifestations of both diseases may overlap in a patient with airway obstruction and cannot be classified as COPD or asthma only. Large population studies show that some of the patients with airway obstruction are classified with more than one diagnosis. Therefore, overlapping diagnoses of asthma and COPD has been proposed and it is called COPD and Asthma Overlap Syndrome (ACOS) [1].

Epidemiology of COPD

COPD is a leading cause of morbidity and mortality worldwide. The prevalence and burden of COPD is increasing now. It is due to continued exposure of risk factors especially smoking and aging population. Estimate of prevalence and incidence of COPD is different according to the study population and diagnostic criteria [2, 3].

Y.S. Kim
Division of Pulmonology, Department of Internal Medicine, Severance Hospital, Yonsei University College of Medicine, Seoul, South Korea
e-mail: ysamkim@yuhs.ac

S.-D. Lee (ed.), *COPD*, DOI 10.1007/978-3-662-47178-4_1

Prevalence

Prevalence of COPD shows remarkable variation due to differences in study population, survey method, and diagnostic criteria [4]. Meta-analysis of 62 studies published between 1990 and 2004 that included prevalence estimates from 28 different countries reported a pooled prevalence of COPD of 7.6%. The prevalence estimate increased to 8.9% from epidemiologic studies using spirometry data. Consistent with previous observations, COPD prevalence was higher among studies using GOLD criteria to define COPD compared with other classification methods. Prevalence was low when it is calculated from self-reporting or physician diagnosis of COPD.

In the USA, data from the Third National Health and Nutrition Examination Survey (NHANES III) estimated that 23.6 million adults (13.9%) met GOLD definition of COPD (stage 1 or higher) in 2000 [1]. According to NHANES data from 2007 to 2010, the prevalence of airway obstruction was 13.5% for adults aged 20–79 years old, comprising 28.9 million people. Among them, 15.9 million had mild degree of obstruction and 12.9 million showed moderate to severe obstruction [5].

The Latin American Project for the Investigation of Obstructive Lung Disease (PLATINO) examined the prevalence of post-bronchodilator airflow limitation among persons over age 40 in five major Latin American cities. The prevalence of COPD ranged from 7.8 to 20.0%. The prevalence is higher in men, in older people, and in those with lower education, lower body-mass index, and greater exposure to smoking [6].

In 2002, the Burden of Obstructive Lung Disease (BOLD) project has been proposed to estimate prevalence globally. This is standardized and population-based epidemiologic studies. Post-bronchodilator FEV_1/FVC ratio of less than 0.7 was used to define the presence of COPD [1]. Participants from 12 countries included in the BOLD study and performed post-bronchodilator spirometry testing and questionnaire survey. The prevalence of COPD that was GOLD stage I or higher varied across countries and was generally greater in men than in women. The prevalence of stage II or higher COPD was 1–10% overall, 8–11% for men, and 5–8% for women [7].

In Asia, Nippon COPD Epidemiology (NICE) Study was performed to estimate prevalence of COPD in Japanese adults. Prevalence of airflow limitation was 10.9%. Among them, 56% of cases were classified to mild, 38% moderate, 6% severe degree of airway obstruction. Airflow limitation was more common in males [8]. In South Korea, nationwide epidemiologic survey called Korean National Health and Nutrition Examination Survey III (KNHANES III) was performed in 2001. The prevalence of airflow limitation by GOLD criteria was 17.2% (men, 25.8%; women, 9.6%) among adults older than 45 years. Most of these cases were mild in degree, and only a minority of these subjects had received physician diagnosis or treatment [9]. According to the data from the fourth Korean National Health and Nutrition Survey, prevalence of airway obstruction was detected in 8.8% of subjects over age 19 and 13.4% of adults older than 40 years (19.4% of men and 7.9% of women) [10]. According to population-based survey data from seven China provinces/cities, overall prevalence of COPD over 40 years old was 8.2% (men, 12.4%; women, 5.1%). COPD was more common in rural residents, elderly patients, smokers, and in those who were exposed to occupational dusts or biomass fuels [11].

In Africa, median prevalence of COPD based on spirometry in persons aged 40 years or older was 13.4%. When applied to the appropriate age group (40 years or more), which accounted for 196.4 million people in Africa in 2010, the estimated prevalence translates into 26.3 million (18.5–43.4 million) cases of COPD [12].

BOLD and PLATINO study which applied standardized survey methods and used same definition of COPD demonstrate a variable prevalence estimates ranging from 5.1% in Chinese women to 22.2% in South African men [2]. In developed countries, prevalence of COPD is 8–10% among adults 40 years of age and older; whereas, in developing countries, prevalence varies significantly among countries and is difficult to estimate. Recent studies which estimate prevalence change of COPD revealed that prevalence has been decreased or stabilized in some developed countries. But most of the world population is still exposed to smoking, biomass fuels, and other environmental risk factors, and prevalence is still high and increasing in the later part of last century [1]. The pooled prevalence of COPD was 7.6% from 37 studies. Prevalence of CB alone was 6.4% and of emphysema alone was 1.8%. The pooled prevalence from spirometric survey data was 8.9% [4]. According to NHANES III study of USA, 70% of adults with airflow obstruction had never received the diagnosis of COPD. The IBERPOC study in Spain also reported that there was no previous diagnosis of COPD in 78% of identified cases. Underdiagnosis and undertreatment is still a significant problem worldwide [13].

Incidence

In this large population-based cohort study of the general Dutch population of 40 years and older, the overall incidence rate of physician-diagnosed COPD was 2.92/1000 person-year. Based on these data, the risk to be diagnosed with COPD in the coming 40 years was 12.7% for a 40-year-old male and 8.3% for a 40-year-old female. The incidence increased with age, and was higher in men than in women. Known risk factors of COPD were confirmed such as smoking status, male gender, and increasing age [14]. Incidence rate of COPD is reported from 2000 to 13,500/100,000 person-year worldwide (Table 1.1) [15–18].

Mortality

Due to inconsistent COPD coding at the report of death and different use of diagnostic criteria, mortality data must be interpreted cautiously. Mortality may be underestimated because of underdiagnosis problem. However, it is clear that COPD is one of the most important causes of death in most countries [13]. According to the World Health Organization, COPD is the fourth leading cause of death in the world. Approximately 2.7 million deaths from COPD occurred in 2000, half of them in the Western Pacific Region especially in China. Annually 400,000 deaths occur in developed countries [3]. In Europe, mortality rates are variable ranging from 20 to 80 per 100,000 population [19]. A report of global burden of disease study that included mortality between 1990 and 2010 demonstrates that COPD is now the third leading cause of mortality in the world, although the number of deaths attributed to COPD decreased from 3.1 to 2.9 million annually.

Table 1.1 Incidence rate of COPD

Author	Nation (City)	Year	Cohort size	Follow-up period	Number of COPD case	Age (years)	Incidence rate
Van Durme et al.	Netherlands (Rotterdam)	1990–2004	7983	11	648	≥55	9.2/1000 person-year
Krzyzanowski et al.	Poland (Cracow)	1968–1981	4612	13	1864	19–70	5.0/1000 person-year
Huhti et al.	Finland (Harjavalta)	1961–1971	1476	10	1163	40–64	2.0/1000 person-year and 10.0/1000 person-year for smokers
Lindberg et al.	Sweden (Norrbotten)	1996–2003	963	7	45 (>Gold II), 91 (>Gold I)	46–77	6.7/1000 person-year for >Gold II and 13.5/1000 person-year for >Gold I

In the period of 1965–1998, death rates from coronary heart disease, strokes, and other cardiovascular diseases decreased but deaths from COPD increased by 163% [13]. However, according to the data from the NHANES I and NHANES III follow-up studies, mortality rate is decreased by 15.8% for participants with moderate or severe COPD and 25.2% for those with mild COPD. Overall mortality of COPD in the USA may be decreasing recently [1]. In China, COPD ranks as the fourth leading cause of death in urban areas and third leading in rural areas. Both crude and age-adjusted COPD mortality rates have fluctuated but have displayed a decreasing trend from 1990 [20]. The World Health Organization (WHO) has predicted that COPD will become the third most common cause of death in the world by 2030 [1]. Other study reports that COPD will become the fourth leading cause of death and 7.8% of death worldwide [21]. Mortality was high especially in very severe COPD patients in whom 26% died after 1 year of follow-up, whereas 2.8% died among the non-COPD subjects [14]. This increased mortality of COPD is mainly caused by worldwide epidemic of smoking and aging of the world population [13].

Economic and Social Burden

COPD is associated with significant economic burden. In the USA, economic burden of COPD was estimated to be US $15.5 billion in 1993. Some studies have shown that the cost of hospital stay represents 40–57% of the total direct costs generated by patients with COPD, reaching up to 63% in severe patients. In the USA, the mean cost of hospital admission by COPD in a cohort of patients with severe COPD was estimated to be US $7100 [13]. In terms of direct medical costs of COPD in 2005, the cost per patient was estimated at US $2700–5900 for attributable costs and to US $6100–6600 for excess costs [22]. Recently estimated direct costs of COPD are $29.5 billion and the indirect costs $20.4 billion. In a cohort study of 413 patients with COPD, direct healthcare costs were US $1681 for mild COPD patients, US $5037 for patients with moderate COPD, and US $10,812 for severe COPD patient. COPD exacerbations account for the greatest proportion of the total cost. In a pharmaco-economic study of COPD patient treated in the outpatient clinic, the average direct cost of acute exacerbation was US $159 [13]. In the European Union, the total direct costs of respiratory disease are estimated to be about 6% of the total cost. Medical cost of COPD accounts for 56% of this cost of respiratory disease. Direct cost of COPD tends to increase in the elderly age above 65 years old because of frequent use of acute healthcare services due to COPD exacerbations [23]. The DALYs for a specific condition are the sum of years lost because of premature mortality and years of life lived with disability, adjusted for the severity of disability. In 1990, COPD was the 12th leading cause of DALYs lost in the world, responsible for 2.1% of the total. According to the projects, COPD will be the seventh leading cause of DALYs lost worldwide in 2030. In the Global Burden of Disease Study 2013 (GBD 2013), migraine, hearing loss, COPD, anxiety, and diabetes are included in the top ten cause of DALYs lost [24].

References

1. Diaz-Guzman E, Mannino DM. Epidemiology and prevalence of chronic obstructive pulmonary disease. Clin Chest Med. 2014;35(1):7–16.
2. Rosenberg SR, Kalhan R, Mannino DM. Epidemiology of chronic obstructive pulmonary disease: prevalence, morbidity, mortality, and risk factors. Semin Respir Crit Care Med. 2015;36(4):457–69.
3. Lopez AD, et al. Chronic obstructive pulmonary disease: current burden and future projections. Eur Respir J. 2006;27(2):397–412.
4. Halbert RJ, et al. Global burden of COPD: systematic review and meta-analysis. Eur Respir J. 2006; 28(3):523–32.
5. Ford ES, et al. Trends in the prevalence of obstructive and restrictive lung function among adults in the United States: findings from the National Health and nutrition examination surveys from 1988-1994 to 2007-2010. Chest. 2013;143(5):1395–406.
6. Menezes AM, et al. Chronic obstructive pulmonary disease in five Latin American cities (the PLATINO study): a prevalence study. Lancet. 2005;366(9500):1875–81.

7. Buist AS, et al. International variation in the prevalence of COPD (the BOLD study): a population-based prevalence study. Lancet. 2007;370(9589):741–50.
8. Fukuchi Y, et al. COPD in Japan: the Nippon COPD epidemiology study. Respirology. 2004;9(4):458–65.
9. Kim DS, et al. Prevalence of chronic obstructive pulmonary disease in Korea: a population-based spirometry survey. Am J Respir Crit Care Med. 2005; 172(7):842–7.
10. Yoo KH, et al. Prevalence of chronic obstructive pulmonary disease in Korea: the fourth Korean National Health and nutrition examination survey, 2008. Respirology. 2011;16(4):659–65.
11. Zhong N, et al. Prevalence of chronic obstructive pulmonary disease in China: a large, population-based survey. Am J Respir Crit Care Med. 2007; 176(8):753–60.
12. Adeloye D, et al. An estimate of the prevalence of COPD in Africa: a systematic analysis. COPD. 2015; 12(1):71–81.
13. Chapman KR, et al. Epidemiology and costs of chronic obstructive pulmonary disease. Eur Respir J. 2006;27(1):188–207.
14. Afonso AS, et al. COPD in the general population: prevalence, incidence and survival. Respir Med. 2011; 105(12):1872–84.
15. van Durme YM, et al. Prevalence, incidence, and lifetime risk for the development of COPD in the elderly: the Rotterdam study. Chest. 2009;135(2):368–77.
16. Krzyzanowski M, Jedrychowski W, Wysocki M. Factors associated with the change in ventilatory function and the development of chronic obstructive pulmonary disease in a 13-year follow-up of the Cracow study. Risk of chronic obstructive pulmonary disease. Am Rev Respir Dis. 1986;134(5):1011–9.
17. Huhti E, Ikkala J, Hakulinen T. Chronic respiratory disease, smoking and prognosis for life. An epidemiological study. Scand J Respir Dis. 1977;58(3):170–80.
18. Lindberg A, et al. Seven-year cumulative incidence of COPD in an age-stratified general population sample. Chest. 2006;129(4):879–85.
19. Raherison C, Girodet PO. Epidemiology of COPD. Eur Respir Rev. 2009;18(114):213–21.
20. Fang X, Wang X, Bai C. COPD in China: the burden and importance of proper management. Chest. 2011;139(4):920–9.
21. Mathers CD, Loncar D. Projections of global mortality and burden of disease from 2002 to 2030. PLoS Med. 2006;3(11):e442.
22. Mannino DM, Buist AS. Global burden of COPD: risk factors, prevalence, and future trends. Lancet. 2007;370(9589):765–73.
23. Bustacchini S, et al. The economic burden of chronic obstructive pulmonary disease in the elderly: results from a systematic review of the literature. Curr Opin Pulm Med. 2011;17(Suppl 1):S35–41.
24. Vos T, et al. Global, regional, and national incidence, prevalence, and years lived with disability for 301 acute and chronic diseases and injuries in 188 countries, 1990–2013: a systematic analysis for the global burden of disease study 2013. Lancet. 2015;386(9995):743–800.

Risk Factors: Factors That Influence Disease Development and Progression

2

Ji Ye Jung

Genes

The most well-known genetic factor related with COPD is a severe hereditary deficiency of alpha-1 antitrypsin (AAT). AAT is the prototypic member of the serine protease inhibitor superfamily of proteins, which have a major role in inactivating neutrophil elastase and other proteases to maintain protease–antiprotease balance. Smoking is most important risk factor for accelerating the airflow obstruction and the onset of dyspnea in those with deficiency of AAT [1]. In nonsmokers with AAT deficiency, lung function declined faster in male and those with increasing age (especially after 50 years old), asthmatic symptoms, and occupations exposure to airway irritants [2].

Familial aggregation of COPD has been reported in a few studies [3, 4]. In Danish and Swedish Twin Registry, genetic factor was related with approximately 60% of the individual susceptibility to develop severe COPD [5]. Various other genes are being investigated in relation to development and progression of COPD in different ethnicities.

J.Y. Jung
Division of Pulmonary, Department of Internal Medicine, Severance Hospital, Yonsei University College of Medicine, Seoul, South Korea
e-mail: stopyes@yuhs.ac

Gender

COPD has been far more frequent in men than in women in regard to patterns of smoking and occupational exposures. However, COPD-related deaths among women continued to increase and it surpassed the number among men by 2000 in the United States [6]. Several studies suggested that women are more susceptible to smoking-related decline in lung function than men [7–12], and women were at a higher risk of hospitalization for COPD [10]. Globally, women are more exposed to biomass fuels related with cooking over open fires compared with men, and women exposed to smoke for cooking had a higher risk of COPD [13–17].

Lung Growth and Development

Lung growth and development starts from the period of gestation, at the birth, and during the childhood and adolescence. Airflow limitation persisted from mid-childhood to adulthood after extreme preterm birth, most evident in those with neonatal bronchopulmonary dysplasia. They may experience an earlier and steeper decline in lung function during adulthood [18, 19]. In relation to birth weight, a meta-analysis reported positive association between birth weight and FEV_1 [20]. Low birth weight was associated with worse adult lung function and higher rate of death from COPD in adult life [21]. Poor airway function

S.-D. Lee (ed.), *COPD*, DOI 10.1007/978-3-662-47178-4_2

shortly after birth was a risk factor for airflow obstruction in young adults [22]. People with early life disadvantages (e.g., maternal asthma, paternal asthma, childhood asthma, maternal smoking, and childhood respiratory infections) have permanently lower lung function and showed no catch-up with age with slightly larger decline in lung function increasing the risk of COPD [23].

Exposure to Particles

Cigarette Smoking

Among the smokers, the proportion of patients with COPD varies from 12 to 35% with dose response to smoking amount [24, 25]. However, recent data reported development of COPD in up to 50% of elderly smokers in Sweden [26]. Among the patients with COPD, ever smokers account for two-third of the prevalence globally [24, 27–30]. Other type of tobacco such as water pipe negatively affects lung function and marijuana is associated with increased respiratory symptoms suggestive of obstructive lung disease [31, 32]. Children whose mothers smoked during pregnancy had significantly lower lung function than did children whose mothers never smoked. Moreover, effects of exposure to tobacco smoking by the mother during pregnancy and/or environmental tobacco smoke exposure in the first few years of life persist into childhood and may affect the pulmonary function attained throughout the child's life [33, 34].

Smoking cessation brought a small recovery in pulmonary function, but ceased to low pulmonary function at an accelerated rate [35–38]. However, reduction in smoking amount did not demonstrate linear relationship in reduction in the rate of lung function decline in continuing smokers in the Lung Health Study [37].

In the study of 50-year trend in smoking-related mortality in the United States, male and female current smokers with 55 years of age or older showed similar relative risks for death from COPD (25.6 for men and 22.4 for women) in the contemporary cohorts between 2000 and 2010 [39]. The hazard ratio for mortality in the usual care group compared with the smoking cessation program intervention group was 1.18 (95% CU, 1.02–1.37) during 14.5 years of follow-up of COPD patients in the Lung Health Study [40].

Occupational Exposures to Dusts, Chemical Agents, Fumes

Occupational exposure contributed to the development and influenced clinical course of COPD. According to ecological analysis of international data using BOLD (Burden of Obstructive Lung Disease), PLATINO (Project for Investigation of Obstructive Lung Disease), and ECRHS (European Community Respiratory Health Survey follow-up study), 0.8% of COPD prevalence increased as 10% of exposure prevalence increased [41]. The model predicted 20% relative reduction in COPD prevalence (i.e., 3.4–2.7%) by 8.8% reduction in prevalence of occupational exposure. The occupational effect was higher in women than in males [41]. Self-reported exposure to vapors, gas, dust, or fumes on the longest held job was associated with an increased risk of COPD (OR = 2.11) [42]. Biological dust increased risk of chronic obstructive bronchitis (OR = 3.19), emphysema (OR = 3.18), and COPD (OR = 2.70). The risk was higher in women than in men, and no significant increased risks for COPD were found for mineral dust or gases/fumes [43]. Joint exposure to both smoking and occupational factors markedly increased the risk of COPD (OR 14.1) [42]. Besides causing COPD, occupational exposure affected decline of lung function in COPD. In men with early COPD, continued fume exposure was associated with a 0.25% predicted reduction in FEV_1% predicted every year [44]. Occupational exposure is also related with mortality in COPD. Construction workers exposed to inorganic dusts demonstrated increased mortality compared to other unexposed construction workers [45].

Indoor Air Pollution

Burning biomass fuel (wood, animal dung, and crop waste) for cooking and heating in poorly ventilated homes is the major source of indoor air pollution. In rural area where the smoking is less common, indoor pollutants from biomass fuels is an important risk factor for COPD [46, 47]. Exposure to wood smoke could equal up to 20 pack-years of active exposure to cigarette smoke [48]. According to meta-analysis, consistent evidence was found that exposure to indoor air pollution is a risk for COPD (OR = 2.80) and chronic bronchitis (OR = 2.32), with at least a doubling of risk, despite of marked heterogeneity by both county and fuel type [49]. At present, a dose–response relationship and differential toxicity for different fuel types cannot be defined because of insufficient information although this analysis shows with wood smoke being associated with the greatest effect [49]. In contrast to that biomass fuel exposure is well-known risk factor for COPD in the developing countries with low socioeconomic status, association between wood and charcoal exposure (OR = 4.5) and COPD was reported in European societies, such as Spain [50]. Higher level of indoor particulate matter less than 2.5 μm was associated with worse health status of patients with severe COPD [51].

Outdoor Air Pollution

A few cross-sectional studies consistently reported that acute increases in air pollution was related with acute exacerbation of COPD [52]. Increased mortality and higher rates of hospitalization or admission to emergency departments were observed [52]. Association of air pollution with the development of COPD has not been established clearly. However, in large samples of representative of the English population, increase in particulate matter less than 10 μm (PM_{10}) level, nitrogen dioxide (NO) and sulfur dioxide (SO_2) of 10 $\mu g/m^3$ was associated with 3 and 0.7% reduction in adult FEV_1 [53]. Similar relationship was also observed in Switzerland where PM_{10}, NO_2, and SO_2 affected both FEV_1 and FVC [54]. In children, changes in air quality (PM_{10}) caused by relocation and urban traffic/pollutant exposure during adolescent growth years have a measurable and potentially important effect on lung function growth and performance [55–57]. According to cross-sectional study in Germany, 55-year-old women living less than 100 m from a busy road were at the higher risk of developing COPD than those living farther away (OR = 1.79, 95% CI 1.06–3.02) [58]. However, to determine the relationship between chronic exposure to outdoor air pollution and COPD risk, more precise measurement of pollutants and longer duration of study are needed.

Socioeconomic Status

The low socioeconomic status is one of the risk factors for COPD and it is also associated with less COPD-related health care utilization [24, 25, 59]. However, its impact on symptoms, lung function, and other indices of COPD such as morbidity and mortality seems to be second only to smoking. Moreover, it is not clear yet whether indoor/outdoor air pollutants, poor nutrition, infections related with low socioeconomic status are the risk factors or low socioeconomic status itself is the significant factor for COPD [60].

Asthma/Bronchial Hyperactivity

Despite distinctive clinical and pathophysiologic characteristics at initial diagnosis, epidemiologic studies of asthma and COPD have demonstrated that similar feature may develop in two diseases [61]. Asthmatic patient is known to be susceptible to rapid lung function decline. In a longitudinal Copenhagen City Heart Study of general population, adults with self-reported asthma had substantially greater declines in FEV_1 over time than those without (38 mL/year vs. 22 mL/year) [62]. Airway hyperresponsiveness and irreversible airway obstruction are cardinal features of asthma. In European Community Respiratory Health Survey of young adults (20–44 years), airway hyperresponsiveness was the second strongest attributable factor (15% of population) with fourfold greater risk of developing COPD [63]. Irreversible airway obstruction ($FEV_1 < 80\%$ predicted and reversibility <9% predicted) was developed in 16% of subjects with asthma and 23% had a reduced postbronchodilator transfer coefficient (carbon monoxide transfer factor/ alveolar volume < 80% predicted) during 21–33 years of follow-up [64]. Among non-smoker males with asthma during 10-year follow-up study, 23% fulfilled the criteria for irreversible airway obstruction and had a steeper decline in FEV_1 than those without irreversible airway obstruction (53 mL/year vs. 36 mL/year) [65]. Asthmatic patients with incomplete reversibility of airflow obstruction ($FEV_1 \leq 75\%$ predicted despite optimal corticosteroid treatment) show more severe asthma and asthma of longer duration than asthmatic subjects with complete reversibility of airflow obstruction ($FEV_1 > 80\%$ of predicted) suggesting that incomplete reversibility of airflow obstruction may result from long-standing airway inflammation and associated structural changes [66]. In Tucson long-term cohort study of airway obstructive disease, active asthmatics were ten times higher risk for acquiring symptoms of chronic bronchitis, 17 times higher risk for being diagnosed with emphysema, and 12.5 times higher risk for fulfilling COPD criteria during 20-year follow-up study [61]. The degree of airflow limitation and hyperinflation is related to the duration of asthma [66, 67].

However, despite similar fixed airflow obstruction, those with a history of asthma and those with a history of COPD show different functional and pathologic airway inflammation suggesting that asthmatic airway inflammation does not change and does not become similar to the airway inflammation characteristics of COPD after development of fixed airflow obstruction. Therefore, asthma and COPD should be identified and treated separately [68].

Infections

The contribution of infection on development and progression of airflow limitation is becoming more important. Respiratory infection in infancy or childhood reduced adult lung function and was a risk factor for COPD [21, 63]. The incidence of COPD was 20.3 per 1000 person-years among HIV-infected patients compared with 17.5 per 1000 person-years among HIV-uninfected patients [69]. The pathogenesis of COPD and other chronic lung diseases in HIV remains unclear. Multiple interacting factors including increased systemic and lung oxidative stress, recurrent respiratory tract infections and colonization in the setting of aging are likely to be involved [69–73]. According to meta-analysis, despite marked heterogeneity, past history of tuberculosis was associated with chronic airflow obstruction independent of cigarette smoking (OR 1.37–3.13) [74–77]. Delay in antituberculosis treatments was associated with higher risk for COPD [78]. Moreover, patients with COPD treated with inhaled corticosteroid are at risk of tuberculosis and NTM pulmonary disease [79, 80].

References

1. Janus ED, Phillips NT, Carrell RW. Smoking, lung function, and alpha 1-antitrypsin deficiency. Lancet. 1985;1:152–4.
2. Piitulainen E, Tornling G, Eriksson S. Effect of age and occupational exposure to airway irritants on lung function in non-smoking individuals with alpha 1-antitrypsin deficiency (PiZZ). Thorax. 1997;52:244–8.
3. Silverman EK, Chapman HA, Drazen JM, et al. Genetic epidemiology of severe, early-onset chronic obstructive pulmonary disease. Risk to relatives for airflow obstruction and chronic bronchitis. Am J Respir Crit Care Med. 1998;157:1770–8.
4. McCloskey SC, Patel BD, Hinchliffe SJ, Reid ED, Wareham NJ, Lomas DA. Siblings of patients with severe chronic obstructive pulmonary disease have a significant risk of airflow obstruction. Am J Respir Crit Care Med. 2001;164:1419–24.
5. Ingebrigtsen T, Thomsen SF, Vestbo J, et al. Genetic influences on chronic obstructive pulmonary disease—a twin study. Respir Med. 2010;104:1890–5.
6. Mannino DM, Homa DM, Akinbami LJ, Ford ES, Redd SC. Chronic obstructive pulmonary disease surveillance—United States, 1971-2000. MMWR Surveill Summ. 2002;51:1–16.
7. Chen Y, Horne SL, Dosman JA. Increased susceptibility to lung dysfunction in female smokers. Am Rev Respir Dis. 1991;143:1224–30.
8. Gan WQ, Man SF, Postma DS, Camp P, Sin DD. Female smokers beyond the perimenopausal

period are at increased risk of chronic obstructive pulmonary disease: a systematic review and meta-analysis. Respir Res. 2006;7:52.
9. Langhammer A, Johnsen R, Gulsvik A, Holmen TL, Bjermer L. Sex differences in lung vulnerability to tobacco smoking. Eur Respir J. 2003;21:1017–23.
10. Prescott E, Bjerg AM, Andersen PK, Lange P, Vestbo J. Gender difference in smoking effects on lung function and risk of hospitalization for COPD: results from a Danish longitudinal population study. Eur Respir J. 1997;10:822–7.
11. Xu X, Weiss ST, Rijcken B, Schouten JP. Smoking, changes in smoking habits, and rate of decline in FEV1: new insight into gender differences. Eur Respir J. 1994;7:1056–61.
12. Sorheim IC, Johannessen A, Gulsvik A, Bakke PS, Silverman EK, DeMeo DL. Gender differences in COPD: are women more susceptible to smoking effects than men? Thorax. 2010;65:480–5.
13. Dossing M, Khan J, Al-Rabiah F. Risk factors for chronic obstructive lung disease in Saudi Arabia. Respir Med. 1994;88:519–22.
14. Dennis RJ, Maldonado D, Norman S, et al. Wood smoke exposure and risk for obstructive airways disease among women. Chest. 1996;109:55S–6S.
15. Perez-Padilla R, Regalado J, Vedal S, et al. Exposure to biomass smoke and chronic airway disease in Mexican women. A case-control study. Am J Respir Crit Care Med. 1996;154:701–6.
16. Ekici A, Ekici M, Kurtipek E, et al. Obstructive airway diseases in women exposed to biomass smoke. Environ Res. 2005;99:93–8.
17. Peabody JW, Riddell TJ, Smith KR, et al. Indoor air pollution in rural China: cooking fuels, stoves, and health status. Arch Environ Occup Health. 2005; 60:86–95.
18. Carraro S, Filippone M, Da Dalt L, et al. Bronchopulmonary dysplasia: the earliest and perhaps the longest lasting obstructive lung disease in humans. Early Hum Dev. 2013;89(Suppl 3):S3–5.
19. Vollsaeter M, Roksund OD, Eide GE, Markestad T, Halvorsen T. Lung function after preterm birth: development from mid-childhood to adulthood. Thorax. 2013;68:767–76.
20. Lawlor DA, Ebrahim S, Davey SG. Association of birth weight with adult lung function: findings from the British women's heart and health study and a meta-analysis. Thorax. 2005;60:851–8.
21. Barker DJ, Godfrey KM, Fall C, Osmond C, Winter PD, Shaheen SO. Relation of birth weight and childhood respiratory infection to adult lung function and death from chronic obstructive airways disease. BMJ. 1991;303:671–5.
22. Stern DA, Morgan WJ, Wright AL, Guerra S, Martinez FD. Poor airway function in early infancy and lung function by age 22 years: a non-selective longitudinal cohort study. Lancet. 2007;370:758–64.
23. Svanes C, Sunyer J, Plana E, et al. Early life origins of chronic obstructive pulmonary disease. Thorax. 2010;65:14–20.
24. Kim DS, Kim YS, Jung KS, et al. Prevalence of chronic obstructive pulmonary disease in Korea: a population-based spirometry survey. Am J Respir Crit Care Med. 2005;172:842–7.
25. Yoo KH, Kim YS, Sheen SS, et al. Prevalence of chronic obstructive pulmonary disease in Korea: the fourth Korean National Health and nutrition examination survey, 2008. Respirology. 2011;16:659–65.
26. Lundback B, Lindberg A, Lindstrom M, et al. Not 15 but 50% of smokers develop COPD?—Report from the obstructive lung disease in northern Sweden studies. Respir Med. 2003;97:115–22.
27. Celli BR, Halbert RJ, Nordyke RJ, Schau B. Airway obstruction in never smokers: results from the third National Health and nutrition examination survey. Am J Med. 2005;118:1364–72.
28. Bridevaux PO, Probst-Hensch NM, Schindler C, et al. Prevalence of airflow obstruction in smokers and never-smokers in Switzerland. Eur Respir J. 2010;36:1259–69.
29. Lamprecht B, McBurnie MA, Vollmer WM, et al. COPD in never smokers: results from the population-based burden of obstructive lung disease study. Chest. 2011;139:752–63.
30. Zhou Y, Wang C, Yao W, et al. COPD in Chinese nonsmokers. Eur Respir J. 2009;33:509–18.
31. Raad D, Gaddam S, Schunemann HJ, et al. Effects of water-pipe smoking on lung function: a systematic review and meta-analysis. Chest. 2011;139:764–74.
32. Tetrault JM, Crothers K, Moore BA, Mehra R, Concato J, Fiellin DA. Effects of marijuana smoking on pulmonary function and respiratory complications: a systematic review. Arch Intern Med. 2007;167:221–8.
33. Cunningham J, Dockery DW, Speizer FE. Maternal smoking during pregnancy as a predictor of lung function in children. Am J Epidemiol. 1994;139:1139–52.
34. Gilliland FD, Berhane K, McConnell R, et al. Maternal smoking during pregnancy, environmental tobacco smoke exposure and childhood lung function. Thorax. 2000;55:271–6.
35. Xu X, Dockery DW, Ware JH, Speizer FE, Ferris BG Jr. Effects of cigarette smoking on rate of loss of pulmonary function in adults: a longitudinal assessment. Am Rev Respir Dis. 1992;146:1345–8.
36. Sherrill DL, Holberg CJ, Enright PL, Lebowitz MD, Burrows B. Longitudinal analysis of the effects of smoking onset and cessation on pulmonary function. Am J Respir Crit Care Med. 1994;149:591–7.
37. Simmons MS, Connett JE, Nides MA, et al. Smoking reduction and the rate of decline in FEV(1): results from the lung health study. Eur Respir J. 2005;25:1011–7.
38. Scanlon PD, Connett JE, Waller LA, et al. Smoking cessation and lung function in mild-to-moderate chronic obstructive pulmonary disease. The Lung Health Study. Am J Respir Crit Care Med. 2000;161:381–90.
39. Thun MJ, Carter BD, Feskanich D, et al. 50-Year trends in smoking-related mortality in the United States. N Engl J Med. 2013;368:351–64.

40. Anthonisen NR, Skeans MA, Wise RA, Manfreda J, Kanner RE, Connett JE. The effects of a smoking cessation intervention on 14.5-year mortality: a randomized clinical trial. Ann Intern Med. 2005;142:233–9.
41. Blanc PD, Menezes AM, Plana E, et al. Occupational exposures and COPD: an ecological analysis of international data. Eur Respir J. 2009;33:298–304.
42. Blanc PD, Iribarren C, Trupin L, et al. Occupational exposures and the risk of COPD: dusty trades revisited. Thorax. 2009;64:6–12.
43. Matheson MC, Benke G, Raven J, et al. Biological dust exposure in the workplace is a risk factor for chronic obstructive pulmonary disease. Thorax. 2005; 60:645–51.
44. Harber P, Tashkin DP, Simmons M, Crawford L, Hnizdo E, Connett J. Effect of occupational exposures on decline of lung function in early chronic obstructive pulmonary disease. Am J Respir Crit Care Med. 2007;176:994–1000.
45. Bergdahl IA, Toren K, Eriksson K, et al. Increased mortality in COPD among construction workers exposed to inorganic dust. Eur Respir J. 2004;23:402–6.
46. Liu S, Zhou Y, Wang X, et al. Biomass fuels are the probable risk factor for chronic obstructive pulmonary disease in rural South China. Thorax. 2007; 62:889–97.
47. Salvi SS, Barnes PJ. Chronic obstructive pulmonary disease in non-smokers. Lancet. 2009;374:733–43.
48. Smith KR, Aggarwal AL, Dave RM. Air pollution and rural biomass fuel in developing countries: a pilot village study in India and implications for research and policy. Atmos Environ. 1983;17:2343–62.
49. Kurmi OP, Semple S, Simkhada P, Smith WC, Ayres JG. COPD and chronic bronchitis risk of indoor air pollution from solid fuel: a systematic review and meta-analysis. Thorax. 2010;65:221–8.
50. Orozco-Levi M, Garcia-Aymerich J, Villar J, Ramirez-Sarmiento A, Anto JM, Gea J. Wood smoke exposure and risk of chronic obstructive pulmonary disease. Eur Respir J. 2006;27:542–6.
51. Osman LM, Douglas JG, Garden C, et al. Indoor air quality in homes of patients with chronic obstructive pulmonary disease. Am J Respir Crit Care Med. 2007;176:465–72.
52. Sunyer J. Urban air pollution and chronic obstructive pulmonary disease: a review. Eur Respir J. 2001; 17:1024–33.
53. Forbes LJ, Kapetanakis V, Rudnicka AR, et al. Chronic exposure to outdoor air pollution and lung function in adults. Thorax. 2009;64:657–63.
54. Ackermann-Liebrich U, Leuenberger P, Schwartz J, et al. Lung function and long term exposure to air pollutants in Switzerland. Study on air pollution and lung diseases in adults (SAPALDIA) team. Am J Respir Crit Care Med. 1997;155:122–9.
55. Avol EL, Gauderman WJ, Tan SM, London SJ, Peters JM. Respiratory effects of relocating to areas of differing air pollution levels. Am J Respir Crit Care Med. 2001;164:2067–72.
56. Nicolai T, Carr D, Weiland SK, et al. Urban traffic and pollutant exposure related to respiratory outcomes and atopy in a large sample of children. Eur Respir J. 2003;21:956–63.
57. Sugiri D, Ranft U, Schikowski T, Kramer U. The influence of large-scale airborne particle decline and traffic-related exposure on children's lung function. Environ Health Perspect. 2006;114:282–8.
58. Schikowski T, Sugiri D, Ranft U, et al. Long-term air pollution exposure and living close to busy roads are associated with COPD in women. Respir Res. 2005;6:152.
59. Jung JY, Kang YA, Park MS, et al. Chronic obstructive lung disease-related health care utilisation in Korean adults with obstructive lung disease. Int J Tuberc Lung Dis. 2011;15:824–9.
60. Prescott E, Vestbo J. Socioeconomic status and chronic obstructive pulmonary disease. Thorax. 1999; 54:737–41.
61. Silva GE, Sherrill DL, Guerra S, Barbee RA. Asthma as a risk factor for COPD in a longitudinal study. Chest. 2004;126:59–65.
62. Lange P, Parner J, Vestbo J, Schnohr P, Jensen G. A 15-year follow-up study of ventilatory function in adults with asthma. N Engl J Med. 1998; 339:1194–200.
63. de Marco R, Accordini S, Marcon A, et al. Risk factors for chronic obstructive pulmonary disease in a European cohort of young adults. Am J Respir Crit Care Med. 2011;183:891–7.
64. Vonk JM, Jongepier H, Panhuysen CI, Schouten JP, Bleecker ER, Postma DS. Risk factors associated with the presence of irreversible airflow limitation and reduced transfer coefficient in patients with asthma after 26 years of follow up. Thorax. 2003;58:322–7.
65. Ulrik CS, Backer V. Nonreversible airflow obstruction in life-long nonsmokers with moderate to severe asthma. Eur Respir J. 1999;14:892–6.
66. Hudon C, Turcotte H, Laviolette M, Carrier G, Boulet LP. Characteristics of bronchial asthma with incomplete reversibility of airflow obstruction. Ann Allergy Asthma Immunol. 1997;78:195–202.
67. Cassino C, Berger KI, Goldring RM, et al. Duration of asthma and physiologic outcomes in elderly nonsmokers. Am J Respir Crit Care Med. 2000;162:1423–8.
68. Fabbri LM, Romagnoli M, Corbetta L, et al. Differences in airway inflammation in patients with fixed airflow obstruction due to asthma or chronic obstructive pulmonary disease. Am J Respir Crit Care Med. 2003;167:418–24.
69. Crothers K, Huang L, Goulet JL, et al. HIV infection and risk for incident pulmonary diseases in the combination antiretroviral therapy era. Am J Respir Crit Care Med. 2011;183:388–95.
70. George MP, Kannass M, Huang L, Sciurba FC, Morris A. Respiratory symptoms and airway obstruction in HIV-infected subjects in the HAART era. PLoS One. 2009;4:e6328.

71. Pacht ER, Diaz P, Clanton T, Hart J, Gadek JE. Alveolar fluid glutathione decreases in asymptomatic HIV-seropositive subjects over time. Chest. 1997;112:785–8.
72. Cole SB, Langkamp-Henken B, Bender BS, Findley K, Herrlinger-Garcia KA, Uphold CR. Oxidative stress and antioxidant capacity in smoking and nonsmoking men with HIV/acquired immunodeficiency syndrome. Nutr Clin Pract. 2005;20:662–7.
73. Morris AM, Huang L, Bacchetti P, et al. Permanent declines in pulmonary function following pneumonia in human immunodeficiency virus-infected persons. The pulmonary complications of HIV infection study group. Am J Respir Crit Care Med. 2000;162:612–6.
74. Allwood BW, Myer L, Bateman ED. A systematic review of the association between pulmonary tuberculosis and the development of chronic airflow obstruction in adults. Respiration. 2013;86:76–85.
75. Lam KB, Jiang CQ, Jordan RE, et al. Prior TB, smoking, and airflow obstruction: a cross-sectional analysis of the Guangzhou Biobank cohort study. Chest. 2010;137:593–600.
76. Menezes AM, Hallal PC, Perez-Padilla R, et al. Tuberculosis and airflow obstruction: evidence from the PLATINO study in Latin America. Eur Respir J. 2007;30:1180–5.
77. Lee SW, Kim YS, Kim DS, Oh YM, Lee SD. The risk of obstructive lung disease by previous pulmonary tuberculosis in a country with intermediate burden of tuberculosis. J Korean Med Sci. 2011;26:268–73.
78. Lee CH, Lee MC, Lin HH, et al. Pulmonary tuberculosis and delay in anti-tuberculous treatment are important risk factors for chronic obstructive pulmonary disease. PLoS One. 2012;7:e37978.
79. Andrejak C, Nielsen R, Thomsen VO, Duhaut P, Sorensen HT, Thomsen RW. Chronic respiratory disease, inhaled corticosteroids and risk of nontuberculous mycobacteriosis. Thorax. 2013;68: 256–62.
80. Kim JH, Park JS, Kim KH, Jeong HC, Kim EK, Lee JH. Inhaled corticosteroid is associated with an increased risk of TB in patients with COPD. Chest. 2013;143:1018–24.

3 Pathology of Chronic Obstructive Pulmonary Diseases

Rubin M. Tuder

Introduction

In this modern age of in-depth molecular and genetic focus on diseases, it is pressing that we revisit the fundamental pathology underlying chronic pulmonary obstructive diseases—forgetting the past limits our ability to make the best from the present. This review seeks to integrate, when possible, what is known about the pathology of chronic obstructive pulmonary diseases (COPD) with key pathogenetic data. However, to move the field forward, investigators dedicated to COPD are required to understand the normal and diseased lung structure (qualitatively and quantitatively), including on how best determine these key parameters; there was a time, approximately more than a half a decade ago, in which these were the most exciting and hopeful developments to understand COPD. They form the foundation to better appreciate the challenge to understand COPD and, most importantly, give proper credit to key studies that, in the past 50 years, shaped our current understanding of this highly challenging disease.

COPD, refers to a complex disease, with varying clinical phenotypes, largely resulting from the impact of socioeconomic development and their ensuing environmental impact that have occurred over the past 500 years. Smoking is a critical determinant of COPD development in more than 90% of patients; environmental pollution and, infrequently, genetic causes account for a growing number of patients. Within this background of epidemiological and clinical complexity, COPD reflects intricate structural alterations within the lung, often the focus of pathologists over decades. These pathological descriptions have contributed to forming the foundation of our attempts to understand the disease. We seek to provide a timely and necessary review of the pathology of COPD, as many of today's scholars have limited understanding of the scope of the pathological data accumulated in the past decades. Investigations in the broad angles of COPD require an understanding of the structural lung alterations in COPD, the structure of the normal and aged lungs, and on how quantitative measures aid in describing both the normal and COPD lung. However, the "bar" for the description of the pathology of COPD is high: William Thurlbeck provides a superlative assessment of role of pathological changes underlying chronic airway obstruction, with a particular emphasis on how they relate function [1]. We will refer to this publication often, as it provides valuable insights into the pathology of COPD, with reference to studies covering investigations initiated in the 1950s and extending by the time of its publication in 1985. The readers are strongly encouraged to read this summary to better appreciate the advances made in the field by the

R.M. Tuder, M.D.
Program in Translational Lung Research, Division of Pulmonary Sciences and Critical Care Medicine, University of Colorado School of Medicine, Aurora, CO 80045, USA
e-mail: Rubin.Tuder@Ucdenver.edu

S.-D. Lee (ed.), *COPD*, DOI 10.1007/978-3-662-47178-4_3

mid-1980s and the challenges that still remain up to this date.

It is highly instructive to go over the extensive literature of COPD, particularly of the pathology of the disease. While in the late 1950s and early 1960s, there was a more qualitative attempt to describe the pathological alterations of the lung aimed at understanding the clinical manifestations of the disease [2]. This early effort translated into the need to better quantification of structural parameters, as means to relate more closely the alterations in lung structure with the clinical manifestations, ultimately providing a clear rationale for treatment and insights into natural history. Stereology was then incorporated into the analysis of the normal lung, led by Weibel, and expanded to the COPD field by Dunnill and Thurlbeck. The accumulated knowledge of quantitative pathology of COPD eventually came to a standstill, as it became apparent that the age of tissue quantification of COPD would not lead to breakthroughs in the understanding of the disease, as it lagged behind the development of pathobiological insights—the field was largely tied up by the protease/antiprotease hypothesis; this is starkly delineated in the historical publication by Snider and colleagues about the definition of emphysema in the middle eighties [3]. In the late 1990s and clearly into the new century, the field of pathogenesis of COPD witnessed a "revolution," breaking the conceptual constrains provided by the protease/antiprotease imbalance. This is apparent in several chapters of this book. But once again, quantitative pathological examination of the diseased human lung, with the benefit of improved lung imaging (like computer tomography) and a growing body of knowledge regarding inflammation, cell signaling, cell death, among others, has provided a major step forward in our understanding of COPD. As outlined below, we also owe James Hogg for his vision, leadership, creativity, and ability to interface through all these domains, the largest contribution in the evolving insights into the pathology of the disease, which span almost 5 decades.

It is our goal in this review to revisit what is known about the normal lung that informs the reader about COPD; we underscore which stereological methods provide the most accurate data not only on the human lung, but that also is required for proper experimental modeling. We then review studies in the pathology of COPD.

Lung Volumes in Lung Stereology

Determination of lung volumes is a key parameter in lung stereology and to properly interpret quantitative lung pathology. It allows to express quantities in relation to the whole lung rather than fractions (like percentages), correct the values for the "real volume," and minimize important biases (errors) that most histological estimates impose. Lung volumes can be estimated from pulmonary function tests when available. However, in most studies involving human disease and animal modeling, the lungs are removed and the lung volumes estimated by water displacement or the Cavaliere's method. An extension of water displacement method is the determination of volume (mL) based on weight in air – weight in water (g) (which is better suited for the lung, which may float and not displace water correctly). Another alternative is the determination of the weight of the lung in water, which when divided by the specific density of tissue of 0.96 (g/mL) should provide the lung volume; the Cavaliere's method involves slicing through the lung at specific thickness, calculating the sum of the area of opposing sides of the sectioned slices and multiplying this sum by the thickness.

One of the most instructive studies referencing lung volumes obtained by water displacement is that of Thurlbeck [4]. He studied 25 individuals with ages ranging from 25 to 79 years. The lung volumes ranged between 3.3 and 7.5 L (mean of 4.9 L ± 1.4 SD). They correlated very closely with body length (Pearson's *r*: .772), but not with age. However, Thurlbeck also used the predicted total lung capacity (TLC), estimated on age, gender, and body length. As the lung volume depends on body length, total lung volume (TLV) and TLC correlated very closely. In his study, TLC ranged between 3.3 and 7.5 L, with a mean of 5 L. Thurlbeck underscores that it is difficult to achieve accurate and reproducible inflation in different lungs; however, inflation with formalin offers several advantages, with a close correlation with lung volume and measurements obtained with different methods. We discuss below key quantitative parameters to describe normal and diseased alveolar structure, including the mean linear intercept (Lm) and internal surface area (ISa), which are defined largely reliant on the measured lung volumes.

Overall, lung volumes obtained after inflation with 10% formalin at 25–30 cmH_2O pressure approximate closely those obtained by X-ray at total lung capacity [5], with a correlation coefficient of .82. On average, lung volumes are 8% higher than those obtained by X-ray.

Normal Lung

Overall Structure

The lung can be broadly divided in large, cartilaginous airways, dividing from mainstem bronchus for six generations and usually larger than 2 mm in diameter (Fig. 3.1a, b); terminal bronchioles (Fig. 3.1c–e), which do not have cartilage, are lined by pseudostratified epithelium overlying a submucosa with connective tissue and outside rim of smooth muscle cells. They give rise to intermediate structures with alveoli in their wall called respiratory bronchioles; each respiratory bronchiole branches 1–3 times prior to giving rise to alveolar ducts (Fig. 3.1d–e) (alveolated conduits, flanked proximally and distally by other alveolar ducts), and ending in a single alveolar sac (which has a blunt end, and is lined by alveoli). The primary lobule is considered to represent the alveolar duct and alveoli it supplies in the alveolar sac; the acinus corresponds to the respiratory bronchiole, alveolar ducts, and alveoli (Fig. 3.1c–e). The secondary lobule, which is largely relevant to radiological imaging, consists of 15–150 primary lobules, measures 1–3 cm, and is supplied by a terminal bronchiole, which branches 5–6 times with its accompanying pulmonary artery. It is often delineated peripherally by connective tissue projecting from the pleura. The respiratory zone contributes to 90% of the lung volume, with conductive airways and large blood vessels (often hilar) making up the remaining 10% [6]. Table 3.1 summarizes key structural characteristics of the normal lung, detailed below.

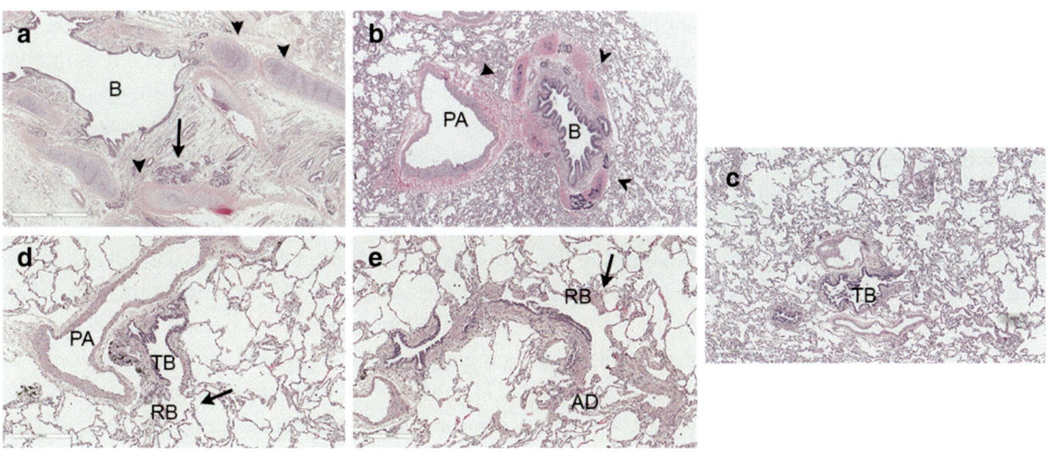

Fig. 3.1 Normal adult human lung. (**a**) Bronchus (*B*) with submucosal glands (*arrow*), seen between the luminal lining and inner surface of cartilage (*arrowheads*). (**b**) Intraparenchymal bronchus (*B*) flanked by a similar size pulmonary artery (PA). (**c**) Periphery of the lung, with a terminal bronchiole (*TB*), which does not have cartilage and contains epithelial lining and a layer of muscle. Note the partly collapsed normal alveoli. (**d**, **e**) Transition between *TB*, respiratory bronchiole (*RB*), and alveolar duct (*AD* in **e**). RB is lined by an interrupted airway epithelial cell layer with alveolated tissue within its walls

Table 3.1 Key structural characteristic of normal lung

Lung volumes
3.3–7.5 L (mean of 4.9 L ± 1.4 SD) (inflation with 10% formalin, Ref. [4])
Number of alveoli
250–450 × 10^6 Ref. [6]
480 × 10^6 Ref. [7]
Mean linear intercept
Mean 289 μm (Ref. [4])
226–350 μm (mean 271 ± 33 μ; Ref [6])
Internal alveolar surface area
Approximately 80 m^2 (range 40–100 m^2, Ref. [9])
Mean 65 ± 16.5 SD m^2 (range 40–100 m^2, Ref. [13])
Number of bronchiole profiles (per cm^2 lung tissue)
0.89 (Ref. [6])
0.84 (Ref. [15])

Alveolar Tissue

It is important to revisit some of the key findings of Weibel and Gomez in their classic reporting of lung structure using stereology [6]. They summarized the relative volume contribution of alveoli to approximately 60% of total lung volume, air ducts to approximately 26%, and tissue to about 4%. They studied five lungs, ranging in age from 8 to 74 years of age, with lung volumes between 2.5 and 7 L. The lung contains approximately 300 × 10^6 (range 250–450 × 10 [6], pending stature) alveoli; alveolar ducts and sacs would account for approximately 14 × 10^6 structures. More recently and using newly developed stereological approaches to directly count alveolar structures, Ochs and collaborators estimated that an adult (between 18–41 years of age) has 480 × 10^6 alveoli [7]. Interestingly, the overall alveolar diameter was lower for younger lungs (around 200 μm) and close to 290 μm in the older lungs (these measurements correspond to lung inflation to 75% of total lung capacity).

The average length of alveolar capillaries ranged between 8.2 and 13 μm; there are approximately 277 billion capillaries with an average diameter of 8 μm. The capillary exchange area would be 10% lower than the alveolar area, accommodating 140 mL of blood. Overall, the pulmonary arteries follow closely the airway branching (for approximately 23 branches), but extending further with a total of about 38 generations down to the precapillary level of approximately 15–25 μm in diameter. A summary of the structure and branching pattern of pulmonary arteries is available in reference [8].

The mean linear intercept (Lm) is determined by the calculation of number of alveolar intercepts crossing a linear grid system. As it reflects the interalveolar septal distance, Lm is the most used tool to express and quantify airspace enlargement in emphysema (see below). It correlates with age and does not correlate with body length. However, Weibel has pointed out that Lm is affected by inflation pressures and the intercept score includes alveolar ducts and small airways [9]. However, the data presented in the subsequent sections argue strongly for the validity of Lm to assess human emphysema. Verbeken et al. studied normal lungs, with a mean age of 49 years [10]. They found an emphysema score of 1.2 (minimal airspace enlargement in selected cases). Other interesting measures from their study consisted of delineation of Lm of 289 μm with a mean of 5.49 intercepts. The coefficient of variation of intercepts was 60%. This study provided quantification of the structural components that contribute to Lm; the airspace proper measured on average 265 μm, while the septal wall measured 24 μm. Verbeken et al. counted alveolar attachments of 6.72/mm of airways; the number of terminal bronchioles per surface tissue was 0.85, with 800 μm diameter in average. In this study, Lm correlated inversely with height (which is in contrast to data from Thurlbeck, see below), and positively with weight, with added regression power when combined with age [11].

Lm according to Thurlbeck has a dispersion of about 20% around the mean in a normal lung, i.e., in excess of this limit, it would be considered abnormal. His study of 25 nonemphysematous lungs (described in more detail below) showed an Lm ranging from 226 to 350 μm, with a mean of 271 μM ± 33. The upper limit, based on the mean + 2 SD, would be 337 μm (or 333 if corrected for predicted lung capacity) [4]. Verbeken and collaborators established this upper limit of normality to 380 μm. Importantly, Lm correlates with age but not with body length [4]. Based on data from Weibel and Gomez, the size of alveoli was estimated to be in the order of 250–290 μm (i.e., close to the range seen with Lm, pending correction for lung volumes and contraction of tissue after formalin inflation and contraction of tissue after paraffin embedding) [6].

An important measurement derived from the studies by Weibel and Gomez was the alveolar internal surface area (ISa), representing the overall gas exchange area of the lung provided by the interface of alveolar septa and alveolar space. The ISa can be determined by the number of intercepts with a grid of lines. Weibel and Gomez determined alveolar surface area of approximately 80 m^2 (range 40–100 m^2 [9]), or akin the size of a tennis court [12]; it is therefore related to Lm, with a relationship defined by the formula ISa = 4 × volume alveolar parenchyma/Lm.

Thurlbeck reassessed the ISa in 25 nonemphysematous (possibly normal) lungs, which were inflated with formalin at 25 cmH_2O pressure [4]. Like in the work targeted at emphysematous lungs [13], Thurlbeck introduced some adjustments to measurements of Lm and ISa. The total lung volumes (TLV) were determined after inflation, by water displacement, therefore including both aerated and tissue parenchyma of the lung. He also corrected the TLV by the total lung capacity (TLC), which represents (only) the aerated volume of the lung based on predicted values, derived from data that included age, gender, and height. The corrective factor was the ratio of TLC/TLV, at 2/3 power for ISa and 1/3 power for Lm. Nonemphysematous lungs showed a wide variation of ISa, ranging from 40 to 100 m^2 (mean 65 ± 16.5 SD m^2) largely derived from the scatter of height. This meant that it is anticipated that a tall individual may have a large ISa while a short individual may have an ISa of 40 m^2. In contrast to Lm, ISa correlates closely with height, with an R^2 of 0.83, adding a potent confounder when to be used in studies involving emphysema. Lung volumes have a greater impact on ISa as MLI does not correlate with ISa (Pearson's r: −0.07).

Small Airways

Airways can be broadly divided based on structure and diameter. Bronchi have cartilage in their walls and have diameters larger than 2 mm. Small airways or terminal bronchioles have less than 2 mm, do not have cartilage in their walls, and are completely surrounded by an epithelium, basal lamina, and bundles of muscle (Fig. 3.1c–e).

Given the orientation dependency of airways and pulmonary arteries, elucidation of these structures (branching, size, etc.) requires either casting or imaging in three dimensions after a radiopaque substance is injected [14]. This approach allows to divide the lung into three compartments pending their role in gas transport and potential for gas exchange: a conducting zone, a transition zone, responsible for conduction and gas exchange, and a respiratory zone, involved in gas exchange. While Weibel assumed the airways branching symmetrically from the trachea, Horsfield proposed that they could be asymmetric as well. Weibel counted 16 generations, leading to 2^{16} or 65,536 terminal bronchioles and 131,071 conducting airways [14]; however, Horsfield predicted half of this number based on asymmetric arrangement of airway branching (rather than a given more proximal branch giving rise consistently to two symmetrical branches). The concept of asymmetry is important as it can explain a lower dead space than the symmetrical dichotomous branching pattern, with gases reaching alveolar units located at much shorter distances from the trachea. The average distance for the gas to travel from the larynx to the gas exchange units is approximately 25 cm, largely covered by convective gas movement. The final 2.6 mm from the alveolar ducts to alveoli is covered by oxygen diffusion (in nitrogen, estimated to be 0.25 cm^2/s). The final step involves the passage of oxygen from the alveolar space to capillaries, largely within water (diffusion constant for oxygen of 0.00193/cm^2/s, i.e., 1.3 log slower than in nitrogen). Despite the slower diffusion rate, oxygen would be required to traverse a shorter distance in the distal lung (respiratory bronchioles, alveolar ducts, and alveolar sacs) before reaching the capillaries.

Matsuba and Thurlbeck investigated the number and internal diameter of membranous airways, less than 2 mm, in twenty normal lungs [15]. The number of small airways was approximately 0.84/cm^2 of lung tissue and the internal diameter was 0.756 mm (please compare below with the measurements in 12 COPD individuals, with number of airways of 0.638/cm^2 and internal diameter of 0.738). The number of airways/area of lung tissue decreases with height, consistent with the conclusion that the total number of airways is constant in different height individuals. Indeed, Matsuba and Thurlbeck, based on several studies, stated that terminal airways would not be affected by overall distension of the lung (i.e., increased TLC in COPD or with age).

Lung Cellular Composition

The study of Crapo and collaborators continues being the seminal reporting of key stereological data regarding the composition of the alveolated lung [16]. The study was based on eight autopsied lungs; they were fixed in glutaraldehyde and sampled for electron microscopy. Type I cells covered 93% of the alveolar surface, with a cell surface area of 5000 μm [2]. Alveolar type II cells are 14-fold thicker than type I cells with 183 μm [2] surface area (i.e., approximately 1.5 log less than type I cells), i.e., covering 7% of the alveolar surface area. Both type I and II accounted for 24% of all cells in the lung parenchyma and 21% of the total alveolar tissue volume. Capillary endothelial cells are much smaller than type I cells; they each cover an equivalent 27% of the alveolar surface area covered by individual type I cells; the total number of capillary endothelial cells is 3.6-fold higher than type I cells, collectively covering almost a similar surface area. Overall, capillary endothelial cells account for 30% of the cells in the alveolus and just 14% of alveolar tissue volume. The remaining interstitial cells (fibroblasts, macrophages, pericytes, inflammatory cells, etc.) accounted for 37% of all alveolar cells.

Lung Growth

A central aspect of lung structure is the developmental growth of the lung. A newborn lung contains approximately 20×10^6 alveoli, with Dunnill proposing that alveolar expansion would occur during the first 8 years, followed by a significant decrease afterwards. However, pending the height of the child, additional significant alveolar number increase occurs into early adulthood. A recent report [17] using stringent stereological approaches as recommended by the American Thoracic Society (ATS) [18] re-examined whether alveolar numbers increase into adulthood. Their approach was based on randomly (done systematically using methods to give all regions the same probability to be chosen for analyses) selecting approximately eight blocks representative of the right or left lung of 11 subjects, with ages ranging from 1 month to 15 year and 11 months. Alveoli were determined and counted by defining their openings in two parallel sections of predetermined thickness (as reported by Ochs et al. [7]). Between 2 and 4 months of age, the number of alveoli increased progressively from approximately 100×10^6 to around 200×10^6 ($n = 8$ individuals). The log of number of alveoli increased with a two-parameter power function with a fast increase in the first two years of age; it tapered off by adolescence, but with continual expansion to the age of about 16 years (an individual with 583×10^6 alveoli). The log number of alveoli correlated closely with weight and height.

Aged Lung

The increase in alveoli associated with age has been interpreted as "single alveolar enlargement." This interpretation stems from the perceived lack of inflammation or other marks of destructive components, including marked fragmentation of elastic fibers, or remodeling of small airway, or disorganization of alveolar airway attachments [3].

Weibel and Gomez's assessments of alveolar surface area were dependent on age, as the older individuals had a decrease in the fractional volume of alveoli from 57% in the younger vs. 52% in the older lungs, while air ducts increased from 27% in younger vs. 32% in older lungs [6]; the aged lungs had a decrease in alveolated lung.

Importantly, this change is paralleled by a decrease in surface area with loss of alveoli. Of interest, this was ascribed to the loss of capillaries by some investigators [19], a concept rediscovered 25 years later to explain the pathogenesis of emphysema [20].

Verbeken and collaborators studied group of senile lungs of individuals aging 69 years. These lungs showed an enlargement of Lm by 60% over controls, with an emphysema score of 9.1 (vs. 1.2 in controls) [11]. The Lm exceeded the upper normal limit of 380 μm (defined in control lungs). The coefficient of variation of Lm increased to 60%; the mean septal component of Lm also increased by about 50%; no difference in alveolar attachments was noted, tough there was a decrease in the numerical density of small airway/area of lung. In their aging group, the expansion of airspaces was uniform. Moreover, it appears that this enlargement occurs without a decrease in alveolar attachments to the bronchiolar wall, which is often seen with more advanced destructive (centri- and panlobular) emphysema. Thurlbeck determined that Lm of 25 normal lungs was 275 μm ± 32, confirming that it increases with age (Pearson's r: 0.575) [13].

Data concerning alveolar internal surface area (ISa) in normal individuals is discussed in regard to emphysema below [21]. Of note is the progressive loss of ISa with age after early adulthood, at an estimated rate of 2.7 m^2/year [13]. These data are largely confirmatory of Thurlbeck's study on nonemphysematous lungs [4], which correlated inversely with age (Pearson's r: −0.5).

Of interest is the correlation of physiological parameters (obtained after death in isolated lungs) with structural endpoints [22]. In senile emphysema, there is a marked increase in minimal air (ma, air remaining after the air has been removed from the lung)/Total Lung Capacity (TLC), though less than in emphysema. Moreover, there is a shift for the pressure volume curves, being intermediate between normals and emphysematous. The measures of FEV1, FEV1/FVC, and airflow were not different between normals and the lungs with senile emphysema. Moreover, the key physiological parameters of ma/TLC and those of airflow did not correlate with morphological parameters.

As with centrilobular emphysema, there is a reduction of membranous bronchiole density in senile lung [10].

COPD

There was an extensive focus of investigations in the pathology of COPD in the period extending from the 1950s through the early 1990s. It is apparent that this effort followed in the footsteps of the studies by Weibel and Gomez revealing structural investigations of the human lung (outlined above [6]) and the need to better understand a frequent and complex disease. Driving this endeavor was the hope that assessments of structural alterations underlying the pathology of disease would provide key explanations regarding on how best diagnose and treat COPD. Despite this intense effort, Thurlbeck recognized the discrepancy between structure and function of COPD, in particular in regards to airflow limitation [1], or in other words, inability to explain the chronic airflow limitation with structural data. He listed several strong reasons behind this realization, particularly those related to difficulties involving the pathological nature of the studies. In fact, he postulated that every known pathological alteration in COPD can explain or contribute to chronic airway obstruction, most notably mucus gland enlargement, intraluminal mucus accumulation, alterations in terminal bronchioles, and emphysematous destruction of the respiratory units, the acini; however, how each of these specific components limits lung function remains unknown. We provide a summary of key points below, emphasizing some key publications.

Chronic Bronchitis

The increase in mucus gland mass has been linked to COPD for more than 50 years and semi-quantitatively assessed by the Reid index [23]: normal individuals would have mucus glands in less than 50% of the bronchial surface area

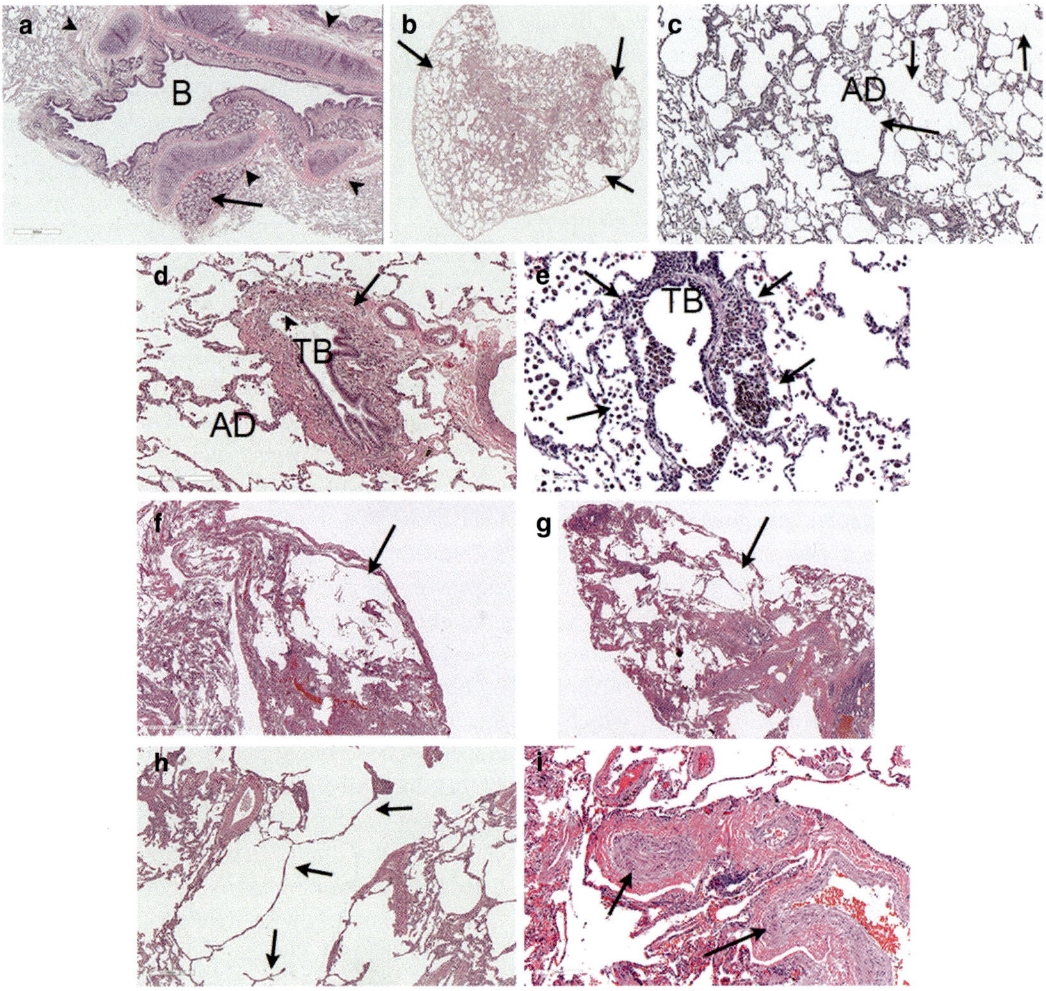

Fig. 3.2 COPD lung. (**a**) Large bronchus (*B*) with chronic bronchitis. Note the expansion of glands (glands) beyond the outer rim of cartilage (*arrowheads*). (**b**) Low magnification of mild emphysema with notable airspace enlargement in the subpleural region (arrows). (**c**) Centrilobular emphysema with enlargement of alveolar duct (*AD*) (*arrows*). (**d**) Chronic bronchiolitis in a terminal bronchiole (*TB*) (*arrow*). Note the increased thickening of the airway wall, largely due to chronic inflammatory cells. There is a focal loss of epithelial lining (*arrowhead*). The adjacent alveolar duct (*AD*) shows enlargement characteristic of emphysema. (**e**) Respiratory bronchiolitis with thickened terminal bronchiole (*TB*) with clusters of pigmented intra-alveolar macrophages (*arrows*). (**f**) Subpleural bullae (*arrow*) with absence of alveolar septa. (**g**) Marked subpleural airspace enlargement (*arrow*). (**h**) Characteristic thinning of alveolar septa in severe centrilobular emphysema, which appears virtually avascular (*arrows*). (**i**) Pulmonary artery thickening in severe COPD (*arrows*)

(Fig. 3.2). In her classic description of chronic bronchitis, Lynne Reid underscored that in early cases, there is hypertrophy of mucus elements and airway luminal accumulation [24]; in advanced cases, she highlighted the finding of purulent inflammation in large and small airways, with associated dilation of airways and sometimes obliterative changes.

Thurlbeck suggested that these airways contribute significantly to chronic airflow limitation. The pathological counterpart of the clinical characteristics of chronic bronchitis represents the excessive mucus production. He proposed that airflow limitation would (also) ensue due to hypertrophy of mucus glands and luminal accumulation of mucus. These would correlate with clinical history of chronic bronchitis and sputum production. However, the Reid index follows a modal distribution, with a right shift in normal and left shift in COPD; but, there is significant overlap. The extremes of both curves are informative in that Reid index less than 0.36 would be only seen in normal while higher than .55 only in COPD specimens [1].

The interaction between mucus gland enlargement and emphysema is of interest, possibly reflecting that cigarette smoke triggers both events. The increase in mucus gland mass occurred with age in COPD patients and age matched controls (mean age of 65 years) to a similar extent; the mean percentage thickness in the control group was approximately 8% vs.12% in the aged groups. There is evidence that the frequency of chronic mucus hypersecretion increases with emphysema severity score (obtained pathologically). However, it is unclear whether the extent of mucus gland hypertrophy relates to the clinical symptoms of chronic bronchitis, like mucus production or cough. A prior study of 353 patients at autopsy showed, based on point counting morphometry, that mucus glands amounted to 17.6% in smokers and 14.5% in nonsmokers [25]; however, no differences were noted with age. Also interestingly, the authors state a lack of direct correlation between mucus gland hypertrophy and emphysema in this cohort of 219 lungs yet the percent mucus gland was higher in emphysematous (18.3%) vs. non-emphysematous lungs (14.8%). These findings led the investigators to question whether chronic bronchitis might result from alterations other than mucus gland hypertrophy [26].

Overall, mucus gland enlargement shows some degree of correlation with flow rates, but the correlation is weak at best, if not existent.

Small Airways

Thurlbeck proposed that small airway disease contributes to mild airflow limitation [27]. He also raised the contribution of inflammation, possibly leading to collapse of bronchioles; fibrosis and muscle hypertrophy could also have a role in obstructing small airways (Fig. 3.2). Additional contributors consist of goblet cells, which might undergo hyperplasia. An overall replacement of luminal contents, displacing surfactant, would result in airway instability. However, distortion of the small airways and obliteration would also contribute to severe airflow limitation; these would follow extensive emphysema. The discussion that follows largely confirms Thurlbeck's predictions of the main contributors for chronic airflow limitation, including some more recent studies involving COPD lungs.

Hogg and collaborators provided key physiological data that supported that the main site of increased airway resistance in COPD (seven emphysematous, one with bronchiectasis, and one with bronchiolitis) was the small airways, in the range of 2 mm in diameter. The increase in peripheral resistance was about fourfold when compared with control lungs [28]. The authors concluded that the increase in resistance in COPD lungs could be derived from mucus-obstructed small airways, narrowing, or occlusion by fibrosis, as emphasized by Thurlbeck.

Inflammation of airways has been recognized since the early description of the pathology of COPD by Leopold and Gough in 1957 [29]. Inflammation in small airways correlates with mild alterations in pulmonary function [1], being perhaps more important in anteceding airway fibrosis and squamous metaplasia. With worsening COPD, the number of airways with inflammatory cells including polymorphonuclear cells, macrophages, eosinophils, CD4, CD8, and B cells increases [30]. Many airways contain lymphoid follicles, most notably in GOLD stage 3 and 4 (most severe disease), contributing to overall airway thickness by 3–4-fold when compared with lungs with GOLD0/1 [30].

Studies by Matsuba and Thurlbeck addressed the question whether there was a change in numbers and internal diameter of small airways, defined as those less than 2 mm in diameter. This study involved 12 individuals with mild COPD based on the Ryder score of 17.8 ± 1.2. As compared with a control cohort [15], they found a significant decrease in numbers per unit area and when corrected for anticipated lung volume at age of 20 years. When both cohorts were adjusted to body length, there were no significant differences. Moreover, there were no differences in internal diameter. Also, they did not find any correlation between measurements of small airways with those of emphysema or flow rates. Of interest, the authors noted a small shift of terminal bronchioles measuring 200–400 μm in diameter while there was a deficit of small airways between 400 and 600 μm in diameter. However, when they analyzed the ratio of small airway to total lung volumes (small airway luminal volume density), they found a significant reduction in emphysema vs. normal. This decrement was accounted by a decrease in the number of small airways and reduction of their size. However, Matsuba and Thurlbeck considered these small airway changes not to have a significant role in increased airway resistance and air flow limitation.

The reduction of the density of membranous bronchioles was noted by Verbeken and referenced as noted previously. They also noted that with increased MLI in emphysema, there is a negative relation with airway diameter (as there is an increase in density of airway less than 600 μm particularly in the lower lobes). Verbeken and collaborators also verified a decrease in numerical densities (per unit area of lung tissue) of terminal bronchioles (0.85–0.51/cm^2) [10]. The airspace is more heterogeneous than due to aging, with increased alveolar septal thickening, usually with mild fibrosis. Small airway density decreased in emphysema lungs; there was a negative interaction between MLI and alveolar attachments, i.e., the higher the MLI, with more severe emphysema, the lower the number of alveolar attachments. This supports a causal relation between small airway remodeling and degree of emphysema.

This reduction in selective diameter size ranges in COPD lungs (vs. normal lungs) might reflect progressive airway narrowing; however, there are important pitfalls in most of the measurements performed thus far, as they relied largely in planimetric assessments, or via stereology (which cannot resolve measures of changes in diameter and numbers of fractal structures, like airways). No studies have used casting or three-dimension reconstruction to define how a specific segment behaves in COPD lungs (or branching, as outlined by Horsfield studies) of the normal lung. However, narrowing of terminal bronchioles, assessed by multiple approaches including volume proportion, bronchiolar diameter, or frequency of airways less than 350 μm in diameter, correlates with airflow limitation. This correlation is however not as strong as between degree of emphysema and chronic airway obstruction [1].

The topic of small airway pathology in COPD was more recently revisited by Hogg and collaborators. Using lung resection specimens aimed at removal of tumors or from patients enrolled in the National Emphysema Therapy Trial (NETT), Hogg et al. found that with worsening of COPD (assessed by the GOLD score, reflecting worse FEV1 [31]) correlated inversely with small airway (less than 2 mm in diameter) occlusion by mucus and debris ($R = 0.5$) [30]. In line with earlier studies on the behavior of small airway in COPD and their association with airflow limitation, Hogg et al. showed that total airwall thickness was strongly associated with worsening of COPD [30].

In a recent study, Hogg and collaborators used a sophisticated CT-based approach to study 2 mm and smaller airways, while relying on histology to further validate their data [32]. They found a progressive decrease in the number of airways of 2–2.5 mm with worsening of GOLD stage. Moreover, there was a dramatic reduction of terminal bronchiole cross-sectional area and a decrease in 89% of terminal bronchiole number. This reduction also happened in regions with Lm of less than 489 μm, the upper limit of the normal Lm values obtained in this study. The residual airways had increased wall thickness. The authors suggest that emphysema might in reality start with the disappearance of terminal bronchioles [32], which might ultimately account for the increase in 4–40-fold the peripheral airway resistance observed previously by the authors [28].

Mucus in terminal bronchioles is increased approximately 15-fold in lungs of patients with chronic bronchitis with severe emphysema, while it is increased only fourfold in lungs of bronchitis with no emphysema [1]. In combination with exudates, mucus plugging can contribute to chronic airflow limitation, which was confirmed more recently by Hogg and collaborators [30].

Another potential contributor for chronic flow limitation could be bronchiole tortuosity, potentially leading to stenotic lesions. The basis of this finding could be related to inflammation or decrease in alveolar attachments (aa) to airways. Based on the study of 41 lungs, Nagai et al. correlated aa (both as absolute numbers and in reference to airway diameter) to emphysema parameters (score and Lm) and measures of airflow [33]. In summary, they delineated that aa/airway diameter were directly related to the degree of emphysema, which would be the most proximal cause of airflow limitation. They also determined that the aa correlated with airway deformity. No associations were detected with airway inflammation. This has been confirmed in more recent studies, with the finding that aa decreased from 6.72 to 5.76 [10]. The diameter of membranous bronchioles correlates with FEV1/FVC in the emphysema group.

Emphysema

The present definition of emphysema was introduced in 1985 in a report of a National Heart, Lung, and Blood Institute workshop [3]. The authors' brief introduction referenced the early definitions by the World Health Organization and American Thoracic Society, which stated that emphysema involved enlargement of the acinus (anatomic unit formed a respiratory bronchiole, 3–4 alveolar ducts, and the alveolar sac) (Fig. 3.2). The committee recognized the importance of the concept of "destruction" in the definition, which was however not defined in their prior statement (note the thinning of alveolar septa in emphysema, Fig. 3.2h). Moreover, the document expresses concern with the frequent finding of increase in airspaces in processes associated with prominent fibrosis, like granulomas (rather than in emphysema, where there is minimal fibrosis). Importantly, the report states that there are forms of alveolar enlargement that are not "destructive" like in age-related enlargement or overdistension after unilateral pneumectomy (referenced as "simple airspace enlargement"). There was an attempt to better define the term "destruction" as a reduction in amount of a specific tissue; others interpreted destruction as disorganization of the alveolar attachments to the terminal and respiratory bronchiole [34] (Fig. 3.2d, e). As discussed below, more refined attempts to characterize "tissue destruction" involved the introduction of destructive index [35] or alveolar septal holes [36]. These somewhat rudimentary and overly simplistic definitions probably reflect the knowledge of the times, prior to clarification on how cell and tissues can "disappear"; in the present days, these processes have been linked to necrosis, apoptosis, and autophagy, all of which have been shown to be involved in emphysema.

The etiology of emphysema has remained largely undetermined, though recognized in the 1960s that it involved a unique form of tissue destruction, labeled as "necrosis" [37]. It was also recognized that, in distinction to other forms of lung necrosis or injury, in emphysema there was mild inflammation and, importantly, a scarring process. The purported etiological agent could arrive to the centrilobular regions via the airflow (like documented at the time with nitrogen dioxide) or via the blood vessels. The latter was considered despite a lack of morphological evidence at the time of precapillary or capillary occlusion [37] (Fig. 3.2h). In advanced COPD, large areas of alveolar destruction lead to increased subpleural airspaces, which can form subpleural bullae (Figs. 3.2f, g).

In the time spanning the 1960s, 1970s, and into the 1980s, there was an apparent impetus to introduce quantitative measures of alterations in lungs of COPD patients so to relate structural changes to clinical presentation and, hopefully, to pathophysiology of the disease.

Quantification of Emphysema

We recommend several excellent introductory texts regarding stereology [6, 9, 18, 38–40], which are necessary for all investigators interested in the lung, including COPD. A critical requirement is the randomization for unbiased selection of regions for analysis. This means that all fields have to be given an equal chance of being represented, which is accomplished by specifically designed sampling approaches. The systematic uniform random sampling (SURS) may provide the best and most stringent sampling design [38]. The main approaches to quantify emphysema in lung slices involved two main methods. The first consisted of stereological determination of the relative contribution of enlargement of air ducts and sacs to the overall lung volume [39] and, the second, involved grading of severity of emphysema on paper mounts of lung slices based on comparisons with a range of severities of emphysema [41]. Two methods are available based on the latter approach: The Thurlbeck system involves radiating segments from a center point positioned in the major fissure, usually in the third sagittal slice of lung; each segment is scored between 0 and 3 pending the severity of emphysema, with an overall score ranging between 0 and 30. The method by Ryder involves matching a paper mount slice to standards ranging from 0 to 100. The advantages of the point counting approach consist of its accuracy, simplicity of use, and independence of shape or complexity of the counting objects. It is important to keep in mind that there is need to increase sampling if there is significant variability of the parameter in question; this applies in particular to centrilobular emphysema. These three approaches have been compared for reproducibility [41]; Thurlbeck's and Ryder's scoring are fast and provide a low intraobserver variation but with a wide interobserver variation [42]. The point counting is the one that takes the longest (3–4 min per read), but with difficulties of calling a point hit with mild lesions.

Table 3.2 Key structural characteristic of emphysematous lung

Lung volumes
Mean for centrilobular emphysema: 6.3 L (range 4.8–7 L); mean for panlobular emphysema: 7.6 L (range 6–10 L), (Ref. [43])
Number of alveoli
Mean in centrilobular emphysema 218 × 10^6 (CI: 126–310); mean in panlobular emphysema 96 × 10^6 ± 23 (Ref. [43])
Parenchyma density
Centrilobular emphysema: 50% alveolar density; 18.5% alveolar duct density; 19.5% centrilobular space density, 12% tissue and blood vessel density, in (Ref. [43])
Mean linear intercept
Mean 598 μm (range: 472–791 μm; Ref. [44])
Mean 279 μm, 304 μm, 369 μm, and 517 μm in normal, mild, moderate, and severe emphysema lungs, respectively (Ref. [13])
Internal surface area
Mean 52 m^2 ± 16.2 SD (range: 28–105); ISA corrected 5 L: 50.8 m^2 ± 13.2 (range: 25–96) (Ref. [13])
Small airways
Number of bronchiole profiles (per cm^2 lung tissue): 0.638 (Ref. [15]), 0.51 (Ref. [10]), 90% reduction over controls (Ref. [32])
Internal diameter: 0.738 μm (Ref. [15])
Increase in terminal bronchioles measuring 200–400 μm in diameter
Deficit of small airways between 400 and 600 μm in diameter

Microscopic Assessments of Emphysema

A summary of key changes in emphysema is included in Table 3.2. The use of the point count method, as performed by Dunnill, provided interesting data [43]. In five lungs with severe centrilobular emphysema (three with cor pulmonale), lungs volumes averaged 6.3 L; alveolar and duct air amount to a mean of about 68% with centrilobular spaces occupying 20% of lung parenchyma. All these lungs had mucus gland enlargement with mucus mass of approximately 0.42. In 18 lungs with panlobular emphysema, the lung volumes averaged 7.6 L (range 6.2–10.5 L); the emphysema volume density was 47% (range 30–60%), largely at the expense of a reduction of alveoli and ducts [43]. Emphysema was found in 219 of 353 autopsied lungs subjected to point counting morphometry [25]. Emphysema was present in 21/73 nonsmokers, with a percentage volume of parenchyma involved by emphysema being 1.7% vs. 10.8% in smokers.

One of the most popular methods of measuring airspaces is the mean linear intercept or Lm.

Lm may provide the best measurement related to panlobular emphysema as its Lm was 598 μm (range: 472–791 μm) in 11 lungs with severe respiratory failure [44]. However, as Thurlbeck recognized in a 1991 report, MLI is insensitive in measuring emphysema, being generally normal in mild and even moderate emphysema [33]. On the other hand, in panlobular emphysema (10 lungs [43]), the Lm was 592 μm ± 23.7 (i.e., increased about twofold over control value).

Internal surface area (ISa): Given the potential importance of alveolar surface area for gas exchange, it is reasonable to propose that this is a key measurement of emphysema. In an early study of five lungs with severe centrilobular emphysema [43], the surface area averaged 62.2 m^2, close to the normal range, which was surprising given the severity of the disease. These five lungs had a somewhat increased lung volume (mean of 6.3 L ± 0.85, vs. normal of 6 L). This compensation of ISa is therefore probably due to the increased lung volumes (suggesting that the ratio of surface/volume may be more accurate in measuring milder forms of emphysema). In ten lungs with panlobular emphysema, the ISa was 48.7 m^2 ± 9.6, therefore reduced by about 50% vs. control.

ISa was determined in a study of 29 pairs of normal lungs. The lungs were inflated at 25 cmH_2O and the lung volume determined by volume displacement, after correction for inflation, or corrected by antemortem total lung capacity assessed by pulmonary testing, or a fixed processed lung volume of 5 L. In normal lungs, the ISa ranged between 40 and 100 m^2.. When the total lung capacity and volume of tissue was set at 5 L (ISa corrected or ISa 5 L), then the effect of body length was decreased [13]. In 44 pairs of emphysematous lungs, the ISa and corrected ISa were significantly decreased, down to 28 m^2. Point counting correlated very closely with semiquantitative assessments of emphysema based on paper lung mounts, either scored by the Thurlbeck method (scores ranging 0–30) or average of the grading between 0 and 3 by eight pathologists. The correlation of Lm was also very good, around Pearson's coefficient of 0.8. ISa (or if corrected by TLC) did not correlate well with a coefficient around 0.5. Only the ISa for 5 L showed improved correlations, around 0.83 [44]. It is remarkable that of nine lungs with mild emphysema based on semiquantitative scoring, eight had normal ISa 5 L. Thurlbeck summarized that ISa is significantly reduced in the severe emphysema group, to levels below 80% of predicted. In fact, the data provided in the tables regarding this study demonstrate that Lm varies more in tune with the emphysema score, registering 279 μm, 304 μm, 369 μm, and 517 μm in normal, mild, moderate, and severe emphysema lungs, respectively [13]. Thurlbeck agreed with Dinnill's postulate that ISa may not accurately reflect centrilobular emphysema as the lung volumes increase *pari passu* with increases in Lm, possibly due to loss of elastic recoil. Interestingly, based on the balance of data, Thurlbeck recommended the use of Lm, because of ease of use, reproducibility, and independence of height and age [13], though recognizing the merits (and accuracy—despite the lack of a gold standard for emphysema) of so-called semiquantitative (called by him as subjective) assessments [13].

Number of alveoli is an infrequently used parameter in emphysema. Dunnill counted a mean number of 218 × 10^6 (CI: 126–310) [43]. Interestingly, only one lung would have a higher number than the normal established by Weibel and Gomez [6], yet still lower than the alveolar number of 480 × 10^6 of Ochs et al. In ten cases of panlobular emphysema, Dunnill reported 96 × 10^6 ± 23 alveoli (i.e., reduced by a 60% over control numbers); the mean alveolar volume increased by twofold vs. normal values [43].

Some other parameters of interest might involve the number of centrilobular spaces and their diameters. Dunnill found that these numbers ranged between 10,600 and 35,000 (mean of 18,600), with 3 logs increased volume when compared with alveoli in the same lungs. Their average diameter was 3.7 mm (i.e., tenfold larger than a normal alveolus).

Destructive index (DI): The DI originated from the need to better define the concept of alveolar destruction in emphysema [35]. DI was defined as interruptions of the alveolar septa; two or more disruptions qualified as a destroyed alveolus. The original study reported that the DI was higher in smokers' lungs and correlated with pulmonary function testing; DI correlated with Lm only in smokers with an "r" of 0.61 [35]. This assessment appears to be reproducible and of similar extent in upper and lower lobes. In a second study led by Thurlbeck and collaborators, they also found that overall, DI increases with Lm (correlation coefficient of 0.64). When the DI is in areas with frank emphysema, the score correlates well with emphysema scoring. DI increases but not significantly in mild emphysema; however, DI increases significantly in moderate and severe emphysema [34]. DI correlated with lung volumes at 30 cm water transpulmonary pressure. The concordance between DI and Lm in nonemphysematous and mild emphysematous lungs suggests that these two parameters change concordantly.

A potentially related finding to DI in emphysema is the presence of "holes" detected by scanning electron microscopy [36]. In normal lung, the holes are largely represented by pores of Kohn, measuring less than 10 μm in diameter. In emphysema, these spaces increase in size and occurrence, reflecting the formation of fenestrae. Interestingly, normal regions in between areas of emphysema have an increase in the diameter and frequency of holes. These holes may be the early event of destruction in emphysema.

Other Forms of Emphysema

In simple pneumoconiosis of coal workers, there is heavy accumulation of coal dust around the bronchioles, forming the spidery macula. Its relationship to centrilobular emphysema is unclear as miners may also have COPD. One interpretation is that simple pneumoconiosis may be due to enlargement while centrilobular emphysema involves tissue destruction [1]. This is supported by the observation that pneumoconiosis usually involves the respiratory bronchiole while centrilobular emphysema extends distally to involve third-order terminal bronchioles.

Panlobular emphysema, characteristic of α1-antitrypsin deficiency, involves uniformly the lobule; some of the quantifiable pathological characteristics, as compared with centrilobular variant, have been referenced above. More recently, panlobular emphysema has been described in intravenous Ritalin drug abusers, possibly related to alteration of pulmonary arteries occluded by tablet compounds [45].

Panlobular emphysema predominantly involves the lower zones, with an overall symmetrical expansion of both lungs. When compared with centrilobular emphysema, panlobular emphysema has less bronchiolar abnormalities, including less muscle and fibrosis [46]; when extreme examples of centrilobular vs. panlobular are compared, the centrilobular has a lower compliance; the increased compliance is more apparent when the Lm is in excess of 360 μm in panlobular emphysema. Given the extent and uniformity of loss of alveolar tissue, it is conceivable that panlobular emphysema has a more sustained and reproducible loss of elastic recoil (than centrilobular emphysema), therefore account for airflow limitation in this group of patients.

Other forms include distal acinar emphysema. It is also called paraseptal, possibly leading to spontaneous pneumothoraces in younger individuals. Irregular emphysema is a common pathological finding associated with the lung parenchyma adjacent to fibrotic processes.

Involvement of Cellular Compartments in Emphysema

More detailed studies of the relative contribution of type I, type II, endothelial cell, and interstitial collagen and elastin in emphysema became available on two decades later than these earlier studies [47]. Vlahovic et al. studied lobes obtained from cancer resection, including mild and moderate emphysema. Five random blocks were processed for morphometric assessment of these compartments, with an overall 35 blocks being analyzed. Lm in the normal lungs was between 200 and 260 μm (13 blocks); in mild emphysema, it increased to 260–390 μm, and in moderate emphysema, the Lm was in excess of 390 μm. The key findings involved a decrease in alveolar and capillary surface area (normalized by basement membrane surface area). The dropout of alveolar epithelial (about 50% in moderate emphysema vs. control lungs) and endothelial cells (reduced by 66% in moderate vs. normal lung) appeared to be equivalent with an increase in Lm, consistent with a synchronous loss of alveolar septal structures; the remaining septa in emphysematous lungs remained constant when compared with normal lungs. Interestingly, the volume of type I and endothelial cells did not differ in all three groups (after normalization with basement membrane surface area). The most dramatic change between control vs. emphysema lungs was the thickening of interstitium (from 0.8 volume density for normals vs. 3.1 in moderate emphysema); the thickening involved both elastin and collagen associated with increase in volume density of fibroblasts and macrophages. These findings suggest that the loss of alveolar septa in emphysema involves the simultaneous disappearance of epithelial and endothelial cells [20] and that residual septa undergo some form of scarring (a finding not registered by early pathological studies).

Physiological–Pathological Correlations

Investigations in the past 5 decades have shown a low correlation between pulmonary physiology and degree of emphysema assessed by Lm or emphysema score. This is particularly apparent on the basis of a study of 48 well-characterized patients from the NIH Intermittent Positive Pressure Clinical Trial [48]. Perhaps illustrating the limitations imposed by studying lung lobes resected during cancer resection in smokers, an extensive study of 407 lungs failed to correlate FEV1 with number of alveolar septa anchored on peripheral airways, small airway remodeling, and airway inflammation [49]. Not surprisingly, lungs from patients with less than 50% predicted FEV1 had a significant increase in Lm (which ranged from 125 to 175 μm (in severe COPD). However, macroscopic assessment of emphysema, based on emphysema score, failed to correlate with the extent of decrease in FEV1. These data imply that more subtle anatomical and pathophysiological alterations in small airways can explain their contribution to increased airway resistance [28].

Notwithstanding the limitations described above, there is evidence that most patients with chronic airflow limitation have severe emphysema. However, several patients with moderate/severe emphysema do not show severely impaired airflow, and there is no clear parallel between degrees of emphysema and severity of airflow limitation.

Occurrence of cor pulmonale or hypertrophy of the right ventricle also correlates with emphysema severity; Thurlbeck describes that less than 1% of patients without emphysema have cor pulmonale, while the complication occurs in 5%, 15%, and 40% in patients with mild, moderate, and severe emphysema, respectively [1].

Assessments of ISa 5 L correlate with DLCO and to some degree with the ratio of residual volume/TLC. The concordance of ISa 5 L and DLCO is apparent with measurements in the range of cutoffs of 75% for ISa 5 L. However, there are more exceptions in regard to the anticipated correlation when DLCO is less than 80% of predicted with up to 40% of patients showing relatively preserved ISa 5 L [3].

Pulmonary Vascular Structure and Function

It is apparent that in normal smokers and patients with COPD, the pulmonary arteries undergo remodeling (Fig. 3.2I). Intima thickening and medial hypertrophy in COPD is more prominent vs. normals, however to a limited extent [50]; lungs of patients with mild to moderate COPD, with no evidence of pulmonary hypertension, had mostly intima remodeling, possibly due to thinning of the media. These data confirm a prior study that focused on pulmonary arteries of 100 μm in diameter or less [51], which found an increase in muscularized pulmonary arteries in COPD lungs based on replicated elastic layers in vessels containing a double layer elastic tissue. The percentage of thick pulmonary arteries was greater in COPD lungs of patients with right ventricular hypertrophy vs. no hypertrophy, and extent of centri- and panlobular emphysema [51]. Using angiograms of patients with and without

COPD, Horsfield and Thomas reconstructed the pulmonary vascular tree larger than 1 mm vascular segments. The hierarchical branching order was then established, for three-order generations [52] (for a review of pulmonary artery branching in normal pulmonary arteries, please refer to the review in Ref. [8]). The most significant pulmonary vascular changes occurred in segments of orders 2–4, with significantly decreased pulmonary artery diameters. Interestingly, this study confirmed a prior finding of increased diameter of the first order pulmonary artery in the hilum. Interestingly, the more severe the pulmonary artery remodeling, the less responsive are the arteries to supplemental oxygen [53].

Conclusions

We owe to several past and current investigators for detailed insights into the pathology of COPD. These investigations developed in the footsteps of the highly innovative and needed developments in lung stereology. The fast speed of research in the present days may obviate the need to grasp these data and incorporate state-of-the-art methods in the assessment of pathology in human and experimental disease, particularly related to COPD. As apparent by the ATS statement on using stereology for measuring parameters in lung tissue using sections [18], it is timely that these methods be used by current investigators. This chapter sought to highlight several key morphological parameters as they relate to the pathogenesis of COPD. They serve as a guide on how best to interpret them and incorporate the most significant alterations present in humans in our understanding of the disease and how to best approach it in animal models.

References

1. Thurlbeck WM. Chronic airflow obstructions: correlation of structure and function. In: Petty TL, editor. Chronic obstructive pulmonary disease. New York: Marcel Decker; 1985. p. 129–203.
2. Mitchell RS, Toll G, Filley GF. The early lesions in pulmonary emphysema. Am J Med Sci. 1962;243:409–19.
3. Snider GL, Kleinerman LJ, Thurlbeck WM, Bengali ZH. The definition of emphysema: report of a National, Heart, Lung and Blood Institute. Division of Lung Diseases Workshop. Am Rev Respir Dis. 1985:182–5.
4. Thurlbeck WM. The internal surface area of nonemphysematous lungs. Am Rev Respir Dis. 1967;95:765–73.
5. Thurlbeck WM. Post-mortem lung volumes. Thorax. 1979;34:735–9.
6. Weibel ER, Gomez DM. Architecture of the human lung. Use of quantitative methods establishes fundamental relations between size and number of lung structures. Science. 1962;137:577–85.
7. Ochs M, Nyengaard JR, Jung A, Knudsen L, Voigt M, Wahlers T, Richter J, Gundersen HJ. The number of alveoli in the human lung. Am J Respir Crit Care Med. 2004;169:120–4.
8. Tuder RM, Stacher E, Robinson J, Kumar R, Graham BB. Pathology of pulmonary hypertension. Clin Chest Med. 2013;34:639–50.
9. Weibel ER. A retrospective of lung morphometry: from 1963 to present. Am J Physiol Lung Cell Mol Physiol. 2013;305:L405–8.
10. Verbeken EK, Cauberghs M, Mertens I, Clement J, Lauweryns JM, van de Woestijne KP. The senile lung. Comparison with normal and emphysematous lungs. 1. Structural aspects. Chest. 1992;1992(101):793–9.
11. Verbeken EK, Cauberghs M, Lauweryns JM, van de Woestijne KP. Anatomy of membranous bronchioles in normal, senile and emphysematous human lungs. J Appl Physiol. 1994;1994(77):1875–84.
12. Weibel ER. Design and structure of human lung. In: Fishman AP, editor. Pulmonary diseases and disorders. New York: McGraw-Hill; 1980. p. 224–81.
13. Thurlbeck WM. Internal surface area and other measurements in emphysema. Thorax. 1967;22:483–96.
14. Horsfield K. Quantitative morphology and structure: functional correlations in the lung. Monogr Pathol. 1978;19:151–9.
15. Matsuba K, Thurlbeck WM. The number and dimensions of small airways in emphysematous lungs. Am J Pathol. 1972;67:265–75.
16. Crapo JD, Young SL, Fram EK, Pinkerton KE, Barry BE, Crapo RO. Morphometric characteristics of cells in the alveolar region of mammalian lungs. Am Rev Respir Dis. 1983;128:S42–6.
17. Herring MJ, Putney LF, Wyatt G, Finkbeiner WE, Hyde DM. Growth of alveoli during postnatal development in humans based on stereological estimation. Am J Physiol Lung Cell Mol Physiol. 2014;307:L338–44.
18. Hsia CC, Hyde DM, Ochs M, Weibel ER. An official research policy statement of the American Thoracic Society/European Respiratory Society: standards for quantitative assessment of lung structure. Am J Respir Crit Care Med. 2010;181:394–418.
19. Liebow AA, Gough J. Pulmonary emphysema with special reference to vascular changes. Am Rev Respir Dis. 1959;80:67–93.
20. Tuder RM, Yoshida T, Fijalkowka I, Biswal S, Petrache I. Role of lung maintenance program in the

heterogeneity of lung destruction in emphysema. Proc Am Thorac Soc. 2006;3:673–9.
21. Thurlbeck WM. Internal surface area of normal and emphysematous lungs. Aspen Emphysema Conf. 1967;10:379–93.
22. Verbeken EK, Cauberghs M, Mertens I, Lauweryns JM, van de Woestijne KP. Tissue and airway impedance of excised normal, senile, and emphysematous lungs. J Appl Physiol. 1992;72:2343–53.
23. Reid LM. Pathology of chronic bronchitis. Lancet. 1956:275–81.
24. Reid LM. Pathology of chronic bronchitis. Lancet. 1954;266:274–8.
25. Dunnill MS, Ryder R. A quantitative study of the relationship between chronic bronchitis, emphysema and smoking. Chest 1971;59: Suppl 35S+.
26. Bedrossian CW, Anderson AE Jr, Foraker AG. Bronchial morphometry in emphysema and senescence. Exp Mol Pathol. 1977;27:44–50.
27. Thurlbeck WM. The pathology of small airways in chronic airflow limitation. Eur J Respir Dis Suppl. 1982;121:9–18.
28. Hogg JC, Macklem PT, Thurlbeck WM. Site and nature of airway obstruction in chronic obstructive lung disease. N Engl J Med. 1968;278:1355–60.
29. Leopold JG, Gough J. The centrilobular form of hypertrophic emphysema and its relation to chronic bronchitis. Thorax. 1957;12:219–35.
30. Hogg JC, Chu F, Utokaparch S, Woods R, Elliott WM, Buzatu L. The nature of small-airway obstruction in chronic obstructive pulmonary disease. N Engl J Med. 2004;350:2645–53.
31. Pauwels RA, Buist AS, Calverley PM, Jenkins CR, Hurd SS. Global strategy for the diagnosis, management, and prevention of chronic obstructive pulmonary disease. NHLBI/WHO Global Initiative for Chronic Obstructive Lung Disease (GOLD) Workshop summary. Am J Respir Crit Care Med. 2001;163:1256–76.
32. McDonough JE, Yuan R, Suzuki M, Seyednejad N, Elliott WM, Sanchez PG, Wright AC, Gefter WB, Litzky L, Coxson HO, Pare PD, Sin DD, Pierce RA, Woods JC, McWilliams AM, Mayo JR, Lam SC, Cooper JD, Hogg JC. Small-airway obstruction and emphysema in chronic obstructive pulmonary disease. N Engl J Med. 2011;365:1567–75.
33. Nagai A, Yamawaki I, Takizawa T, Thurlbeck WM. Alveolar attachments in emphysema of human lungs. Am Rev Respir Dis. 1991;144:888–91.
34. Saito K, Cagle P, Berend N, Thurlbeck WM. The "destructive index" in nonemphysematous and emphysematous lungs. Morphologic observations and correlation with function. Am Rev Respir Dis. 1989;1989(139):308–12.
35. Saetta M, Shiner RJ, Angus GE, Kim WD, Wang NS, King M, Ghezzo H, Cosio MG. Destructive index: a measurement of lung parenchymal destruction in smokers. Am Rev Respir Dis. 1985;131:764–9.
36. Nagai A, Inano H, Matsuba K, Thurlbeck WM. Scanning electronmicroscopic morphometry of emphysema in humans. Am J Respir Crit Care Med. 1994;150:1411–5.
37. Wright GW, Kleinerman J. The J. Burns Amberson Lecture: A consideration of the etiology of emphysema in terms of contemporary knowledge. Am Rev Respir Dis 1963; 88: 605–620
38. Hyde DM, Harkema JR, Tyler NK, Plopper CG. Design-based sampling and quantitation of the respiratory airways. Toxicol Pathol. 2006;34:286–95.
39. Dunnill MS. Evaluation of a simple method of sampling for quantitative histological analysis. Thorax. 1964;19:443–8.
40. Dunnill MS. Quantitative methods in the study of pulmonary pathology. Thorax. 1962;17:320–8.
41. Thurlbeck WM, Dunnill MS, Hartung W, Heard BE, Heppleston AG, Ryder RC. A comparison of three methods of measuring emphysema. Hum Pathol. 1970;1:215–26.
42. Dunnill MS. The recognition and measurement of pulmonary emphysema. Pathol Microbiol (Basel). 1970;35:138–45.
43. Dunnill MS. Quantitative observations on the anatomy of chronic non-specific lung disease. Med Thorac. 1965;22:261–74.
44. Thurlbeck WM. Measurement of pulmonary emphysema. Am Rev Respir Dis. 1967;95:752–64.
45. Schmidt RA, Glenny RW, Godwin JD, Hampson NB, Cantino ME, Reichenbach DD. Panlobular emphysema in young intravenous Ritalin abusers. Am Rev Respir Dis. 1991;143:649–56.
46. Kim WD, Eidelman DH, Izquierdo JL, Ghezzo H, Saetta MP, Cosio MG. Centrilobular and panlobular emphysema in smokers. Two distinct morphologic and functional entities. Am Rev Respir Dis. 1991;144:1385–90.
47. Vlahovic G, Russell ML, Mercer RR, Crapo JD. Cellular and connective tissue changes in alveolar septal walls in emphysema. Am J Respir Crit Care Med. 1999;160:2086–92.
48. West WW, Nagai A, Hodgkin JE, Thurlbeck WM. The National Institutes of Health Intermittent Positive Pressure Breathing trial—pathology studies. III. The diagnosis of emphysema. Am Rev Respir Dis. 1987;135:123–9.
49. Hogg JC, Wright JL, Wiggs BR, Coxson HO, Opazo SA, Pare PD. Lung structure and function in cigarette smokers. Thorax. 1994;49:473–8.
50. Magee F, Wright JL, Wiggs BR, Pare PD, Hogg JC. Pulmonary vascular structure and function in chronic obstructive pulmonary disease. Thorax. 1988;43:183–9.
51. Scott KW. Quantitation of thick-walled peripheral lung vessels in chronic airways obstruction. Thorax. 1976;31:315–9.
52. Horsfield K, Thomas M. Morphometry of pulmonary arteries from angiograms in chronic obstructive lung disease. Thorax. 1981;36:360–5.
53. Barbera JA, Riverola A, Roca J, Ramirez J, Wagner PD, Ros D, Wiggs BR, Rodriguez-Roisin R. Pulmonary vascular abnormalities and ventilation-perfusion relationships in mild chronic obstructive pulmonary disease. Am J Respir Crit Care Med. 1994;149:423–9.

Pathogenesis of COPD

4

Ji-Hyun Lee

COPD Is an Inflammatory Disease

COPD has been traditionally viewed as a chronic inflammatory disease, which develops in response to noxious particles or gases, most commonly from tobacco smoking. Inflammation related to COPD includes cells and mediators of both innate and adaptive immunity.

Exposure to cigarette smoke leads to activation of several pattern recognition receptors (PRRs), either directly or indirectly by damage-associated molecular patterns (DAMPs) released from injured epithelial cells. Activation of PRRs such as Toll-like receptors (TLRs) and receptor for advanced glycation end products (RAGE) in airway epithelium and alveolar macrophages leads to release of proinflammatory cytokines and to attract circulating neutrophils, monocytes, and lymphocytes into the lung [1, 2].

From these cells, several types of proteases and oxidants are released and, if not sufficiently counterbalanced by antiproteases and antioxidants, further damage will occur [1, 2]. Immature dendritic cells pick up antigens released from damaged tissue and foreign pathogens and present them to naive T cells in the draining lymph nodes [1]. On activation, these antigen-specific $CD4^+$ and $CD8^+$ cells and antibody-producing B cells are drawn to the lungs to neutralize the antigens. $CD8^+$ T cells and natural killer cells contribute to cytotoxicity of lung tissue cells through the release of the proteolytic enzymes perforin and granzyme B [3, 4]. As the disease progresses, tertiary lymphoid aggregates including an oligoclonal selection of the B and T cells develop around the small airways [5, 6].

Even though smoking elicits an inflammatory response in the lungs of all smokers, this response is enhanced and exaggerated in those who develop COPD. This suggests that there is an abnormal amplification of the inflammatory response in the lungs of smokers who develop COPD, and the intensity of infiltration with activated inflammatory cells correlates with the severity of COPD [7–10]. In addition, this inflammation persists for several years even after smoking cessation, suggesting that there was self-perpetuating mechanisms.

Inflammatory Cells in COPD

Airway Epithelial Cells

The normal differentiated airway epithelium is composed of ciliated cells, undifferentiated columnar cells, secretary cells, and basal cells. Ciliated and mucus-producing cells remove microbes and other foreign particles via mucociliary clearance mechanism. Non-mucus

J.-H. Lee
Department of Allergy, Pulmonary and Critical Care Medicine, CHA Bundang Medical Center, CHA University, Pocheon, South Korea
e-mail: plmjhlee@cha.ac.kr

S.-D. Lee (ed.), *COPD*, DOI 10.1007/978-3-662-47178-4_4

secretory cells produce antimicrobial and anti-inflammatory proteins, and basal cells function as stem/progenitor cells to constantly renew the differentiated cell populations. In addition, airway epithelial cells provide a physical barrier against the outside environment via tight- and adherence junctions that keep adjacent epithelial cells physically connected to each other and prevent passage of microbes and xenobiotics across the epithelial layer [11, 12]. Also, epithelial cells are in fact a rich source of cytokines and chemokines molecules involved in modulating inflammation and lung defense mechanisms [13].

Smoking- and COPD-associated functional and architectural changes of the airway epithelial barrier can also contribute to lung inflammation. Smoking causes loss of Clara cells in the small airways, which leads to decreased production of anti-inflammatory protein secretoglobin 1A1 (also known as Clara cell protein). Squamous metaplasia, a common histologic lesion in the airway epithelium of individuals with COPD [14], is associated with increased production of proinflammatory cytokines, interleukin (IL)-1α and IL-1β [15] and decreased expression of antimicrobial factors, such as secretory leukoprotease inhibitor (SLPI) [16]. Further, disorganization of the junctional barrier in the airway of COPD smokers results in increased permeability of the airway epithelium [17, 18], which may allow microbial products or cigarette smoke to diffuse through the epithelial layer and activate inflammatory cells in the airway mucosa [11].

Alveolar Macrophages

Alveolar macrophages reside on the respiratory epithelial surface and thus are directly exposed to the outside environment. Macrophages are responsible for a broad set of host defense including recognition and phagocytosis of pathogenic material and apoptotic cells.

There is a five to tenfold increase in the numbers of macrophages in airways, lung parenchyma, and bronchoalveolar lavage (BAL) fluid in patients with COPD. Macrophage numbers in the airways correlate with the severity of COPD [19] and macrophage numbers in the alveoli correlate with the severity of emphysema [20].

There is a lot of evidence that macrophages play a key role in orchestrating the inflammation of COPD through the release of chemokines that attract neutrophils, monocytes, and T cells, providing a cellular mechanism that links smoking with inflammation in COPD (Fig. 4.1). Increased numbers of macrophages in the lungs of patients with COPD and in the lungs of smokers may result from increased recruitment of monocytes from the circulation in response to monocyte chemotactic chemokines such as monocyte chemotactic peptide (MCP)-1, and other CXC chemokines (CXCL1, CCL2) released by macrophages via interaction with the chemokine receptor CCR2 and CXCR2 expressed on monocytes [21]. Macrophages also attract neutrophils into the lung via CXCL1 and CXCL8 (also known as IL-8), which act on CXCR2 expressed predominantly by neutrophils [22]. Chemokines such as CXCL9, CXCL10, and CXCL11 released from macrophages are chemotactic for $CD8^+$ T cytotoxic (Tc) cells and $CD4^+$ Th1 cells, via interaction with the chemokine receptor CXCR3 expressed on these cells [23]. Macrophages also release transforming growth factor (TGF)-β and connective tissue growth factor (CTGF), which stimulate fibroblast proliferation, resulting in fibrosis in the small airways.

Alveolar macrophages secrete proteases, including matrix metalloproteinase MMP-2, MMP-9, and MMP-12; cathepsins K, L, and S; and neutrophil elastase, taken up from neutrophils, which may contribute to emphysematous alveolar destruction [2]. Alveolar macrophages from patients with COPD are more activated, secrete more inflammatory proteins, and have greater elastolytic activity than those from normal smokers, which is further enhanced by exposure to cigarette smoke [21, 24].

Mechanism of macrophage activation occurs via oxidant-induced inactivation and reduction of histone deacetylase-2 (HDAC2), shifting the balance toward acetylated or loose chromatin, exposing nuclear factor-κB (NF-*k*B) sites, and resulting in transcription of MMPs, proinflammatory cytokines [25]. Corticosteroid resistance in COPD may be linked to the decreased HDAC activity [26, 27].

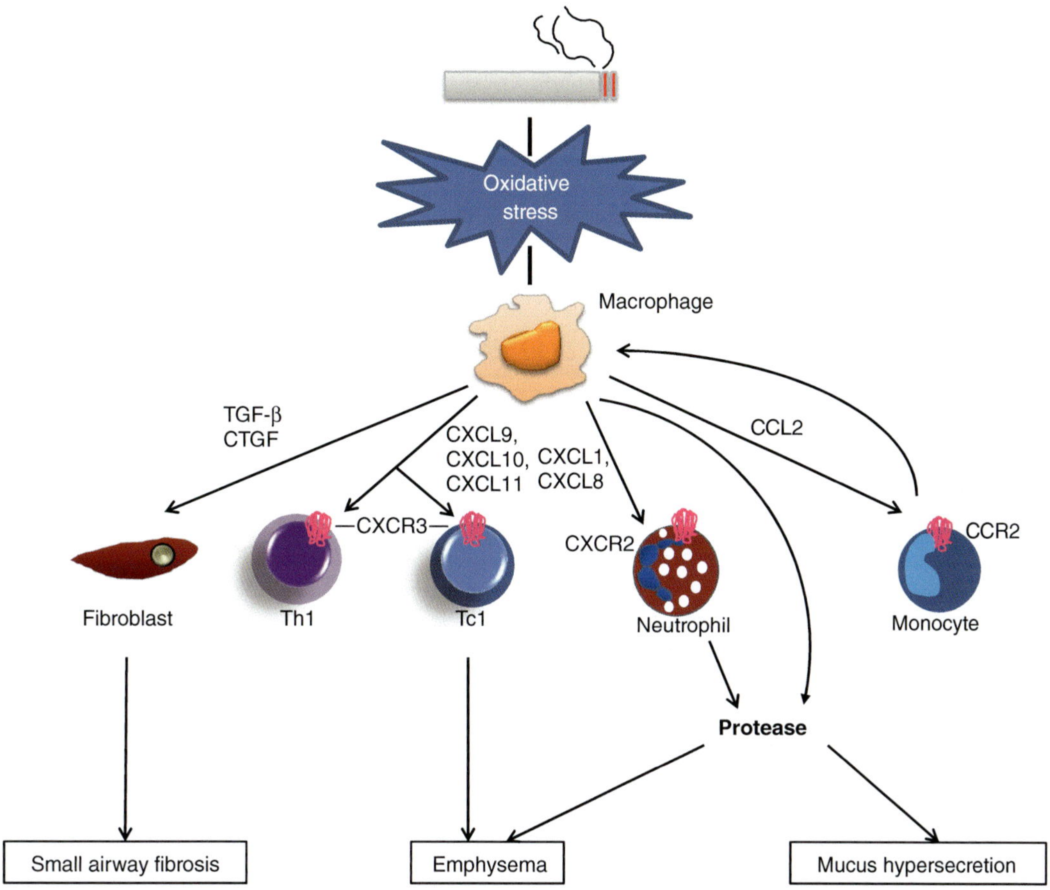

Fig. 4.1 Macrophages play a key role in orchestrating the inflammation of COPD through the release of several chemokines that attract neutrophils, monocytes, and T cells. Release of transforming growth factor (TGF)-β and connective tissue growth factor (CTGF) from macrophage also stimulate fibroblast proliferation

Alveolar macrophages from COPD patients are defective in phagocytic removal of apoptotic cells (efferocytosis), and phagocytic uptake of bacteria, which may contribute to the maintenance of chronic inflammation in COPD [28] and chronic colonization of the lower airways by bacteria such as *Haemophilus influenzae* or *Streptococcus pneumonia* [29]. The bacterial colonization of lower airways may predispose to acute exacerbations or pneumonia in patients with COPD [30].

Neutrophils

There is a lot of data supporting neutrophils as the key effector cells in COPD. Activated neutrophils were increased in number within the sputum of COPD patients [31]. The numbers of neutrophils in bronchial biopsy specimen and induced sputum were correlated with the degree of airflow limitation [32] and the rate of lung function decline in COPD [33].

Smoking stimulates the granulocyte production/release from the bone marrow and prolongs the survival of neutrophils in the respiratory tract, possibly mediated by granulocyte macrophage colony-stimulating factor (GM-CSF) and granulocyte colony-stimulating factor (G-CSF) released from alveolar macrophages [34]. Smoking also causes sequestration of neutrophils in the lung capillaries by decreasing their deformability [35].

Neutrophils migrate and accumulate into the lungs from the circulation under the direction of various neutrophil chemotactic factors, including leukotriene B4, CXCL1, CXCL5 (ENA-78), and CXCL8, which are increased in COPD airways [36].

The migrating neutrophils release proteinases, such as neutrophil elastase, cathepsin G, and proteinase-3, as well as MMP-8 and MMP-9, which may contribute to alveolar destruction and mucus hypersecretion from submucosal glands and goblet cells.

Interestingly, neutrophils from patients with COPD show marked abnormalities in chemotactic response with increased migration but adopted more circuitous pathways [37], which is likely to increase damage to bystander lung tissue and impede bacterial clearance [38].

Dendritic Cells

Dendritic cells are a specialized population of mononuclear cells responsible for recognition and uptake of pathogenic materials. The airways and lungs contain a rich network of immature dendritic cells that are localized near the surface. Airway dendritic cells reside adjacent to epithelial cells and extend cytoplasmic protrusions to sample luminal antigens and interact with environmental signals. Upon recognition of antigen, dendritic cells undergo a maturation process and migrate toward the local lymphoid tissues, such as regional lymph nodes or mucosal lymphoid aggregates. Mature dendritic cells present the processed antigens to naive T lymphocytes, initiating adaptive immune response to pathogens.

There is an increased number of dendritic cells in the airways and alveolar walls of smokers [39]. It is likely that the specific subset of dendritic cells is activated in the lungs of patients with COPD [40] and is linked to disease severity [41]. The role of dendritic cells in COPD is not yet defined, but they may form the crucial link between the innate and adaptive immune responses in COPD.

Lymphocytes

The only significant difference in the inflammatory cell infiltrate in asymptomatic smokers and smokers with COPD is an increase in T cells, mainly $CD8^+$ Tc cells.

The number of lung $CD8^+$ T cells in COPD increases substantially with the severity of airflow limitation and emphysema [3]. On activation, $CD8^+$ Tc cells cause cytolysis and apoptosis of alveolar epithelial cells through release of perforins, granzyme B, and tumor necrosis factor-α (TNF-α), and there is an association between $CD8^+$ Tc cells and apoptotic alveolar cells in emphysema [42].

The numbers of $CD4^+$ T cells are also increased in the airways and lungs of COPD patients. At least two different types of effector $CD4^+$ T cells accumulate in the lungs of patients with stable COPD: Th1 cells and Th17 cells [23, 43].

Th1 cells produce interferon-γ and promote accumulation of inflammatory cells to the lungs. Lung lymphocytes isolated from the patients with COPD have higher percentages of Th1 cells and secrete more interferon-γ than in control smokers [23]. IL-18, which promotes Th1 cell development, is strongly expressed in alveolar macrophages, Tc cells, and epithelial cells in lungs of severe COPD patients [44]. Cytokines of Th1 cells participate in perpetuating autoimmune responses and result in excessive proinflammatory responses that can lead to uncontrolled tissue damage.

Th17 cells are a distinct lineage of activated $CD4^+$ T cells, mediate immunity against extracellular pathogens, but have also been implicated in autoimmunity [45]. Th17 cells, which secrete IL-17A and IL-22, are also increased in airways of patients with COPD and may play a role in orchestrating neutrophilic inflammation [43, 46]. Th17 cells may be regulated by IL-6 and IL-23 released from alveolar macrophages.

Regulatory T cells (Treg) are another subset of $CD4^+$ T cells with immunoregulatory functions, which inhibit autoimmunity and suppress inflammation. Tapering of the immune response by Treg cells protects against uncontrolled inflammation [47], and reduced Treg cell population have been found in the lungs of patients with COPD [48, 49].

In severe and very severe COPD patients, B cells are found in large airways and bronchial-associated lymphoid tissues around small airways [7] and the lung parenchyma [6]. B cells might be activated by bacterial or viral antigens as a consequence of the chronic bacterial colonization or latent viral infection in the airways of these patients. The pathogenic role of the B cell response is controversial; it might be protective against microbial colonization and infection of the lower respiratory tract or it could be directed against lung tissue antigens, suggesting an autoimmune component in the pathogenesis of COPD.

Other Cells

Although mast cells and eosinophils have been traditionally associated with the pathogenetic mechanisms of allergic asthma, evidence suggests that mast cells and eosinophils could be implicated in the pathogenesis of COPD.

Histological studies of human lungs have shown that as COPD progresses to its severe stages, mast cell populations undergo changes in density, morphology, and distribution, including an increase in the number in airway lumen [50]. Even though, not all patients with stable COPD have shown the increased number of eosinophils in the airways [51, 52], many reports have consistently shown that the increased numbers of eosinophils in bronchial biopsies or BAL fluid during acute exacerbations of COPD [53, 54]. The presence of eosinophils in patients with COPD predicts a response to corticosteroids and may indicate coexisting asthma [52, 55].

Natural killer cells are classified as lymphocytes on the basis of their morphology, the expression of lymphoid markers, and their origin from a common lymphoid progenitor cells. However, they are deemed components of innate immunity because they lack antigen-specific cell surface receptors [56]. Natural killer cells act as cytolytic effector lymphocytes, which can directly induce the death not only of virus-infected cells and tumor cells, but also of damaged structural cells in the lungs [4, 57]. Increased cytotoxic activity of natural killer cells expressing both perforin and granzyme B have been shown in induced sputum of patients with COPD compared with healthy smokers [4].

Additionally, natural killer cells cross-talk with dendritic cells and promote the maturation of dendritic cells by producing interferon-γ and TNF-α [58].

Inflammatory Mediators in COPD

A lot of inflammatory cytokines and chemokines have been found to be associated with COPD [2, 59, 60]. Pulmonary epithelial cells when exposed to noxious environmental substances release TNF-α, IL-1β, GM-CSF, TGF-β1, MCP-1, leukotriene B4, and IL-8 [59, 61, 62]. Macrophages also release many kinds of chemokines, such as CCL2, CXCL1, CXCL8, CXCL9, CXCL10, and CXCL11, which are chemotactic to monocytes, neutrophils, and lymphocytes [62]. In addition, proteolytic enzymes, e.g., MMP-2, MMP-9, MMP-12, and cathepsins, are also secreted in response to reactive oxygen species (ROS)-rich environment [63]. Transcription factor NF-κB orchestrates these responses in the cells of patients with COPD [64].

Which cytokines are the major players at each time point along the evolving stage of COPD remains unclear [2, 60].

Similar inflammatory mediators increased in the circulation of patients with COPD may underlie and potentiate systemic comorbidities frequently seen in patients with COPD.

Pathogenesis of Emphysema

Largely due to the greater structural similarity of animal air spaces than airways to human, we know more about mechanisms involved in emphysema than small airway obstruction.

Protease-Antiprotease Imbalance in the Pathogenesis of COPD

The discovery of severe α1-antitrypsin deficiency in early-onset emphysema patients [65], and the induction of emphysema by intratracheal instillation of a proteolytic enzyme in experimental animals [66, 67], led to the protease-antiprotease imbalance hypothesis of emphysema. According to this hypothesis, smoking induces an increased number of neutrophils and macrophages in the lung and the released proteases from these cells are not fully inhibited by antiproteases, which lead to proteolysis of lung connective tissue, particularly elastin and also stimulate inflammation into the lung [68, 69].

A large body of literature has been tested the hypothesis that a protease-antiprotease imbalance is the critical mechanism in the pathogenesis of emphysema in COPD.

Protease-Antiprotease Imbalance in α1-Antitrypsin Deficiency

There is strong evidence to support this hypothesis as the main pathogenic mechanism in emphysema associated with severe α1-antitrypsin deficiency. α1-antitrypsin is a 52-kDa single-chain glycoprotein with a sequence of 394 amino acids that is synthesized predominantly in the liver and functions as the major inhibitor of neutrophil elastase [69].

Several mechanisms are related to deficiency of α1-antitrypsin, including total absence of the gene, frame shift mutations that lead to premature stop codons, as well as point mutations that may lead to no production or production of abnormal α1-antitrypsin phenotypes [70]. Abnormal α1-antitrypsin is accumulated in the hepatocytes and has retained a tendency to form spontaneous polymers both in the serum and tissues, especially the lung. The most common phenotype of α1-antitrypsin is the normal M form. Affected individuals have two genes and these are usually expressed in a codominant form, thus heterozygotes are common. The level of α1-antitrypsin may be key to the susceptibility to develop pulmonary emphysema [69]. MZ heterozygotes have partially reduced serum levels (approximately 60% of normal MM homozygotes), and SZ heterozygotes have levels approximately 40% of the normal MM homozygotes. In contrast, ZZ or Z-null types have levels less than 15% of the normal value.

Elastin is the principal component of elastic fibers. Insoluble elastin fibers are formed by complex mechanisms from the tropoelastin molecules secreted from several cell types. Elastin is an important target for proteolytic enzymes, and its destruction results in emphysematous destruction and loss of elasticity in the lung parenchyma [71].

Neutrophil elastase is a potent elastolytic enzyme and its intratracheal injection in experimental animals induces emphysema [66, 67]. A pathogenic role of neutrophil elastase in α1-antitrypsin-deficient emphysema is supported by the correlation of increased neutrophil elastase concentration with severity of emphysema [72].

Increased elastase activity in patients with COPD may contribute to inflammation because fragments of matrix proteins, generated by protease activity, have chemotactic activity for neutrophils and monocytes and may also be proinflammatory [73]. Neutrophil elastase is also a potent stimulant of mucus secretion in the airways [2].

The classic presentation for individuals with α1-antitrypsin deficiency is early-onset basal panacinar emphysema. However, in recent years α1-antitrypsin deficiency testing has become more widespread, and the variability of the age of presentation has become more apparent as well as variations in the clinical phenotype. Patients may present with bronchiectasis and no emphysema [74], upper zone and centrilobular emphysema [75], as well as the classic lower zone panacinar emphysema.

Protease-Antiprotease Imbalance in COPD Without Antitrypsin Deficiency

Smoking may cause a protease-antiprotease imbalance by reducing the functional activity of α1-antitrypsin and by increasing the amount of elastolytic proteases released in the lung [76, 77]. However, most of the α1-antitrypsin in cigarette smokers remains active and is therefore still capable of protecting against the increased protease burden [78–80].

Therefore, further hypotheses have invoked a contributory role for other proteases and antiproteases imbalance, especially in COPD patients without α1-antitrypsin deficiency.

Pathological studies of accidentally dying young smokers reported an increased number of macrophages in the respiratory bronchioles, where centrilobular emphysema develops in smokers without α1-antitrypsin deficiency [81], suggesting a potential role of macrophages especially in centrilobular emphysema.

Alveolar macrophages may bind and internalize released neutrophil elastase in the lung [82] and alveolar macrophage from smokers with low attenuation area on CT scan showed higher activity of neutrophil elastase [83].

Alveolar macrophage also releases several elastolytic enzymes including MMP-2, MMP-9, MMP-12, cathepsins L and S [84–87], which are not inhibited by α1-antitrypsin. In addition, non-elastolytic enzyme, MMP-1 (collagenase) from macrophages, has been implicated in the pathogenesis of emphysema in transgenic mice [88, 89] by degrading type III collagen [90]. Elastolytic activity of cultured alveolar macrophage from patients with emphysema was increased compared with those of patients with bronchitis or other lung diseases [91]. Emphysematous lung tissue showed significantly higher levels of MMP-2 (gelatinase A) and MMP-9 (gelatinase B) compared with control tissue [92]. A study using immunohistochemistry showed increases in MMP-1, MMP-2, MMP-8, and MMP-9 in lung tissue from COPD patients compared with controls. MMP-9 is also known to activate the latent form of TGF-β to its active form [93], which could provide a link between enhanced elastolytic activity by MMP-9 and the simultaneous airway fibrosis by activation of TGF-β.

In addition, extracellular matrix proteolytic degradation fragments may act as chemokines and promote inflammation [73, 94, 95]. MMP-9 generates a collagen fragment, N-acetyl-proline-glycine-proline tripeptide, which is chemotactic to neutrophils [73]. Laminin and fibronectin fragments are chemotactic to human neutrophils and monocytes [94]. In that way, proteolysis of extracellular matrix generates fragments that may perpetuate inflammation even after smoking cessation.

Human alveolar macrophages also release endogenous inhibitors of MMPs, TIMP1 and TIMP2 [96]. Alveolar macrophages from COPD patients release less TIMP1 in vitro than those from smokers without COPD and nonsmokers [97]. TIMP3 is the only TIMP that binds strongly to the extracellular matrix. TIMP3 knockout mice demonstrate progressive airspace enlargement and enhanced collagen degradation or increased elastin breakdown without inflammation [98].

While extracellular matrix proteolysis by inflammatory cell-derived proteolytic enzymes is a central event in emphysema, it is apparent that it cannot explain the complexity of alveolar destruction in COPD.

Oxidative Stress in the Pathogenesis of COPD

Oxidants include reactive molecules, including free radicals and non-radical reactive species, summarized as reactive species comprising ROS and reactive nitrogen species (RNS). Normal airways are replete with antioxidants, such as glutathione (GSH), urate, ascorbate, and extracellular superoxide dismutase (ECSOD). The balance between oxidants and antioxidants is important to maintain normal physiologic function in the lung. Oxidative stress is a potentially harmful imbalance between oxidants and antioxidants and occurs when the burden of oxidants is not well counterbalanced by the antioxidant defense system [99], which may provoke diverse lung pathologies.

Although inflammation and protease-antiprotease imbalance have been postulated to be critical in cigarette smoke-induced emphysema, there is considerable evidence that oxidative stress plays an important role in COPD [100, 101].

Physiological Roles of Radical Species

Experimental studies have identified mitochondrial ROS as essential for O_2 sensing. Superoxide radicals may aid in maintaining defined redox potentials on the cellular level and so regulate development and differentiation processes of the organism. Tyrosine radicals are part of the subunit of ribonucleoside diphosphate reductase in the synthesis of DNA. Reactive species also contribute to the synthesis of prostaglandins and leukotrienes. Inflammatory cells not only use but also release oxidizing agents (e.g., myeloperoxidase from neutrophils or eosinophilic peroxidase from eosinophils) to destroy microbes and to protect the organs. Some of the reactive species are important signaling mediators; ROS generated by macrophages in inflammatory processes may initiate intracellular signal transduction and then express cytokines and other mediators of inflammation [102]. The function of nitric oxide is well documented as a potent vasodilator, neurotransmitter, and bactericide. In addition, reactive species are closely correlated to cellular apoptosis.

Oxidative Stress in the Pathogenesis of COPD

With a large surface area of 80–100 m^2 and a daily breathing volume of 10,000–20,000 L, the lungs are very susceptible to oxidative stress. Especially in smokers, the situation is drastic because smoking leads to a significant exposure to oxidants [103]. Besides cigarette smoke, urban (biomass fuel), industrial, and occupational air pollution provide various exogenous oxidants that probably are responsible for the high prevalence rates of COPD in nonsmokers in developing countries [102].

The enhanced oxidizing environment can facilitate the binding of pathogens or antigens to effector cells leading to an innate immune system.

Increased expression of multiple inflammatory genes is regulated by acetylation of core histones, and HDAC2 suppresses inflammatory gene expression. Oxidants modify HDAC protein, induce proteosomal degradation of HDAC, and thus decrease HDAC activity [104]. It turns on the redox-sensitive transcription factors (NF-κB and activating protein-1 [AP-1]) resulting in the production of proinflammatory cytokines and chemokines, which further aggravate inflammation and oxidative stress [102].

Oxidants inactivate antiproteases (such as α1-antitrypsin or secretory leukoprotease inhibitor) [105] and activate MMPs [102], resulting in a protease-antiprotease imbalance in the lungs, and damage the lung matrix protein (e.g., elastin and collagen) [106]. In addition, oxidants may interfere with elastin synthesis and repair [101].

In COPD, HDAC2 expression and activity are reduced in peripheral lung and in alveolar macrophages, resulting in amplification of the inflammatory response. Oxidative stress also causes alveolar cell apoptosis in the setting of human and experimental emphysema [107–109]. Moreover, oxidative stress underlies several of the mechanisms thought to participate in aging, which is another suggested mechanism of the pathogenesis of COPD [110].

The defense mechanisms of the cell through the activation of antioxidant system are also significantly defected in COPD patients [111]. A master antioxidant transcription factor, nuclear erythroid-related factor 2 (Nrf2), controls the expression of more than 100 gene products, including many important antioxidant enzymes. Disruption of the Nrf2 gene in mice led to earlier onset and more extensive cigarette smoke-induced emphysema with increased inflammation and apoptosis in the lung [112].

Cell Death and Impaired Repair in COPD

Excess oxidative stress causes cell death by nonphysiological (necrotic) or regulated pathways (apoptosis). Apoptotic death of alveolar structural cells (endothelial and epithelial cells) has been shown to play a crucial role in the development of emphysema.

Alveolar cell apoptosis was induced by the intratracheal instillation of active caspase-3 and caused emphysematous change [113]. Direct instillation of ceramide, oxidative stress-induced proapoptotic molecule, to the lungs of mice cause apoptotic cell death and alveolar enlargement [114]. Superoxide dismutase protected against ceramide-induced alveolar cell apoptosis and alveolar enlargement [115]. These findings indicate that alveolar cell apoptosis and oxidative stress mutually interact to mediate emphysematous alveolar destruction.

Also, vascular endothelial growth factor (VEGF) signaling seems to be important for the maintenance of the integrity of alveolar structure. Decreased VEGF or VEGF signaling could cause experimental emphysema with apoptotic cell death in animals [116, 117]. Decreased expression of

VEGF and VEGF-receptor 2 expressions were demonstrated in human emphysema lungs [118] and cigarette smoke reduced the levels of VEGF-receptor 2 expression in rat lung and in the lungs of smokers and COPD patients [119].

Recently, autophagic cell death prior to apoptosis has been implicated in the pathogenesis of emphysema. Autophagy is a pro-survival mechanism responding to injury. Lung epithelial cells [120], endothelial cells [121], fibroblasts [122], and alveolar macrophages [122, 123] initiate autophagy signaling responding to cigarette smoke exposure. Current evidence suggests that the abnormal persistence of such signaling or the inability to complete a physiological autophagic program may increase cellular stress such as endoplasmic reticulum (ER) stress, leading to caspase activation and apoptosis in diseased lungs [121, 123, 124]. In the specimens of COPD patients, markers of autophagy were upregulated in the early stage of disease progression, while caspase activation was examined at the later stages of COPD. This might indicate that autophagy is attempting to protect during the initial stages from cigarette smoke-induced stress [27].

Although, significant regeneration and repair are possible after physiologic insults, including pneumonectomy and severe respiratory infection [125–128], the ability of the adult lung to repair damaged alveoli appears limited. It is unlikely that the process of septation that is responsible for alveologenesis during lung development can be reinitiated. Also, it appears difficult for an adult human to completely restore an appropriate extracellular matrix, particularly functional elastic fibers.

Some compensatory lung tissue regrowth is possible, for which several factors, such as, thyroid transcription factor 1, VEGF, hypoxia-inducible factor 1, and keratinocyte growth factor are known to be responsible [129–132].

It is well known that the type II alveolar epithelial cells have regenerative capacity. In a recent study, type II epithelial cells can be self-renewed in culture and differentiated into alveolar-like structures "alveolospheres" containing type II and cells expressing type I epithelial cell markers. [133].

In alveolar tissue context, mesenchymal stem cell (MSC) also has been shown to contribute to regeneration in cigarette smoke-induced emphysema in rat lung [134, 135]. Amniotic fluid-derived MSC has generated type II alveolar epithelial cells, integrated at the sites of destruction, and induced local regeneration of the lung alveolar epithelium [134]. Administration of bone marrow-derived cell, MSC, cell free MSC-conditioned media also induced a repair of emphysema and increased the number of small pulmonary vessels [135]. The reparative effects of these stem cells are thought to be achieved due to paracrine effect rather than stem cell engraftment because stem cell engraftment rate was very low and cell-free MSC-conditioned media also induced repair.

Finally, lung fibroblasts are considered crucial for maintenance of the integrity of alveolar structure by producing extracellular matrix proteins, including collagen, elastin, and fibronectin, which are required for attachment, structure, and function of alveolar epithelial cells [136]. Cigarette smoke extract suppresses proliferation [137], apoptotic death [138], senescence [139], and inhibition of collagen gel contraction [140] in lung fibroblasts in vitro. Similarly, lung fibroblasts from patients with COPD showed similar effects [141, 142], suggesting that cigarette smoke may interfere with reparative roles of lung fibroblasts.

The relentless lung injury due to oxidant exposure, disruption of the balance between cell death and replenishment of structural cells along with the potential exhaustion of lung maintenance program ultimately leads to emphysema.

Other Pathogenetic Mechanism of Emphysema

Accelerated Aging

Oxidative stress induce a number of molecular and cellular mechanisms associated with cellular senescence including accumulation of DNA damage [143], impairment of DNA repair [144] epigenetic modifications in nuclear DNA [145], protein damage [146].

There is growing evidence that emphysema may be caused by accelerated aging of the lungs. Emphysema and cellular senescence share some features, inflammation and oxidative stress, which are the main pathogenic mechanisms of COPD [110, 147].

In addition, several aging animal models have been associated with emphysema. The klotho gene encodes a membrane protein that is a regulator of oxidative stress and cell senescence [148]; mice with a defect of the klotho gene develop a syndrome resembling aging including emphysema [149]. Senescent marker protein-30 (SMP-30) is expressed in early life and progressively decreases with age [150]; SMP-30 knockout mice develop distal airspace enlargement indicative of emphysema [151].

Telomeres are DNA caps located at the end of chromosomes, protecting DNA against degradation and remodeling, and preventing gene mutation that may lead to cancerous changes [152]. Owing to the end-replication problem in mature somatic cells, telomere repeats are lost with each replicative cycle until a critical length is reached, at which point cells undergo apoptosis or other disruptive events. This entire process is accelerated by the presence of ROS or inflammation [153], leading to short telomeres and telomere length is well-known biomarkers of biological aging. From patients with COPD, telomeres of blood leukocytes are shorter compared with control subjects [154].

As other cellular senescence markers, expression of senescence-associated β-galactosidase (SA–β-gal) and cyclin-kinase inhibitors p16 and p21, and detection of DNA repair/damage can be used [155]. Cigarette smoke extract leads to increased SA–β-gal expression in cultured type II cells [156] or lung fibroblasts [139]. Lung fibroblasts harvested from emphysematous lungs also showed increased SA–β-gal expression [157]. Alveolar epithelial and endothelial cells in emphysematous lungs showed increased expression of p21 in association with decreased telomere length [158].

Sirtuin I (SIRT-1) is an anti-aging and anti-inflammatory protein, essential for maintaining silent chromatin via metabolic NAD(+)-dependent protein/histone deacetylase. SIRT-1 also regulates NF-κB-dependent transcription and cell survival in response to TNF-α [159]. Environmental stress, such as cigarette smoke exposure, reduced activity and expression of SIRT-1 via increased expression of MMP-9 [160]. SIRT-1 is decreased in lung cells from patients with COPD, compared with smokers without COPD as a result of post-translational oxidative modification [161]. This would accelerate the process of aging and also enhance inflammation.

In conclusion, cellular senescence induced by ROS further impair tissue repair in response to repetitive cigarette smoke-induced injury of the lungs.

Autoimmunity and COPD

Autoimmunity has been proposed as a late pathogenic event in the progressive course of COPD. Cigarette-induced lung injury may uncover previously sequestered autoantigens, or cigarette smoke may damage lung interstitial and structural cells and make them antigenic [57].

Several autoantibodies have been found in the circulation of patients with COPD, particularly in severe disease [162, 163]. Antibodies against primary pulmonary epithelial cells, including anti-Hep-2 epithelial cell IgG autoantibodies, were found more frequently in patients with COPD than in controls [164]. Even though the data are conflicting, antielastin antibodies also have been proposed to drive COPD progression [48, 165].

Lung vascular endothelial cells also can be exposed to autoimmune attacks. Xenogeneic endothelial cells injected in rats induced autoantibody production that subsequently leads to lung emphysema [166]. Corroboratively, another study demonstrated that patients with COPD have significantly higher serum antiendothelial cell antibodies than subjects without COPD [167].

In addition, it was reported that antinuclear autoantibodies were more prevalent in patients with COPD than in healthy controls, but these molecules were not associated with smoking status or FEV_1, even though, the pathological importance of these observations is unclear [168, 169].

Consequences of such self-attack induce lung tissue damage and further lead to structural alterations and creation of neoantigens [170]. Autoimmunity to these modified host molecules could be important in the pathogenesis of emphysema.

Epigenetic Changes in COPD Development

A lot of evidence support that individual susceptibility is important in the development of COPD. Many candidate genes that could be linked to the development of COPD have been examined; however, the results have been quite inconsistent, suggesting that not only genetics, but also other factors, may contribute to the susceptibility of COPD.

Epigenetic regulation can affect the transcriptional activity of specific genes leading to alteration of gene expression patterns upon environmental stimulus without modifying the DNA sequence. Typical epigenetic changes are post-translational modifications of histones, DNA methylation, which modulate gene expression without altering the sequence of the target genes.

There is emerging evidence supporting a role of epigenetics in the regulation of inflammatory genes in COPD.

HDACs are key enzymes in the control of proinflammatory cytokines. Oxidants reduce expression levels/activity of these deacetylases. Therefore, reduced HDAC2 expression and activity in the lung and alveolar macrophages correlated with the disease severity and the intensity of the inflammation in COPD [26]. Overexpression or knockdown of HDAC2 in alveolar macrophages from COPD patients affected not only the inflammatory response but also the corticosteroid responsiveness [27].

SIRT1 is a histone and protein deacetylase, which deacetylates histones (H3 and H4) and non-histone proteins including transcription factors, co-activators, and other signaling molecules (e.g., FOXO, p53, and RelA/p65) [171]. It is recognized that SIRT1 modulates NF-*k*B-dependent transcription [159] and inhibits the activity of NF-*k*B [172]. SIRT1 expression is reduced in the lungs of smokers and COPD patients. Cigarette smoke extracts derived reactive species down-regulated SIRT1 protein level in human monocyte-macrophage cells via post-translational modifications, leading to increased level of pro-inflammatory cytokines [161].

Given their demonstrated modifiable nature, epigenetic mechanisms may open new possibilities for therapeutic intervention.

Pathogenesis of Airway Obstruction

Infiltration of Inflammatory Cells in Small Airways

Progression of COPD is associated with the infiltration of the airway wall by innate and adaptive inflammatory immune cells and the percentage of airways that containing these cells increased as COPD progressed [7]. With increasing disease severity, there is also increased mucus hypersecretion, submucosal gland hypertrophy, peribronchial fibrosis, and an increase in airway smooth muscle mass. Although, it is likely that infiltrating inflammatory cells contribute to the structural abnormalities in airway, evidence linking these processes remains scarce.

Mucus Hypersecretion

The accumulation of mucus exudates in the airway lumen is characteristic in advanced COPD [7]. Cigarette smoke that inhibits the cystic fibrosis transmembrane conductance regulator (CFTR) function provides a mechanistic link between smoking and abnormal mucous secretion by airway epithelial cells [173].

The increased expression of the mucin MUC5B in the bronchiolar lumen and the mucin MUC5AC in the bronchiolar epithelium were showed in the lungs of COPD patients [174]. Activation of a ligand-dependent EGFR signaling mediated by neutrophil elastase or MMP-9 is also responsible for the mucin synthesis [175–177]. Mucus-secreting goblet cells are increased in the small airways of patients with COPD [178]. Goblet cell hyperplasia may be caused by the activation of the epidermal growth factor receptor (EGFR), which may be upregulated by oxidants in cigarette smoke and by cytokines, such as TNF-α, IL-8, or IL-13 [179, 180]. Neutrophils may directly cause degranulation of goblet cells through the release of neutrophil elastase and cathepsin G [181].

Airway Remodeling

Airway wall remodeling is present in the small airways of patients with COPD, consisting of tissue repair and epithelial metaplasia that contribute to airway wall thickening and airflow obstruction.

TGF-β is proposed as an important mediator of airway remodeling in COPD [182]. Increased TGF-β is found in the small airway epithelium of COPD patients, and its levels correlate with the severity of obstruction [183, 184]. Adenoviral transfer of TGF-β1 to murine lung shows increased fibroblast accumulation around airways, and airway epithelial transgenic expression of TGF-β causes peribronchiolar fibrosis [185, 186]. TGF-β also increases the expression of smooth muscle contractile proteins, such as α-smooth muscle actin and calponin, in airway smooth muscle and fibroblasts, which increases airway smooth muscle mass [187, 188].

TGF-β is ubiquitously expressed in three isoforms in all mammalian cell types and tissues but is found almost entirely in a latent form [189, 190]. Thus, a major point of regulation of TGF-β function is through its activation.

Squamous metaplasia actively contributes to airway wall thickening through alteration of epithelial-mesenchymal interactions in COPD. IL-1β released by squamous metaplastic epithelium activates TGF-β in human airway fibroblasts [15].

Smooth muscle mass seen in small airways of COPD patients is inversely correlated with the lung function [3]. However, it is unknown whether increased smooth muscle mass is caused by an increased cell number, an increased cell size, or both [191].

Airway smooth muscle cells also have potential to contribute to the inflammatory and remodeling processes in the small airways [191]. Recent study reported that oxidative stress induces mitochondrial dysfunction in airway smooth muscle cells isolated from COPD patients, which might contribute to inflammation and increased airway smooth muscle mass in COPD [192].

Unanswered Question

Although major progress has been made in understanding COPD, many questions about COPD remain unanswered.

1. Why do not all smokers develop COPD?
2. Why does it take decades to develop COPD?
3. How the underlying inflammatory process is linked to pathophysiology and disease progression?
4. Why inflammation and disease progression persist even after smoking cessation?
5. Why is COPD heterogeneous?

The issues will provide a valuable basis for future research into this devastating disease.

References

1. Brusselle GG, Joos GF, Bracke KR. New insights into the immunology of chronic obstructive pulmonary disease. Lancet. 2011;378(9795):1015–26.
2. Barnes PJ. Cellular and molecular mechanisms of chronic obstructive pulmonary disease. Clin Chest Med. 2014;35(1):71–86.
3. Saetta M, Di Stefano A, Turato G, Facchini FM, Corbino L, Mapp CE, et al. CD8+ T-lymphocytes in peripheral airways of smokers with chronic obstructive pulmonary disease. Am J Respir Crit Care Med. 1998;157(3 Pt 1):822–6. doi:10.1164/ajrccm.157.3.9709027.
4. Urbanowicz RA, Lamb JR, Todd I, Corne JM, Fairclough LC. Enhanced effector function of cytotoxic cells in the induced sputum of COPD patients. Respir Res. 2010;11:76. doi:10.1186/1465-9921-11-76.
5. Sullivan AK, Simonian PL, Falta MT, Mitchell JD, Cosgrove GP, Brown KK, et al. Oligoclonal CD4+ T cells in the lungs of patients with severe emphysema. Am J Respir Crit Care Med. 2005;172(5):590–6. doi:10.1164/rccm.200410-1332OC.

6. van der Strate BW, Postma DS, Brandsma CA, Melgert BN, Luinge MA, Geerlings M, et al. Cigarette smoke-induced emphysema: a role for the B cell? Am J Respir Crit Care Med. 2006;173(7):751–8. doi:10.1164/rccm.200504-594OC.
7. Hogg JC, Chu F, Utokaparch S, Woods R, Elliott WM, Buzatu L, et al. The nature of small-airway obstruction in chronic obstructive pulmonary disease. N Engl J Med. 2004;350(26):2645–53. doi:10.1056/NEJMoa032158.
8. Tetley TD. Inflammatory cells and chronic obstructive pulmonary disease. Curr Drug Targets Inflamm Allergy. 2005;4(6):607–18.
9. Gadgil A, Zhu X, Sciurba FC, Duncan SR. Altered T-cell phenotypes in chronic obstructive pulmonary disease. Proc Am Thorac Soc. 2006;3(6):487–8. doi:10.1513/pats.200603-064MS.
10. Domagala-Kulawik J, Maskey-Warzechowska M, Kraszewska I, Chazan R. The cellular composition and macrophage phenotype in induced sputum in smokers and ex-smokers with COPD. Chest. 2003;123(4):1054–9.
11. Shaykhiev R, Crystal RG. Innate immunity and chronic obstructive pulmonary disease: a mini-review. Gerontology. 2013;59(6):481–9. doi:10.1159/000354173.
12. Shaykhiev R, Otaki F, Bonsu P, Dang DT, Teater M, Strulovici-Barel Y, et al. Cigarette smoking reprograms apical junctional complex molecular architecture in the human airway epithelium in vivo. Cell Mol Life Sci. 2011;68(5):877–92. doi:10.1007/s00018-010-0500-x.
13. Thorley AJ, Tetley TD. Pulmonary epithelium, cigarette smoke, and chronic obstructive pulmonary disease. Int J Chron Obstruct Pulmon Dis. 2007;2(4):409–28.
14. Auerbach O, Forman JB, Gere JB, Kassouny DY, Muehsam GE, Petrick TG, et al. Changes in the bronchial epithelium in relation to smoking and cancer of the lung; a report of progress. N Engl J Med. 1957;256(3):97–104. doi:10.1056/nejm195701172560301.
15. Araya J, Cambier S, Markovics JA, Wolters P, Jablons D, Hill A, et al. Squamous metaplasia amplifies pathologic epithelial-mesenchymal interactions in COPD patients. J Clin Invest. 2007;117(11):3551–62. doi:10.1172/jci32526.
16. Aarbiou J, van Schadewijk A, Stolk J, Sont JK, de Boer WI, Rabe KF, et al. Human neutrophil defensins and secretory leukocyte proteinase inhibitor in squamous metaplastic epithelium of bronchial airways. Inflamm Res. 2004;53(6):230–8. doi:10.1007/s00011-003-1240-x.
17. Kennedy SM, Elwood RK, Wiggs BJ, Pare PD, Hogg JC. Increased airway mucosal permeability of smokers. Relationship to airway reactivity. Am Rev Respir Dis. 1984;129(1):143–8.
18. Heijink IH, Brandenburg SM, Postma DS, van Oosterhout AJ. Cigarette smoke impairs airway epithelial barrier function and cell-cell contact recovery. Eur Respir J. 2012;39(2):419–28. doi:10.1183/09031936.00193810.
19. Russell RE, Culpitt SV, DeMatos C, Donnelly L, Smith M, Wiggins J, et al. Release and activity of matrix metalloproteinase-9 and tissue inhibitor of metalloproteinase-1 by alveolar macrophages from patients with chronic obstructive pulmonary disease. Am J Respir Cell Mol Biol. 2002;26(5):602–9. doi:10.1165/ajrcmb.26.5.4685.
20. Meshi B, Vitalis TZ, Ionescu D, Elliott WM, Liu C, Wang XD, et al. Emphysematous lung destruction by cigarette smoke. The effects of latent adenoviral infection on the lung inflammatory response. Am J Respir Cell Mol Biol. 2002;26(1):52–7. doi:10.1165/ajrcmb.26.1.4253.
21. Capelli A, Di Stefano A, Gnemmi I, Balbo P, Cerutti CG, Balbi B, et al. Increased MCP-1 and MIP-1beta in bronchoalveolar lavage fluid of chronic bronchitics. Eur Respir J. 1999;14(1):160–5.
22. Pappas K, Papaioannou AI, Kostikas K, Tzanakis N. The role of macrophages in obstructive airways disease: chronic obstructive pulmonary disease and asthma. Cytokine. 2013;64(3):613–25. doi:10.1016/j.cyto.2013.09.010.
23. Grumelli S, Corry DB, Song LZ, Song L, Green L, Huh J, et al. An immune basis for lung parenchymal destruction in chronic obstructive pulmonary disease and emphysema. PLoS Med. 2004;1(1):e8. doi:10.1371/journal.pmed.0010008.
24. Lim S, Roche N, Oliver BG, Mattos W, Barnes PJ, Chung KF. Balance of matrix metalloprotease-9 and tissue inhibitor of metalloprotease-1 from alveolar macrophages in cigarette smokers. Regulation by interleukin-10. Am J Respir Crit Care Med. 2000;162(4 Pt 1):1355–60. doi:10.1164/ajrccm.162.4.9910097.
25. Barnes PJ. Role of HDAC2 in the pathophysiology of COPD. Annu Rev Physiol. 2009;71:451–64. doi:10.1146/annurev.physiol.010908.163257.
26. Ito K, Ito M, Elliott WM, Cosio B, Caramori G, Kon OM, et al. Decreased histone deacetylase activity in chronic obstructive pulmonary disease. N Engl J Med. 2005;352(19):1967–76. doi:10.1056/NEJMoa041892.
27. Ito K, Yamamura S, Essilfie-Quaye S, Cosio B, Ito M, Barnes PJ, et al. Histone deacetylase 2-mediated deacetylation of the glucocorticoid receptor enables NF-kappaB suppression. J Exp Med. 2006;203(1):7–13. doi:10.1084/jem.20050466.
28. Hodge S, Hodge G, Scicchitano R, Reynolds PN, Holmes M. Alveolar macrophages from subjects with chronic obstructive pulmonary disease are deficient in their ability to phagocytose apoptotic airway epithelial cells. Immunol Cell Biol. 2003;81(4):289–96. doi:10.1046/j.1440-1711.2003.t01-1-01170.x.
29. Taylor AE, Finney-Hayward TK, Quint JK, Thomas CM, Tudhope SJ, Wedzicha JA, et al.

Defective macrophage phagocytosis of bacteria in COPD. Eur Respir J. 2010;35(5):1039–47. doi:10.1183/09031936.00036709.
30. Mullerova H, Chigbo C, Hagan GW, Woodhead MA, Miravitlles M, Davis KJ, et al. The natural history of community-acquired pneumonia in COPD patients: a population database analysis. Respir Med. 2012;106(8):1124–33. doi:10.1016/j.rmed.2012.04.008.
31. Keatings VM, Collins PD, Scott DM, Barnes PJ. Differences in interleukin-8 and tumor necrosis factor-alpha in induced sputum from patients with chronic obstructive pulmonary disease or asthma. Am J Respir Crit Care Med. 1996;153(2):530–4. doi:10.1164/ajrccm.153.2.8564092.
32. Sparrow D, Glynn RJ, Cohen M, Weiss ST. The relationship of the peripheral leukocyte count and cigarette smoking to pulmonary function among adult men. Chest. 1984;86(3):383–6.
33. Stanescu D, Sanna A, Veriter C, Kostianev S, Calcagni PG, Fabbri LM, et al. Airways obstruction, chronic expectoration, and rapid decline of FEV1 in smokers are associated with increased levels of sputum neutrophils. Thorax. 1996;51(3):267–71.
34. Terashima T, Wiggs B, English D, Hogg JC, van Eeden SF. Phagocytosis of small carbon particles (PM10) by alveolar macrophages stimulates the release of polymorphonuclear leukocytes from bone marrow. Am J Respir Crit Care Med. 1997;155(4):1441–7. doi:10.1164/ajrccm.155.4.9105091.
35. MacNee W, Wiggs B, Belzberg AS, Hogg JC. The effect of cigarette smoking on neutrophil kinetics in human lungs. N Engl J Med. 1989;321(14):924–8. doi:10.1056/nejm198910053211402.
36. Traves SL, Culpitt SV, Russell RE, Barnes PJ, Donnelly LE. Increased levels of the chemokines GROalpha and MCP-1 in sputum samples from patients with COPD. Thorax. 2002;57(7):590–5.
37. Sapey E, Stockley JA, Greenwood H, Ahmad A, Bayley D, Lord JM, et al. Behavioral and structural differences in migrating peripheral neutrophils from patients with chronic obstructive pulmonary disease. Am J Respir Crit Care Med. 2011;183(9):1176–86. doi:10.1164/rccm.201008-1285OC.
38. Stockley JA, Walton GM, Lord JM, Sapey E. Aberrant neutrophil functions in stable chronic obstructive pulmonary disease: the neutrophil as an immunotherapeutic target. Int Immunopharmacol. 2013;17(4):1211–7. doi:10.1016/j.intimp.2013.05.035.
39. Soler P, Moreau A, Basset F, Hance AJ. Cigarette smoking-induced changes in the number and differentiated state of pulmonary dendritic cells/Langerhans cells. Am Rev Respir Dis. 1989;139(5):1112–7. doi:10.1164/ajrccm/139.5.1112.
40. Van Pottelberge GR, Bracke KR, Demedts IK, De Rijck K, Reinartz SM, van Drunen CM, et al. Selective accumulation of langerhans-type dendritic cells in small airways of patients with COPD. Respir Res. 2010;11:35. doi:10.1186/1465-9921-11-35.
41. Freeman CM, Martinez FJ, Han MK, Ames TM, Chensue SW, Todt JC, et al. Lung dendritic cell expression of maturation molecules increases with worsening chronic obstructive pulmonary disease. Am J Respir Crit Care Med. 2009;180(12):1179–88. doi:10.1164/rccm.200904-0552OC.
42. Majo J, Ghezzo H, Cosio MG. Lymphocyte population and apoptosis in the lungs of smokers and their relation to emphysema. Eur Respir J. 2001;17(5):946–53.
43. Di Stefano A, Caramori G, Gnemmi I, Contoli M, Vicari C, Capelli A, et al. T helper type 17-related cytokine expression is increased in the bronchial mucosa of stable chronic obstructive pulmonary disease patients. Clin Exp Immunol. 2009;157(2):316–24. doi:10.1111/j.1365-2249.2009.03965.x.
44. Imaoka H, Hoshino T, Takei S, Kinoshita T, Okamoto M, Kawayama T, et al. Interleukin-18 production and pulmonary function in COPD. Eur Respir J. 2008;31(2):287–97. doi:10.1183/09031936.00019207.
45. Miossec P, Korn T, Kuchroo VK. Interleukin-17 and type 17 helper T cells. N Engl J Med. 2009;361(9):888–98. doi:10.1056/NEJMra0707449.
46. Pridgeon C, Bugeon L, Donnelly L, Straschil U, Tudhope SJ, Fenwick P, et al. Regulation of IL-17 in chronic inflammation in the human lung. Clin Sci (Lond). 2011;120(12):515–24. doi:10.1042/cs20100417.
47. Tang Q, Bluestone JA. The Foxp3+ regulatory T cell: a jack of all trades, master of regulation. Nat Immunol. 2008;9(3):239–44. doi:10.1038/ni1572.
48. Lee SH, Goswami S, Grudo A, Song LZ, Bandi V, Goodnight-White S, et al. Antielastin autoimmunity in tobacco smoking-induced emphysema. Nat Med. 2007;13(5):567–9. doi:10.1038/nm1583.
49. Barcelo B, Pons J, Ferrer JM, Sauleda J, Fuster A, Agusti AG. Phenotypic characterisation of T-lymphocytes in COPD: abnormal CD4+CD25+ regulatory T-lymphocyte response to tobacco smoking. Eur Respir J. 2008;31(3):555–62. doi:10.1183/09031936.00010407.
50. Andersson CK, Mori M, Bjermer L, Lofdahl CG, Erjefalt JS. Alterations in lung mast cell populations in patients with chronic obstructive pulmonary disease. Am J Respir Crit Care Med. 2010;181(3):206–17. doi:10.1164/rccm.200906-0932OC.
51. Turato G, Zuin R, Saetta M. Pathogenesis and pathology of COPD. Respiration. 2001;68(2):117–28. doi:10.1159/000050478.
52. Brightling CE, Monteiro W, Ward R, Parker D, Morgan MD, Wardlaw AJ, et al. Sputum eosinophilia and short-term response to prednisolone in chronic obstructive pulmonary disease: a randomised controlled trial. Lancet. 2000;356(9240):1480–5. doi:10.1016/s0140-6736(00)02872-5.
53. Saetta M, Di Stefano A, Maestrelli P, Turato G, Ruggieri MP, Roggeri A, et al. Airway eosinophilia in chronic bronchitis during exacerbations. Am J Respir Crit Care Med. 1994;150(6 Pt 1):1646–52. doi:10.1164/ajrccm.150.6.7952628.
54. Zhu J, Qiu YS, Majumdar S, Gamble E, Matin D, Turato G, et al. Exacerbations of bronchitis: bronchial

eosinophilia and gene expression for interleukin-4, interleukin-5, and eosinophil chemoattractants. Am J Respir Crit Care Med. 2001;164(1):109–16. doi:10.1164/ajrccm.164.1.2007050.
55. Papi A, Romagnoli M, Baraldo S, Braccioni F, Guzzinati I, Saetta M, et al. Partial reversibility of airflow limitation and increased exhaled NO and sputum eosinophilia in chronic obstructive pulmonary disease. Am J Respir Crit Care Med. 2000;162(5):1773–7. doi:10.1164/ajrccm.162.5.9910112.
56. Vivier E, Raulet DH, Moretta A, Caligiuri MA, Zitvogel L, Lanier LL, et al. Innate or adaptive immunity? The example of natural killer cells. Science (New York, NY). 2011;331(6013):44–9. doi:10.1126/science.1198687.
57. Cosio MG, Saetta M, Agusti A. Immunologic aspects of chronic obstructive pulmonary disease. N Engl J Med. 2009;360(23):2445–54. doi:10.1056/NEJMra0804752.
58. Degli-Esposti MA, Smyth MJ. Close encounters of different kinds: dendritic cells and NK cells take centre stage. Nat Rev Immunol. 2005;5(2):112–24. doi:10.1038/nri1549.
59. Barnes PJ. The cytokine network in chronic obstructive pulmonary disease. Am J Respir Cell Mol Biol. 2009;41(6):631–8. doi:10.1165/rcmb.2009-0220TR.
60. Bagdonas E, Raudoniute J, Bruzauskaite I, Aldonyte R. Novel aspects of pathogenesis and regeneration mechanisms in COPD. Int J Chron Obstruct Pulmon Dis. 2015;10:995–1013. doi:10.2147/copd.s82518.
61. Chung KF, Adcock IM. Multifaceted mechanisms in COPD: inflammation, immunity, and tissue repair and destruction. Eur Respir J. 2008;31(6):1334–56. doi:10.1183/09031936.00018908.
62. Caramori G, Di Stefano A, Casolari P, Kirkham PA, Padovani A, Chung KF, et al. Chemokines and chemokine receptors blockers as new drugs for the treatment of chronic obstructive pulmonary disease. Curr Med Chem. 2013;20(35):4317–49.
63. Barnes PJ. Mediators of chronic obstructive pulmonary disease. Pharmacol Rev. 2004;56(4):515–48. doi:10.1124/pr.56.4.2.
64. Caramori G, Casolari P, Adcock I. Role of transcription factors in the pathogenesis of asthma and COPD. Cell Commun Adhes. 2013;20(1–2):21–40. doi:10.3109/15419061.2013.775257.
65. Laurell CB, Eriksson S. The electrophoretic alpha1-globulin pattern of serum in alpha1-antitrypsin deficiency. 1963. COPD. 2013;10(Suppl 1):3–8. doi:10.3109/15412555.2013.771956.
66. Janoff A, Sloan B, Weinbaum G, Damiano V, Sandhaus RA, Elias J, et al. Experimental emphysema induced with purified human neutrophil elastase: tissue localization of the instilled protease. Am Rev Respir Dis. 1977;115(3):461–78.
67. Senior RM, Tegner H, Kuhn C, Ohlsson K, Starcher BC, Pierce JA. The induction of pulmonary emphysema with human leukocyte elastase. Am Rev Respir Dis. 1977;116(3):469–75.
68. Churg A, Wright JL. Proteases and emphysema. Curr Opin Pulm Med. 2005;11(2):153–9.
69. Stockley RA. Alpha1-antitrypsin review. Clin Chest Med. 2014;35(1):39–50. doi:10.1016/j.ccm.2013.10.001.
70. Dickens JA, Lomas DA. Why has it been so difficult to prove the efficacy of alpha-1-antitrypsin replacement therapy? Insights from the study of disease pathogenesis. Drug Des Devel Ther. 2011;5:391–405. doi:10.2147/dddt.s14018.
71. MacNee W. Pathogenesis of chronic obstructive pulmonary disease. Proc Am Thorac Soc. 2005;2(4):258–66. doi:10.1513/pats.200504-045SR; discussion 90–1.
72. Kidokoro Y, Kravis TC, Moser KM, Taylor JC, Crawford IP. Relationship of leukocyte elastase concentration to severity of emphysema in homozygous alpha1-antitrypsin-deficient persons. Am Rev Respir Dis. 1977;115(5):793–803.
73. O'Reilly P, Jackson PL, Noerager B, Parker S, Dransfield M, Gaggar A, et al. N-alpha-PGP and PGP, potential biomarkers and therapeutic targets for COPD. Respir Res. 2009;10:38. doi:10.1186/1465-9921-10-38.
74. Rodriguez-Cintron W, Guntupalli K, Fraire AE. Bronchiectasis and homozygous (P1ZZ) alpha 1-antitrypsin deficiency in a young man. Thorax. 1995;50(4):424–5.
75. Parr DG, Stoel BC, Stolk J, Stockley RA. Pattern of emphysema distribution in alpha1-antitrypsin deficiency influences lung function impairment. Am J Respir Crit Care Med. 2004;170(11):1172–8. doi:10.1164/rccm.200406-761OC.
76. Gadek JE, Fells GA, Crystal RG. Cigarette smoking induces functional antiprotease deficiency in the lower respiratory tract of humans. Science (New York, NY). 1979;206(4424):1315–6.
77. Carp H, Miller F, Hoidal JR, Janoff A. Potential mechanism of emphysema: alpha 1-proteinase inhibitor recovered from lungs of cigarette smokers contains oxidized methionine and has decreased elastase inhibitory capacity. Proc Natl Acad Sci U S A. 1982;79(6):2041–5.
78. Stone PJ, Calore JD, McGowan SE, Bernardo J, Snider GL, Franzblau C. Functional alpha 1-protease inhibitor in the lower respiratory tract of cigarette smokers is not decreased. Science (New York, NY). 1983;221(4616):1187–9.
79. Boudier C, Pelletier A, Pauli G, Bieth JG. The functional activity of alpha 1-proteinase inhibitor in bronchoalveolar lavage fluids from healthy human smokers and non-smokers. Clin Chim Acta. 1983;132(3):309–15.
80. Abboud RT, Fera T, Richter A, Tabona MZ, Johal S. Acute effect of smoking on the functional activity of alpha1-protease inhibitor in bronchoalveolar lavage fluid. Am Rev Respir Dis. 1985;131(1):79–85.
81. Niewoehner DE, Kleinerman J, Rice DB. Pathologic changes in the peripheral airways of young cigarette smokers. N Engl J Med. 1974;291(15):755–8. doi:10.1056/nejm197410102911503.
82. Campbell EJ, White RR, Senior RM, Rodriguez RJ, Kuhn C. Receptor-mediated binding and inter-

nalization of leukocyte elastase by alveolar macrophages in vitro. J Clin Invest. 1979;64(3):824–33. doi:10.1172/jci109530.
83. Betsuyaku T, Yoshioka A, Nishimura M, Miyamoto K, Kondo T, Kawakami Y. Neutrophil elastase associated with alveolar macrophages from older volunteers. Am J Respir Crit Care Med. 1995;151(2 Pt 1):436–42. doi:10.1164/ajrccm.151.2.7842203.
84. Reilly JJ Jr, Mason RW, Chen P, Joseph LJ, Sukhatme VP, Yee R, et al. Synthesis and processing of cathepsin L, an elastase, by human alveolar macrophages. Biochem J. 1989;257(2):493–8.
85. Reilly JJ Jr, Chen P, Sailor LZ, Wilcox D, Mason RW, Chapman HA Jr. Cigarette smoking induces an elastolytic cysteine proteinase in macrophages distinct from cathepsin L. Am J Physiol. 1991;261(2 Pt 1):L41–8.
86. Shi GP, Munger JS, Meara JP, Rich DH, Chapman HA. Molecular cloning and expression of human alveolar macrophage cathepsin S, an elastinolytic cysteine protease. J Biol Chem. 1992;267(11):7258–62.
87. Shapiro SD, Kobayashi DK, Ley TJ. Cloning and characterization of a unique elastolytic metalloproteinase produced by human alveolar macrophages. J Biol Chem. 1993;268(32):23824–9.
88. Foronjy RF, Okada Y, Cole R, D'Armiento J. Progressive adult-onset emphysema in transgenic mice expressing human MMP-1 in the lung. Am J Physiol Lung Cell Mol Physiol. 2003;284(5):L727–37. doi:10.1152/ajplung.00349.2002.
89. D'Armiento J, Dalal SS, Okada Y, Berg RA, Chada K. Collagenase expression in the lungs of transgenic mice causes pulmonary emphysema. Cell. 1992;71(6):955–61.
90. Shiomi T, Okada Y, Foronjy R, Schiltz J, Jaenish R, Krane S, et al. Emphysematous changes are caused by degradation of type III collagen in transgenic mice expressing MMP-1. Exp Lung Res. 2003;29(1):1–15.
91. Muley T, Wiebel M, Schulz V, Ebert W. Elastinolytic activity of alveolar macrophages in smoking-associated pulmonary emphysema. Clin Investig. 1994;72(4):269–76.
92. Ohnishi K, Takagi M, Kurokawa Y, Satomi S, Konttinen YT. Matrix metalloproteinase-mediated extracellular matrix protein degradation in human pulmonary emphysema. Lab Invest. 1998;78(9):1077–87.
93. Imai K, Hiramatsu A, Fukushima D, Pierschbacher MD, Okada Y. Degradation of decorin by matrix metalloproteinases: identification of the cleavage sites, kinetic analyses and transforming growth factor-beta1 release. Biochem J. 1997;322(Pt 3):809–14.
94. Hautamaki RD, Kobayashi DK, Senior RM, Shapiro SD. Requirement for macrophage elastase for cigarette smoke-induced emphysema in mice. Science (New York, NY). 1997;277(5334):2002–4.
95. Hunninghake GW, Davidson JM, Rennard S, Szapiel S, Gadek JE, Crystal RG. Elastin fragments attract macrophage precursors to diseased sites in pulmonary emphysema. Science (New York, NY). 1981;212(4497):925–7.
96. Shapiro SD, Kobayashi DK, Welgus HG. Identification of TIMP-2 in human alveolar macrophages. Regulation of biosynthesis is opposite to that of metalloproteinases and TIMP-1. J Biol Chem. 1992;267(20):13890–4.
97. Pons AR, Sauleda J, Noguera A, Pons J, Barcelo B, Fuster A, et al. Decreased macrophage release of TGF-beta and TIMP-1 in chronic obstructive pulmonary disease. Eur Respir J. 2005;26(1):60–6. doi: 10.1183/09031936.05.00045504.
98. Leco KJ, Waterhouse P, Sanchez OH, Gowing KL, Poole AR, Wakeham A, et al. Spontaneous air space enlargement in the lungs of mice lacking tissue inhibitor of metalloproteinases-3 (TIMP-3). J Clin Invest. 2001;108(6):817–29. doi:10.1172/jci12067.
99. Sies H. Oxidative stress: oxidants and antioxidants. Exp Physiol. 1997;82(2):291–5.
100. Domej W, Oettl K, Renner W. Oxidative stress and free radicals in COPD—implications and relevance for treatment. Int J Chron Obstruct Pulmon Dis. 2014;9:1207–24. doi:10.2147/copd.s51226.
101. MacNee W. Oxidants and COPD. Curr Drug Targets Inflamm Allergy. 2005;4(6):627–41.
102. Mak JC. Pathogenesis of COPD. Part II. Oxidative-antioxidative imbalance. Int J Tuberc Lung Dis. 2008;12(4):368–74.
103. Eiserich JP, van der Vliet A, Handelman GJ, Halliwell B, Cross CE. Dietary antioxidants and cigarette smoke-induced biomolecular damage: a complex interaction. Am J Clin Nutr. 1995;62(6 Suppl):1490s–500s.
104. Cosio BG, Tsaprouni L, Ito K, Jazrawi E, Adcock IM, Barnes PJ. Theophylline restores histone deacetylase activity and steroid responses in COPD macrophages. J Exp Med. 2004;200(5):689–95. doi:10.1084/jem.20040416.
105. Cavarra E, Lucattelli M, Gambelli F, Bartalesi B, Fineschi S, Szarka A, et al. Human SLPI inactivation after cigarette smoke exposure in a new in vivo model of pulmonary oxidative stress. Am J Physiol Lung Cell Mol Physiol. 2001;281(2):L412–7.
106. Shapiro SD. Proteolysis in the lung. Eur Respir J Suppl. 2003;44:30s–2s.
107. Sussan TE, Rangasamy T, Blake DJ, Malhotra D, El-Haddad H, Bedja D, et al. Targeting Nrf2 with the triterpenoid CDDO-imidazolide attenuates cigarette smoke-induced emphysema and cardiac dysfunction in mice. Proc Natl Acad Sci U S A. 2009;106(1):250–5. doi:10.1073/pnas.0804333106.
108. Yokohori N, Aoshiba K, Nagai A. Increased levels of cell death and proliferation in alveolar wall cells in patients with pulmonary emphysema. Chest. 2004;125(2):626–32.
109. Segura-Valdez L, Pardo A, Gaxiola M, Uhal BD, Becerril C, Selman M. Upregulation of gelatinases A and B, collagenases 1 and 2, and increased parenchymal cell death in COPD. Chest. 2000;117(3):684–94.

110. Tuder RM. Aging and cigarette smoke: fueling the fire. Am J Respir Crit Care Med. 2006;174(5):490–1. doi:10.1164/rccm.200607-924ED.
111. Vlahos R, Bozinovski S. Glutathione peroxidase-1 as a novel therapeutic target for COPD. Redox Rep. 2013;18(4):142–9. doi:10.1179/1351000213y.0000000053.
112. Rangasamy T, Cho CY, Thimmulappa RK, Zhen L, Srisuma SS, Kensler TW, et al. Genetic ablation of Nrf2 enhances susceptibility to cigarette smoke-induced emphysema in mice. J Clin Invest. 2004;114(9):1248–59. doi:10.1172/jci21146.
113. Aoshiba K, Yokohori N, Nagai A. Alveolar wall apoptosis causes lung destruction and emphysematous changes. Am J Respir Cell Mol Biol. 2003;28(5):555–62. doi:10.1165/rcmb.2002-0090OC.
114. Petrache I, Natarajan V, Zhen L, Medler TR, Richter AT, Cho C, et al. Ceramide upregulation causes pulmonary cell apoptosis and emphysema-like disease in mice. Nat Med. 2005;11(5):491–8. doi:10.1038/nm1238.
115. Petrache I, Medler TR, Richter AT, Kamocki K, Chukwueke U, Zhen L, et al. Superoxide dismutase protects against apoptosis and alveolar enlargement induced by ceramide. Am J Physiol Lung Cell Mol Physiol. 2008;295(1):L44–53. doi:10.1152/ajplung.00448.2007.
116. Tuder RM, Yoshida T, Fijalkowka I, Biswal S, Petrache I. Role of lung maintenance program in the heterogeneity of lung destruction in emphysema. Proc Am Thorac Soc. 2006;3(8):673–9. doi:10.1513/pats.200605-124SF.
117. Tang K, Rossiter HB, Wagner PD, Breen EC. Lung-targeted VEGF inactivation leads to an emphysema phenotype in mice. J Appl Physiol. 2004;97(4):1559–66. doi:10.1152/japplphysiol.00221.2004; discussion 49.
118. Kasahara Y, Tuder RM, Cool CD, Lynch DA, Flores SC, Voelkel NF. Endothelial cell death and decreased expression of vascular endothelial growth factor and vascular endothelial growth factor receptor 2 in emphysema. Am J Respir Crit Care Med. 2001;163(3 Pt 1):737–44. doi:10.1164/ajrccm.163.3.2002117.
119. Marwick JA, Stevenson CS, Giddings J, MacNee W, Butler K, Rahman I, et al. Cigarette smoke disrupts VEGF165-VEGFR-2 receptor signaling complex in rat lungs and patients with COPD: morphological impact of VEGFR-2 inhibition. Am J Physiol Lung Cell Mol Physiol. 2006;290(5):L897–908. doi:10.1152/ajplung.00116.2005.
120. Chen ZH, Kim HP, Sciurba FC, Lee SJ, Feghali-Bostwick C, Stolz DB, et al. Egr-1 regulates autophagy in cigarette smoke-induced chronic obstructive pulmonary disease. PLoS One. 2008;3(10):e3316. doi:10.1371/journal.pone.0003316.
121. Csordas A, Kreutmayer S, Ploner C, Braun PR, Karlas A, Backovic A, et al. Cigarette smoke extract induces prolonged endoplasmic reticulum stress and autophagic cell death in human umbilical vein endothelial cells. Cardiovasc Res. 2011;92(1):141–8. doi:10.1093/cvr/cvr165.
122. Hwang JW, Chung S, Sundar IK, Yao H, Arunachalam G, McBurney MW, et al. Cigarette smoke-induced autophagy is regulated by SIRT1-PARP-1-dependent mechanism: implication in pathogenesis of COPD. Arch Biochem Biophys. 2010;500(2):203–9. doi:10.1016/j.abb.2010.05.013.
123. Monick MM, Powers LS, Walters K, Lovan N, Zhang M, Gerke A, et al. Identification of an autophagy defect in smokers' alveolar macrophages. J Immunol. 2010;185(9):5425–35. doi:10.4049/jimmunol.1001603.
124. Kim HP, Wang X, Chen ZH, Lee SJ, Huang MH, Wang Y, et al. Autophagic proteins regulate cigarette smoke-induced apoptosis: protective role of heme oxygenase-1. Autophagy. 2008;4(7):887–95.
125. Kumar PA, Hu Y, Yamamoto Y, Hoe NB, Wei TS, Mu D, et al. Distal airway stem cells yield alveoli in vitro and during lung regeneration following H1N1 influenza infection. Cell. 2011;147(3):525–38. doi:10.1016/j.cell.2011.10.001.
126. Kauffman SL. Cell proliferation in the mammalian lung. Int Rev Exp Pathol. 1980;22:131–91.
127. Butler JP, Loring SH, Patz S, Tsuda A, Yablonskiy DA, Mentzer SJ. Evidence for adult lung growth in humans. N Engl J Med. 2012;367(3):244–7. doi:10.1056/NEJMoa1203983.
128. Wansleeben C, Barkauskas CE, Rock JR, Hogan BL. Stem cells of the adult lung: their development and role in homeostasis, regeneration, and disease. Wiley Interdiscip Rev Dev Biol. 2013;2(1):131–48. doi:10.1002/wdev.58.
129. Takahashi Y, Izumi Y, Kohno M, Kimura T, Kawamura M, Okada Y, et al. Thyroid transcription factor-1 influences the early phase of compensatory lung growth in adult mice. Am J Respir Crit Care Med. 2010;181(12):1397–406. doi:10.1164/rccm.200908-1265OC.
130. Sakurai MK, Lee S, Arsenault DA, Nose V, Wilson JM, Heymach JV, et al. Vascular endothelial growth factor accelerates compensatory lung growth after unilateral pneumonectomy. Am J Physiol Lung Cell Mol Physiol. 2007;292(3):L742–7. doi:10.1152/ajplung.00064.2006.
131. Zhang Q, Bellotto DJ, Ravikumar P, Moe OW, Hogg RT, Hogg DC, et al. Postpneumonectomy lung expansion elicits hypoxia-inducible factor-1alpha signaling. Am J Physiol Lung Cell Mol Physiol. 2007;293(2):L497–504. doi:10.1152/ajplung.00393.2006.
132. Kaza AK, Kron IL, Leuwerke SM, Tribble CG, Laubach VE. Keratinocyte growth factor enhances post-pneumonectomy lung growth by alveolar proliferation. Circulation. 2002;106(12 Suppl 1):I120–4.
133. Barkauskas CE, Cronce MJ, Rackley CR, Bowie EJ, Keene DR, Stripp BR, et al. Type 2 alveolar cells are stem cells in adult lung. J Clin Invest. 2013;123(7):3025–36. doi:10.1172/jci68782.

134. Li Y, Gu C, Xu W, Yan J, Xia Y, Ma Y, et al. Therapeutic effects of amniotic fluid-derived mesenchymal stromal cells on lung injury in rats with emphysema. Respir Res. 2014;15:120. doi:10.1186/s12931-014-0120-3.
135. Huh JW, Kim SY, Lee JH, Lee JS, Van Ta Q, Kim M, et al. Bone marrow cells repair cigarette smoke-induced emphysema in rats. Am J Physiol Lung Cell Mol Physiol. 2011;301(3):L255–66. doi:10.1152/ajplung.00253.2010.
136. Dunsmore SE, Rannels DE. Extracellular matrix biology in the lung. Am J Physiol. 1996;270(1 Pt 1):L3–27.
137. Nakamura Y, Romberger DJ, Tate L, Ertl RF, Kawamoto M, Adachi Y, et al. Cigarette smoke inhibits lung fibroblast proliferation and chemotaxis. Am J Respir Crit Care Med. 1995;151(5):1497–503. doi:10.1164/ajrccm.151.5.7735606.
138. Carnevali S, Petruzzelli S, Longoni B, Vanacore R, Barale R, Cipollini M, et al. Cigarette smoke extract induces oxidative stress and apoptosis in human lung fibroblasts. Am J Physiol Lung Cell Mol Physiol. 2003;284(6):L955–63. doi:10.1152/ajplung.00466.2001.
139. Nyunoya T, Monick MM, Klingelhutz A, Yarovinsky TO, Cagley JR, Hunninghake GW. Cigarette smoke induces cellular senescence. Am J Respir Cell Mol Biol. 2006;35(6):681–8. doi:10.1165/rcmb.2006-0169OC.
140. Carnevali S, Nakamura Y, Mio T, Liu X, Takigawa K, Romberger DJ, et al. Cigarette smoke extract inhibits fibroblast-mediated collagen gel contraction. Am J Physiol. 1998;274(4 Pt 1):L591–8.
141. Holz O, Zuhlke I, Jaksztat E, Muller KC, Welker L, Nakashima M, et al. Lung fibroblasts from patients with emphysema show a reduced proliferation rate in culture. Eur Respir J. 2004;24(4):575–9. doi:10.1183/09031936.04.00143703.
142. Togo S, Holz O, Liu X, Sugiura H, Kamio K, Wang X, et al. Lung fibroblast repair functions in patients with chronic obstructive pulmonary disease are altered by multiple mechanisms. Am J Respir Crit Care Med. 2008;178(3):248–60. doi:10.1164/rccm.200706-929OC.
143. von Zglinicki T, Burkle A, Kirkwood TB. Stress, DNA damage and ageing—an integrative approach. Exp Gerontol. 2001;36(7):1049–62.
144. Lou Z, Chen J. Cellular senescence and DNA repair. Exp Cell Res. 2006;312(14):2641–6. doi:10.1016/j.yexcr.2006.06.009.
145. Fraga MF, Agrelo R, Esteller M. Cross-talk between aging and cancer: the epigenetic language. Ann N Y Acad Sci. 2007;1100:60–74. doi:10.1196/annals.1395.005.
146. Friguet B. Oxidized protein degradation and repair in ageing and oxidative stress. FEBS Lett. 2006;580(12):2910–6. doi:10.1016/j.febslet.2006.03.028.
147. MacNee W. Accelerated lung aging: a novel pathogenic mechanism of chronic obstructive pulmonary disease (COPD). Biochem Soc Trans. 2009;37(Pt 4):819–23. doi:10.1042/bst0370819.
148. Kuro-o M, Matsumura Y, Aizawa H, Kawaguchi H, Suga T, Utsugi T, et al. Mutation of the mouse klotho gene leads to a syndrome resembling ageing. Nature. 1997;390(6655):45–51. doi:10.1038/36285.
149. Suga T, Kurabayashi M, Sando Y, Ohyama Y, Maeno T, Maeno Y, et al. Disruption of the klotho gene causes pulmonary emphysema in mice. Defect in maintenance of pulmonary integrity during postnatal life. Am J Respir Cell Mol Biol. 2000;22(1):26–33. doi:10.1165/ajrcmb.22.1.3554.
150. Fujita T, Shirasawa T, Uchida K, Maruyama N. Gene regulation of senescence marker protein-30 (SMP30): coordinated up-regulation with tissue maturation and gradual down-regulation with aging. Mech Ageing Dev. 1996;87(3):219–29.
151. Maruyama N, Ishigami A, Kuramoto M, Handa S, Kubo S, Imasawa T, et al. Senescence marker protein-30 knockout mouse as an aging model. Ann N Y Acad Sci. 2004;1019:383–7. doi:10.1196/annals.1297.068.
152. Fulop T, Larbi A, Kotb R, de Angelis F, Pawelec G. Aging, immunity, and cancer. Discov Med. 2011;11(61):537–50.
153. von Zglinicki T. Oxidative stress shortens telomeres. Trends Biochem Sci. 2002;27(7):339–44.
154. Savale L, Chaouat A, Bastuji-Garin S, Marcos E, Boyer L, Maitre B, et al. Shortened telomeres in circulating leukocytes of patients with chronic obstructive pulmonary disease. Am J Respir Crit Care Med. 2009;179(7):566–71. doi:10.1164/rccm.200809-1398OC.
155. Jeyapalan JC, Sedivy JM. Cellular senescence and organismal aging. Mech Ageing Dev. 2008;129(7–8):467–74. doi:10.1016/j.mad.2008.04.001.
156. Tsuji T, Aoshiba K, Nagai A. Cigarette smoke induces senescence in alveolar epithelial cells. Am J Respir Cell Mol Biol. 2004;31(6):643–9. doi:10.1165/rcmb.2003-0290OC.
157. Muller KC, Welker L, Paasch K, Feindt B, Erpenbeck VJ, Hohlfeld JM, et al. Lung fibroblasts from patients with emphysema show markers of senescence in vitro. Respir Res. 2006;7:32. doi:10.1186/1465-9921-7-32.
158. Tsuji T, Aoshiba K, Nagai A. Alveolar cell senescence in patients with pulmonary emphysema. Am J Respir Crit Care Med. 2006;174(8):886–93. doi:10.1164/rccm.200509-1374OC.
159. Yeung F, Hoberg JE, Ramsey CS, Keller MD, Jones DR, Frye RA, et al. Modulation of NF-kappaB-dependent transcription and cell survival by the SIRT1 deacetylase. EMBO J. 2004;23(12):2369–80. doi:10.1038/sj.emboj.7600244.
160. Nakamaru Y, Vuppusetty C, Wada H, Milne JC, Ito M, Rossios C, et al. A protein deacetylase SIRT1 is a negative regulator of metalloproteinase-9. FASEB J. 2009;23(9):2810–9. doi:10.1096/fj.08-125468.
161. Rajendrasozhan S, Yang SR, Kinnula VL, Rahman I. SIRT1, an antiinflammatory and antiaging protein,

is decreased in lungs of patients with chronic obstructive pulmonary disease. Am J Respir Crit Care Med. 2008;177(8):861–70. doi:10.1164/rccm.200708-1269OC.
162. Kirkham PA, Caramori G, Casolari P, Papi AA, Edwards M, Shamji B, et al. Oxidative stress-induced antibodies to carbonyl-modified protein correlate with severity of chronic obstructive pulmonary disease. Am J Respir Crit Care Med. 2011;184(7):796–802. doi:10.1164/rccm.201010-1605OC.
163. Nunez B, Sauleda J, Anto JM, Julia MR, Orozco M, Monso E, et al. Anti-tissue antibodies are related to lung function in chronic obstructive pulmonary disease. Am J Respir Crit Care Med. 2011;183(8):1025–31. doi:10.1164/rccm.201001-0029OC.
164. Feghali-Bostwick CA, Gadgil AS, Otterbein LE, Pilewski JM, Stoner MW, Csizmadia E, et al. Autoantibodies in patients with chronic obstructive pulmonary disease. Am J Respir Crit Care Med. 2008;177(2):156–63. doi:10.1164/rccm.200701-014OC.
165. Rinaldi M, Lehouck A, Heulens N, Lavend'homme R, Carlier V, Saint-Remy JM, et al. Antielastin B-cell and T-cell immunity in patients with chronic obstructive pulmonary disease. Thorax. 2012;67(8):694–700. doi:10.1136/thoraxjnl-2011-200690.
166. Taraseviciene-Stewart L, Scerbavicius R, Choe KH, Moore M, Sullivan A, Nicolls MR, et al. An animal model of autoimmune emphysema. Am J Respir Crit Care Med. 2005;171(7):734–42. doi:10.1164/rccm.200409-1275OC.
167. Karayama M, Inui N, Suda T, Nakamura Y, Nakamura H, Chida K. Antiendothelial cell antibodies in patients with COPD. Chest. 2010;138(6):1303–8. doi:10.1378/chest.10-0863.
168. Greene CM, Low TB, O'Neill SJ, McElvaney NG. Anti-proline-glycine-proline or antielastin autoantibodies are not evident in chronic inflammatory lung disease. Am J Respir Crit Care Med. 2010;181(1):31–5. doi:10.1164/rccm.200904-0545OC.
169. Wood AM, de Pablo P, Buckley CD, Ahmad A, Stockley RA. Smoke exposure as a determinant of autoantibody titre in alpha(1)-antitrypsin deficiency and COPD. Eur Respir J. 2011;37(1):32–8. doi:10.1183/09031936.00033710.
170. Enelow RI, Mohammed AZ, Stoler MH, Liu AN, Young JS, Lou YH, et al. Structural and functional consequences of alveolar cell recognition by CD8(+) T lymphocytes in experimental lung disease. J Clin Invest. 1998;102(9):1653–61. doi:10.1172/jci4174.
171. Rajendrasozhan S, Yao H, Rahman I. Current perspectives on role of chromatin modifications and deacetylases in lung inflammation in COPD. COPD. 2009;6(4):291–7.
172. Rajendrasozhan S, Yang SR, Edirisinghe I, Yao H, Adenuga D, Rahman I. Deacetylases and NF-kappaB in redox regulation of cigarette smoke-induced lung inflammation: epigenetics in pathogenesis of COPD. Antioxid Redox Signal. 2008;10(4):799–811. doi:10.1089/ars.2007.1938.
173. Cantin AM, Hanrahan JW, Bilodeau G, Ellis L, Dupuis A, Liao J, et al. Cystic fibrosis transmembrane conductance regulator function is suppressed in cigarette smokers. Am J Respir Crit Care Med. 2006;173(10):1139–44. doi:10.1164/rccm.200508-1330OC.
174. Caramori G, Di Gregorio C, Carlstedt I, Casolari P, Guzzinati I, Adcock IM, et al. Mucin expression in peripheral airways of patients with chronic obstructive pulmonary disease. Histopathology. 2004;45(5):477–84. doi:10.1111/j.1365-2559.2004.01952.x.
175. Kohri K, Ueki IF, Nadel JA. Neutrophil elastase induces mucin production by ligand-dependent epidermal growth factor receptor activation. Am J Physiol Lung Cell Mol Physiol. 2002;283(3):L531–40. doi:10.1152/ajplung.00455.2001.
176. Takeyama K, Jung B, Shim JJ, Burgel PR, Dao-Pick T, Ueki IF, et al. Activation of epidermal growth factor receptors is responsible for mucin synthesis induced by cigarette smoke. Am J Physiol Lung Cell Mol Physiol. 2001;280(1):L165–72.
177. Deshmukh HS, Case LM, Wesselkamper SC, Borchers MT, Martin LD, Shertzer HG, et al. Metalloproteinases mediate mucin 5AC expression by epidermal growth factor receptor activation. Am J Respir Crit Care Med. 2005;171(4):305–14. doi:10.1164/rccm.200408-1003OC.
178. Saetta M, Turato G, Baraldo S, Zanin A, Braccioni F, Mapp CE, et al. Goblet cell hyperplasia and epithelial inflammation in peripheral airways of smokers with both symptoms of chronic bronchitis and chronic airflow limitation. Am J Respir Crit Care Med. 2000;161(3 Pt 1):1016–21. doi:10.1164/ajrccm.161.3.9907080.
179. Shim JJ, Dabbagh K, Ueki IF, Dao-Pick T, Burgel PR, Takeyama K, et al. IL-13 induces mucin production by stimulating epidermal growth factor receptors and by activating neutrophils. Am J Physiol Lung Cell Mol Physiol. 2001;280(1):L134–40.
180. Takeyama K, Dabbagh K, Jeong Shim J, Dao-Pick T, Ueki IF, Nadel JA. Oxidative stress causes mucin synthesis via transactivation of epidermal growth factor receptor: role of neutrophils. J Immunol. 2000;164(3):1546–52.
181. Sommerhoff CP, Nadel JA, Basbaum CB, Caughey GH. Neutrophil elastase and cathepsin G stimulate secretion from cultured bovine airway gland serous cells. J Clin Invest. 1990;85(3):682–9. doi:10.1172/jci114492.
182. Wang RD, Wright JL, Churg A. Transforming growth factor-beta1 drives airway remodeling in cigarette smoke-exposed tracheal explants. Am J Respir Cell Mol Biol. 2005;33(4):387–93. doi:10.1165/rcmb.2005-0203OC.
183. Takizawa H, Tanaka M, Takami K, Ohtoshi T, Ito K, Satoh M, et al. Increased expression of transforming growth factor-beta1 in small airway epithelium from tobacco smokers and patients with chronic

obstructive pulmonary disease (COPD). Am J Respir Crit Care Med. 2001;163(6):1476–83. doi:10.1164/ajrccm.163.6.9908135.
184. de Boer WI, van Schadewijk A, Sont JK, Sharma HS, Stolk J, Hiemstra PS, et al. Transforming growth factor beta1 and recruitment of macrophages and mast cells in airways in chronic obstructive pulmonary disease. Am J Respir Crit Care Med. 1998;158(6):1951–7. doi:10.1164/ajrccm.158.6.9803053.
185. Lee CG, Cho SJ, Kang MJ, Chapoval SP, Lee PJ, Noble PW, et al. Early growth response gene 1-mediated apoptosis is essential for transforming growth factor beta1-induced pulmonary fibrosis. J Exp Med. 2004;200(3):377–89. doi:10.1084/jem.20040104.
186. Sime PJ, Xing Z, Graham FL, Csaky KG, Gauldie J. Adenovector-mediated gene transfer of active transforming growth factor-beta1 induces prolonged severe fibrosis in rat lung. J Clin Invest. 1997;100(4):768–76. doi:10.1172/jci119590.
187. Black PN, Young PG, Skinner SJ. Response of airway smooth muscle cells to TGF-beta 1: effects on growth and synthesis of glycosaminoglycans. Am J Physiol. 1996;271(6 Pt 1):L910–7.
188. Cohen P, Rajah R, Rosenbloom J, Herrick DJ. IGFBP-3 mediates TGF-beta1-induced cell growth in human airway smooth muscle cells. Am J Physiol Lung Cell Mol Physiol. 2000;278(3):L545–51.
189. Annes JP, Munger JS, Rifkin DB. Making sense of latent TGFbeta activation. J Cell Sci. 2003;116(Pt 2):217–24.
190. Rifkin DB. Latent transforming growth factor-beta (TGF-beta) binding proteins: orchestrators of TGF-beta availability. J Biol Chem. 2005;280(9):7409–12. doi:10.1074/jbc.R400029200.
191. Chung KF. The role of airway smooth muscle in the pathogenesis of airway wall remodeling in chronic obstructive pulmonary disease. Proc Am Thorac Soc. 2005;2(4):347–54. doi:10.1513/pats.200504-028SR; discussion 71–2.
192. Wiegman CH, Michaeloudes C, Haji G, Narang P, Clarke CJ, Russell KE, et al. Oxidative stress-induced mitochondrial dysfunction drives inflammation and airway smooth muscle remodeling in patients with chronic obstructive pulmonary disease. J Allergy Clin Immunol. 2015;136(3):769–80. doi:10.1016/j.jaci.2015.01.046.

Part II

Assessment

Pathophysiology of COPD

5

Eun Kyung Kim

Chronic obstructive pulmonary disease (COPD) is a progressive inflammatory disease of the lung that involves complex interaction of cells and mediators. And it involves destruction of various tissue and repair mechanisms leading to structural changes that result in progressive airflow limitation with incomplete reversibility [1].

The pathological changes in patients with COPD occur in the following compartments of the lungs: the central, large airways; the peripheral, small airways; the lung parenchyma; and the pulmonary vasculature. Changes in large airways cause cough and sputum. The relative contribution to the obstruction of the airways was made by the pathological changes in the small airways and alveoli [2]. The pathologic abnormalities of COPD are associated with lung inflammation resulting from an imbalance of proteinases and antiproteinases, and oxidative stress induced by noxious particles and gases in susceptible individuals [2]. The physiologic changes of COPD can be described with mucus hypersecretion, ciliary dysfunction, airflow limitation, pulmonary hyperinflation, gas exchange abnormalities, pulmonary hypertension, and *cor pulmonale*.

Persistent reduction in forced expiratory flow rates is the most typical finding in COPD. The airflow limitation principally results from an increase in the resistance of the small conducting airways and a decrease in pulmonary elastic recoil due to emphysematous lung destruction. Emphysema and small airway pathology are both present in most patients with COPD; however, they do not appear to be mechanistically related to each other, and their relative contributions to obstruction vary from one person to another [1]. Increases in the residual volume and the residual volume/total lung capacity ratio (RV/TLC), non-uniform distribution of ventilation, and ventilation-perfusion mismatching also occur.

The pathophysiology of COPD is complicated and largely undiscovered. This is complicated by the fact that there is heterogeneity of the disease, with some patients showing a predominant emphysema pattern, whereas in others small airway disease predominates, although many patients have a mixed pattern. This chapter provides a general overview of the pathophysiology of COPD.

Mucus Hypersecretion and Ciliary Dysfunction

Innate immune response to inhaled toxic particles and gases in cigarette smoke results in inflammation in the epithelium of the central large airways and in the mucus-producing glands leading to

E.K. Kim
Department of Internal Medicine, CHA Bundang Medical Center, CHA University School of Medicine, Seongnam, South Korea
e-mail: imekkim@hanmail.net, imekkim@cha.ac.kr

S.-D. Lee (ed.), *COPD*, DOI 10.1007/978-3-662-47178-4_5

cough and sputum production that define chronic bronchitis [3]. Chronic mucus hypersecretion may be a reflection of the inflammatory response in the submucosal glands, which is associated with increased mucus production, reduced mucociliary clearance [4, 5]. Inflammatory cells release proteases that are potent secretagogues for mucus [6]. Oxidants derived from cigarette smoke and released from inflammatory leukocytes may also be involved in overproduction of mucin by induction of the *MUC5AC* gene [7]. Bronchi also undergo squamous metaplasia, disrupting mucociliary clearance and predisposing to carcinogenesis. The contribution of mucus hypersecretion to the airflow limitation in COPD is still uncertain. It appears that it contributes little in the early stages of COPD because mucus production in smokers with normal lung function does not appear to predict later development of COPD [8]. However, chronic mucus hypersecretion may contribute in the later stages of the disease because of an increased risk of exacerbations that may accelerate the loss of FEV_1.

Airflow Obstruction

The pathological consequences of the COPD induce series of physiological changes. Elastin proteolysis results in reduction in elastic recoil pressures in the lungs. It results in significant airway narrowing with reduction in air flow in the small airways and air-trapping in the lungs. Fibrotic remodeling of the airways results in fixed airway narrowing causing increased airway resistance which is not fully reversible even with bronchodilators. A major site of airway obstruction in COPD is the smaller conducting airways: membranous and respiratory bronchioles (<2 mm in diameter) [9]. Inflammation and peribronchial fibrosis contribute to the fixed airway obstruction in the small airways in COPD. Extensive alveolar and bronchiolar epithelial cells and pulmonary capillary apoptosis result in histological feature such as emphysema and physiological feature such as decreased surface area of alveoli for gas exchange and ventilation-perfusion (VA/Q) mismatch [10, 11]. Emphysema does not remain small airway patency by destruction of alveolar attachments, also reduces lung elastic recoil pressure which leads to a reduced driving pressure for expiratory flow through narrowed and poorly supported airways in which airflow resistance is significantly increased [12].

Airflow limitation, also known as airflow obstruction, particularly during expiration is cardinal to COPD diagnosis. It is the result of the balance between the elastic recoil of the lungs promoting flow and the resistance of the airways limiting flow. Expiratory flow limitation arises because of the combined effects of airway narrowing (caused by mucosal edema, mucus plugging, airway remodeling, and peribronchial fibrosis); reduced lung elastic recoil (reduced driving pressure for expiratory flow); and disrupted alveolar attachments, which predispose to dynamic airway collapse [13–15].

In normal lungs, as well as in lungs affected by COPD, maximal expiratory flow diminishes as the lungs empty because the lung parenchyma provides progressively less elastic recoil and because the cross-sectional area of the airways falls, raising the resistance to airflow. Due to reduced airway caliber and increased airway resistance, there is reduced airflow during expiration which prolongs the removal of air from the lungs [16]. The volume of air remaining in the lung at the end of spontaneous expiration is increased in COPD compared with healthy person [12]. During spontaneous breathing at rest in patients with COPD, which have airflow limitation, end expiratory lung volume is also "dynamically" determined. In flow-limited patients, the mechanical time constant for lung emptying is increased in most alveolar units, but the expiratory time available is often insufficient. As a result, air-trapping occurs [12, 17].

The physiological feature of COPD is usually determined by spirometry, which detected with forced expiratory maneuvers using spirometric lung volume ratio of volume of air removed in first second (FEV_1) and total volume of air exhaled during the entire spirometric maneuver [forced vital capacity (FVC)] during forceful expiration after maximal inhalation. Patients with airflow obstruction related to COPD have a chronically reduced ratio of FEV_1/FVC (FEV_1/FVC <0.7). In contrast to asthma, the reduced FEV_1 in COPD seldom shows large responses to inhaled bronchodilators although improvements up to 15% are common [18].

Fixed airway obstruction depicts intensity of small airway inflammation (mucosal edema, fibrotic remodeling of the airway, and mucus impaction) and possibly increased cholinergic airway smooth muscle tone [5, 13, 19–21]. Contraction of airway smooth muscle, accumulation of inflammatory cells, mucus, and plasma exudate in airways might explain a part of the mechanism of airflow limitation and can be improved by the treatment.

Hyperinflation

Lung hyperinflation or air-trapping is one of the hallmarks of COPD pathophysiology. Increased residual volume, total lung capacity, functional residual capacity (FRC), and increased RV/TLC are common in COPD.

Hyperinflation is primary cause of dyspnea, poor quality of life, and advertent disease prognosis associated with COPD [12]. Damage to elastin and narrowing of airways are major causes for air-trapping in COPD. The barrel-shaped chest in COPD is attributed to hyperinflation of the lungs.

The inward lung elastic recoil pressures are the primary forces which drive air out of the small airways and alveoli during tidal expiration for which it has to counteract outward recoil pressures generated by thoracic wall. During end tidal expiration, both these forces equally balance each other causing relative airflow stasis and relaxed lung state. The volume of air trapped in the lungs at this equi-pressure stage is physiologically termed as FRC [12, 22].

In COPD, weakening of elastic tissue generates inadequate inward lung elastic recoil pressures to cause movement of air out of the lungs. Therefore to counteract the outward recoil pressures of thoracic cage, the reduced elastic recoil of the lungs generates equi-pressure states with larger FRC resulting in state of hyperinflation [12, 22, 23]. This pushes the equi-pressure point further away from the alveoli. It is believed that the symptomatic improvement produced by bronchodilators is majorly by reduction in lung hyperinflation rather than bronchodilation [23].

Hyperinflation of the thorax during tidal breathing may be beneficial, it preserves maximum expiratory airflow, because as lung volume increases, elastic recoil pressure increases, and airways enlarge so that airway resistance decreases.

Despite compensating for airway obstruction, hyperinflation can push the diaphragm into a flattened position with a number of adverse effects. The zone of apposition between the diaphragm and the abdominal wall is decreased. So, positive abdominal pressure during inspiration is not applied as effectively to the chest wall, hindering rib cage movement and impairing inspiration. Additionally, as the muscle fibers of the flattened diaphragm are shorter than those of a more normally curved diaphragm, they are less capable of generating inspiratory pressures than normal. Furthermore, the flattened diaphragm (with increased radius of curvature, r) must generate greater tension (t) to develop the transpulmonary pressure (p) required to produce tidal breathing (This follows from Laplace's law; $p = 2\,t/r$). Also, because the thoracic cage is distended beyond its normal resting volume, during tidal breathing the inspiratory muscles must do work to overcome the resistance of the thoracic cage to further inflation instead of gaining the normal assistance from the chest wall recoiling outward toward its resting volume [12, 24, 25].

The hyperinflation is dynamic in nature and is present in all stages of the disease, which is usually manifested in hyperventilation states which are outcome of expiratory flow limitation, anxiety, and ventilation perfusion mismatches related to COPD exacerbations or any activity which increases oxygen demand. In hyperventilation during each breath, inhalation commences before full exhalation is achieved, this results in air-trapping which enhances with each breath. With every breath FRC increases and inspiratory capacity reduces. When the rising FRC encroaches inspiratory reserve volumes further increase in inspiratory muscle activation produce little or no additional ventilation [26].

Also, FRC no longer occurs at the passive point of equilibrium between chest wall and lung recoil, but occurs at a positive end-expiratory pressure (PEEP) before exhalation has achieved the relaxation volume [26]. The increasing intrinsic-PEEP during dynamic hyperinflation places diaphragm in a mechanical disadvantaged position shortens its operating length and alters the mechanical linkage between its various parts. This progressively diminishes the tension and resulting trans-diaphragmatic pressure generated by diaphragmatic contraction [12]. These altered actions of diaphragm can potentially cause disability and impending respiratory failure during COPD exacerbations.

Abnormality of Gas Exchange

COPD is the most common chronic respiratory disease state associated with chronic and/or acute respiratory insufficiency. The partial pressure of oxygen in arterial blood (PaO_2) usually remains near normal until the FEV_1 is decreased to ~50% of predicted, and even much lower FEV_1 values can be associated with a normal PaO_2, at least at rest. An elevation of arterial level of carbon dioxide ($PaCO_2$) is not expected until the FEV_1 is <25% of predicted and even then may not occur [1, 27]. Hypoxemia occurs only during exercise in the early stage of the disease. However, it appears to be at rest as the disease progress.

Uneven distribution of both alveolar ventilation and pulmonary blood flow, namely, VA/Q mismatch, remains the most important cause of arterial hypoxemia, with or without hypercapnia, in both stable and exacerbated COPD [28].

Non-uniform ventilation and VA/Q mismatching are characteristic of COPD, reflecting the heterogeneous nature of the disease process within the airways and lung parenchyma. Physiologic studies are consistent with multiple parenchymal compartments having different rates of ventilation due to regional differences in compliance and airway resistance. Among patients with COPD, those with predominant emphysema have high VA/Q areas within the lungs, whereas those with predominant chronic bronchitis have low VA/Q regions as a result of small airways distortion and mucus plugging [29, 30].

In mild-to-moderate COPD, Barbera and colleagues [31] and Rodriguez-Roisin and colleagues [29] have demonstrated that significant VA/Q mismatching and loss of protective hypoxic vasoconstriction can occur while breathing at rest. Thus, the resting alveolar-to-arterial oxygen tension gradient was abnormally widened (>15 mmHg) in most of a small sample of patients with milder COPD who also had predominantly low regional VA/Q ratios measured by multiple inert gas elimination techniques [31].

The attendant abnormalities in arterial blood gases, if sustained, stimulate integrated compensatory adaptations over time. Thus, activation of neurohumoral, renal, and hemodynamic homeostatic mechanisms, together with modulation of the central respiratory controller, combine to preserve critical arterial oxygenation and acid-base status.

Preservation of arterial oxygenation during exercise suggests that compensatory increases in ventilation in the setting of a normal increase in cardiac output ensure improved overall VA/Q relations during exercise in mild-to-moderate COPD [31]. Ultimately, in advanced COPD, the compensations may fail and reduced alveolar ventilation at a given CO_2 production leads to CO_2 retention.

Pulmonary Arterial Hypertension

Pulmonary arterial hypertension (PAH) is a known independent prognostic marker of COPD. Structural changes in COPD initiate instability in pulmonary hemodynamics. Most moderate-to-severe COPD patients develop some degree of mild PAH (25–35 mmHg) over the course of time, and rarely severe PAH (>45 mmHg) [32]; however, it may be rare in mild-moderate COPD.

Pathophysiological consequences of COPD such as hypoxia, emphysema, hyperinflation, hypoxia-induced polycythemia, inflammation of lung and systemic inflammation can induce pulmonary capillary muscularization, plexiform lesions, intimal-wall thickenings, endothelial dysfunctions, and apoptosis which can potentially generate enhanced pulmonary vascular resistance which predisposes PAH [32]. Increased intrathoracic pressures in emphysema induce positive pressures on right ventricle which results in increased pulmonary artery wedge pressure. Left ventricular diastolic dysfunction associated with cardiovascular morbidities in COPD can also cause back pressure changes in pulmonary vasculature and right ventricles.

Chronic severe pulmonary hypertension increases right ventricular afterload and leads to the clinical syndrome (*cor pulmonale*) of right heart failure with systemic congestion and the inability to adapt right ventricular output to peripheral vascular demands. Pulmonary hypertension severe enough to cause *cor pulmonale* and right ventricular failure due to COPD typically occurs in individuals who have marked decreases in FEV_1 (<25% of predicted) and chronic hypoxemia ($PaO_2 < 55$ mmHg); however, recent evidence suggests that some patients will develop significant pulmonary hypertension independent of COPD severity [33, 34]. A recent prospective study with a large number of patients with COPD who underwent right heart catheterization during exercise found abnormal elevations in pulmonary artery pressures as a function of cardiac output, even in those without resting pulmonary hypertension [35].

Pathophysiology of COPD Exacerbation

Acute exacerbation is one of the most common complications in the evolution of COPD. These episodes are characterized by worsening of pulmonary gas exchange that results in severe hypoxemia with or without hypercapnia irrespective of the precipitating factor [28]. Altered gas exchange during exacerbation of COPD results from the increased VA/Q mismatch together with a reduced oxygen content of mixed venous blood, which is associated with greater consumption of oxygen by the respiratory muscles.

Abnormality of ventilation during acute exacerbation of COPD was the result of greater narrowing of the airways by inflammation of the airway, bronchospasm, or hypersecretion of mucus [20]. Pulmonary vasoconstriction due to hypoxemia changed distribution of perfusion. During exacerbations, the oxygen demands of the respiratory muscles increase considerably due to greater airway resistance and to the additional efforts of inspiratory muscles to overcome dynamic hyperinflation [31].

Minute ventilation did not decrease during exacerbation. Instead, a slight increase was shown when compared with stable conditions [28]. This finding reinforces the concept that the development of hypercapnia during exacerbations of COPD is essentially due to increased VA/Q mismatch rather than hypoventilation.

Another thing should be considered in exacerbation of COPD. Airflow limitation during expiration is a pathophysiological hallmark of COPD. In patients with exacerbated COPD, the time available for lung emptying (expiratory time) during spontaneous breathing is often insufficient to allow end expiratory lung volume to decline to its natural relaxation volume, which leads to lung overinflation [36]. Thus, in those patients, end expiratory lung volume becomes dynamically rather than statically determined. Dynamic hyperinflation refers to acute and variable increase in end expiratory lung volume above its baseline value. Dynamic hyperinflation occurs during exercise in COPD patients as inspired tidal volume increases and expiratory time decreases, and is associated with severe mechanical constraints on ventilation and perceived respiratory discomfort. In this setting, the reduction in inspiratory capacity (IC), which reflects the increase in end expiratory lung volume, correlates strongly with the perception of inspiratory difficulty. During COPD exacerbations, airway resistance is abruptly increased (due to bronchospasm, narrowing of the airways by inflammation of the airway, or hypersecretion of mucus) and this worsens airflow limitation during expiration. Therefore, the time constant for lung emptying is prolonged and end expiratory lung volume is dynamically increased. Furthermore, during an exacerbation, patients tend to adopt a rapid shallow breathing pattern which further limits the time available for lung emptying, thus promoting dynamic hyperinflation in a vicious cycle. In fact, any acute increase in ventilation can be associated with dynamic hyperinflation in patients with COPD. There is evidence that acute dynamic hyperinflation may be life threatening and requiring mechanical ventilation during severe exacerbations of asthma or COPD [37].

References

1. Pauwels RA, Buist AS, Calverley PM, Jenkins CR, Hurd SS. Global strategy for the diagnosis, management, and prevention of chronic obstructive pulmonary disease. NHLBI/WHO global initiative for chronic obstructive lung disease (GOLD) workshop summary. Am J Respir Crit Care Med. 2001;163(5):1256–76. doi:10.1164/ajrccm.163.5.2101039.
2. Hogg JC. Lung structure and function in COPD. Int J Tuberc Lung Dis. 2008;12(5):467–79.
3. Hogg JC. Pathophysiology of airflow limitation in chronic obstructive pulmonary disease. Lancet (London, England). 2004;364(9435):709–21. doi:10.1016/s0140-6736(04)16900-6.
4. Fletcher C, Peto R. The natural history of chronic airflow obstruction. Br Med J. 1977;1(6077):1645–8.
5. Mullen JB, Wright JL, Wiggs BR, Pare PD, Hogg JC. Reassessment of inflammation of airways in chronic bronchitis. Br Med J (Clin Res Ed). 1985;291(6504):1235–9.
6. Sommerhoff CP, Nadel JA, Basbaum CB, Caughey GH. Neutrophil elastase and cathepsin G stimulate secretion from cultured bovine airway gland serous cells. J Clin Invest. 1990;85(3):682–9. doi:10.1172/jci114492.
7. Shao MX, Nakanaga T, Nadel JA. Cigarette smoke induces MUC5AC mucin overproduction via tumor necrosis factor-alpha-converting enzyme in human airway epithelial (NCI-H292) cells. Am J Physiol Lung Cell Mol Physiol. 2004;287(2):L420–7. doi:10.1152/ajplung.00019.2004.
8. Vestbo J, Lange P. Can GOLD stage 0 provide information of prognostic value in chronic obstructive pulmonary disease? Am J Respir Crit Care Med. 2002;166(3):329–32. doi:10.1164/rccm.2112048.
9. Hogg JC, Macklem PT, Thurlbeck WM. Site and nature of airway obstruction in chronic obstructive lung disease. N Engl J Med. 1968;278(25):1355–60. doi:10.1056/nejm196806202782501.
10. Tuder RM, Petrache I, Elias JA, Voelkel NF, Henson PM. Apoptosis and emphysema: the missing link. Am J Respir Cell Mol Biol. 2003;28(5):551–4. doi:10.1165/rcmb.F269.
11. Kasahara Y, Tuder RM, Cool CD, Lynch DA, Flores SC, Voelkel NF. Endothelial cell death and decreased expression of vascular endothelial growth factor and vascular endothelial growth factor receptor 2 in emphysema. Am J Respir Crit Care Med. 2001;163(3 Pt 1):737–44. doi:10.1164/ajrccm.163.3.2002117.
12. O'Donnell D, Laveneziana P. Physiology and consequences of lung hyperinflation in COPD. Eur Respir Rev. 2006;15(100):61–7.
13. McDonough JE, Yuan R, Suzuki M, Seyednejad N, Elliott WM, Sanchez PG, et al. Small-airway obstruction and emphysema in chronic obstructive pulmonary disease. N Engl J Med. 2011;365(17):1567–75. doi:10.1056/NEJMoa1106955.
14. Black LF, Hyatt RE, Stubbs SE. Mechanism of expiratory airflow limitation in chronic obstructive pulmonary disease associated with 1-antitrypsin deficiency. Am Rev Respir Dis. 1972;105(6):891–9.
15. Leaver DG, Tatterfield AE, Pride NB. Contributions of loss of lung recoil and of enhanced airways collapsibility to the airflow obstruction of chronic bronchitis and emphysema. J Clin Invest. 1973;52(9):2117–28. doi:10.1172/jci107396.
16. Fry DL, Hyatt RE. Pulmonary mechanics: a unified analysis of the relationship between pressure, volume and gasflow in the lungs of normal and diseased human subjects. Am J Med. 1960;29(4):672–89.
17. Vinegar A, Sinnett EE, Leith DE. Dynamic mechanisms determine functional residual capacity in mice, *Mus musculus*. J Appl Physiol Respir Environ Exerc Physiol. 1979;46(5):867–71.
18. Mannino DM, Buist AS. Global burden of COPD: risk factors, prevalence, and future trends. Lancet. 2007;370(9589):765–73.
19. Cosio M, Ghezzo H, Hogg JC, Corbin R, Loveland M, Dosman J, et al. The relations between structural changes in small airways and pulmonary-function tests. N Engl J Med. 1978;298(23):1277–81. doi:10.1056/nejm197806082982303.
20. Kuwano K, Bosken CH, Pare PD, Bai TR, Wiggs BR, Hogg JC. Small airways dimensions in asthma and in chronic obstructive pulmonary disease. Am Rev Respir Dis. 1993;148(5):1220–5. doi:10.1164/ajrccm/148.5.1220.
21. Matsuba K, Wright JL, Wiggs BR, Pare PD, Hogg JC. The changes in airways structure associated with reduced forced expiratory volume in one second. Eur Respir J. 1989;2(9):834–9.
22. Brashier BB, Kodgule R. Risk factors and pathophysiology of chronic obstructive pulmonary disease (COPD). J Assoc Physicians India. 2012;60(Suppl):17–21.
23. Ferguson GT. Why does the lung hyperinflate? Proc Am Thorac Soc. 2006;3(2):176–9. doi:10.1513/pats.200508-094DO.

24. Minh V, Dolan GF, Konopka RF, Moser KM. Effect of hyperinflation on inspiratory function of the diaphragm. J Appl Physiol. 1976;40(1):67–73.
25. Decramer M. Hyperinflation and respiratory muscle interaction. Eur Respir J. 1997;10(4):934–41.
26. Calverley PMA. Dynamic hyperinflation. Proc Am Thorac Soc. 2006;3(3):239–44. doi:10.1513/pats.200508-084SF.
27. Lane DJ, Howell JB, Giblin B. Relation between airways obstruction and CO_2 tension in chronic obstructive airways disease. Br Med J. 1968;3(5620):707–9.
28. Barbera JA, Roca J, Ferrer A, Felez MA, Diaz O, Roger N, et al. Mechanisms of worsening gas exchange during acute exacerbations of chronic obstructive pulmonary disease. Eur Respir J. 1997;10(6):1285–91.
29. Rodriguez-Roisin R, Drakulovic M, Rodriguez DA, Roca J, Barbera JA, Wagner PD. Ventilation-perfusion imbalance and chronic obstructive pulmonary disease staging severity. J Appl Physiol (1985). 2009;106(6):1902–8. doi:10.1152/japplphysiol.00085.2009.
30. Wagner PD, Dantzker DR, Dueck R, Clausen JL, West JB. Ventilation-perfusion inequality in chronic obstructive pulmonary disease. J Clin Invest. 1977;59(2):203–16. doi:10.1172/jci108630.
31. Barbera JA, Riverola A, Roca J, Ramirez J, Wagner PD, Ros D, et al. Pulmonary vascular abnormalities and ventilation-perfusion relationships in mild chronic obstructive pulmonary disease. Am J Respir Crit Care Med. 1994;149(2 Pt 1):423–9. doi:10.1164/ajrccm.149.2.8306040.
32. Chaouat A, Naeije R, Weitzenblum E. Pulmonary hypertension in COPD. Eur Respir J. 2008;32(5):1371–85. doi:10.1183/09031936.00015608.
33. Wright JL, Levy RD, Churg A. Pulmonary hypertension in chronic obstructive pulmonary disease: current theories of pathogenesis and their implications for treatment. Thorax. 2005;60(7):605–9. doi:10.1136/thx.2005.042994.
34. Sabit R, Bolton CE, Fraser AG, Edwards JM, Edwards PH, Ionescu AA, et al. Sub-clinical left and right ventricular dysfunction in patients with COPD. Respir Med. 2010;104(8):1171–8. doi:10.1016/j.rmed.2010.01.020.
35. Hilde JM, Skjorten I, Hansteen V, Melsom MN, Hisdal J, Humerfelt S, et al. Haemodynamic responses to exercise in patients with COPD. Eur Respir J. 2013;41(5):1031–41. doi:10.1183/09031936.00085612.
36. O'Donnell DE, Parker CM. COPD exacerbations. 3: pathophysiology. Thorax. 2006;61(4):354–61. doi:10.1136/thx.2005.041830.
37. Calverley PM. Respiratory failure in chronic obstructive pulmonary disease. Eur Respir J Suppl. 2003;47:26s–30s.

Diagnosis and Assessment of COPD

6

Yong Bum Park

Introduction

A clinical diagnosis of COPD should be considered in patients over the age of 40 who present with dyspnea, chronic cough or sputum production, and a history exposure to risk factors for the disease. Spirometry is fundamental to making a diagnosis of COPD, and the presence of a post-bronchodilator $FEV_1/FVC < 0.70$ confirms the presence of persistent airflow limitation. COPD assessment is to determine the severity of disease, including the severity of airflow limitation, the impact on the patient's health status, and the future risk. COPD assessment is important for therapy and prognosis. COPD often coexists with comorbidities that may have significant impact on mortality and prognosis. At the initial assessment and follow-up visits should include a discussion of symptoms, particularly any new or worsening symptoms and physical examination.

Y.B. Park
Division of Pulmonary, Allergy and Critical Care Medicine, Hallym University Medical Center, Seoul, South Korea

Department of Internal Medicine, Hallym University Kangdong Sacred Heart Hospital, Seoul, South Korea

Lung Research Institute of Hallym University College of Medicine, Seoul, South Korea
e-mail: bfspark2@gmail.com

Diagnosis

A clinical diagnosis of COPD should be considered in patients over the age of 40 who present with dyspnea, chronic cough or sputum production, and a history exposure to risk factors for the disease. Spirometry is fundamental to making a diagnosis of COPD, and the presence of a post-bronchodilator $FEV_1/FVC < 0.70$ confirms the presence of persistent airflow limitation. The spirometric criteria for airflow limitation remains a post-bronchodilator fixed ratio of $FEV_1/FVC < 0.70$.

The use of the fixed FEV_1/FVC ratio to define airflow limitation is not perfect. Using this cutoff may lead to an overdiagnosis of COPD in the elderly [1], and an underdiagnosis in young adults [2]. Because of these imperfections in the FEV_1/FVC ratio, there have been several alternate methods proposed to diagnose obstruction. One proposal is to use the lower limit of normal (LLN) for the cutoff of FEV_1/FVC ratio. The LLN takes into consideration the age, height, and gender for each individual. This minimizes the age-related changes in the FEV_1/FVC ratio and may reduce the misclassification of airway obstruction [2]. However, it also may be more difficult for primary care clinicians to perform and interpret. In addition, using this cutoff may not improve clinical care.

It may be difficult for some patients to perform a forced exhalation maneuver for several reasons, including poor mental status and coughing. Another option is the FEV_1/FEV_6 ratio. The FEV_1/FEV_6 ratio has been shown to be an

S.-D. Lee (ed.), *COPD*, DOI 10.1007/978-3-662-47178-4_6

acceptable surrogate for the FEV_1/FVC ratio [3]. It is also thought to be an easier test for patients to perform than the FVC maneuver.

Unfortunately, a considerable number of subjects had not been diagnosed [4, 5]. Frequently the disease will not be diagnosed until it is quite progressed. Targeted screening of symptomatic patients with risk factors for COPD results in better diagnosis rates and more appropriate therapy [6].

Symptoms

The characteristic symptoms of COPD are chronic and progressive dyspnea, cough, and sputum production that can be variable from day to day and from individual to individual. Chronic cough and sputum production may precede the development of airflow limitation by many years. Conversely, significant airflow limitation may develop without chronic cough and sputum production. In the early stages, COPD may produce minimal or no symptoms and as the disease progresses the symptoms in individual patients vary. Symptoms should be assessed as objectively as possible by using questionnaires such as the mMRC, CCQ, and CAT. In general, dyspnea is the symptom which causes them most concern. A person may seek medical facility either because of chronic symptoms or because of a first exacerbation.

Dyspnea is major cause of disability and anxiety associated with the disease. Dyspnea is typically present only with exertion until late in the course of the disease. Cough may be the presenting symptom and may be very troublesome and can compromise quality of life significantly. However, cough is frequently neglected by the patient as an expected result of smoking or environmental exposure. Initially, the cough may be intermittent, but later is present every day. In some cases, significant airflow limitation may develop without the presence of a cough. Sputum is insidious in the majority of patients. Regular production of sputum for 3 or more months in 2 consecutive years (in the absence of any other conditions that may explain it) is the epidemiological definition of chronic bronchitis. Patients producing large volumes of sputum may have underlying bronchiectasis. The presence of purulent sputum reflects an increase in inflammatory conditions, and its development may identify the onset of bacterial exacerbation [7]. Wheezing and chest tightness are nonspecific symptoms that may vary between days. An absence of wheezing and chest tightness does not exclude a diagnosis of COPD, nor does the presence of these symptoms confirm a diagnosis of asthma. Fatigue, weight loss, and anorexia are common problems in patients with severe and very severe COPD. Ankle swelling can be a sign of cor pulmonale. Symptoms of depression and/or anxiety occur and are associated with increased risk of exacerbations and poorer health status.

Medical History

A detailed medical history in a patient with COPD should assess:

Exposure to risk factors	Smoking and occupational and environmental exposures including biomass fuel
Past medical history	Asthma, atopy, bronchial hyperresponsiveness; respiratory infection in childhood
	Other respiratory infections including tuberculosis
Family history of COPD	COPD, asthma, alpha-1 antitrypsin deficiency
Symptom	Cough, sputum, dyspnea
	Progressive, chronic
	Typically develops in adult life
	More frequent or prolonged "winter colds"
Recent medical history	History of exacerbations and previous hospitalization for respiratory disorder
Presence of comorbidities	Cardiovascular disease, osteoporosis, musculoskeletal disorder, malignancy
Impact of disease on patient's life	Limitation of activity, missed work and economic impact, effect on family routines, feeling on depression and anxiety, well-being and sexual activity
Support for the patient	Family, society, and daycare
Possibilities for reducing risk factors	Especially smoking cessation

Physical Examination

Since the typical physical findings in COPD usually do not appear until the disease has become severe, the absence of abnormal findings does not rule out the possibility of COPD. When COPD becomes severe, patients present more apparent physical signs. These include the barrel shaped chest, purse-lipped breathing, and debility. Pulmonary hypertension may develop in patients with COPD and may be worse during exercise. It may be suspected with a loud pulmonary component of the second heart sound and heart sounds may be displaced to the midline due to hyperinflation.

Introduction to Pulmonary Function Testing

Pulmonary function testing has three basic components: (1) spirometry, (2) lung volumes, and (3) diffusing capacity of the lung for carbon monoxide (DLCO). Each of these components can be affected by COPD. The most important test is spirometry. Measurement of lung volume and diffusion capacity may be helpful, particularly whether airflow limitation is due to emphysema or airway disease.

Spirometry

Spirometry is the most important test to diagnose COPD. Peak expiratory flow measurement may significantly underestimate the severity of the airflow limitation. Spirometry should measure the volume of air forcibly exhaled from the point of maximal inspiration (forced vital capacity, FVC) and the volume of air exhaled during the first second of this maneuver (forced expiratory volume in one second, FEV_1) and the ratio of these two measurements (FEV_1/FVC) should be calculated. A reduction in FEV_1/FVC ratio is diagnostic of airway obstruction. An FEV_1/FVC ratio of <0.70 after bronchodilator is typically considered diagnostic of COPD. The FEV_1/FVC ratio can establish a diagnosis of obstruction but is not useful to monitor disease progression and severity of COPD. Along with spirometry, a flow-volume loop is also typically generated. A flow-volume loop plots flow on the y-axis and volume on the x-axis. A normal flow-volume loop has a characteristic shape (Fig. 6.1a). In obstructive lung disease such as COPD, the expiratory limb takes on a coved shape (Fig. 6.1b).

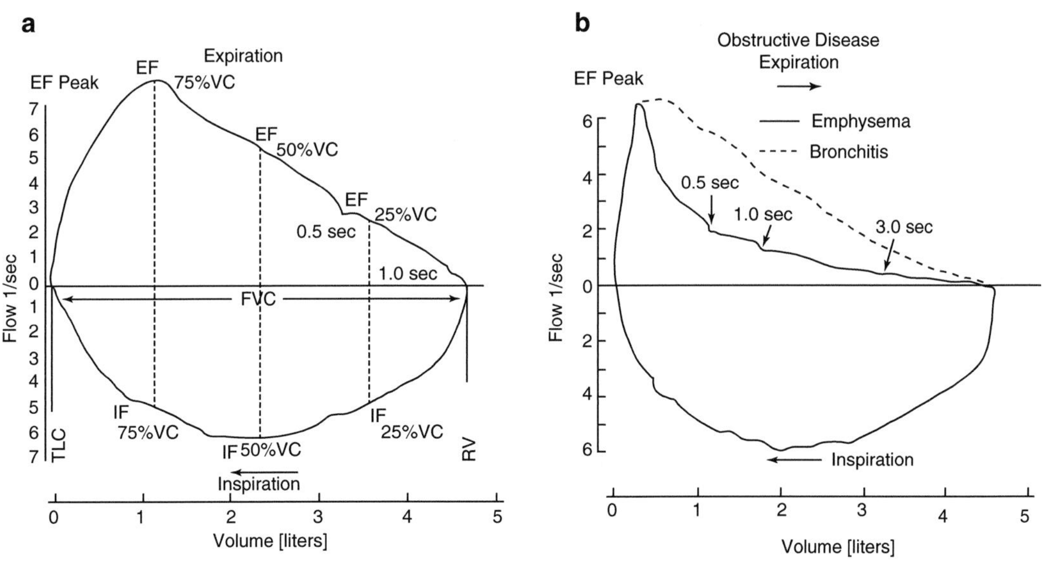

Fig. 6.1 Flow-volume curve for healthy person (**a**) and patients with airflow obstruction (**b**)

Lung Volumes

In addition to spirometry, lung volumes can also be measured. Lung volumes consist of total lung capacity (TLC), residual volume (RV), and functional residual capacity (FRC). The TLC is the volume of air contained in the lung after a full inhalation. The RV is the volume of air left in the lung after a full exhalation. The FRC is the volume of gas left in the lungs after a tidal breath.

The most commonly used method is the body plethysmography. Emphysema destroys lung tissue, leading to loss of elastic recoil. Loss of elastic recoil allows the lungs to be stretched to abnormally large volumes, resulting in an increased TLC. RV and FRC can also be increased in COPD when disease progression destroys the elastic tethers. This leads to premature closing of the airways, which causes abnormal amounts of air to be trapped in the lung. In some patients, there is also inflammation of the small airways, which causes narrowing, further contributing to air trapping and the increase in RV.

Air trapping can lead to hyperinflation. There is both a static and dynamic component of hyperinflation. Static hyperinflation refers to the baseline level of air trapping seen at rest. This is due to the loss of elastic recoil properties of the lung and fixed airway obstruction. Dynamic hyperinflation occurs during exercise or times of rapid respiratory rate. In these situations, the patient is unable to finish exhaling before the next breath starts. With each breath, the patient becomes progressively more hyperinflated. This causes inefficient respiratory muscles function and increases the work of breathing.

Diffusing Capacity of the Lung for Carbon Monoxide

The diffusing capacity of the lung for carbon monoxide (DLCO) is a measure of how easily carbon monoxide (CO) molecules transfer from the alveolar gas to the hemoglobin of the red cells in the pulmonary circulation. To measure the DLCO, the patient inhales a single breath containing a minute amount of CO and holds it for 10 s. The breath is then exhaled and the exhaled breath is analyzed for CO. The change in the concentration of the CO is then multiplied by the single breath TLC to calculate the DLCO. Some patients with severe COPD may have difficulty performing the breath hold required to measure DLCO.

The DLCO is decreased in proportion to the severity of emphysema of the destruction of the alveoli and the loss of capillary bed. It is also reduced in other diseases that destroy the alveolar capillary bed.

Assessment of the Disease

COPD is heterogeneous, so no single measure can give an adequate assessment of the severity of the disease in an individual patient. However, severity assessment is important because it has significances for therapy and relates to prognosis. COPD assessment is to determine the severity of disease, including the severity of airflow limitation, the impact on the patient's health status, and the future risk (such as exacerbation, hospital admission, or death).

Global initiative for chronic obstructive lung disease (GOLD) [8] documents that COPD assessment must consider the following aspects of the disease separately to achieve these goals.

- Current levels of patient's symptoms.
- Severity of spirometric abnormality.
- Exacerbation risk.
- Presence of comorbidity.

The Assessment of Symptoms

A simple measurement of dyspnea such as the Modified British Medical Research Council (mMRC) Questionnaire was considered adequate for assessment of symptoms, as the mMRC relates well to other measures of health status [9] and predicts future mortality risk [10]. However, it is now recognized that COPD has broad range of effects on health status. For this reason, a comprehensive symptom assessment is recommended rather than just a measure of dyspnea.

The most comprehensive disease-specific health-related quality of life or health status questionnaires such as CRQ and SGRQ are too complex to use in routine practice, but two shorter comprehensive measures (COPD Assessment Test, CAT and COPD Control Questionnaire, CCQ) have been developed and are suitable. To find more about symptomatic assessment tool, refer to the next section (Symptomatic assessment of COPD).

Spirometric Assessment

The table shows the classification of airflow limitation severity in COPD.

Classification of severity of airflow limitation in COPD (post-bronchodilator FEV_1 in patients with $FEV_1/FVC < 0.70$)	
GOLD 1: Mild	$FEV_1 \geq 80\%$ predicted
GOLD 2: Moderate	$50\% \leq FEV_1 < 80\%$ predicted
GOLD 3: Severe	$30\% \leq FEV_1 < 50\%$ predicted
GOLD 4: Very severe	$FEV_1 < 30\%$ predicted

Spirometry should be performed after the administration of a short-acting inhaled bronchodilator. However, there is only a weak correlation between FEV_1, symptoms, and patient's health-related quality of life.

Assessment of Exacerbation Risk

An exacerbation of COPD is defined as an acute event characterized by a worsening of the patient's respiratory symptoms that is beyond normal day-to-day variations and leads to a change in medication [11–13]. The rate of exacerbations varies between patients. Exacerbations of COPD are important, since they have a serious negative impact on health status, and are associated with accelerated lung function decline and increased mortality. Although exacerbations are considered to become more frequent as the severity of the underlying COPD increases, the most reliable predictor of exacerbation appears to be a history of exacerbations.

Classification of exacerbations was assessed according to Anthonisen et al. [14]. A type I exacerbation is defined by the presence of three major symptoms (worsening dyspnea with increased sputum volume and purulence), type II by the presence of two major symptoms and type III exacerbations as the presence of one major symptom present on the worst day of an exacerbation. Definitions of exacerbations vary between clinical studies that evaluate drugs to prevent exacerbations. Recent clinical trials define moderate exacerbations as those that require treatment with systemic corticosteroids or antibiotics (or both) and severe exacerbations as those that require hospital admission.

Exacerbations of chronic pulmonary disease tool (EXACT) was a single, standardized instrument of collecting patient-reported outcome (PRO) data, which helps to capture not only the frequency of exacerbations but also the severity and the time-course [15, 16].

Additional Investigations

Oximetry and Arterial Blood Gas Measurement

Pulse oximetry should be used to assess all stable patients with $FEV_1 < 35\%$ predicted or with clinical signs suggestive of respiratory failure or right heart failure. If peripheral saturation is <92%, arterial blood gases should be assessed. Arterial blood gases show mild or moderate hypoxemia without hypercapnia in the early stage of COPD. In the later stages of the disease, hypoxemia tends to become more severe and may be accompanied by hypercapnia with increased serum bicarbonate levels. Blood gas abnormalities worsen during acute exacerbations and may also worsen during exercise and sleep.

Alpha-1 Antitrypsin Deficiency Screening

Mutation in alpha-1 protease inhibitor represents the only proven genetic abnormality that predisposes to COPD. The typical patient tends to present at a younger age (<45 years) with lower lobe emphysema. A serum concentration of alpha-1 antitrypsin below 15–20% of the normal value is highly suggestive of homozygous alpha-1 antitrypsin deficiency.

Exercise Testing

Exercise tests are useful for evaluating exercise tolerance, identifying factors that limit exercise, and assessing the effectiveness of pulmonary rehabilitation. Exercise disability is a predictor of prognosis and marker of health status. Both the paced shuttle walk tests and the 6-min walk test can be used. Cardiopulmonary exercise test using cycle or treadmill can identify coexisting or alternative conditions such as cardiac diseases or neuromuscular diseases.

Composite Scores

Several variables including low FEV_1, a low functional exercise capacity, a high degree of dyspnea, low body-mass index, and presence of hypoxemia or hypercapnia are associated with an increased risk for mortality. A relatively simple approach to identifying disease severity using a combination of most of the above variables has been proposed. All these approaches need validation across a wide range of disease severities and in different clinical settings to confirm that they are suitable for routine clinical use.

Summary table of multidimensional index of COPD:

	PFT	Dyspnea	BMI	Exercise capacity	Smoking	Exacerbation	QoL	Co-morbidity	Age
BODE	O	O	O	O					
mBODE	O	O	O	O					
eBODE	O	O	O	O		O			
BODEx	O	O	O			O			
uBODE	O	O	O	O					
ADO	O	O							O
CPI	O	O	O	O		O	O	O	O
SAFE	O			O			O		
DOSE	O	O			O	O			

BODE: the body-mass index (B), the degree of airflow obstruction (O) and dyspnea (D), and exercise capacity (E), measured by the 6-min walk test
mBODE: modified BODE
eBODE: exacerbation + BODE
BODEx: the body-mass index (B), the degree of airflow obstruction (O) and dyspnea (D), and severe exacerbation (Ex)
uBODE: updated BODE
ADO: age (A), dyspnea (D), and the degree airflow obstruction (O)
CPI: COPD prognostic index
SAFE: SGRQ score, air-flow limitation and exercise tolerance
DOSE: dyspnea (D), airflow obstruction (O), smoking status (S), and exacerbation frequency (E)

The Classification of COPD

The GOLD consensus report proposed a new classification for COPD in 2011 to more comprehensively assess disease severity [17]. This new classification system combined the symptoms in addition to COPD exacerbation history and airflow limitation measured by FEV_1.

- Patient Group A—Low risk, Less symptoms
- Patient Group B—Low risk, More symptoms
- Patient Group C—High risk, Less symptoms
- Patient Group D—High risk, More symptoms

In GOLD Report 2017, it has been revised and ABCD groups are derived from patients' symptoms and their history of exacerbation. Spirometry still has its role for diagnosis and prognostication but out of classification criteria.

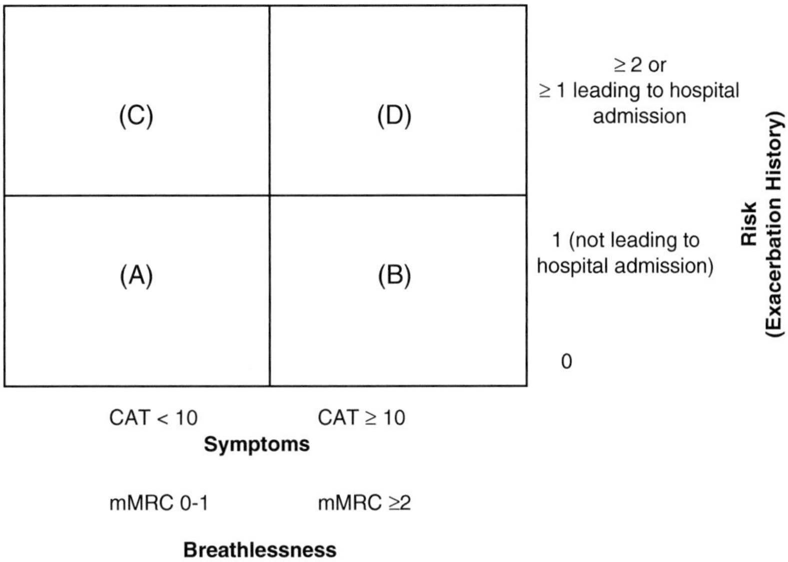

In Korea, a revised COPD guideline was released in 2012 and updated in 2014 by the Korean Academy of Tuberculosis and Respiratory diseases [18]. The new Korean COPD guideline also emphasized the combined assessment for COPD patients. However, there were some differences between the Korean guideline and GOLD consensus report. The Korean guideline classified the COPD patients into three groups. The Korean guideline combined GOLD C, D group into one group and used the spirometry cutoff value for the high risk of exacerbation different from that of GOLD report. The Korean COPD guideline stratified first on the basis of risk of exacerbation with either FEV_1 (<60% or ≥60%) or exacerbation history (0–1 vs. ≥2) or history of hospitalization due to exacerbation (0 vs. ≥1) in the previous year resulting in low risk or high risk group (group "da"). The low risk group then stratified with mMRC or CAT like in GOLD report resulting in low symptom (group "ga") or high symptom (group "na") group.

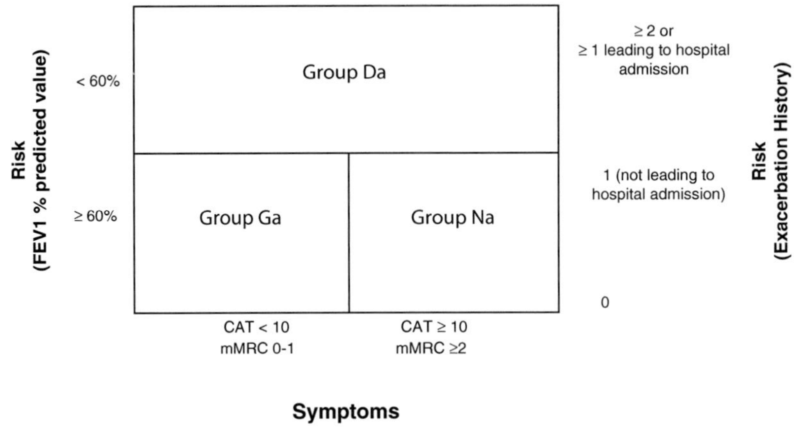

Korean COPD classification system

In Spanish COPD guideline, it was proposed that four different phenotypes of prognostic and therapeutic relevance characterized by the combination of the classical types of emphysema, chronic bronchitis, exacerbators, and patients with overlap COPD-asthma be defined [19]. The proposed phenotypes are: (A) infrequent exacerbators with either chronic bronchitis or emphysema; (B) overlap COPD-asthma; (C) frequent exacerbators with emphysema predominant; and (D) frequent exacerbators with chronic bronchitis predominant (Fig. 6.1).

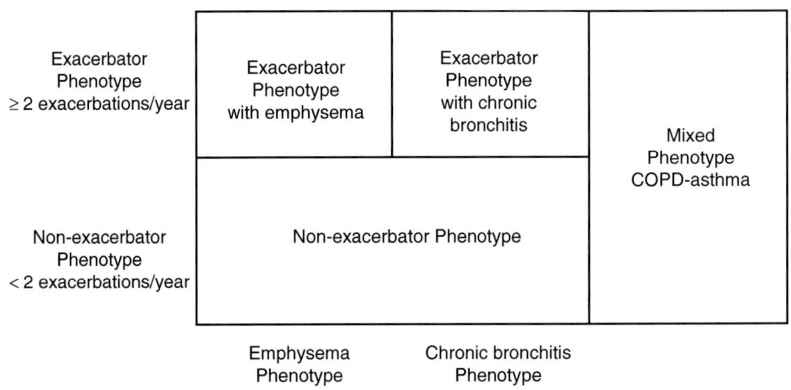

Clinical phenotypes proposed by GesEPOC

Differential Diagnosis

The most difficult clinical problem is to distinguish asthma from COPD. Spirometry and clinical characteristics are the useful method. Improvement in lung function and clinical course is the characteristic feature of asthma. Improvement into the normal range excludes a diagnosis of COPD. In some patients with chronic asthma, a clear distinction from COPD is not possible using current imaging and physiological examination, and it is assumed that asthma and COPD coexist in these patients. Other potential diagnoses are usually easier to distinguish from COPD.

COPD and its differential diagnoses	
COPD	Onset in mid-life
	Symptoms slowly progressive
	History of smoking or exposure to occupational and environmental exposures including biomass fuel
Asthma	Onset early in life (often childhood)
	Symptoms vary widely from day to day
	Symptoms worse at night/early morning
	Allergy, rhinitis, and/or eczema also present
	Family history of asthma
Congestive heart failure	Chest radiography shows enlarged heart and pulmonary edema
	Pulmonary function test indicated restrictive ventilatory defect
Bronchiectasis	Large volumes of purulent sputum
	Commonly associated with bacterial infection
	Chest radiography shows bronchial dilatation and bronchial wall thickening
Tuberculosis	Onset all ages
	Chest radiography shows lung infiltration and/or cavity formation
	Microbiological confirmation
	High prevalence of tuberculosis

Monitoring

Routine follow-up is essential in COPD. However, there are no data to guide decisions on how frequently patients should be reviewed but clearly this will vary according to individual circumstances and the severity of the patient's disease. Symptoms and objective measures of airflow limitation should be monitored to determine when to modify therapy and to identify complications that may develop. At the initial assessment and follow-up visits should include a discussion of symptoms, particularly any new or worsening symptoms and physical examination.

Monitor Disease Progression and Development of Complications

Some patients with COPD deteriorate faster than others and it is important to identify these individuals who may need specialist referral and investigation. Decline in lung function is best tracked by spirometry performed at least once a year or more frequently if indicated. Questionnaires such as the CAT can be performed every 2 or 3 months; trends and changes are more valuable than single measurements.

At each visit, ask about changes in symptoms since the last visit, including cough and sputum, breathlessness, fatigue, activity limitation, and sleep disturbances.

At each visit, identify current smoking status and offer smoking cessation advice. Encouraging patients with COPD to stop smoking is one of the most important components of their management.

Monitor Pharmacotherapy and Other Medical Treatment

Adherence to the maintenance treatment, inhaler technique, effectiveness of the current regimen, and side effects of treatment should be monitored.

Monitor Exacerbation History

The assessment of an exacerbation is based on the patient's medical history and clinical signs of severity and some laboratory test, if available. Assessthe frequency, severity, and possible causes of any exacerbations. Unscheduled visits, use of emergency care, and hospitalization are important. Severity of exacerbation can be estimated by the increased need for bronchodilator or corticosteroids and by the need for antibiotic treatment. Hospitalizations should be documented, including duration of stay, and any use of intensive care unit or mechanical ventilator support.

Monitor Comorbidities

COPD often coexists with other disease that may have a significant impact on prognosis. Comorbidities are common at any severity of COPD. The focus should be on identification and management of these individual problems in line with local treatment guidance.

References

1. Hardie JA, Buist AS, Vollmer WM, Ellingsen I, Bakke PS, Morkve O. Risk of over-diagnosis of COPD in asymptomatic elderly never-smokers. Eur Respir J. 2002;20(5):1117–22.
2. Swanney MP, Ruppel G, Enright PL, Pedersen OF, Crapo RO, Miller MR, et al. Using the lower limit of normal for the FEV1/FVC ratio reduces the misclassification of airway obstruction. Thorax. 2008;63(12):1046–51.
3. Jing JY, Huang TC, Cui W, Xu F, Shen HH. Should FEV1/FEV6 replace FEV1/FVC ratio to detect airway obstruction? A metaanalysis. Chest. 2009;135(4):991–8.
4. Yoo KH, Kim YS, Sheen SS, Park JH, Hwang YI, Kim SH, Yoon HI, Lim SC, Park JY, Park SJ, Seo KH, Kim KU, Oh YM, Lee NY, Kim JS, Oh KW, Kim YT, Park IW, Lee SD, Kim SK, Kim YK, Han SK. Prevalence of chronic obstructive pulmonary disease in Korea: the fourth Korean National Health and nutrition examination survey, 2008. Respirology. 2011;16(4):659–65.
5. Mannino DM, Gagnon RC, Petty TL, Lydick E. Obstructive lung disease and low lung function in adults in the United States: data from the National Health and nutrition examination survey, 1988-1994. Arch Intern Med. 2000;160(11):1683–9.
6. Walker PP, Mitchell P, Diamantea F, Warburton CJ, Davies L. Effect of primary-care spirometry on the diagnosis and management of COPD. Eur Respir J. 2006;28(5):945–52.
7. Stockley RA, O'Brien C, Pye A, Hill SL. Relationship of sputum color to nature and outpatient management of acute exacerbations of COPD. Chest. 2000;117(6):1638–45.
8. Global Initiative for Chronic Obstructive Lung Disease. Global strategy for the diagnosis, management and Prevent of chronic obstructive pulmonary disease, updated 2015. http://www.goldcopd.org.
9. Bestall JC, Paul EA, Garrod R, Garnham R, Jones PW, Wedzicha JA. Usefulness of the Medical Research Council (MRC) dyspnoea scale as a measure of disability in patients with chronic obstructive pulmonary disease. Thorax. 1999;54(7):581–6.
10. Nishimura K, Izumi T, Tsukino M, Oga T. Dyspnea is a better predictor of 5-year survival than airway obstruction in patients with COPD. Chest. 2002;121(5):1434–40.
11. Rodriguez-Roisin R. Toward a consensus definition for COPD exacerbations. Chest. 2000;117(5 Suppl 2):398S–401S.
12. Burge S, Wedzicha JA. COPD exacerbations: definitions and classifications. Eur Respir J Suppl. 2003;41:46s–53s.
13. Celli BR, Barnes PJ. Exacerbations of chronic obstructive pulmonary disease. Eur Respir J. 2007;29(6):1224–38.
14. Anthonisen NR, Manfreda J, Warren CP, Hershfield ES, Harding GK, Nelson NA. Antibiotic therapy in exacerbations of chronic obstructive pulmonary disease. Ann Intern Med. 1987;106:196–204.
15. Leidy NK, Wilcox TK, Jones PW, et al. Development of the EXAcerbations of chronic obstructive pulmonary disease tool (EXACT): a patient-reported outcome (PRO) measure. Value Health. 2010;13:965–75.
16. Jones PW, Chen WH, Wilcox TK, et al. Characterizing and quantifying the symptomatic features of COPD exacerbations. Chest. 2011;139:1388–94.
17. Global Initiative for Chronic Obstructive Lung Disease. Global strategy for the diagnosis, management and Prevent of chronic obstructive pulmonary disease, revised 2011. http://www.goldcopd.org.
18. Korean Academy of Tuberculosis and Respiratory Diseases. COPD guideline revised 2014. http://www.lungkorea.org/thesis/guide.php.
19. Miravitlles M, Soler-Cataluña JJ, Calle M, Molina J, Almagro P, Quintano JA, Riesco JA, Trigueros JA, Piñera P, Simón A, Rodríguez-Hermosa JL, Marco E, López D, Coll R, Coll-Fernández R, Lobo MÁ, Díez J, Soriano JB, Ancochea J. Spanish guideline for COPD (GesEPOC). Arch Bronconeumol. 2014;50(Suppl 1):1–16. doi:10.1016/S0300-2896(14)70070-5.

7 Symptomatic Assessment of COPD

Paul W. Jones

Introduction

This chapter is mainly about formal assessment and quantification of symptoms, rather the elements of eliciting a clinical history, although the latter can be informed by the scientific analysis needed to create an instrument that can measure symptoms. Whilst measurement has become a fundamental part of medicine, it has come only slowly into that most basic clinical assessment—assessing symptoms and their impact on the patient's daily life and sense of well-being. The latter statement may trigger the question—'Why should I measure symptoms, since I am already trained to assess a patient from their history and form a clinical judgement?' There is a general set of answers to this question that apply to any clinical measurement: formal should remove observer bias; numbers can be recorded more easily than descriptions; formal assessment with a common language can aid communication between healthcare professional (and between healthcare professional and patients); perhaps most importantly, it allows a reliable record to be made of changes over time, since formal numerical assessments should be independent of whoever is making them.

Another statement that is still sometimes heard is: 'I can measure lung function, so I don't need to measure symptoms'. That argument is now difficult to sustain because there is a large body of evidence to show that the FEV_1 is only weakly correlated with other clinically important outcomes such as breathlessness, exercise tolerance, exacerbations, and health status. This is illustrated very well by data from the ECLIPSE study [1]. Whilst there is a statistically significant correlation between FEV_1 and these other outcomes at a population level, these associations are much too weak to be of value when assessing individual patients (Fig. 7.1). For example, a patient with moderate airflow limitation (e.g. 70% predicted) may have very good exercise capacity, as measured by their 6-min walking distance (6MWD), and very good health status, measured using the St George's Respiratory Questionnaire (SGRQ), but equally they could have very poor 6MWD and SGRQ score.

It goes without saying that a measurement is only as good as the reliability of the instrument used and the manner in which it is used. Symptomatic assessment in pulmonary medicine was first used in clinical studies, using well-validated instruments that were too complex for routine use, but these have provided a lot of insight into the health status of patients with COPD and factors that influence it, together with its response to treatment and progression over

P.W. Jones, Ph.D., F.R.C.P., F.E.R.S.
Institute for Infection and Immunity,
St George's, University of London,
Cranmer Terrace, London SW170RE, UK
e-mail: pjones@sgul.ac.uk

S.-D. Lee (ed.), *COPD*, DOI 10.1007/978-3-662-47178-4_7

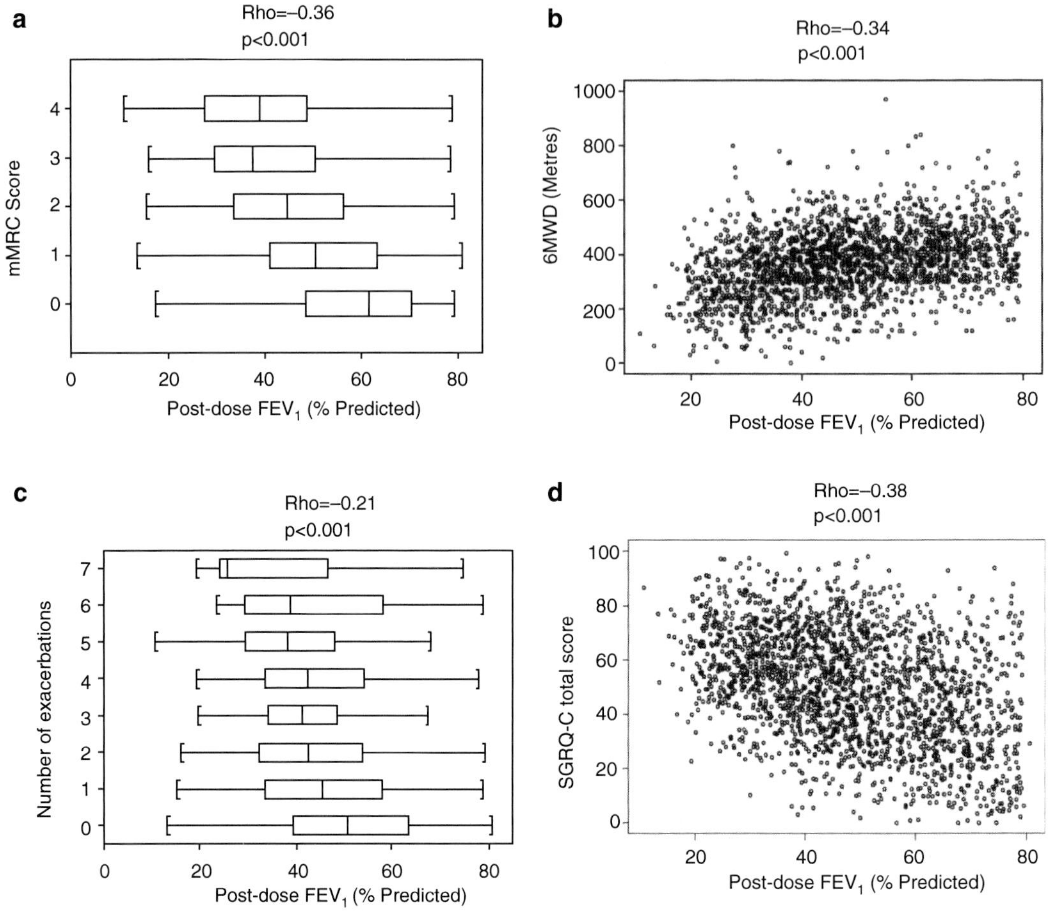

Fig. 7.1 Correlation between post-bronchodilator FEV_1 and: (**a**) mMRC score; (**b**) 6-min walking distance; (**c**) number of exacerbations and (**d**) SGRQ. From [1]

time. Newer health status instruments are simpler to use and can be used reliably in routine clinical practice.

Breathlessness

It is appropriate to begin with breathlessness, since this is a core symptom in COPD that leads to impaired exercise capacity and poor quality of life; it was also the first symptom to be measured in a standardized way, through the Medical Research Council (MRC) Dyspnoea Scale that was developed 60 years ago. Confusingly when modified by the American Thoracic Society for use in the USA, the scaling range was changed from 1–5 to 0–4. For that reason, it is important to be clear which version is being used, the modified version being abbreviated to mMRC. Throughout the rest of this section, the generic name MRC will be used. The original MRC scale is shown in Fig. 7.2, and it will be seen that it might be better described as a measure of disability associated with breathlessness. It is not a direct measure of breathlessness such as the visual analogue scale (VAS) and Borg scale.

The MRC scale was initially developed as an epidemiological tool and was only fully validated as a measure of COPD severity many years later [2]. Studies showing that the MRC was a better predictor of mortality than the FEV_1 [3], led to its

MRC dyspnoea scale

Grade 1:	Breathless on strenuous exercise
Grade 2:	Short of breath when hurrying or walking up a slight hill
Grade 3:	Walk slower than others or stop when walking at own pace on level ground
Grade 4:	Stop every 100 m or after a few minutes
Grade 5:	Too breathless to leave the house or breathless on washing/dressing

Fig. 7.2 MRC dyspnoea scale

incorporation into the BODE prognostic instrument [4]. The chief disadvantage of the MRC scale is that the intervals between the different grades are very large and, at an individual patient level, few patients will improve with treatment by one grade and fortunately few patients will deteriorate by one grade over months to years of follow-up.

The relative insensitivity of the MRC led to the development of the Baseline and Transition Dyspnea Indices (BDI and TDI), like the MRC scale they are indirect measures of breathlessness since they link dyspnoea to activity [5]. Interestingly, the simple direct measures of breathlessness, such as the VAS and Borg scales, have not found application in routine pulmonary medicine, outside the exercise laboratory, unlike scales for pain which commonly use that type of methodology. A more recent 12-item dyspnoea scale (the Dyspnoea-12) was developed with modern psychometric methods using descriptions used by patients to describe their breathlessness [6]. It has been validated, but has not yet found its way into routine clinical practice, although it is short enough to be practical in that setting.

Respiratory Symptoms

No standardized measures of respiratory symptoms have been developed for use in routine practice; in fact, until recently they hadn't even been developed for clinical trials. Now a daily diary card has been created, which is now called the Evaluating Respiratory Symptoms in COPD (E-RS), although when first developed it was known as the EXACT-RS [7]. It has 11 items that provide a total score and three domains: Breathlessness (five items); Cough and Sputum (three items) and Chest Symptoms (three items). The latter includes factors such as chest tightness. The E-RS has been validated [8] and full details are available from the website although users will have to register to get full details (http://www.exactproinitiative.com/instrument-descriptions/). Whilst daily diaries are not practical for routine use, the finding that there are three scientifically determined domains within stable COPD symptoms provides useful confirmation of established clinical experience. The E-RS has recently been shown to be responsive to pharmacological treatment [9].

Exacerbations

It is appropriate to include exacerbations in a chapter devoted to assessment of symptoms because exacerbations are symptomatic events. Furthermore, the patient's history of exacerbations appears to be the single best predictor of future risk of exacerbations [10], so clinical assessment and standardization are important.

Like respiratory symptoms, exacerbations have only recently been subject to rigorous scientific analysis [11] this supported the development of the EXACT diary card [12] http://www.exactproinitiative.com/instrument-descriptions/. The E-RS symptom diary, described above, was developed from the 14-item EXACT, so it is perhaps not surprising that it has the same three domains: breathlessness, chest symptoms, and cough and sputum. Until the development of the EXACT, the consensus definition of an exacerbation was: 'a sustained worsening of the patient's condition, from the stable state and beyond normal variation, that is acute in onset' [13]; later 'and leads to a change in treatment' was added [14]. It will be noted that the 'worsening' and 'day-to-day variation' are not defined and neither is 'sustained' although the common definition in clinical trials requires symptoms to have worsened for 2–3 days. The criterion about change in symptoms necessitating a change in treatment led to the creation of a severity grading: mild (use of extra routine medication such short-acting bronchodilator), moderate (use of systemic corticosteroid and/or antibiotics), severe (moderate plus hospital admission or emergency room attendance). Though very widely used, these severity grades have never been validated. In contrast, the EXACT has strict criteria for determining that an acute change in symptom score is an exacerbation.

Although it is a research tool, the development of the EXACT has been important for routine practice for two main reasons. First, it has emphasized that there are distinct symptomatic components of an exacerbation, not just an increase in cough with sputum production. Furthermore, the contribution of each component to the patients worsening may vary between exacerbations and patients; indeed, an exacerbation may meet the EXACT criteria for an exacerbation without the patient having a worsening of cough and sputum. A second and perhaps even more important contribution of the EXACT has been to show that patients experience frequent unreported exacerbations that appear to have similar short-term (6 months) consequences as those that are reported [15]. The reasons for the lack of reporting are ill-understood. Unreported exacerbations may occur in patients who are a little less severe than those patients who do report them, but a more striking observation is that there are big differences in reporting rates between countries that may not be related to differences in severity. A possible reason for under-reporting may be that patients do not understand that worsening of chest symptoms with a viral upper respiratory tract infection is not a feature of a cold, but is in fact a worsening of their chest condition. This suggests that physicians should enquire specifically for symptoms of exacerbations (not just cough and sputum), and a simple severity guide would be to ask whether the worsening of chest symptoms and breathlessness was sufficient to disturb the patient's daily routine.

Health Status—Complex Questionnaires

COPD is a very complex disease and health status questionnaires attempt to quantify its overall impact on a patient's daily life and well-being. Health status scores provide a marker of a person's health-related quality of life (HRQoL), but they should not be called HRQoL scores. The distinction between health status and HRQoL is important. HRQoL is a *clinical outcome* that is unique to each person, since the factors that determine his or her quality of life will differ, depending on their personality and circumstances. For the same reason, illness will affect HRQoL in a way that is unique to each person. It is not possible to make standardized measurements that allow comparisons between patients and treatments because the components of the scale will differ between patients. In contrast, a health status questionnaire is *standardized marker* of impaired HRQoL that is made up of items that should be common (at least potentially) to every patient; this means that they assess each patient as if he/she was a 'typical' patient—in the same way that % predicted FEV^1 treats every patient as being typical of someone of the same age, height, sex and race.

The first health status measure to be developed was the Chronic Respiratory Questionnaire (CRQ) [16]. It is widely used although largely in the context of rehabilitation. It is too complex for routine clinical use although it is often used to monitor and evaluate rehabilitation programmes. It has four domains and through these it drew attention to two important aspects of COPD that had been largely under-recognized; these are fatigue and mastery, the latter being the patient's sense of being in control of their condition. One of the challenges with questionnaires designed to measure overall health status is the production of a valid total score. Interestingly, the CRQ's developer never approved the calculation of a total score, but researchers often calculate one, although its validity has never been established.

The SGRQ was developed and validated in both asthma and COPD [17], but its use has largely been confined to COPD, although recently it has been used successfully to assess the response to treatment in patients with severe asthma [18]. To address the problem of creating a valid total score, each item has specific weight, which means that its score is best calculated using a computer. A revised and slightly shorter 40-item set was created and termed the SGRQ for COPD (SGRQ-C) [19]. Manuals and over 60 language versions are available for download (www.healthstatus.sgul.ac.uk). A user-friendly scoring system for both versions is now available for a number of platforms (www.sgrq.github.io).

Health Status—Insights from Research Studies

The SGRQ is too complex for routine use, but much has been learnt from its application to research studies that is applicable to routine care. There is a large body of data from clinical trials about a range of different treatments. For example, a recent network meta-analysis has shown quite large differences between different bronchodilators in SGRQ scores (and breathlessness measured by the TDI) [20]. A significant contribution has been the demonstration that SGRQ scores may detect a worthwhile patient benefit in the absence of large improvements in objective physical measurements. For example, following placement of endobronchial coils for severe emphysema, the improvement in SGRQ was twice the minimum clinically important difference (MCID), despite there being only small improvements in FEV_1 and 6MWD [21]. The ability of the SGRQ to quantify health status improvements from the patient's perspective has now been recognized by the Food and Drugs Administration (FDA) in the USA which has qualified it for use as a co-primary outcome in new drug registration trials.

At this point, it should be appreciated that health status questionnaires are designed to be 'treatment agnostic'—i.e. a change in score should indicate the same health status benefit, regardless of the therapeutic mechanism of action. The large improvement seen in the study of endobronchial coils, just described, reflects similarly large improvements seen with lung volume reduction for emphysema [22], but it should be appreciated that both of these treatments are invasive and are only used for patients at the severe end of the disease-spectrum. In the much larger population of less severe COPD patients, the benefits with inhaled therapy is smaller, although modern once-daily long-acting bronchodilators appear to be more effective than older twice-daily agents and show average improvements that are at the level of the MCID [20]. In contrast, pulmonary rehabilitation, which is a treatment that is appropriate to all COPD patients, produces an average improvement in SGRQ score that is approximately 1.5 times the MCID [23]. The benefits from these complementary treatment modalities are likely to be additive, so effective bronchodilation followed by rehabilitation should, on average, lead to a patient achieving a good improvement in their HRQoL.

One of the interesting observations that has come from pharmacological treatment trials in COPD has come from the placebo arms of the trials. These typically shows an improvement in SGRQ score that is around half the MCID. This 'clinical trial effect' is not understood. It is not immediate in onset; the patients slowly improve, typically for up to 6 months, and the improvement is maintained for 1 year (Fig. 7.3). The mechanisms are not understood. One factor may be a Hawthorne effect, in which the patient, their physician or both of them, change their behaviour when a patient enters a trial. This could include better compliance with concomitant therapy, lifestyle changes and perhaps earlier intervention if there were any worsening. There may be something in the doctor–patient relationship that also improves the patient's sense of well-being; perhaps giving the patient greater confidence in managing their condition, lessening the effect that it has on their lives. One randomized trial of antidepressant therapy has shed a little light on this phenomenon since it showed a bigger improvement in patients who were seen regularly in the trial compared to those who were seen only at the beginning and the end [24]. Whatever the mechanism, these observations suggest that patients do receive benefit just from regular medical review.

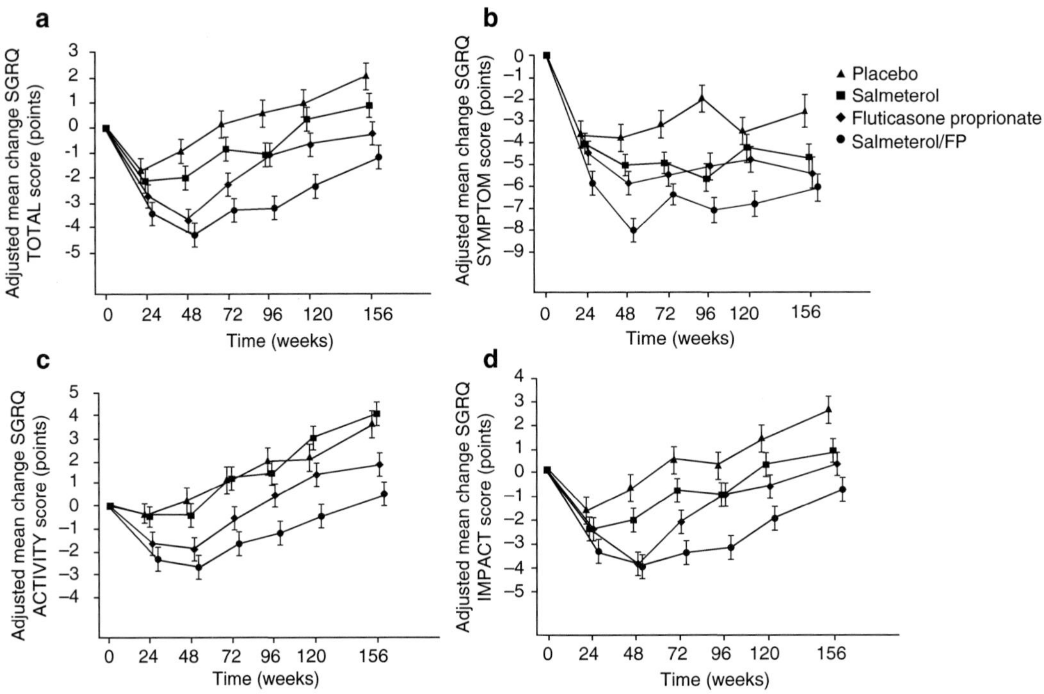

Fig. 7.3 Changes in SGRQ score over 156 weeks in the TORCH trial. (**a**) Total score; (**b**) Symptoms score; (**c**) Activity score; (**d**) Impacts score. Data from [26]

Apart from quantifying therapeutic benefit, perhaps the most significant contribution of health status measurement has been to provide a better understanding of changes in the patients' health over time. This has been seen and measured with both disease-specific questionnaires and with generic physical and mental health, as measured with the SF-36 [25]. At least two disease factors are known to be associated with worsening health status: decline in FEV_1 [26] and frequency of exacerbations [27]. Patients do not deteriorate at the same rate and two cohort studies from Japan provide useful insights into the relationship between worsening FEV_1 and worsening health status. In one, there was no deterioration in health status over the first 18 months, but thereafter the SGRQ score deteriorated progressively, whilst the FEV_1 showed little consistent directional change [28]. The initial period of health status stability may be due, not only to the impact of treatment when the patient joined the clinic, but also due to the effect of keeping them under review in the clinic (analogous to the clinical trial effect described earlier). The second study showed different patterns of worsening in patients related to their change in FEV_1 over time. Patients who were fast FEV_1 decliners showed the fastest deterioration in SGRQ, exceeding the MCID after 4 years; whereas slow decliners showed little worsening [29]. Most interestingly, those patients whose FEV_1 was maintained actually showed an improvement in SGRQ that exceed the MCID by 4 years. In the latter study and in the TORCH clinical trial ([26] and Fig. 7.3), there was a different pattern of disease progression across the domains of the SGRQ; the symptoms domain score showed a sustained improvement regardless of change in FEV_1 (in the cohort study) or treatment group (TORCH trial), whereas there was a worsening in the Activity and Impacts scores across treatment groups in TORCH and, if the FEV_1 deteriorated, in the cohort study. In the latter study, the Activity component did not improve, even if FEV_1 did not worsen, in fact there was a general trend for Activity to worsen. These findings all point to heterogeneity of the pattern of health status worsening, both in the degree and character of that change. Finally, deterioration in SGRQ score may be a predictor of worse health in the future since an analysis of the ECLIPSE study suggests that patients who deteriorate by more than the MCID have a greater risk of hospitalization and death 2 years later [30].

There is evidence that pharmacological treatment can have an impact on worsening in health status. The ISOLDE study showed that inhaled corticosteroid (ICS) alone could alter the rate of worsening of SGRQ and general health status scores [25]. More recently, the TORCH study (long-acting beta$_2$-agonist (LAMA) plus ICS) and UPLIFT (long-acting anti-muscarinic (LAMA)) showed that maintenance treatment can produce improvements in health status that may be maintained for 3 years or more [26, 31]. The true size of the effect may have been underestimated in these trials because of differential drop out of the sickest patients who had the worst health status, an effect that was greatest in the placebo arm [32].

Health Status—Shorter Questionnaires

Whilst a great deal has been learnt from health status measurement in clinical studies, the complexity of the questionnaires prevented them from being used in routine clinical practice, but there are now two that are suitable for use in that setting. The first to be developed was the Clinical COPD Questionnaire (CCQ) [33]. It has ten items, exists in daily and weekly versions, and is available in 60 languages. A website gives more details (http://www.ccq.nl). The 8-item COPD Assessment Test (CAT) (Fig. 7.4) was developed to facilitate communication between doctor and patient, but with good measurement properties so that it would be suitable for use in clinical trials [34]. The website contains a user guide and allows online completion and scoring in 64 languages (www.CATestonline.org). Mean CAT scores appear to be very consistent across countries (Fig. 7.5). The CAT has shown good correlations with the established measures such as the CRQ [35], SGRQ [36] and CCQ [37]. It has also been proven to be a good predictor of exacerbations in patients who were already at higher risk of exacerbations because of an exacerbation in the preceding year.

There are many publications about the CAT that further tested its validity and responsiveness to treatment, and these are detailed in two recent systematic reviews [38, 39]. Data summarized in these reviews suggest that it appears to be as responsive to rehabilitation as the CRQ and SGRQ, with a change in score, compared to usual care, that is $\approx$1.5 times the MCID (note: the individual patient MCID for the CAT = 2 units [40]). In terms of pharmacological treatment, the CAT has been shown to be as sensitive as the SGRQ in response to ICS/LAMA and LAMA/LABA treatment [41]; the mean improvement with both treatments was 2.2–2.4 units, i.e. well above the MCID.

Symptomatic Assessment in Routine Practice

There are perhaps three broad areas in COPD management where formal assessment of symptoms has a place: baseline assessment, evaluating the response to treatment and monitoring.

The simplest assessment of a COPD patient is to ask about the severity of their disease; however, there is good evidence that this may lead to an under-estimated of the true impact of the disease. For example, 36% of patients who said that their disease was only mild or moderate also indicated that they were MRC Grade 5, i.e. they were breathless when washing and dressing or too breathless to leave the house [42]. In 2011, the Global Initiative for Chronic Obstructive Pulmonary Disease (GOLD) revision of its assessment scheme (www.goldcopd.org) recommended, for the first time, a process based on symptoms and risk of exacerbations. It suggested use of either the mMRC or the CAT, recommending the maintenance treatment should be started with a mMRC score ≥ 2, or CAT ≥ 10 for the CAT. Unfortunately, it made an error in equating

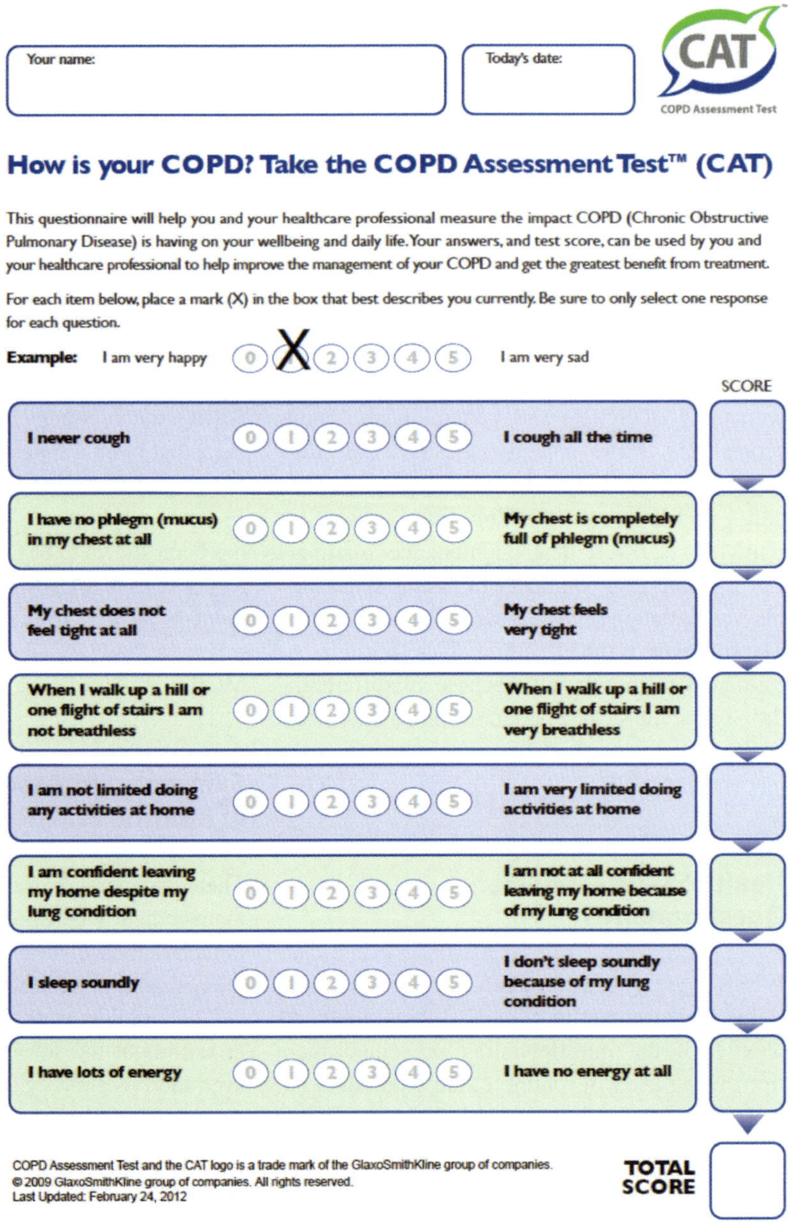

Your name: Today's date:

CAT COPD Assessment Test

How is your COPD? Take the COPD Assessment Test™ (CAT)

This questionnaire will help you and your healthcare professional measure the impact COPD (Chronic Obstructive Pulmonary Disease) is having on your wellbeing and daily life. Your answers, and test score, can be used by you and your healthcare professional to help improve the management of your COPD and get the greatest benefit from treatment.

For each item below, place a mark (X) in the box that best describes you currently. Be sure to only select one response for each question.

Example: I am very happy (0) (X) (2) (3) (4) (5) I am very sad

			SCORE
I never cough	0 1 2 3 4 5	I cough all the time	
I have no phlegm (mucus) in my chest at all	0 1 2 3 4 5	My chest is completely full of phlegm (mucus)	
My chest does not feel tight at all	0 1 2 3 4 5	My chest feels very tight	
When I walk up a hill or one flight of stairs I am not breathless	0 1 2 3 4 5	When I walk up a hill or one flight of stairs I am very breathless	
I am not limited doing any activities at home	0 1 2 3 4 5	I am very limited doing activities at home	
I am confident leaving my home despite my lung condition	0 1 2 3 4 5	I am not at all confident leaving my home because of my lung condition	
I sleep soundly	0 1 2 3 4 5	I don't sleep soundly because of my lung condition	
I have lots of energy	0 1 2 3 4 5	I have no energy at all	

COPD Assessment Test and the CAT logo is a trade mark of the GlaxoSmithKline group of companies.
© 2009 GlaxoSmithKline group of companies. All rights reserved.
Last Updated: February 24, 2012

TOTAL SCORE

Fig. 7.4 COPD Assessment Test (CAT). Available from www.CATestonline.org

these thresholds because subsequently it has been shown that mMRC ≥ 2 equates to CAT > 20 [43], which is a 'severe impact' according to the CAT handbook (www.CATestonline.org). In fact, CAT ≥ 10 corresponds approximately to mMRC Grade 0 (breathless on strenuous exercise). More recently, GOLD has emphasized the importance of the CAT since it measures much more than just breathlessness, in fact only 25% of the items in the CAT are concerned with activity limitation. The mMRC can be used if the CAT is not available, but with the caveat that the available evidence suggests that the equivalent threshold is mMRC 0, not >1. Confusingly, mMRC Grade 0 does not mean the absence of symptoms (which would be zero on the original MRC scale), it is breathlessness with strenuous exercise. In this, we see an example in which some degree of breathlessness is seen as being 'normal' in COPD.

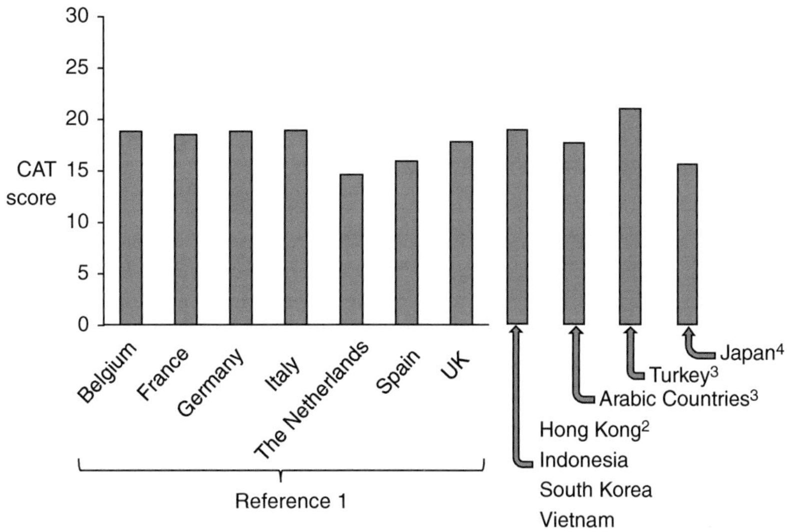

Fig. 7.5 CAT scores from clinics in different countries. Data from the following references: Country 1 [45]; Country 2 [36]; Country 3 [46]; Country 4 [47]

The assessment of the response to treatment requires special consideration. The limits of day-to-day repeatability of most measurements in COPD (including the FEV_1) are wider than the size of the MCID, so pairs of measurements before and after treatment may give a misleading indication of the size of change in an individual patient. However, there is evidence that patients' global ratings of treatment efficacy may, on average, provide a reliable measure of the overall treatment effect. In a 16-week study of salmeterol in COPD, a 4-unit change in SGRQ (the MCID for the SGRQ) was associated with a global estimate of 'effective' treatment and an 8-unit change was 'very effective' [44]. In contrast, a response that was 'satisfactory' was associated with a change that was less than two units. Thus, the patient's global estimate of a treatment effect has some scientific validity! Questionnaires are not the right way to assess an individual's response to treatment, however, because each patient may respond to treatment and notice benefit in a different way. For example, a woman may once again be able to play nine rounds of golf, whilst a man may find that he can clean his apartment without having to stop for breath. A traditional clinical history-taking approach is required to evaluate benefit. The method used by this author illustrated in Fig. 7.6. It should be emphasized that the most important component is that the patient should be able to specify one activity or symptomatic aspect of their disease that has noticeably improved. If they can't do that, it is reasonable to assume that they haven't had a worthwhile benefit.

A quick assessment of response to treatment

- Have you noticed a difference?
- What have you noticed, for example*
  - Are you less breathless?
  - Can you do more?
  - Can you do things more easily or quickly?
  - Can you sleep better?
- Tell me one thing that you have noticed is better

Fig. 7.6 A simple method of evaluating response to symptomatic treatment in COPD patients

Perhaps the most useful application of health status questionnaires is in routine monitoring. Since the CAT and the SGRQ are closely correlated, a picture of the different patterns of change in CAT score may be created from a number of sources discussed earlier. These are illustrated in Fig. 7.7. A combination of effective bronchodilation and rehabilitation should produce a total improvement of at least 3–4 units, which should be maintained within a 2-unit range. On average, the worsening should be ≤1 unit per year. A cause should be sought if there is any worsening beyond that range. For example: less adherence

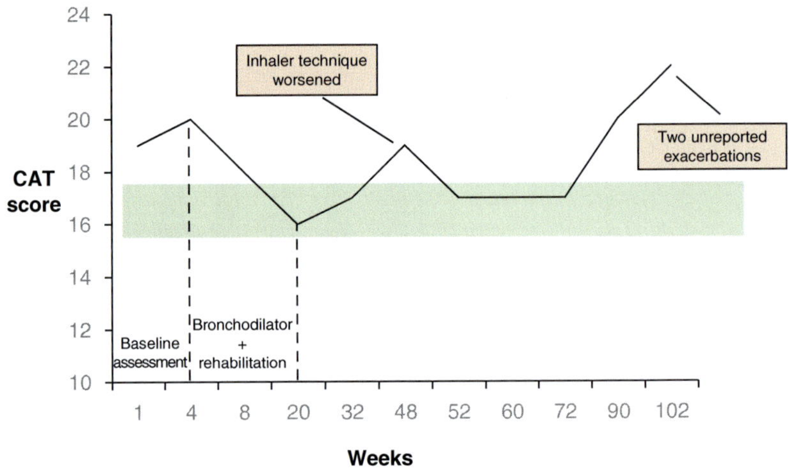

Fig. 7.7 A schematic of changes in CAT score that may be seen in an individual with COPD. The *green shaded area* shows the range of usual between visit variations that might be expected. If a worsening outside that range is seen, enquiries should be made to identify a cause

to treatment, failure of inhaler technique, frequent exacerbations (reported or unreported) and rapid decline of lung function. Monitoring with the CAT is much easier than spirometry which is more time consuming and may be sensitive to a wider range of disease factors.

Summary

Formal symptom assessment is now an established place in COPD management. The introduction of simple health status instruments such as the CAT has made it possible to make reliable, routine and valid assessments of the overall impact of COPD on a patient's health. They do not replace clinical assessment or lung function, but add to the information available to the clinician in deciding management of their patient.

References

1. Agusti A, Calverley PMA, Celli B, Coxson HO, Edwards L, Lomas D, et al. Characterisation of COPD heterogeneity in the ECLIPSE cohort. Respir Res. 2010;11(1):122.
2. Bestall JC, Paul EA, Garrod R, Garnham R, Jones PW, Wedzicha JA. Usefulness of the Medical Research Council (MRC) dyspnoea scale as a measure of disability in patients with chronic obstructive pulmonary disease. Thorax. 1999;54(7):581–6.
3. Nishimura K, Izumi T, Tsukino M, Oga T. Dyspnea is a better predictor of 5-year survival than airway obstruction in patients with COPD. Chest. 2002;121(5):1434–40.
4. Celli BR, Cote CG, Marin JM, Casanova C, Montes de Oca M, Mendez RA, et al. The body-mass index, airflow obstruction, dyspnea and exercise capacity index in chronic obstructive pulmonary disease. NEJM. 2004;350:1005–12.
5. Mahler DA, Weinberg DH, Wells CK, Feinstein AR. Measurements of dyspnea. Contents, interobserver correlates of two new clinical indices. Chest. 1984;85:751–8.
6. Yorke J, Moosavi SH, Shuldham C, Jones PW. Quantification of dyspnoea using descriptors: development and initial testing of the Dyspnoea-12. Thorax. 2010;65(1):21–6.
7. Leidy NK, Sexton CC, Jones PW, Notte SM, Monz BU, Nelsen L, et al. Measuring respiratory symptoms in clinical trials of COPD: reliability and validity of a daily diary. Thorax. 2014;69(5):443–9.
8. Leidy NK, Murray LT, Monz BU, Nelsen L, Goldman M, Jones PW, et al. Measuring respiratory symptoms of COPD: performance of the EXACT- Respiratory Symptoms Tool (E-RS) in three clinical trials. Respir Res. 2014;15(1):124.
9. Jones PW, Leidy NK, Hareendran AR, Lamarca, Chuecos F, Garcia Gil E. The effect of aclidinium bromide on daily respiratory symptoms of COPD, measured using the Evaluating Respiratory Symptoms in COPD (E-RS: COPD) diary: pooled analysis of two 6-month phase III studies. Respir Res. 2016;17(1):61.
10. Hurst JR, Vestbo J, Anzueto A, Locantore N, Müllerova H, Tal-Singer R, et al. Susceptibility to exacerbation in chronic obstructive pulmonary disease. N Engl J Med. 2010;363(12):1128–38.
11. Jones PW, Chen W-H, Wilcox TK, Sethi S, Leidy NK, Group E-PS. Characterizing and quantifying the

symptomatic features of COPD exacerbations. Chest. 2011;139(6):1388–94.
12. Leidy NK, Wilcox TK, Jones PW, Roberts L, Powers JH, Sethi S, et al. Standardizing measurement of chronic obstructive pulmonary disease exacerbations. Am J Respir Crit Care Med. 2011;183(3):323–9.
13. Rodriguez-Roisin R. Toward a consensus definition for COPD exacerbations. Chest. 2000;117(5 Suppl 2):398S–401S.
14. Burge S, Wedzicha JA. COPD exacerbations: definitions and classifications. Eur Respir J. 2003;21(41 suppl):46s–53s.
15. Jones PW, Lamarca R, Chuecos F, Singh D, Agustí A, Bateman ED, et al. Characterisation and impact of reported and unreported exacerbations: results from ATTAIN. Eur Respir J. 2014;44(5):1156–65.
16. Guyatt GH, Berman LB, Townsend M, Pugsley SO, Chambers LW. A measure of quality of life for clinical trials in chronic lung disease. Thorax. 1987;42:773–8.
17. Jones PW, Quirk FH, Baveystock CM, Littlejohns P. A self-complete measure for chronic airflow limitation—the St George's respiratory questionnaire. Am Rev Respir Dis. 1992;145:1321–7.
18. Ortega HG, Liu MC, Pavord ID, Brusselle GG, FitzGerald JM, Chetta A, et al. Mepolizumab treatment in patients with severe eosinophilic asthma. N Engl J Med. 2014;371(13):1198–207.
19. Meguro M, Barley EA, Spencer S, Jones PW. Development and validation of an improved COPD-specific version of the St George's respiratory questionnaire. Chest. 2007;132:456–63.
20. Cope S, Donohue JF, Jansen JP, Kraemer M, Capkun-Niggli G, Baldwin M, et al. Comparative efficacy of long-acting bronchodilators for COPD—a network meta-analysis. Respir Res. 2013;14(1):100.
21. Sciurba FC, Criner GJ, Strange C, et al. Effect of endobronchial coils vs usual care on exercise tolerance in patients with severe emphysema: the renew randomized clinical trial. JAMA. 2016;315(20):2178–89.
22. National Emphysema Treatment Trial Research Group. Cost effectiveness of lung-volume-reduction surgery for patients with severe emphysema. NEJM. 2003;348:2092–102.
23. Bernard M, Dympna C, Declan D, Kathy M, Edel M, Yves L. Pulmonary rehabilitation for chronic obstructive pulmonary disease. Cochrane Database Syst Rev. 2015;2:CD003793.
24. McCarney R, Warner J, Iliffe S, van Haselen R, Griffin M, Fisher P. The Hawthorne effect: a randomised, controlled trial. BMC Med Res Methodol. 2007;7(1):30.
25. Spencer S, Calverley PMA, Burge PS, Jones PW. Health status deterioration in patients with chronic obstructive pulmonary disease. Am J Respir Crit Care Med. 2001;163:122–8.
26. Jones P, Anderson J, Calverley P, Celli B, Ferguson G, Jenkins C, et al. Health status in the TORCH study of COPD: treatment efficacy and other determinants of change. Respir Res. 2011;12(1):71.
27. Spencer S, Calverley PMA, Burge PS, Jones PW. Impact of preventing exacerbations on deterioration of health status in COPD. Eur Respir J. 2004; 23(5):698–702.
28. Oga T, Nishimura K, Tsukino M, Sato S, Hajiro T, Mishima M. Longitudinal deteriorations in patient reported outcomes in patients with COPD. Respir Med. 2007;101(1):146–53.
29. Nagai K, Nishimura M, Makita H, Suzuki M, Shimizu K, Konno S, et al. Differential changes in quality of life components over 5 years in chronic obstructive pulmonary disease patients. COPD. 2015;10(1):745–57.
30. Wilke S, Jones PW, Mullerova H, Vestbo J, Tal-Singer R, Franssen FME, et al. One-year change in health status and subsequent outcomes in COPD. Thorax. 2015;70(5):420–5.
31. Tashkin DP, Celli B, Senn S, Burkhart D, Kesten S, Menjoge SS, et al. A 4-year trial of tiotropium in chronic obstructive pulmonary disease. N Engl J Med. 2008;359(15):1543–54.
32. Vestbo J, Anderson JA, Calverley PMA, Celli B, Ferguson GT, Jenkins C, et al. Bias due to withdrawal in long-term randomised trials in COPD: evidence from the TORCH study. Clin Respir J. 2011;5(1):44–9.
33. van der Molen T, Willemse BWM, Schokker S, ten Hacken NHT, Postma DS, Juniper EF. Development, validity and responsiveness of the clinical COPD questionnaire. Health Qual Life Outcomes. 2003;1(1):13.
34. Jones PW, Harding G, Berry P, Wiklund I, Chen WH, Kline LN. Development and first validation of the COPD assessment test. Eur Respir J. 2009; 34(3):648–54.
35. Jones PW, Harding G, Wiklund I, Berry P, Tabberer M, Yu R, et al. Tests of the responsiveness of the COPD assessment test following acute exacerbation and pulmonary rehabilitation COPD assessment test responsiveness. Chest J. 2012;142(1):134–40.
36. Kwon N-H, Amin M, Hui DS, Jung K-S, Lim SY, Ta HD, et al. Validity of the chronic obstructive pulmonary disease assessment test (CAT) translated into local languages for Asian patients. Chest. 2013; 143:703–10.
37. Ställberg B, Nokela M, Ehrs P-O, Hjemdal P, Jonsson EW. Validation of the clinical COPD questionnaire (CCQ) in primary care. Health Qual Life Outcomes. 2009;7(1):1–9.
38. Gupta N, Pinto LM, Morogan A, Bourbeau J. The COPD assessment test: a systematic review. Eur Respir J. 2014;44(4):873–84.
39. Karloh M, Mayer AF, Maurici R, Pizzichini MMM, Jones PW, Pizzichini E. The COPD assessment test: what do we know so far?: a systematic review and meta-analysis about clinical outcomes prediction and classification of patients into gold stages. Chest. 2016;149(2):413–25.
40. Kon SSC, Canavan JL, Jones SE, Nolan CM, Clark AL, Dickson MJ, et al. Minimum clinically

important difference for the COPD assessment test: a prospective analysis. Lancet Respir Med. 2014;2(3):195–203.
41. Singh D, Worsley S, Zhu C-Q, Hardaker L, Church A. Umeclidinium/vilanterol versus fluticasone propionate/salmeterol in COPD: a randomised trial. BMC Pulm Med. 2015;15:91.
42. Rennard S, DeCramer M, Calverley PMA, Pride NB, Soriano JB, Vermeire PA, et al. Impact of COPD in North America and Europe in 2000: subjects' perspective of confronting COPD international survey. Eur Respir J. 2002;20:799–805.
43. Jones PW, Adamek L, Nadeau G, Banik N. Comparisons of health status scores with MRC grades in COPD: implications for the GOLD 2011 classification. Eur Respir J. 2013;42(3):647–54.
44. Jones PW, Bosh TK. Changes in quality of life in COPD patients treated with salmeterol. Am J Respir Crit Care Med. 1997;155:1283–9.
45. Jones PW, Brusselle G, Dal Negro RW, Ferrer M, Kardos P, Levy ML, et al. Properties of the COPD assessment test in a cross-sectional European study. Eur Respir J. 2011;38(1):29–35.
46. Jones PW, Shahrour N, Nejjari C, Lahlou A, Doble A, Rashid N, et al. Psychometric evaluation of the COPD assessment test: data from the BREATHE study in the Middle East and North Africa region. Respir Med. 2012;106(Suppl 2):S86–99.
47. Tsuda T, Suematsu R, Kamohara K, Kurose M, Arakawa I, Tomioka R, et al. Development of the Japanese version of the COPD assessment test. Respir Invest. 2012;50(2):34–9.

Imaging of COPD

8

Sang Min Lee, Song Soo Kim, Hye Jeon Hwang, and Joon Beom Seo

Computed Tomography (CT)

CT Basic Physics

Computed tomography (CT) of the thorax is a very quick and the most advanced imaging technique. CT scanner is designed to use a form of gantry which allows rotation of the X-ray tube and the detector around the patient during breath hold. With the development of CT technology, single breath-hold scanning of the thorax can be achieved, and image reconstruction of sagittal and coronal planes is also feasible with minimal loss of spatial resolution. During the decades, the fan beam of a CT scanner is broadened along the *Z*-axis and two-dimensional detectors are developed, acquisition of a number of slices per rotation is possible. Recently developed multi-slice and multi-detector CT allows cone beam CT and volumetric imaging. After CT scan, the X-ray attenuation, called tissue density, is expressed as a Hounsfield Units (HU). The scale of HU values range from −1000 HU (attenuation value of air) to 3000 HU, and 0 HU corresponds to the attenuation of water (Fig. 8.1). Generally, normal lung has an attenuation value around −850 HU on inspiratory CT because normal lung attenuation reflects the mixed attenuation of intrapulmonary air and lung parenchyma.

S.M. Lee, M.D. • J.B. Seo, M.D., Ph.D. (✉)
Division of Cardiothoracic Radiology, Department of Radiology, Asan Medical Center, University of Ulsan College of Medicine, Seoul, South Korea
e-mail: sangmin.lee.md@gmail.com; asellion@hanmail.net, joonbeom.seo@gmail.com

S.S. Kim, M.D.
Department of Radiology, Chungnam National University Hospital, Chungnam National University School of Medicine, Daejeon, South Korea
e-mail: haneul88@hanmail.net

H.J. Hwang, M.D.
Department of Radiology, Hallym University College of Medicine, Hallym University Sacred Heart Hospital, Seoul, South Korea
e-mail: umttette@hanmail.net

Radiation Dose of COPD CT

The radiation dose during CT scan is presented as the gray or mGy unit, which is proportional to the amount of energy that the irradiated body part is expected to absorb. The Sievert (Sv) unit is used in the report of the effective dose. Regarding chest CT scan for evaluation of chronic obstructive pulmonary disease (COPD), acceptable low dose screening and standard dose of CTs can be performed at effective dose of approximately 2 and 7 mSv, respectively [1].

CT Protocol

Optimization of CT protocol and quality control of image acquisition are critical for assessment of COPD [2, 3]. Ideally, single CT protocol using dedicated single CT scanner and software system based on exactly the same parameters of image

S.-D. Lee (ed.), *COPD*, DOI 10.1007/978-3-662-47178-4_8

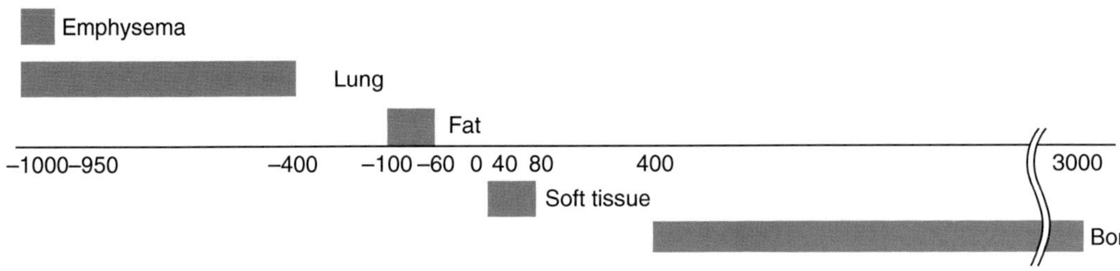

Fig. 8.1 Hounsfield unit on CT images. The Hounsfield unit (HU) is a quantitative value for describing attenuation on CT images. Zero HU and −1000 HU are defined as attenuation of distilled water and air at standard pressure and temperature. CT images can be appropriately displayed according to target organs adjusting window width and level. Window width describes the range of HU on CT image and window level is the median HU of window width. In the thorax, lung, mediastinum, and bone window setting are usually used

acquisition and reconstruction should be used. Nevertheless, it is impossible in most cases, particularly for multicenter trials. There are several important issues to be considered for the optimization of CT protocol which include kilovoltage setting, tube currents, respiration level, image thickness, reconstruction kernel, and so on (Table 8.1). Generally speaking, the volumetric CT acquisition obtained at maximal inspiration with standardized breathing instruction is essential for accurate COPD assessment using CT. Thin-section CT reconstructions (even or less than 1 mm in thickness) are required for proper characterization and quantification of emphysema and airway change in COPD. It has been known that CT estimates of emphysema severity increase as section thickness decreases and that higher frequency (edge-enhancing, sharper) image reconstruction kernel results in higher CT measurements of emphysema than lower frequency resolution (smoothing) kernel [4–6]. Low radiation dose CT scan allows the visual evaluation of emphysema, however, which trade off relatively high image noise, resulting in overestimation of emphysema extent. Relatively higher dose CT is also necessary for the accurate measurement of airway dimensions. Recently, further reduction of CT dose can be possible with the use of novel technique of iterative reconstruction [7–9]. However, it is not recommended for the quantitative assessment of COPD CT because the influence of changing reconstruction method has not been fully studied. Dose modulation technique to reduce radiation dose is not recommended. Expiratory CT is gradually regarded as an important part of COPD evaluation for the presence and distribution of air trapping on visual and quantitative assessment [10]. Expiratory CT scan may be obtained at relatively low dose after inspiratory CT acquisition. However, different noise level between inspiratory and expiratory CT is potential problem for the quantitative analysis. Expiratory scan can be obtained at the end of a tidal expiration, which corresponds to functional residual capacity, or after full expiration, which is in residual volume status.

Diagnosis of Morphologic Change in COPD

Emphysema: Definition of CT Finding, Subtype, Pathologic Correlation

Pulmonary emphysema is defined as an abnormal permanent enlargement of the airspaces distal to the terminal bronchioles, which results in lower CT attenuation values than those of normal healthy lung areas. Although pulmonary function test (PFT) is useful for clinical severity assessment of COPD, it does not represent the type and range of heterogeneous pathophysiologic abnormalities in COPD [11, 12]. In addition, it tends to be relatively insensitive to both early stages and small changes in COPD [13]. CT scan may be ideal for the detection and characterization of COPD in that it allows for an in vivo analysis of morphologic characteristics and distribution of emphysema. Visual assessment is also useful to

Table 8.1 General principle of CT protocol for COPD evaluation

	Inspiratory CT	Expiratory CT (optional)
Scan type, mode	Spiral (volumetric)	Spiral (volumetric)
Rotation time (s)	As short as possible, usually no greater than 0.5 s	As short as possible, usually no greater than 0.5 s
Detector configuration	More than 16 channels × submillimeter collimation	More than 16 channels × submillimeter collimation
Pitch	Usually smaller than 1.0	Usually smaller than 1.0
kVp	120	120
mA	40 mAs (low dose) up to 200 mAs (moderate dose)	40 mAs (low dose) up to 200 mAs (moderate dose)
Dose modulation	Not recommended	Not recommended
Reconstruction I for visual assessment		
Algorithm	Sharp or high-frequency kernel	Sharp or high-frequency kernel
Thickness (mm)	Submillimeter (0.5–0.75 mm)	Submillimeter (0.5–0.75 mm)
Interval (mm)	0.5	0.5
DFOV (cm)	To cover the whole lung	To cover the whole lung
Reconstruction II for QCT		
Algorithm	Neutral, smooth kernel	Neutral, smooth kernel
Thickness (mm)	Submillimeter (0.5–0.75 mm)	Submillimeter (0.5–0.75 mm)
Interval (mm)	0.5	0.5
DFOV (cm)	To cover the whole lung	To cover the whole lung

subtype the emphysema into centrilobular, panlobular, and paraseptal types. Centrilobular emphysema is the most common morphologic subtype of pulmonary emphysema. Pathologically, it begins near the center of the secondary pulmonary lobule (the most fundamental structural component of the lung containing parenchyma, airways, lymphatics, and vasculature) in the region of the proximal respiratory bronchiole. Parenchymal destruction starts in the center of secondary pulmonary lobule results in the characteristic apposition of normal and emphysematous lung (area of low attenuated destruction surrounded by normal tissue). On CT, small round low attenuated holes are evenly distributed with ill-defined borders in early stage and these low attenuated areas become confluent and inseparable with paucity of pulmonary vascularity in late stage (Fig. 8.2). Panlobular emphysema is characterized by permanent destruction of the entire acinus distal to the respiratory bronchiole, and its pathogenesis relates to alpha-1 antitrypsin deficiency. Parenchymal destruction involving entire acinus, which is contrast to centrilobular subtype, affects the lower lobes more severely (Fig. 8.2). Paraseptal emphysema tends to be limited in extent and occurs most commonly along the subpleural portion of the upper lung, often coexisting with other types of emphysema and fibrosis. Small focal lucencies, up to 10 mm in size, can be seen on CT (Fig. 8.2). Bullae or blebs, termed interchangeably, are focal regions of emphysema with no discernible wall, usually more than 1 cm in diameter at subpleural location. In some cases, they can be very large and may result in pneumothorax in COPD patients (Fig. 8.3).

Airway Change: Bronchus, Trachea

Bronchial wall thickening, bronchial luminal irregularity, and bronchiectasis are commonly seen in patients with COPD with mixed findings of emphysema. Bronchial wall thickening is regarded as a sign of chronic bronchitis, easily identified in heavy cigarette smokers. Pathophysiologically, irreversible and progressive histologic changes in airways show diffuse hyperplasia of mucous glands associated with hypersecretion and bronchial wall thickening. Traditionally, bronchial wall is regarded to be

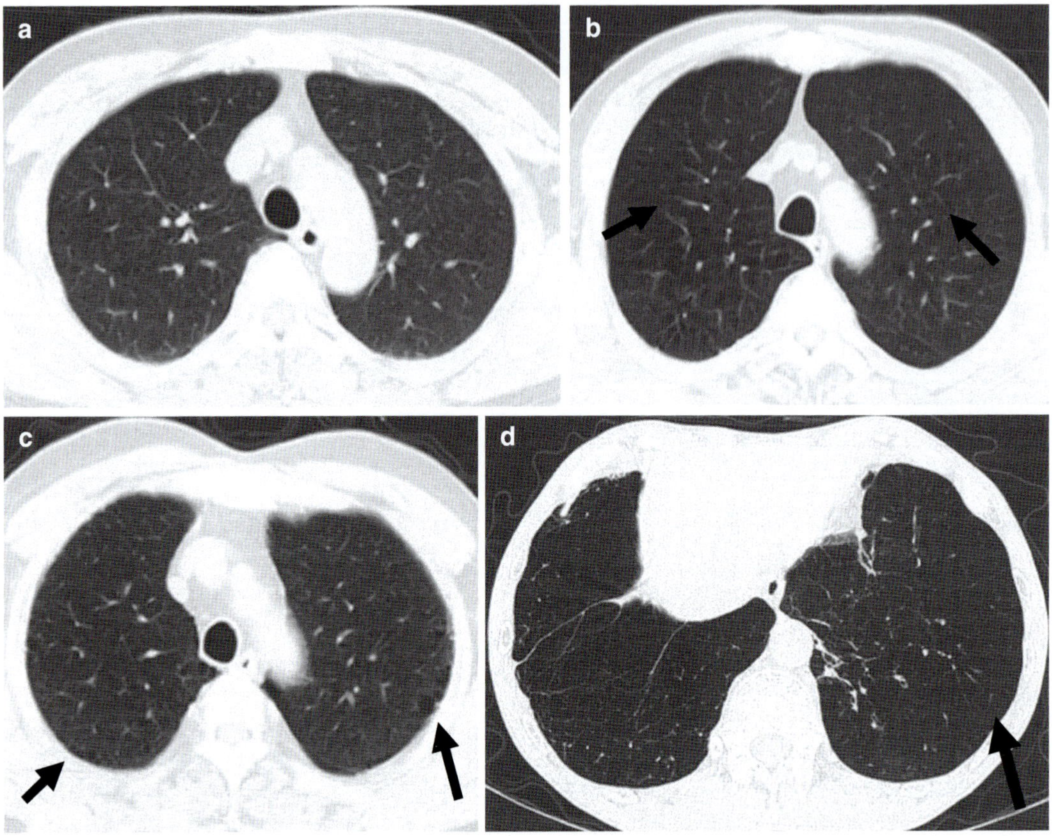

Fig. 8.2 Emphysema subtypes on CT images. (**a**) Normal lung parenchyma. (**b**) Centrilobular emphysema. Scattered small focal lucencies (parenchymal destruction) in upper lobes, measuring more or less than 1 cm in diameter. (**c**) Paraseptal emphysema. Small focal lucencies, up to 1 cm in diameter, are located in subpleural ar8ea adjacent to the pleura and septal lines. (**d**) Panlobular emphysema. Secondary pulmonary lobules area completely replaced with emphysema with showing uniform and relatively homogeneous lucencies across parts of the secondary pulmonary lobules

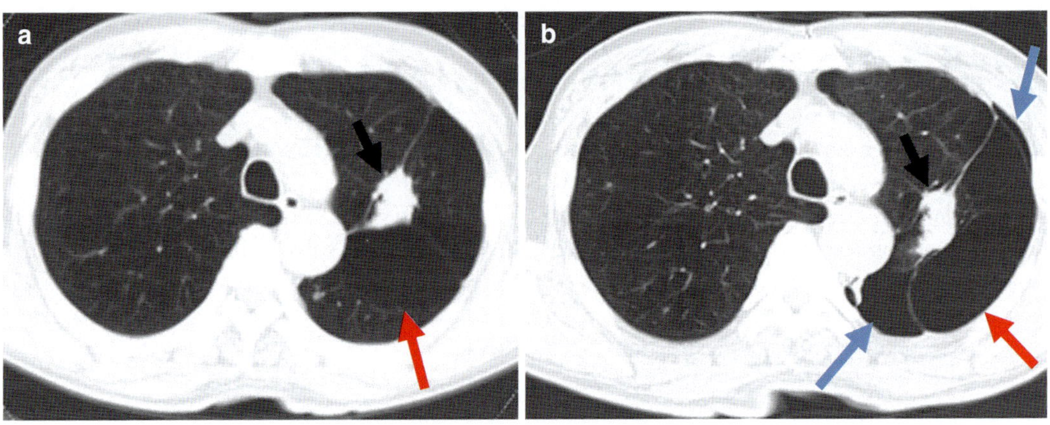

Fig. 8.3 Large bullae and pneumothorax in a COPD patients. A 71-year-old male with COPD complaint of sudden dyspnea. (**a**) CT image at 3 month ago showed large subpleural bullae with collapsed central lung. (**b**) Left pneumothorax was noted with collapsed lung and large bullae

thick if the diameter ratio of inner to outer lumen of bronchus is greater than 0.8. Nevertheless, the diagnosis of bronchial wall thickening of COPD with naked eyes on CT is subjective and still limited (Fig. 8.4). Moreover, it is virtually impossible to differentiate bronchial wall thickening of COPD from acute bronchitis or asthma. Bronchiectasis can be accompanied in COPD patients and may represent severe airflow obstruction [14, 15]. Trachea and main bronchus abnormalities can be visually defined on CT in COPD patients. Tracheobronchomalacia, saber-sheath deformity of trachea, and outpouching of trachea and main bronchus can be seen in advanced COPD (Fig. 8.5). Tracheobronchomalacia is traditionally defined as a more than 50% collapse of the trachea and main bronchus at end-expiratory CT. Saber-sheath deformity is seen as coronal narrowing and sagittal widening of the intrathoracic tracheal diameter. Tracheal outpouching is defined as a focal herniation of mucosa through the tracheal wall.

Air Trapping

It has been understood that small airway airflow resistance is the major site of obstruction in patients with COPD and precede the onset of emphysematous destruction in both centrilobular and paraseptal emphysema phenotypes of COPD [16]. Therefore, early detection and diagnosis of small airway disease in COPD is fundamental for early diagnosis of COPD. The small airways are referred to as airway lumen less than 2 mm, which cannot be visualized directly using even recently developed CT scanners. Thus, the finding of air or gas trapping, which appears to decrease lung attenuation on expiratory CT, can be used as indirect sign of small airway dysfunction in COPD because this finding is thought to be caused by early collapse of small airway on expiration. Expiratory CT is increasingly regarded as an essential tool for the evaluation of air trapping as an obstructive pattern of small airway disease in COPD patients. In many cases, especially in emphysema dominant COPD patients, the detection of small airway dysfunction may be hampered by the presence of emphysema because the lung density of emphysema area on expiration CT can be low without small airway dysfunction. In such situation, side-by-side comparison of inspiratory and expiratory CT images is necessary to detect lack of normal increase of lung attenuation and decrease of lung volume on expiration (Fig. 8.6).

Others: Chest Wall, Diaphragm, Heart, Pulmonary Vessel, and Bone

Morphologic changes secondary to pulmonary hyperinflation in COPD include chest wall

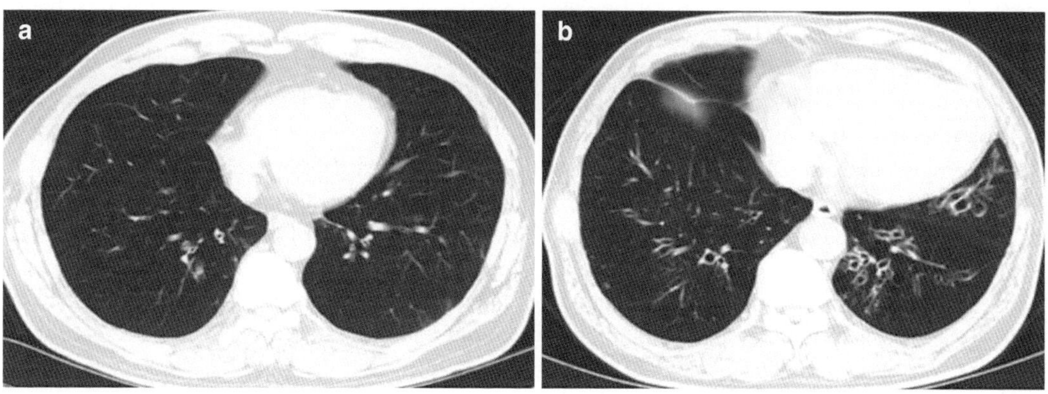

Fig. 8.4 Airway changes in COPD. (**a**) Example of bronchial wall thickening. Typical and severe thickening of wall of entire segmental bronchi in both lower lobes is noted. The diameter ratio of inner to outer lumen is smaller than 0.8. (**b**) Example of bronchiectasis. Marked dilatation of bronchial lumen in both lower lungs is noted. The inner luminal diameter of bronchus is greater than the diameter of the accompanying pulmonary artery. There are also loss of normal tapering with bronchial wall thickening

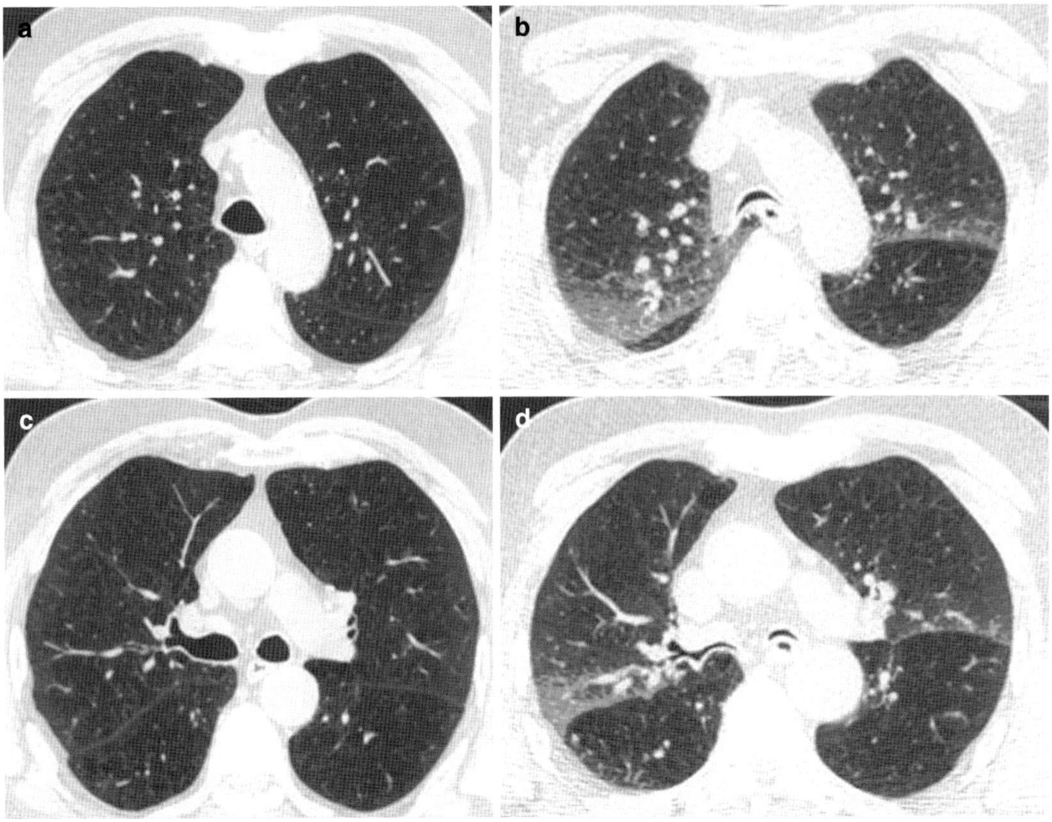

Fig. 8.5 Tracheobronchomalacia. Tracheobronchomalacia is defined as abnormal collapse of airway lumen on expiration. This abnormal finding can be seen in COPD patients. CT images on inspiration (**a**) and expiration (**b**) demonstrate severe lumen narrowing of the trachea on expiration (**b**) and CT images on inspiration (**c**) and expiration (**d**) also depicted severe lumen narrowing of both bronchi (**d**). In addition, severe air trapping is seen in both lower lobes

deformity, diaphragmatic change, changes in the heart, and pulmonary vasculatures. Barrel chest deformity is the well-known chest wall deformity of COPD and depression of diaphragm indicates the flattening of the domes of the diaphragm due to hyperinflation of the lung in COPD (Fig. 8.7). As the progression of COPD, the heart tends to be more vertically oriented due to hyperinflation of the lung. In later stage, right ventricular and atrial dilatation, dilatation of central pulmonary arteries, and acute tapering of distal pulmonary vessels can be seen as a finding of pulmonary hypertension. Osteoporosis is also one of the systemic effects associated with COPD attributed by inactivity, COPD-related systemic inflammation, the use of systemic corticosteroids, and vitamin D deficiency. Bone fracture related to osteoporosis, in turn, may also reduce pulmonary function or even cause COPD exacerbations [17].

Severity Assessment of COPD

Extent of Emphysema: Visual Assessment

Visual assessment of COPD is relatively simple, cheap, and independent from variation of CT machine or reconstruction algorithms. Furthermore, comprehensive visual emphysema assessment of CT in COPD allows assessment of the pattern, subtype, regional location, and degree of emphysema. It also has an advantage for detecting lots of accompanying pathologic changes in the parenchyma as well as in the small

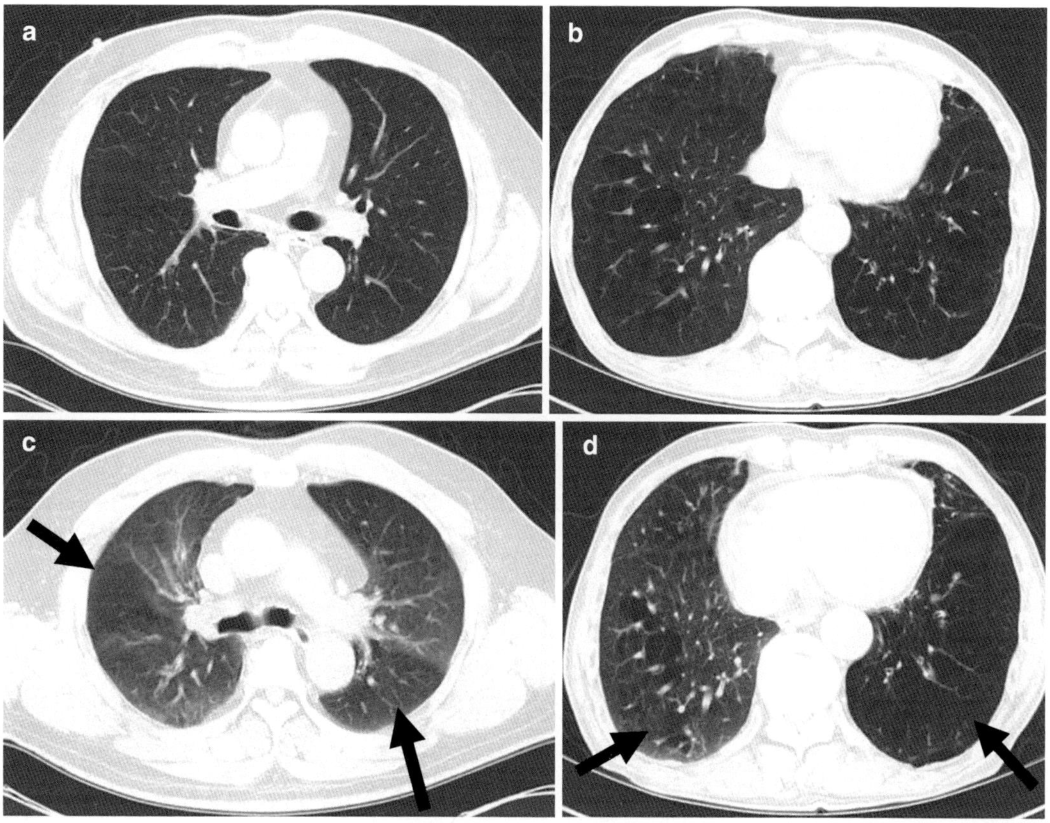

Fig. 8.6 Air trapping assessment using inspiration- and expiration CT images. Air trapping should be assessed by side-by-side comparison of inspiration (**a**, **b**) and expiration (**c**, **d**) CT images. Expiratory air trapping can be defined as areas showing lack of normal increase of lung attenuation and decrease of lung volume on expiration image (**c**, **d**). The areas of air trapping are marked in *arrows*

and large airways. Visual assessment allows for the detection of early emphysema in asymptomatic smokers even before the development of airflow limitation, which is essential for the diagnosis of COPD. It is also useful to follow the progression of emphysema over time. For the optimal evaluation of emphysema with CT images in COPD patients, thin-section, high-resolution CT images should be used at recommended window settings (usually with a window level of −700 and window width of 1000–1500). On visual assessment, emphysema is classified as centrilobular, panlobular, and paraspetal emphysema (Fig. 8.2). The extent of emphysema has been assessed by using visual scoring system [18]. Typically, the extent of emphysema in each lobe can be assessed by using a six-point scale system: 0, 1–5%, 6–25%, 26–50%, 51–75%, and greater than 75% [19]. However, main limitation of visual assessment has been the relatively low inter-reader agreement [20, 21]. The inter-reader agreement was moderate for the presence or absence of emphysema and for the presence of panlobular emphysema; fair for the presence of centrilobular and paraseptal subtypes [22]. In an effort to improve the inter-reader agreement, usage of standardized reference images has been attempted with promising results [19].

Extent of Emphysema: Computer-Based Quantification

For the objective and reproducible assessment of emphysema, computer-based quantification method, the so-called quantitative CT (QCT), has

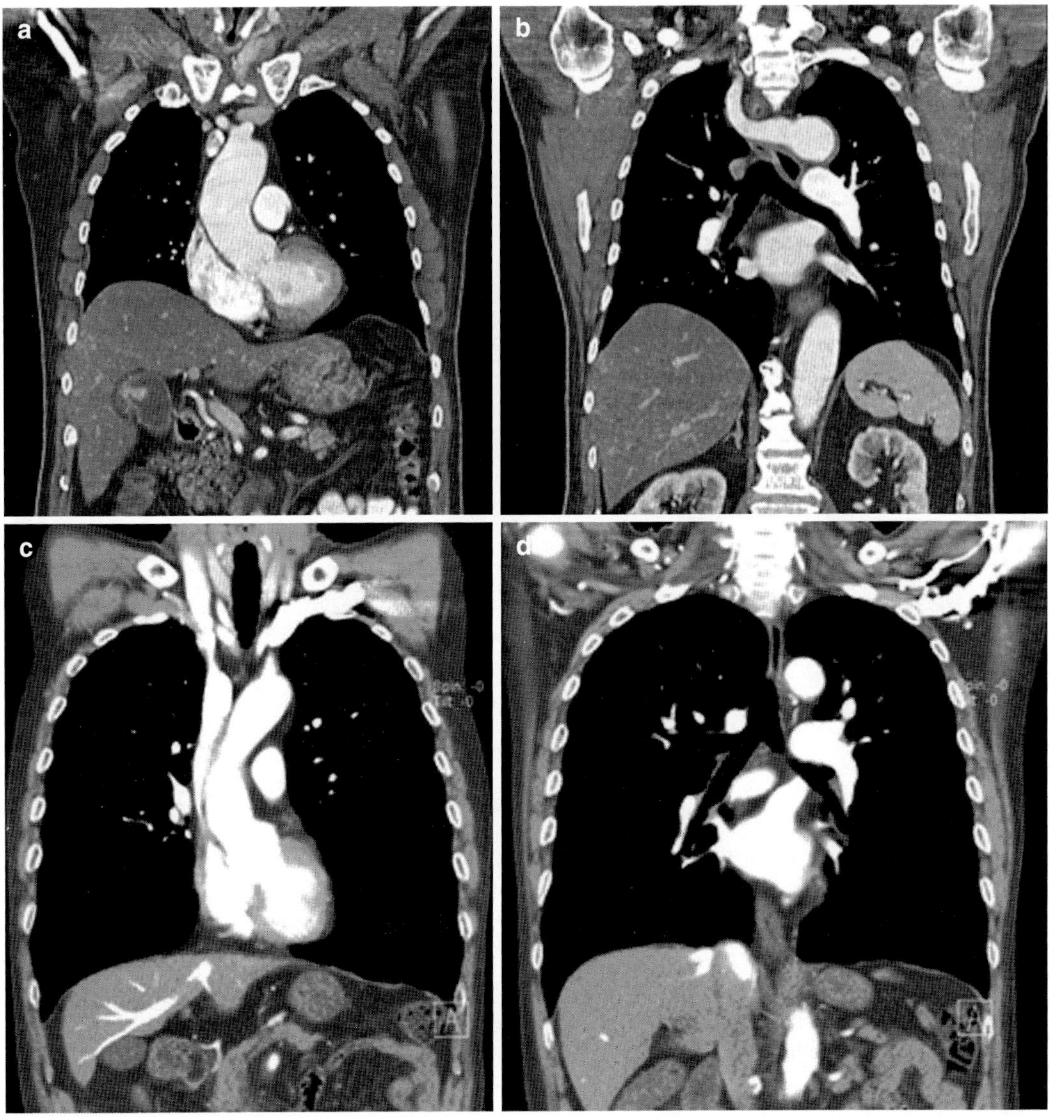

Fig. 8.7 Morphologic change of the diaphragm in COPD patients. Compared with CT images in a normal individual (**a**, **b**), coronal CT images (**c**, **d**) in a 74-year-old male with COPD shows depressed and flattened shape of the diaphragm. This change is due to hyperinflation of the lung in COPD

been introduced. As briefly explained in "CT Basic Physics" section, emphysema area on CT with relatively increased air fraction in inspiration lung is shown as area of decreased CT attenuation approaching air attenuation of −1000 HU, compared with normal lung CT attenuation around −850 HU [23]. Accordingly, if a certain threshold value is applied, the area of emphysema with decreased CT attenuation can be objectively divided from normal lung area. This method is called as "density mask" and the threshold of −910 HU was initially applied [24]. Recent studies using thin-section, multi-detector CT scanners showed that the highest correlation between QCT and histology is found when the threshold set at −960 or −970 HU [25]. However, the lower the thresholds, the more sensitive the image noise; therefore, the threshold of −950 HU is now most commonly used. When the correction for lung volume changes influenced by degree of inspiration is applied, this quantitative method for emphysema is near perfectly reproducible method. The term of percent of emphysema (emphysema index, EI or $\%LAA_{-950}$) stands for the relative area of lung less than −950 HU (Figs. 8.8 and 8.9). Another method is using the nth cutoff percentile in the attenuation distribution curve using the CT attenuation at a certain percentile along the frequency histogram of pulmonary parenchymal attenuation (density value in HU under which n% of frequency histogram) (Fig. 8.8). This value is called as "percentile index," and it is reported that it has an advantage on longitudinal evaluation and less sensitive to lung volume changes [26–28]. The first percentile value is much optimal for correlation with histology; however, it is known to be sensitive to an artifact from image noise and truncation effect. Instead, the 15th percentile threshold is commonly used [28, 29]. The last method is to assess the mean of the whole lung attenuation (mean lung density, MLD). Regional heterogeneity of emphysema can be assessed quantitatively to assess the regional distribution of emphysema. Most available QCT methods can divide each lung into upper, mid, and lower zones of equal height or volume, and ratios between the extent of emphysema in upper and lower lung can be computed. Newer methods can also permit segmentation of lobes to compute lobar volumes and extent of emphysema objectively (Fig. 8.9).

Comparison Between Visual Assessment and CT Quantification

In the assessment of emphysema in COPD patients, although QCT measures correlate with the severity of visual CT assessment, the level of correlation is only moderate [22]. Especially in less severe categories of emphysema, visual assessment by radiologists tends to be usually underestimated for the extent of emphysema when compared to QCT measures, while in those with more severe emphysema, the radiologists tend to relatively overestimate the emphysema extent [30]. Therefore, visual assessment and QCT measures should be used complementarily and performed independently for the assessments of severity of emphysema.

Correlation Between the Extent of Emphysema and Clinical Parameters

Visual, subjective assessment of the emphysema using contiguous 10-mm thick CT started in 1986, there were significant correlations between CT visual scores and macroscopic emphysema. However, even with the development of high-resolution CT, visual grading assessment is not really a quantitative measure but just grading the degree of emphysema according to categories of emphysema severity. Recently, using pulmonary lobe-by-lobe visual assessment, severity of emphysema correlates quite well with physiologic parameters (FEV_1 and FEV_1/FVC) and GOLD stage [19]. The correlation coefficient ranges between 0.67 (for GOLD stage) and −0.74 (for FEV_1/FVC) and notably the range of correlation coefficients are similar to the correlations between extent of emphysema on QCT and each physiologic parameter (0.62 for GOLD stage and −0.70 for FEV_1/FVC). However, inter-reader agreement regarding severity of emphysema on visual assessment tends to be variable, so QCT is preferred for assessing disease severity of emphysema. Moreover, QCT measurements have shown to correlate better than visual CT assessment with macroscopic measurement of emphysema [21].

Regional Heterogeneity of Emphysema

Severity and distribution of emphysema differs in lung regions such as core (inner) vs. rind (outer), upper vs. lower, even among each lobe (Fig. 8.10). There have been several reports regarding regional variation of emphysema. Basal distribution of emphysema is associated with greater impairment of FEV_1 but less impairment of gas exchange (PaO_2) and alveolar-arterial oxygen gradient than the apical distribution of emphysema [31]. Emphysema areas on CT are more often found in the inner segment of the lung than in the outer segment and the extent of emphysema in inner segment of the lower lung in QCT is much more clearly correlated with airflow limitation than those in outer segment [32]. In another report applying the slope of the EI in the upper-lower, anterior-posterior, and central-peripheral direction in both side lung, the heterogeneity of emphysema distribution in

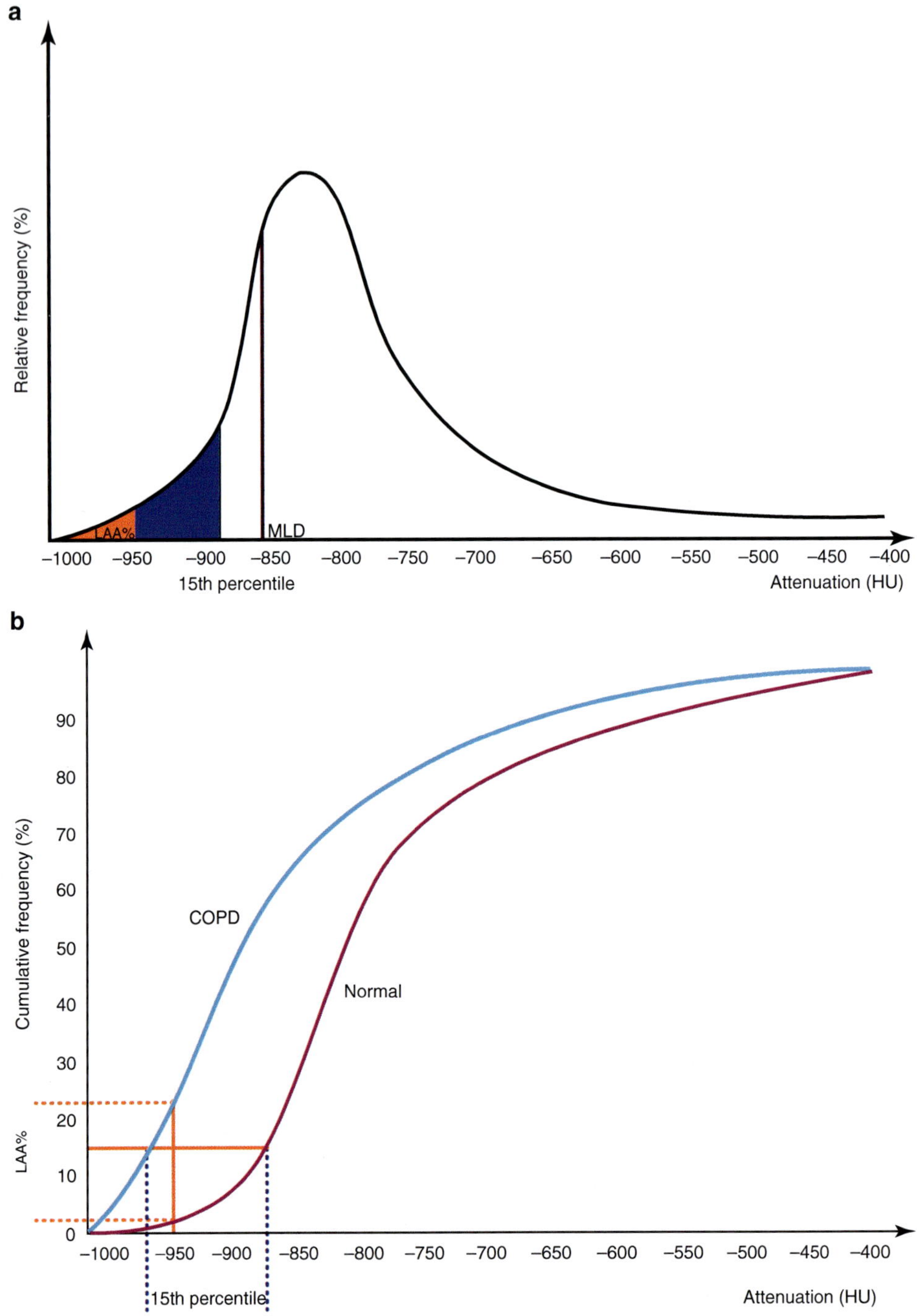

Fig. 8.8 Quantitative CT measurements of emphysema regarding LLA%, percentile index, and mean lung density (MLD). The concept of QCT measurement is illustrated in Fig. (**a**). Frequency distribution curves are plotted according to the apparent X-ray attenuation values. The threshold of −400 HU is to define lung area. Threshold (LAA %) technique uses a predefined threshold of HU (i.e., −950 HU) is chosen and the percentage of lung less than this value can be calculated. Contrary to this, the percentile index method uses a certain percentile point (i.e., lowest 15th percentile) and the HU value for that percentile is calculated. The last index is the mean of lung density (MLD). Left side shift of frequency curve in patient with emphysema is demonstrated in Fig. (**b**). As a result of the shift, LAA % increases and percentile index decreases in patients with emphysema. The area of emphysema can be overlaid on the CT images to highlight the emphysema lesion (**c**, **d**)

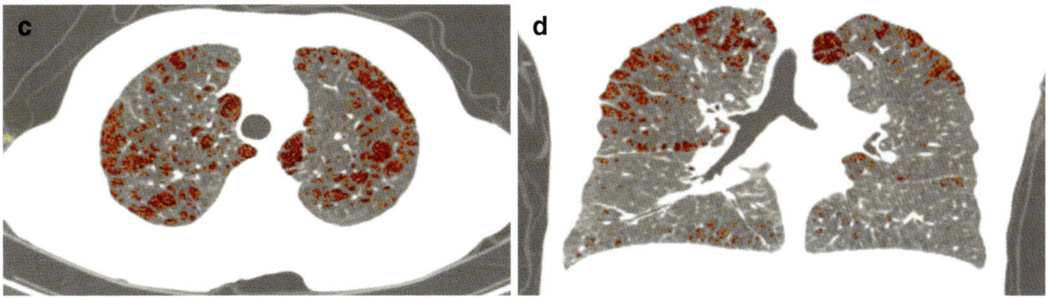

Fig. 8.8 (continued)

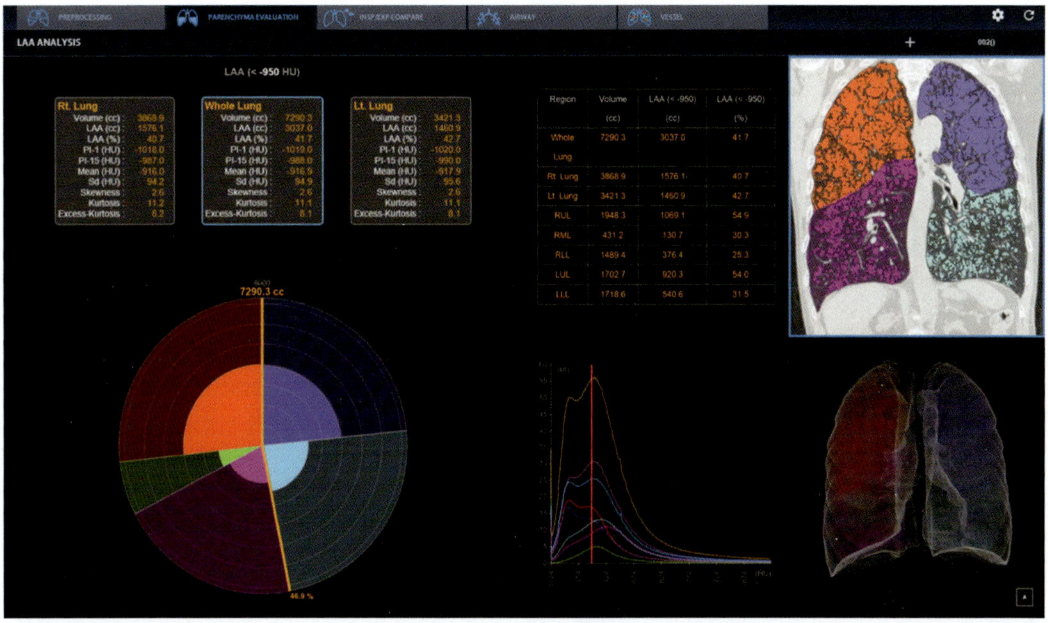

Fig. 8.9 Lobar-specific quantification of emphysema. Example of software providing automatic segmentation of lobes and quantitative assessment of extent of emphysema at the whole lung and lobar level

anterior-posterior and upper-lower direction was independent determinants of FEV_1 and FEV_1/FVC and the lower and posterior regional dominant emphysema is associated with a decrease in FEV_1 and FEV_1/FVC [33]. Regional assessment using QCT helps in selecting candidates for lung volume reduction surgery (LVRS) and provides rationale for the mechanisms of improvement after LVRS (Fig. 8.11). The extent of emphysema of the upper-rind region of the lungs is a significant predictor for improvement of pulmonary function after LVRS [34].

Airway Change: Visual Assessment

Although visual assessment of large airways is a subjective process, the presence of airway wall thickening or dilation of large airways can represent bronchial inflammation with remodeling, and it also contributes to the symptomatic exacerbation in COPD patients. Bronchial wall thickening

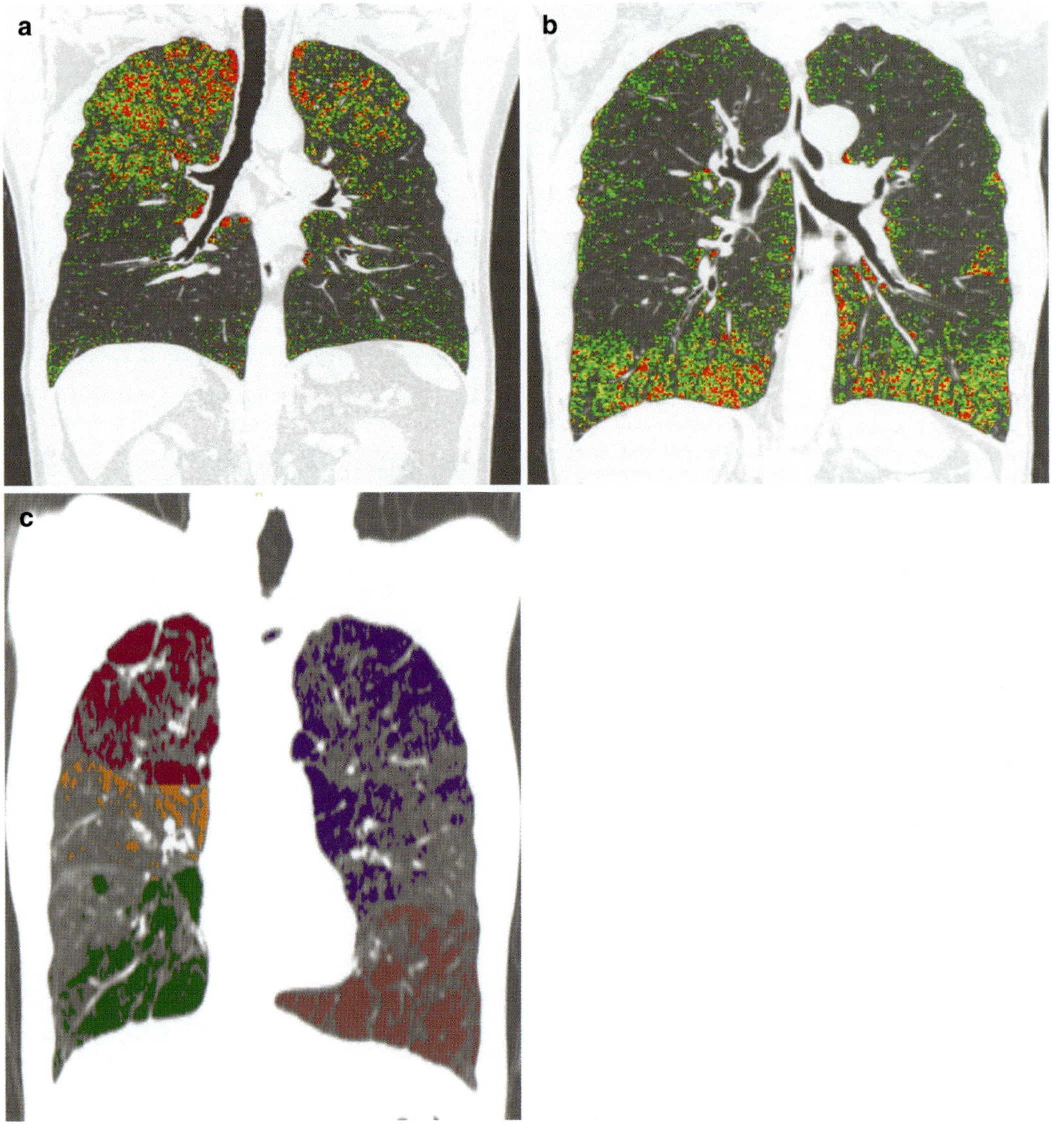

Fig. 8.10 Regional heterogeneity. CT images with color mapping (**a**, **b**) show different predominance of emphysema in two patients with similar emphysema index (17.56 and 23.27%). This regional heterogeneity can also be quantified by emphysema on each lobes (**c**)

is commonly found in heavy cigarette smokers with a sign of chronic bronchitis (Fig. 8.4). Bronchiectasis is also a common finding in COPD associated with severe airflow obstruction and risk for COPD exacerbation [14, 15, 35].

Airway Change: Computer-Based Quantification

With the current development of available software permitting multiplanar reconstruction of airways from thin-section volumetric datasets, CT scan seems to be well positioned to become the method of choice to noninvasively measuring airway wall dimensions of luminal diameter and wall thickness to the level of segmental and subsegmental airways. The simple analysis of "full-width at half maximum" algorithm is commonly used to evaluate the airways including absolute measures (bronchial luminal diameter or area, bronchial wall thickness or area, and total

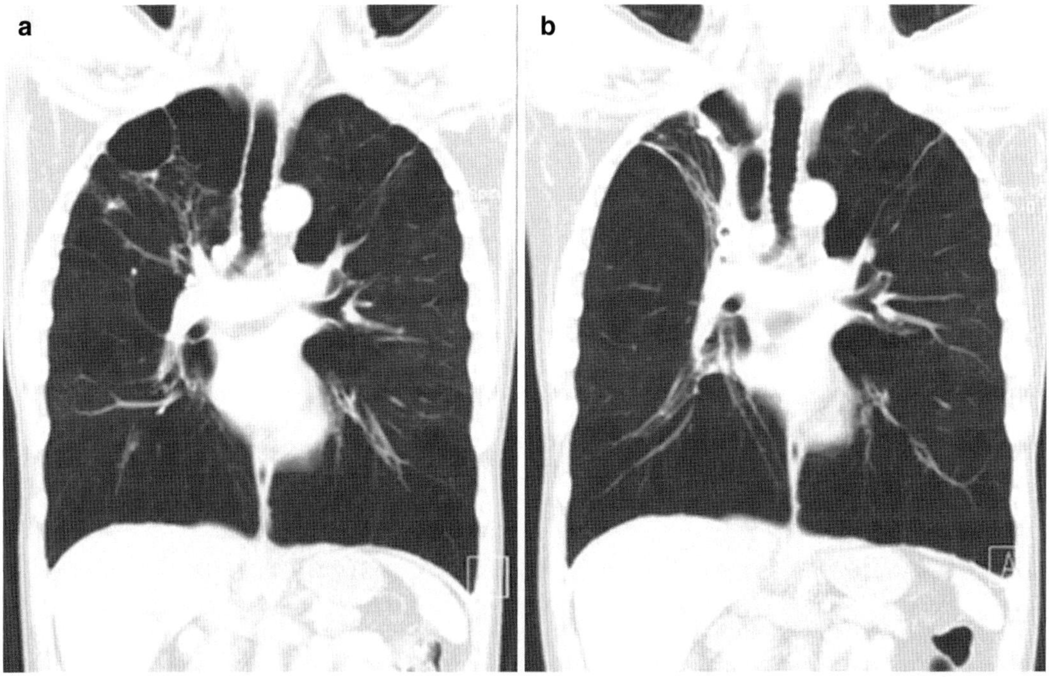

Fig. 8.11 Effect of lung volume reduction procedure. (**a**) CT image in a 61-year-old male showed severe and regional heterogeneity of emphysema. Endobronchial L was performed to collapse the RUL which was most severely affected by emphysema. (**b**) After the procedure, RUL was near totally collapsed on CT and pulmonary function of this patient much improved (FEV1, 0.46 L —> 0.82; mMRC, Gr4 —> 1)

bronchial area) and relative measures (bronchial wall area %, WA%: 100 × (wall area)/(lumen + wall area)) (Fig. 8.12). Variable software algorithms to define the boundaries of airway wall have been proposed and tested. Another commonly used measure is the square root of wall area of a hypothetical bronchus having internal perimeter of 10 mm (Pi10) [36].

Correlation Between Airway Measures and Clinical Parameters

Many studies showed that patients with the greatest WA% had the lowest FEV_1 expressed as a percent predicted [37]. The WA% has been considered as the most commonly employed metric for clinical investigation, and there are modest correlations between airway WA% and lung physiologic impairment [10, 38]. Moreover, central airway remodeling apparent on CT may reflect the distal histopathologic remodeling of the small airways, so the greater the central airway wall thickening, the more small the airway disease [39]. Moderate correlations ($-0.56 < r < -0.62$) between airway wall measurements and airflow obstruction (FEV_1 and FEV_1% predicted) have been reported and stronger correlations were noted when only small airways were analyzed [40]. In recent report, bronchial wall thickening as well as severity of emphysema measured on QCT is associated with exacerbation frequency, independently; bronchial predominant and emphysema predominant subtypes of COPD can be defined [41].

Other Large Airway Changes in COPD

Among the large airway changes in COPD, Saber-sheath trachea is not an uncommon finding in COPD (Fig. 8.5). It defines as the ratio of the sagittal to coronal diameter is greater than 2 and the extra-thoracic portion of the trachea is not narrowed. By comparison with normal healthy persons, COPD patients show that this tracheal morphologic change of the elongation of the sagittal diameter correlated with the severity of

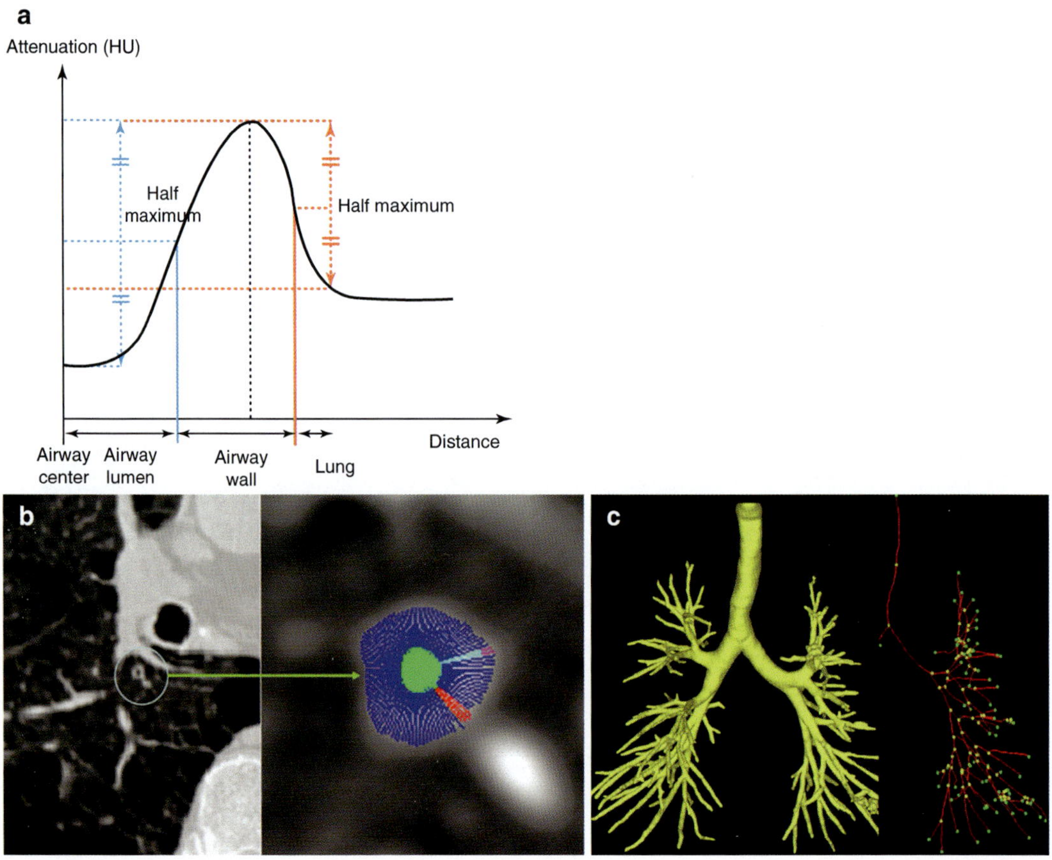

Fig. 8.12 Quantification of airway wall thickening using computerized method principle for full-width-at-half-maximum (FWHM) method. In the attenuation profile along an outward flowing ray from the luminal center-point through the airway wall, the inner and outer airway wall boundaries are assumed halfway to the maximum on the lumen side and halfway to the minimum on the parenchymal side, respectively. (**a**) After the detection of boundaries, the airway wall area can be highlighted with color overlay (**b**). This method is called as full-width-at-half-maximum method and is most common method to quantify wall thickness. The airway dimensions of the whole airway trees can be assessed using automatic airway segmentation, centerline extraction, followed by airway quantification (**c**)

emphysema and QCT indices, reflecting airflow limitation and air trapping [42]. Furthermore, expiratory tracheal collapse in obese COPD patients shows greater quality of life impairment and worse exercise performance than expected based on functional measures [43].

Small Airway Disease: Visual Assessment

The small airways are referred to as airway lumen less than 2 mm, those cannot be visualized using current CT scanners. The presence of air trapping on expiratory CT scan can be identified as an indirect sign to evaluate small airway remodeling. However, accurate discrimination between emphysematous area and air trapping area is difficult and challenging, and even normal healthy person can show minimal air tapping area in both basal lobes. Recently, there have been introduced several methods to evaluate the degree of pathologic air trapping in COPD patients using QCT.

Small Airway Disease: Computer-Based Quantification

With the usage of expiratory CT images, quantitative assessment of air trapping is possible.

However, there are severe inborn limitations when only expiratory CT is used because it is impossible to separate trapped air area from air remaining in emphysematous spaces. Moreover, air trapping phenomenon can also be seen in healthy smokers and healthy individuals with normal lung physiology. However, even with these drawbacks, many studies have evaluated the presence of air trapping in COPD by assessing the area fraction of the lung lesion having CT values lower than the threshold of −856 or −850 HU (LAA_{exp856} or LAA_{exp850}) in expiration [44]. With this simple method, they reported that high correlations were noted between LAA_{exp850} and FEV_1/FVC and FEV_1 percent predicted. As an effort to overcome this single threshold method of combining air trapping and emphysema quantification into single measure, quantifying air trapping outside the emphysematous area is possible through the density-based quantification method [45, 46]. With excluding emphysema portion of all voxels with attenuation lower than −950 HU from inspiration and expiration scans and calculating the relative volumes for whole lung with attenuation value less than −860 HU on each inspiratory CT (inspiratory relative $volume_{<-860\ HU}$) and expiratory CT (expiratory relative $volume_{<-860\ HU}$), the relative volume change between −860 and −950 HU can be calculated as follows: Relative volume change $_{<-860\ HU}$ (%) = expiratory relative volume $_{<-860\ HU}$— inspiratory relative $volume_{<-860\ HU}$. Results from this method show that air trapping correlates with lung physiologic parameters significantly ($r = 0.50–0.80$). Other methods for measuring air trapping have been addressed as an index of air trapping including the ratio of inspiratory to expiratory lung volume ($E/I\text{-}ratio_{LV}$) and the expiratory to inspiratory ratio of mean lung density ($E/I\text{-}ratio_{MLD}$) [47, 48]. $E/I\text{-}ratio_{MLD}$ correlates with clinical parameters of COPD such as BODE-index ($0.48 < r < 0.68$) and $E/I\text{-}ratio_{LV}$ shows almost perfect correlation with $E/I\text{-}ratio_{MLD}$ ($r = 0.95$, $p < 0.001$). All of these values have a limitation that it can't represent regional distribution of air trapping. Recently, new approach of air trapping assessment has been proposed [49, 50]. By using software techniques, anatomical correspondence of lung region between inspiration and expiration CT images can be assessed and both images can be co-registered. By direct assessment of density difference between inspiration and expiration CT, the density change map can be generated and the areas with decreased density change can be defined as the area of air trapping. By using this method, in addition to the global assessment, regional assessment of air trapping is possible (Fig. 8.13) [49, 50].

Other Components of COPD: Correlation with Clinical Parameters

Texture-Based Emphysema Assessment

With an effort to discriminate various obstructive lung diseases from normal lung, more sophisticated automatic classification system based on the texture and shape features of CT images has been introduced. Using this method, further differentiation of lung areas, for example, into normal lung, small airway disease, centrilobular emphysema and panlobular emphysema, is possible. This quantification method showed comparable correlation with the pulmonary function test results when compared with conventional density-based quantification [51, 52]. This method can also be used for the assessment of combined pulmonary fibrosis.

Pulmonary Vascular Change

Pulmonary vascular change is also one of the characteristic features of COPD and the extent of emphysema, rather than airway obstruction, is responsible for pulmonary endothelial dysfunction in COPD [53]. After volumetric CT scans of the lung, pulmonary vasculature was automatically segmented from the parenchyma using software [54, 55] (Fig. 8.14). With the usage of QCT measuring the cross sectional area (CSA) of small pulmonary vessels (sub-subsegmental level, CSA less than 5 mm^2), the total CSA of small pulmonary vessels in COPD shows strong (negative) correlation with the extent of emphysema ($\%LAA_{-950}$), whereas weak correlation with airflow obstruction [56]. The anatomic extent of emphysema instead of airway obstruction is responsible for impairment of pulmonary

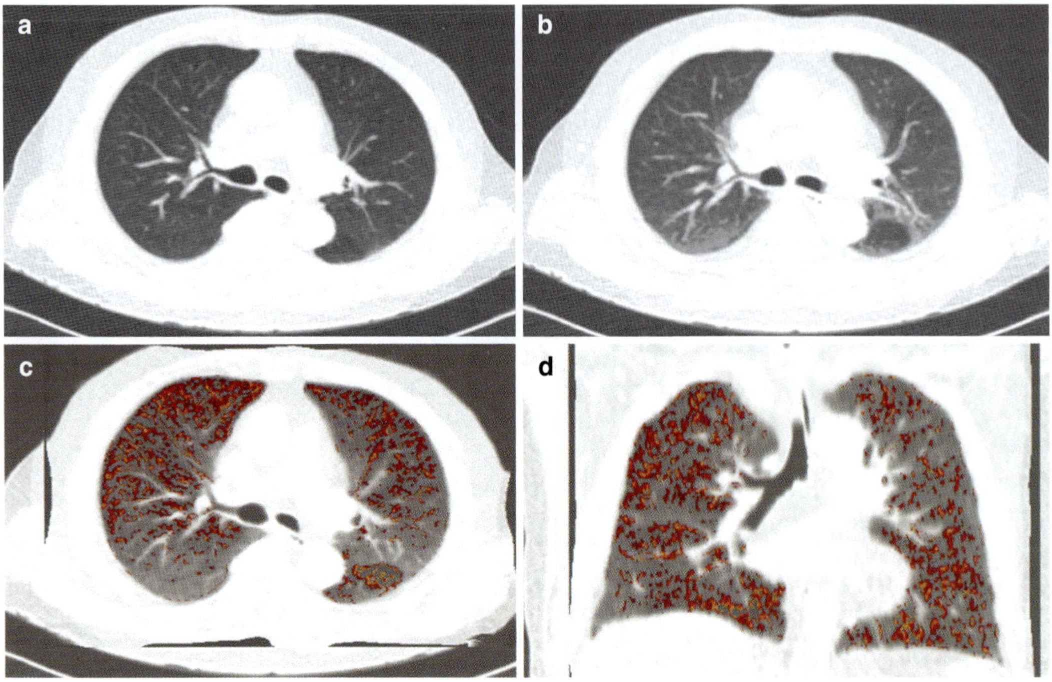

Fig. 8.13 Subtraction image from co-registered inspiratory and expiratory images. Image maps (**c**, **d**) derived from co-registered inspiratory (**a**) and expiratory (**b**) images depict changes in lung attenuation from inspiration to expiration. Using image registration technique, the expiration CT image is deformed to match with the corresponding anatomical area on inspiration CT (**c**). By comparing CT attenuation between inspiration CT and registered expiration CT, area of air trapping with little change in CT attenuation can be extracted and visualized in color overlay (**c**). This process is applied in the whole lung and coronal distribution of air trapping can be visualized (**d**)

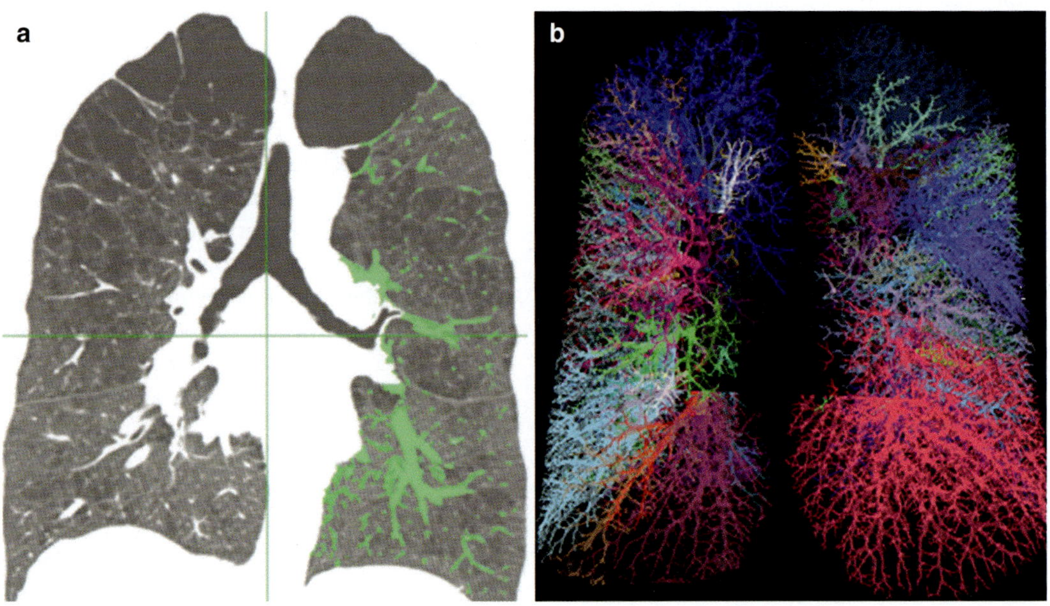

Fig. 8.14 Vascular subbranches of lung. (**a**) Extraction vessels in CT and (**b**) Vascular tree reconstruction; random coloring; each color represents one vascular branch and mediastinal region is cropped

vascular structure. Moreover, the percentage of the total CSA for the lung area is significantly higher in airway dominant phenotype than emphysema dominant phenotype.

Osteoporosis

Osteoporosis should be considered as one of the important pathology of COPD, because it may cause vertebral compression fractures, which can also deteriorate FEV_1 and decrease in vital capacity. Actually, the loss of vertebral bone mineral density on CT is closely related to the severity of emphysema showing many risk factors of low BMI, decreased activity, systemic inflammation, and use of corticosteroids [17, 57, 58] (Fig. 8.15). There has been reported that the decrease in thoracic vertebral bone mineral density is greater in patients with a history of exacerbations than in those without a history of exacerbations. Indeed, osteoporosis progression should be checked in COPD patients, especially in those with a history of frequent exacerbations [59].

Chest Wall and Diaphragm

COPD is also characterized by progressive impairment of respiratory function and dysfunction of respiratory muscle. There have been reports that the depletion of peripheral muscle mass is a better predictor of mortality than BMI in patients with COPD [60, 61]. Thoracic respiratory muscles are unique and crucial for alveolar ventilation and weakness of respiratory muscle results in dyspnea and respiratory failure associated with mortality in COPD patients. It is reported that intercostal mass and intercostal attenuation measured by QCT are significantly correlated with FEV_1 and extent of emphysema of QCT measurement [62]. A decrease in thoracic muscle mass with increasing intercostal fat is associated with worsening of COPD (Fig. 8.16). Hyperinflation in COPD makes diaphragm to be flatter and shorter. As the progression of COPD, breathing becomes gradually more dependent on the thoracic intercostal muscles than diaphragm (Fig. 8.7).

Atherosclerosis

In COPD patients, reduced FEV_1 has known to be an increased risk factor for cardiovascular diseases and mortality, independent of smoking [63, 64]. In other words, systemic inflammation in COPD patients may accelerate the rates of cardiovascular disease, and this degree or status of atherosclerosis may be associated with impaired lung function and emphysema in COPD patients. There has been an attempt to demonstrate the

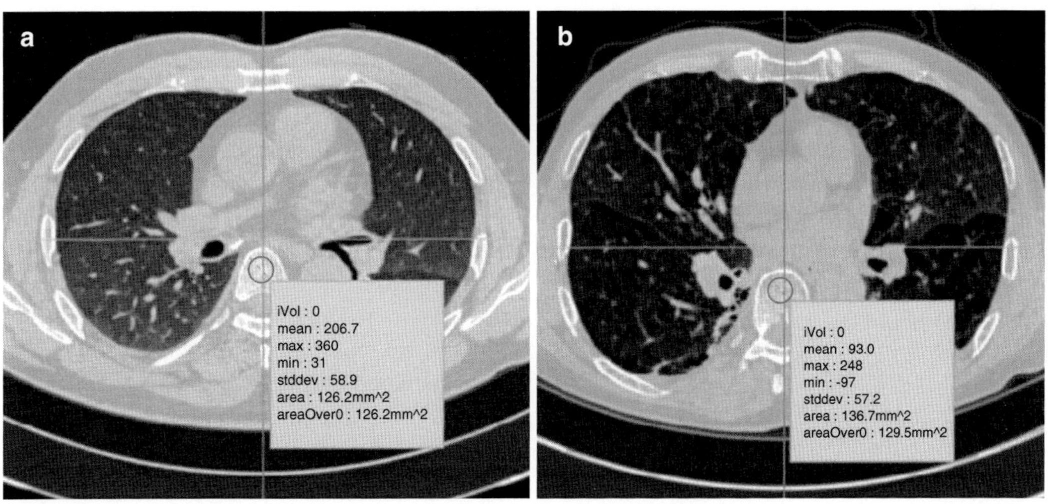

Fig. 8.15 Thoracic bone density on CT image. Vertebral bone mineral density on CT is closely related to the severity of emphysema. (**a**) CT image of a 59-year-old male with 6.2% of emphysema index shows 206.7 HU on thoracic vertebra. (**b**) CT image of a 79-year-old male with 52.2% of emphysema index shows 93.0 HU on thoracic vertebra

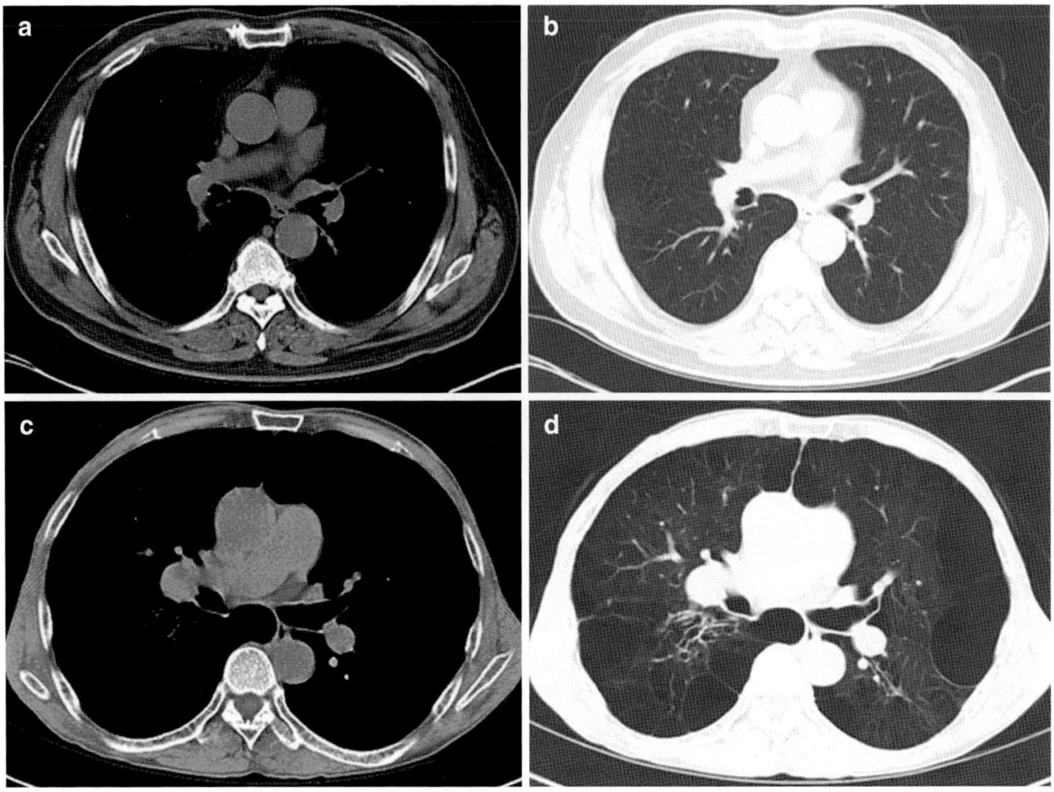

Fig. 8.16 Thoracic muscle mass on CT image. Thoracic muscle mass and intercostal fat are associated with severity of COPD. (**a**, **b**) CT images of a 75-year-old male with 7.4% of emphysema index shows more prominent thoracic muscle mass than CT images of a 62-year-old male with 54.8% of emphysema index

association of the total amount of calcification in coronary artery, thoracic aorta, mitral and aortic annuli, and the extent of emphysema on QCT and lung physiology [65]. Calcium score as a measurement for degree of atherosclerosis shows weak but significant correlation with volume fraction of emphysema on QCT, FEV_1/FVC, and diffusion capacity, independent of age, BMI, and smoking amount. The degree of atherosclerosis is associated with impaired lung function and the extent of emphysema.

Imaging Studies of Treatment Monitoring and Disease Progression

Predicting Tool in Treatment Outcome

COPD is a heterogeneous condition featuring both parenchymal destruction (emphysema) and small airway disease (obstructive bronchiolitis); its relative contributions vary in each COPD patient. Previous studies already have suggested that different spirometric response patterns to bronchodilator exist in patients with obstructive lung disease showing improvement in expiratory flow (FEV_1) or lung volume (FVC) [66, 67]. Therefore, QCT measurements can be used as a longitudinal evaluation of treatment monitoring based on the fact of a significant correlation between QCT measurement indices and lung physiologic indices. Notably, in the assessment of different spirometric response patterns to bronchodilator treatment, the extent of emphysema in QCT measurement shows a significant negative correlation with postbronchodilator FEV1 change and the E/I-ratio_{MLD} also shows a significant positive correlation with postbronchodilator FVC change [68]. In case of lung volume reduction therapy in regions with severe emphysema, QCT can be used as a predictor of improvement of lung function after surgical or bronchoscopic approaches [34].

Disease Progression

There have been several efforts to evaluate the progression of emphysema using QCT measurement and QCT is useful in demonstrating the change in extent of emphysema directly (Fig. 8.17). However, the main drawback of QCT measurement is a variation of inspiration level on each CT scan. Studies showed that the change in the 15th percentile CT density after the correction of lung volume difference was found to be more sensitive as an index of progression compared with measures of physiology or healthy status [69]. Recently, new single unified approach using a voxel-wise imaging analysis can be used in diagnosing disease extent and phenotype of COPD, detailed spatial distribution and location. This method allows us to distinguish the relative contributions of functional small airway disease component and emphysema in COPD in the course of disease progression [49].

Quality Control and Standardization

Emphysema Quantification

There are several sources of variation in quantification of emphysema in COPD including scanner, software, and patient factors. Thinner slice thickness and the lower CT dose setting result in overestimation of emphysema extent on QCT due to increasing image noise [4]. Inter- and intra-scanner variation due to calibration error and beam hardening effects should also be considered, and there have been attempt to demonstrate that density correction of volumetric CT

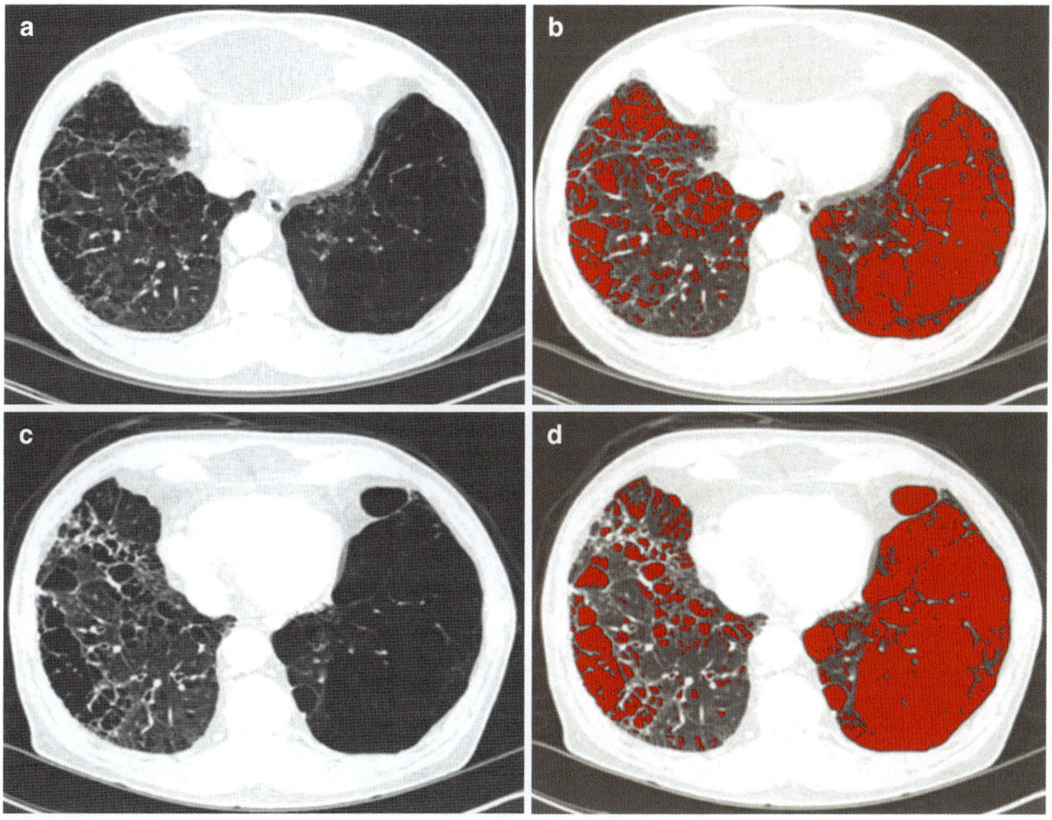

Fig. 8.17 Follow-up emphysema quantification (LAA, %) in same subject. Initial emphysema index (EI, %) was measured to 41.8% on CT image (**a**) and matched color coding image (**b**). Three years hence, EI has increased and measured to 56.2% on CT image (**c**) and matched color coding image (**d**)

data based on air (reference value: −1000 HU in tracheal air or outside patient air) will improve the correlation between emphysema quantification and pulmonary function test [70, 71]. This correction method may be useful to decrease the variation of measured results when multiscanners are involved. Second, a smooth reconstruction algorithm is usually recommended for the emphysema quantification using QCT because a strong or overenhancing algorithm can result in overestimation of emphysema [6]. Regarding patient factors, variation in lung volume, which is influenced by degree of inspiration, can be a major source of variation in clinical practice. Measurements of emphysema can be different at varying inspiration levels. However, quantitative measurement of differences in emphysema would not be significant when scans are obtained above 90% of vital capacity [72]. Current smoking status or coexisting air trapping or parenchymal fibrosis can also alter the quantitative emphysema measurements. Measured extent of emphysema in current smokers appears to be lower than those in former smokers, probably due to increased attenuation induced by smoking-related infiltration of inflammatory cells in the lungs in current smokers [73, 74]. Therefore, for accurate and precise quantitative assessment of emphysema extent, it is important to consider and control all the factors discussed above.

Airway Quantification

In quantitative airway measurements, considering factors about the source of variation are similar to emphysema measurements. Because airway is small, it is easily influenced by partial volume averaging and reconstruction algorithm than in quantitative measurement of emphysema. Appropriate radiation dose to overcome image noise during reconstruction and submillimeter section will reduce the variation in airway measurements. In addition, there are varieties of suggested software algorithms to measure airway dimension, resulting in different measurement values. Accordingly, usage of same software method is essential in multicenter trial or for following up the patients.

Magnetic Resonance Imaging (MRI)

The MRI can obtain morphologic and functional imaging without ionizing radiation. However, there are some reasons of difficulty in imaging the lung with MRI. The lung consists of the low density tissue, so it contains a relatively small number of protons which generate signal in MRI. In the lung, these are fast decay of signal due to susceptibility artifacts from countless air-tissue interfaces. The fast imaging, triggering, and gating techniques are needed due to respiratory, vascular, and cardiac motions. The major advantage of MRI is combination of morphological and functional lung imaging, such as perfusion, ventilation, blood flow, gas exchange, and respiratory motion, with high spatial and temporal resolution [75].

Morphologic Evaluation of COPD

Simply speaking, there are two different types in COPD. The airway type relates to chronic bronchitis and airflow obstruction. The emphysema type shows the parenchymal destruction with severe airflow obstruction and distal airspace enlargement. The morphologic evaluation in COPD using MRI is always compared to CT. MRI is technically more challenging due to hyperinflation and loss of lung tissue [76]. So, there are only a few publications on morphologic evaluation of COPD using MRI.

Imaging Technique

Many MRI sequences can be used for visualization of the lung: balanced steady-state free precession (bSSFP), volumetric interpolated breath-hold examination (VIBE), half-Fourier-acquired single-shot turbo spin-echo (HASTE), and ultra-short echo time (UTE) [77–79]. Three-dimensional (3D) T1-weighted gradient-echo sequences are used for the assessment of mediastinum and lung parenchymal tissues. T2-weighted fast spin-echo with half-Fourier acquisition sequence can visualize bronchial wall thickening and mucus plugging. Respiratory, vascular, and cardiac motions can be overcome by using fast imaging, gating, and triggering techniques. Half-Fourier acquisition or ultra-short echo times are recommended.

Emphysema

It is a major role of T1- and T2-weighted images to differentiate inflammation from muscular hypertrophy, edema, and mucus plugging in bronchial wall [80]. Emphysematous change of lung cannot be easily diagnosed by a loss of signal. However, hyperinflation can be easily detected by increased lung volume and reduced blood volume. There is one study about the change of signal intensity of lung parenchyma between inspiration and expiration MRIs, which is correlated with FEV_1 [81]. The MR signal can be improved and emphysema can be quantified by using the UTE pulse sequences [82]. Using fast radiofrequency (RF) excitation pulses, compressed sensing and parallel imaging in UTE pulse sequence, MR signal decay, and motion artifacts can be minimized [83]. UTE pulse sequences improve contrast-to-noise ratio, signal-to-noise ratio, and signal intensity with strong relationship between signal intensity and tissue density. Using UTE pulse sequence, pulmonary emphysema [84, 85], lobar fissures and airways [86], inflammation and peribronchial abnormalities [87] can be estimated.

Airway

There are several factors, such as bronchial level, diameter, wall thickness, and signal from bronchus, to detect bronchiectasis [88]. MRI usually visualizes central and peripheral bronchiectasis and central bronchi, whereas poorly visualizes normal peripheral bronchi. Using 3D volume interpolated gradient-echo sequence (VIBE) with high spatial resolution, the airway can be visualized [89]. T2-weighted sequences can visualize inflammation, mucus, edema, and fluid collections. Active inflammation can be represented by increased fluid, which shows high signal of the bronchial wall on T2-weighted sequences. Inflammatory activity has relation with contrast enhancement of thickened bronchial wall on contrast-enhanced T1-weighted sequence. Therefore, airway inflammation can be visualized by high signal on T2-weighted and contrast-enhanced T1-weighted sequences [90]. In contrast, mucus plugging on peripheral bronchi shows high signal intensity of fluid content on T2-weighted sequence without contrast enhancement on T1-weighted sequence on MRI.

Perfusion MRI

Using perfusion MRI, perfusion information of lung can be acquired without ionizing radiation. One of the advantages using perfusion MRI in COPD is combination of perfusion and morphologic information about parenchymal destruction and cause of perfusion changes. Several imaging techniques have been introduced.

Imaging Techniques

For assessment of pulmonary vasculature and perfusion, both of non-contrast-enhanced and contrast-enhanced sequences are available. Non-contrast-enhanced perfusion MRI can be acquired using arterial spin labeling technique, which is to mark a specific part of spins magnetically using radiofrequency (RF) excitation [91]. Using the electrocardiogram (ECG) gating technique, signal differences between systolic phase and diastolic phase can make perfusion images of the lung without contrast injection [92]. However, one of the limitations of ECG-gated perfusion MRI is that the image subtraction process is sensitive to misregistration due to bulk respiratory motion [91]. Contrast-enhanced 2D and 3D MRI, which is based on dynamic acquisition of lung tissue during contrast injection, can assess lung perfusion and quantify pulmonary perfusion [93, 94]. The advantage of contrast-enhanced perfusion MRI is high signal-to-noise ratio [95]. For evaluation of whole lung perfusion during peak enhancement period, 3D technique should be needed. For improvement of spatial resolution and reduce of the total acquisition time, k-space sampling techniques such as parallel imaging techniques or echo sharing techniques can be used [96, 97].

Quantification

Using MR perfusion technique, pulmonary blood flow can be assessed quantitatively [98, 99]. The indicator-dilution theory using the maximum of signal intensity and the temporal course of the signal change is base of quantification of pulmonary perfusion. If linear relation can be assumed between the concentration of contrast agent and the signal, concentration-time curves can be made by conversion of signal-time curves. The relationship among the perfusion parameters—pulmonary blood flow (PBF, mL/100 mL lung tissue/min), pulmonary blood volume (PBV, mL/100 mL lung tissue), and mean transit time (MTT, s0) is as follows:

$$MTT = \frac{PBV}{PBF}$$

Normalizing the area under the tissue concentration-time curve to the integral of the arterial input function can calculate PBV. Figure 8.18 shows quantification images of lung perfusion using perfusion MRI technique.

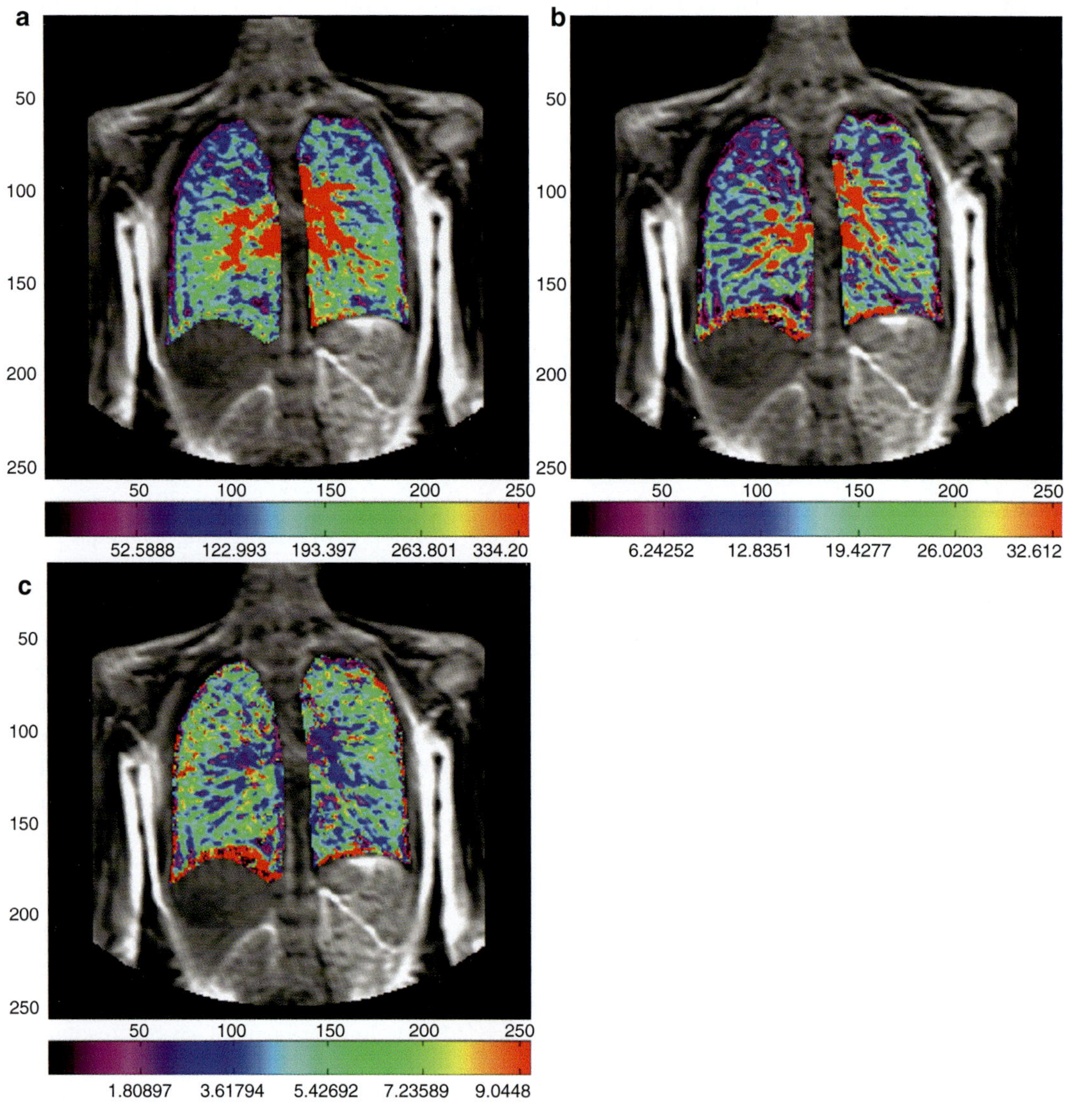

Fig. 8.18 Lung perfusion quantification image. Using perfusion MRI technique, PBF map (**a**), a PBV map (**b**), and an MTT map (**c**) are generated

COPD Studies Using Perfusion MRI

In COPD, chronic inflammation is thought to lead to intimal wall thickening and smooth muscle hypertrophy of pulmonary arteries. Hyperinflation and air trapping can make hypoxic vasoconstriction. Perfusion MRI shows high accuracy in detecting perfusion abnormalities in patients with emphysema [100, 101]. The perfusion abnormalities in COPD usually show a low degree of inhomogeneous contrast enhancement, especially in the area of severe emphysema [102] and decreased peak signal intensity. In COPD patients with severe emphysema, visual assessment of perfusion using 3D perfusion MRI shows high agreement with parenchymal destruction [103]. With quantitative analysis, decreased perfusion parameters on MRI correlate with worsening of FEV_1/FVC and increased emphysema index on CT [104]. Quantitative perfusion MRI in COPD shows decreased value and heterogeneous change in mean pulmonary blood flow (PBF), pulmonary blood volume (PBV), and mean transit time (MTT) than those in normal volunteer [105].

Ventilation MRI

For assessment of lung ventilation, several methods of MRI, such as oxygen-enhanced MRI and hyperpolarized noble gas MRI, are developed. Repeated or time-resolved measurements of lung dynamics can be obtained using ventilation MRI.

Oxygen-Enhanced MRI

Oxygen-enhanced MRI can visualize lung ventilation. Oxygen couples to hemoglobin and is present as dissolved oxygen in blood during oxygen exchange between capillary beds and alveoli [106]. Paramagnetic property of deoxyhemoglobin makes little T1 shortening effect with T2* shortening effect [107, 108]. Dissolved oxygen makes shortening of T1 relaxation time of blood in pulmonary vein due to paramagnetic property of oxygen [107]. This shortening leads to increased signal intensity on oxygen-enhanced MRI [109, 110]. Several sequences, such as centrically reordered phase-encoding scheme on HASTE sequence and single-shot rapid acquisition with relaxation enhancement (RARE) or HASTE sequences, can make oxygen-enhanced MRI [111]. Respiratory gating techniques are preferred because pulmonary physiology and physiopathology can be affected by breath hold despite decreased misregistration. Oxygen-enhanced MRI is used to assess ventilation abnormalities in pulmonary emphysema [112]. Regional changes in ventilation on oxygen-enhanced MRI reflect the regional lung function [113]. Figure 8.19 shows ventilation of patients with severe COPD using dynamic oxygen-enhanced MRI. FEV_1 and DLco well correlate with slope of oxygen-enhancement time-course curve and degree of oxygen-enhancement, respectively. Dynamic oxygen-enhanced MRI reflects DLco and provides diffusing capacity maps [112].

Hyperpolarized Noble Gas MRI

Using hyperpolarized noble gas MRI with ^{3}He or ^{129}Xe gas, ventilation MRI can be acquired [110, 114, 115]. These techniques visualize the ^{3}He or ^{129}Xe gas in airway and airspaces, so it can be used for regional mapping of airflow and assessment of diffusion in airspace [116, 117]. For these techniques, specialized laser equipment and specialized RF transmitter and receiver coils are mandatory. Four different techniques are used for hyperpolarized ^{3}He MRI [118]. Static ventilation imaging generally uses 2D or 3D fast low-angle single-shot or bSSFP sequences [119]. Diffusion imaging uses gradient-echo pulse sequence with bipolar diffusion-sensitizing gradient waveform between the excitation RF pulse and data acquisition [120]. Dynamic ventilation imaging uses the ultrafast pulse sequences such as interleaved spiral pulse sequence with good balance between spatial and temporal resolution [121]. Oxygen partial pressure imaging uses the paramagnetic effect of oxygen on polarization of ^{3}He [122]. Single-acquisition and single breath-hold technique improves temporal resolution and reduces error due to second breath hold. MRI with this technique can directly measure the regional ventilation and perfusion distribution [123]. Because ^{129}Xe is naturally richer than ^{3}He

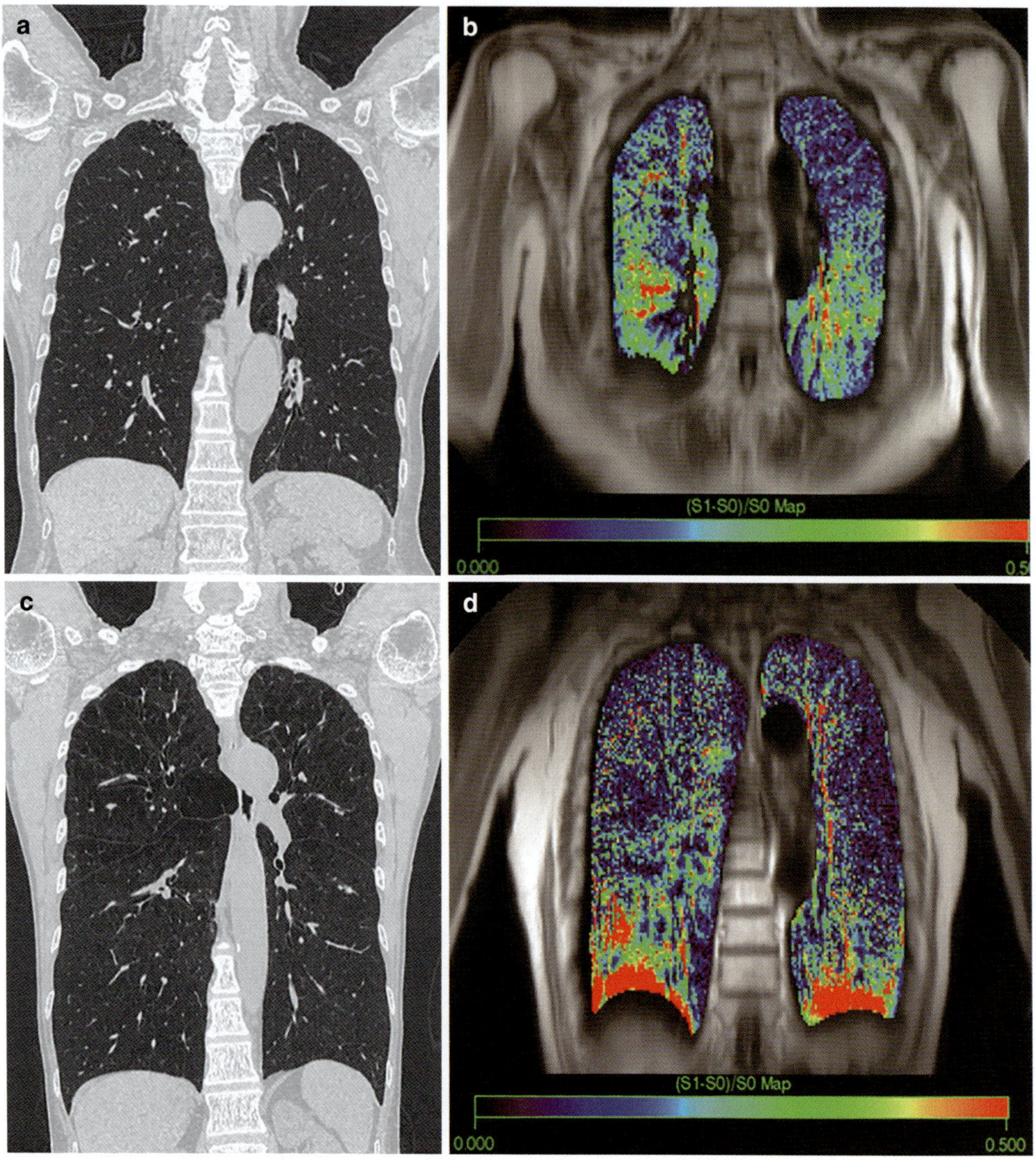

Fig. 8.19 Oxygen-enhanced MRI in COPD patients. (**a**, **b**) A 75-year-old female smoker with mild COPD (**a**: thin-section coronal multiplanar reformatted (MPR) CT image shows centrilobular emphysema in the left upper lung field, **b**: relative enhancement (RER) map from oxygen O_2-enhanced MRI demonstrates heterogeneously decreased oxygen-enhancement in the both lung, especially left upper lung filed.) (**c**, **d**) a 56-year-old female smoker with severe COPD (**c**: thin-section coronal MPR CT image demonstrates panlobular emphysema in bilateral upper and middle lung field. **d**: RER map from oxygen O_2-enhanced MRI demonstrates heterogeneously decreased oxygen-enhancement in the both lung, especially upper lung fields.) Image courtesy of Yoshiharu Ohno, Kobe University Graduate School of Medicine

and ^{129}Xe MRI shows comparable quality to ^{3}He MRI with recent advances in polarization and imaging methods; many methods of ^{3}He are translated for ^{129}Xe. However, ^{129}Xe MRI differs from ^{3}He MRI due to difference of gas distribution. In stage III COPD, ventilation defect volume (VDV) was sensitive to minimal changes during short-term follow-up [114]. Percentage of ventilation volume was significantly different among three groups (healthy volunteers, healthy asymptomatic smokers, and COPD patients). COPD patients are separated from healthy subjects by apparent diffusion coefficient (ADC) map [124]. Using diffusion-weighted hyperpolarized ^{129}Xe MRI, ADC was significantly correlated with PFTs (FEV_1, FEV_1/FVC, and DLco) [115]. Ventilation defect percentages in ^{3}He MRI show significant correlations with ventilation defect percentages in ^{129}Xe MRI and ventilation defect percentages show strong correlations with FEV_1 [125]. ADC can measure airspace size sensitively. In COPD, airspace dimensions are increased compared to non-smokers [126]. ADCs in emphysema show regional variations and significantly larger than those of healthy volunteers, which is homogeneous [127].

Fourier Decomposition MRI for Combined V-Q Imaging

Non-contrast-enhanced ventilation and perfusion MRI, known as Fourier decomposition MRI, uses a short echo dynamic SSFP acquisition with subsequent compensation for respiratory motion by using non-rigid image registration [128, 129]. Peaks at the respiratory and cardiac frequencies can be identified by spectral analysis of the image time series. Deformation of lung parenchyma and pulmonary blood flow leads to regional proton density change, which is related to amplitude of these peaks [130]. With image post-processing, ventilation- and perfusion-weighted maps are generated for regional assessment of lung function from a single acquisition series [131].

Dynamic Respiration MRI

Diaphragmatic geometry is affected by hyperinflation of the lung. Dynamic respiration MRI with fast-acquisition technique can visualize complex interaction between chest wall and diaphragmatic motion with high spatial and temporal resolution [132]. Using dynamic respiration MRI, the change in lung volume during the respiratory cycle can be assessed. In emphysema patients, motion of the diaphragm and chest wall is reduced, irregular or asynchronous [133]. Emphysema in lower lung shows significant correlation with diaphragmatic flattening, abnormal chest wall motion, and severe airflow limitation [134]. Although both normal and paradoxical diaphragmatic motion is restricted by severe hyperinflation, the paradoxical diaphragmatic motion shows significant correlation with hyperinflation [135].

Other Imaging for COPD

Dual-Energy CT

Introduction of Dual-Energy CT

Dual-energy CT refers to CT that uses two different energy spectra (usually 80 and 140 kVp). With the knowledge about the X-ray attenuation change of a particular substance at two different X-ray energies, the material differentiation and elemental decomposition of tissues are possible in dual-energy CT [136, 137]. Therefore, with single contrast CT scanning at two different energies, the CT images used for structural evaluation are created by combination of the CT images from the low- and high-energy CT data, and the material-specific images such as iodine map or xenon map for functional evaluation are created by the material-decomposition algorithms in the postproccessing of dual-energy datasets (Fig. 8.20). Three different designs of dual-energy CT for the acquisition of dual-energy data have been proposed. Firstly, dual-source CT system has two separate X-ray tubes and two corresponding detectors, which are placed with an angular off-set of 90° on the rotating gantry. Each X-ray tube can be operated at different kilovoltage and milliamperage settings. Secondly, in rapid kVp switching, the single X-ray source is used and X-ray tube electronically switches the tube voltage between higher energy and lower energy in about 0.5 ms. Lastly, the energy-sensitive sandwich detector is now commercially available. This system uses a layered detector and single X-ray tube with the polychromatic

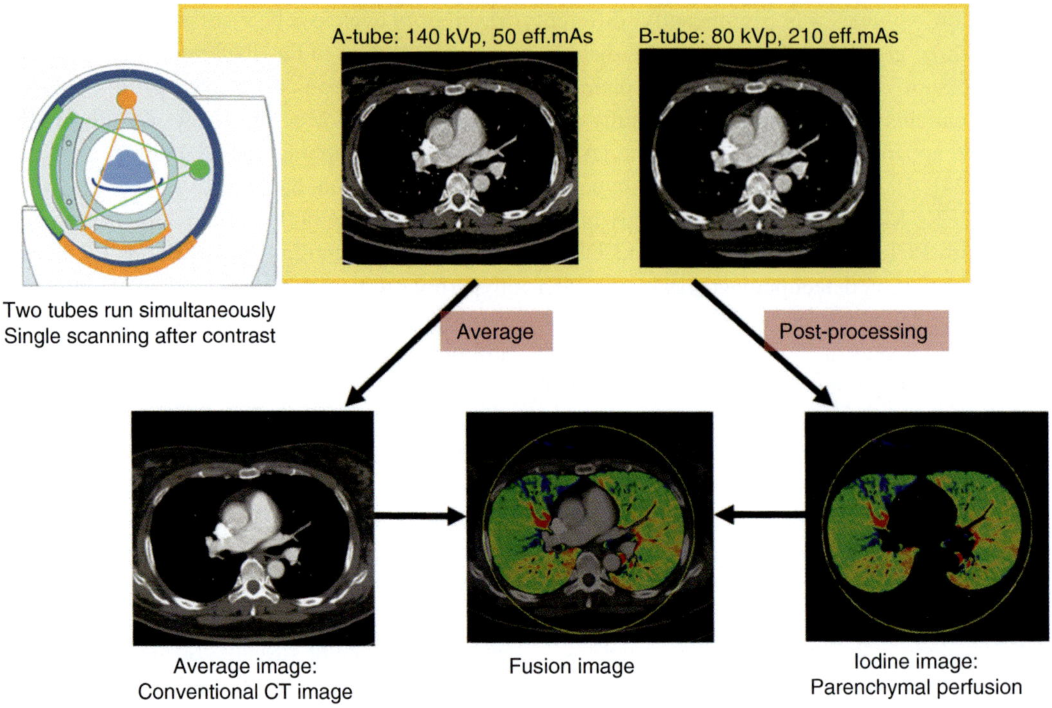

Fig. 8.20 Iodine perfusion imaging using dual-source CT. CT image data is generated in dual-energy acquisition mode of dual-source CT. Axial CT image is obtained at 140 kVp and 50 mAs from A-tube and at 80 kVp and 210 mAs from B-tube. And conventional CT image (approximate 120 kVp image) is generated from combination of the 140 and 80 kVp datasets. Iodine image is obtained with extraction of iodine component with material-decomposition theory in post-processing. Fusion image with conventional CT image and iodine image is generated for the evaluation of lung parenchymal perfusion

spectrum. The layered detector comprises two layers: a thin top scintillator that absorbs low energy photons and a bottom scintillator that absorbs the higher mean energy photons.

For COPD patients, which is characterized by airway obstruction and emphysematous alveolar destruction, pulmonary vascular changes are also produced, which are characterized by hypoxic vasoconstriction, numeric reduction, and endothelial dysfunction of the small pulmonary arteries [138–140]. These characteristic anatomic changes influence and impair alveolar gas exchange, and the uneven distribution of alveolar ventilation and pulmonary blood flow (V/Q mismatch) is the most important cause of arterial hypoxemia in the COPD patients [141, 142]. Therefore, evaluating COPD patients should focus on not only the extent and severity of anatomic destruction of the lung parenchyma but also the functional changes and impairment such as alveolar ventilation changes or parenchymal perfusion changes.

Perfusion Dual-Energy CT

Dual-energy CT-derived iodine map represents the iodine content of the capillary bed, i.e., pulmonary blood volume at the time of CT scanning rather than pulmonary blood flow. However, it has been demonstrated that the similarity of the dynamic CT-derived pulmonary blood flow and dual-energy CT-derived pulmonary blood volume [143]. Therefore, pulmonary blood volume, assessed with dual-energy CT, can be used for the evaluation of lung perfusion as a surrogate for dynamic CT-derived pulmonary blood flow with simpler protocol while maintaining quantitative similarity (Fig. 8.21).

In COPD, the regional lung perfusion impairment occurs due to the hypoxic vasoconstriction of the area with decreased ventilation

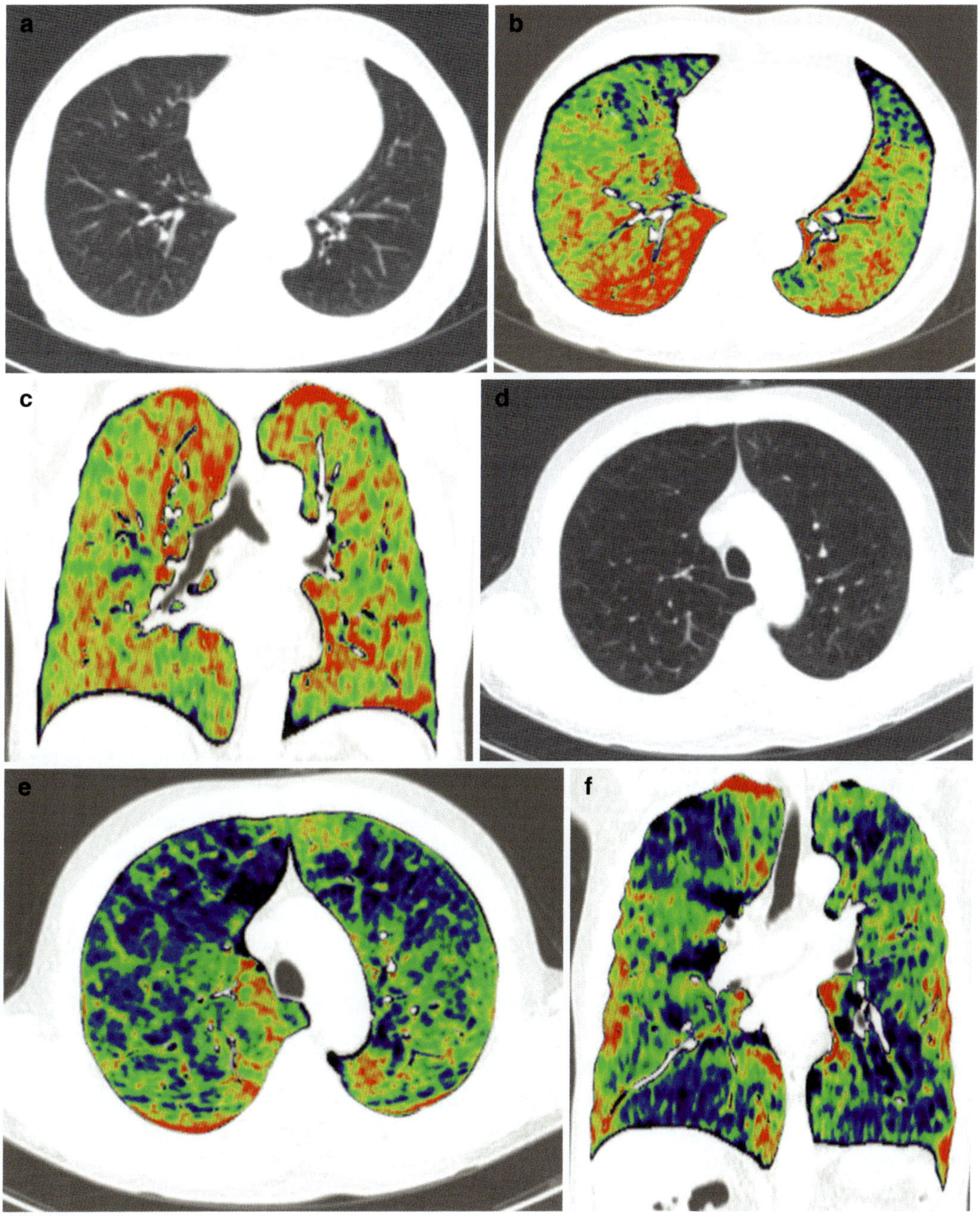

Fig. 8.21 Iodine perfusion image with dual-energy CT in COPD patient. (**a–c**) Dual-energy CT in COPD patient with mild emphysema. (**d–f**) Dual-energy CT in COPD patient with severe emphysema. From iodine perfusion CT using dual-energy CT, (**a**, **d**) weighted conventional CT image and (**b**, **c**, **e**, **f**) iodine perfusion map are generated. Lung parenchymal destruction in COPD patient can be assessed on high-resolution conventional CT image (**a**, **d**), and anatomically matched parenchymal perfusion information can be evaluated on perfusion map (**b**, **c**, **e**, **f**). In the area of confluent emphysema of both lower lobes, parenchymal perfusion is decreased (displayed with *blue color*)

and reduction of the pulmonary capillary by the chronic inflammation of pulmonary artery [144]. Moreover, alveolar surface destruction is accompanied by the reduction of the pulmonary capillary bed. Thus, considerable attention has been paid to the evaluation of lung perfusion alterations in COPD patients because the severity of parenchymal destruction and the alteration of lung perfusion determine the functional effect of emphysematous changes. Lung parenchymal perfusion has been assessed by perfusion scintigraphy, single-photon emission CT and MR. However, the distribution of perfusion impairment does not match with the area of parenchymal destruction [145]. Dynamic multi-detector CT perfusion imaging also can provide the regional perfusion. It has been demonstrated that smokers with subtle CT findings of centrilobular emphysema and normal findings at spirometry has increased regional heterogeneity of lung perfusion compared with never smoked subjects and smokers with normal CT image [146]. However, dynamic multi-detector CT perfusion imaging necessitates a central high-pressure bolus of contrast material and scanning a limited axial extent of the lung during a cardiac-gated scan.

Pansini et al. have demonstrated that regional alteration of lung perfusion can be assessed by dual-energy CT, matching parenchymal destruction in 47 smokers with predominant emphysema [147]. Moreover, Lee et al. have shown that the contrast-enhanced dual-energy CT can be used for the quantification of emphysema and regional perfusion evaluation by using the virtual non-contrast images and iodine map, simultaneously [148]. Assessing the distribution of pulmonary emphysema and anatomically matched parenchymal perfusion information is particularly applicable in the patient and target lobe selection for lung volume reduction surgery or bronchoscopic lung volume reduction. Data from National Emphysema Treatment Trial with more than 1000 patients undergoing lung volume reduction surgery showed that lung volume reduction surgery reduces mortality in patients with upper-lobe predominant emphysema only if there is low perfusion to the upper lobe on scintigraphy [149]. Park et al. used dual-energy CT with lung perfusion imaging for target lobe selection of bronchoscopic lung volume reduction by endobronchial valves. In that study, the target lobe was selected, if it was most hyperinflated and least perfused, and if it had no collateral ventilation with other lobes on perfusion image with dual-energy CT [150].

Ventilation Dual-Energy CT

In clinical practice, the evaluation of COPD severity is based on the result of pulmonary function test; however, pulmonary function test provides global status of lung function and does not show the regional distribution of functional abnormality. For evaluation of regional lung parenchymal ventilation, radionuclide scintigraphy or MR is used, but it is limited by its low spatial resolution. CT also can be used to depict lung ventilation with inhalation of xenon gas [151, 152]. Xenon is a radio-opaque gas and xenon gas concentration in alveolar space can be measured based on the attenuation changes on CT image (Fig. 8.22). However, because of variability in baseline lung attenuation between images due to misregistration artifacts and different respiration levels, the accurate measurement of lung ventilation function is limited, triggering great attention in the simultaneous structural and functional evaluation with single CT scanning accessible to dual-energy CT. Two stable gases, xenon and krypton, with high atomic numbers (54 for xenon and 36 for krypton) are eligible for ventilation imaging with dual-energy CT. For xenon ventilation imaging with dual-energy CT, the patient usually inhales 30% stable xenon (a mixture of 30% xenon and 70% oxygen) for 1 min to 1 min 30 s with use of a xenon gas inhalation system (Zetron V; Anzai Medical, Tokyo, Japan).

The first clinical report with xenon ventilation imaging with dual-energy CT was reported by Chae et al., investigating eight healthy volunteers and four patients with COPD. The authors have demonstrated the direct visualization of the degree of xenon gas enhancement in the lung parenchyma as a color overlay on a conventional thin-section chest CT image by material decomposition [153]. Park et al. performed two phase

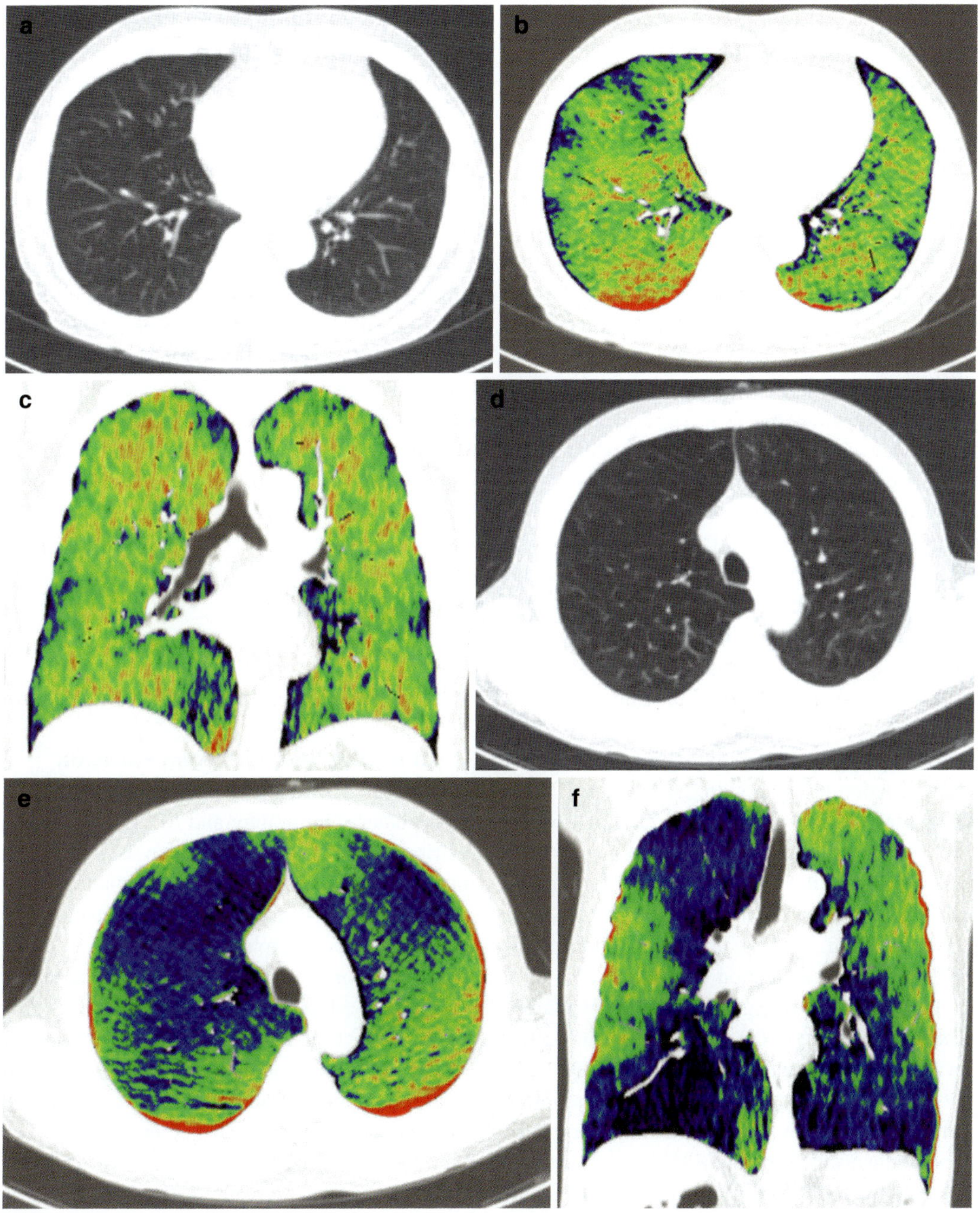

Fig. 8.22 Xenon ventilation image with dual-energy CT in COPD patient. (**a**–**c**) Dual-energy CT in COPD patient with mild emphysema. (**d**–**f**) Dual-energy CT in COPD patient with severe emphysema. (**a**, **d**) Conventional CT image and (**b**, **c**, **e**, **f**) xenon ventilation map image obtained from xenon ventilation dual-energy CT. On weighted average image (**a**, **d**), centrilobular emphysema and bronchial wall thickening in both lower lobes are noted. (**b**, **c**, **e**, **f**) In right upper lobe and left upper lobe, decreased xenon ventilation is identified, while xenon ventilation is preserved in left upper lobe posterior segment

(wash-in and wash-out phase) xenon ventilation dual-energy CT in 32 patients with COPD. And regional quantified value of xenon enhancement in abnormally low attenuating lung area on xenon-enhanced images with wash-out phase showed inverse correlation with pulmonary function test, and it showed better correlation with pulmonary function test than CT attenuation parameters [154]. Similar approaches were also reported in asthma patients. Investigating 22 asthma patients, Chae et al. have demonstrated the ventilation defects that appeared on xenon ventilation imaging with dual-energy CT in asthma patients with severe airflow limitation and airway wall thickening. And the extent of the ventilation defects on xenon-enhanced CT showed correlations with parameters of pulmonary function test [155]. Demonstration of the reversibility of airflow obstruction after inhalation of bronchodilator has been reported, and it suggested that xenon-enhanced dual-energy CT may be feasible for visualizing the changes of airflow in response to drugs in asthma patients [156–158].

Stable krypton can be an alternative to xenon for ventilation imaging with dual-energy CT due to its high atomic number, and lack of toxicity and anesthetic properties. Hachulla et al. have firstly reported the krypton ventilation imaging using dual-energy CT in COPD patients. Single CT acquisition covering the whole thorax was performed after inhalation of a mixture of 80% krypton and 20% oxygen with five respiratory maneuvers through the mask. The maximum level of krypton enhancement within the lung was 18.5 HU, which is lower than that reported with xenon, with an average maximum degree of xenon enhancement of 23.78 HU, is sufficient to detect ventilation abnormalities [159]. This single static approach in phantoms and volunteers also has been reported recently using xenon gas after a single vital capacity inhalation [160]. The single static evaluation delivers a lower radiation dose and a few or single inhalation method is more easily implementable for radiologists and patients, without side effects. However, different ventilation dynamics can be evaluated regarding the scanning method and gas inhalation method.

Combined Ventilation and Perfusion Assessment with Dual-Energy CT

Pulmonary parenchymal perfusion change or ventilation impairment was evaluated with dual-energy CT separately in COPD patients. However, the pulmonary parenchymal ventilation and perfusion are changed concurrently, and the imbalance between ventilation and perfusion is the important characteristics in the patients with COPD. Investigating ten patients with various diseases from an anesthesiological intensive care unit, Thieme et al. have reported the potential of dual-energy CT to provide both pulmonary ventilation and perfusion imaging [161]. Zhang et al. applied combined ventilation and perfusion imaging with dual-energy CT in patients with suspected pulmonary embolism [162]. Combined ventilation and perfusion imaging with dual-energy CT in patients with COPD has not yet been reported (Fig. 8.23).

Nuclear Medicine Imaging

Scintigraphy, Single-Photon Emission Computed Tomography (SPECT)

Both planar scintigraphy and SPECT image the distribution of radiotracer which is introduced into the body, and the emitted radiation from radiotracer is detected by external detectors. In contrast to scintigraphy which forms a single two-dimensional image, analogous to a planar X-ray scan, SPECT provides three-dimensional imaging about the distribution of a radiotracer by combining scintigraphic and computed tomographic technique, and allows the functional information from SPECT to be easily combined with the high-resolution anatomic information from CT. Perfusion scanning is generally performed using 99 m-technetium-labeled macroaggregated albumin (99 m Tc-MAA), which lodges in the pulmonary circulation after peripheral injection. In an animal study using pigs, perfusion SPECT has been shown to be more sensitive than HRCT to detect mild physiologic changes of elastase-induced pulmonary emphysema [163]. Moreover, Suga et al. have been demonstrated that perfusion abnormalities on breath-hold

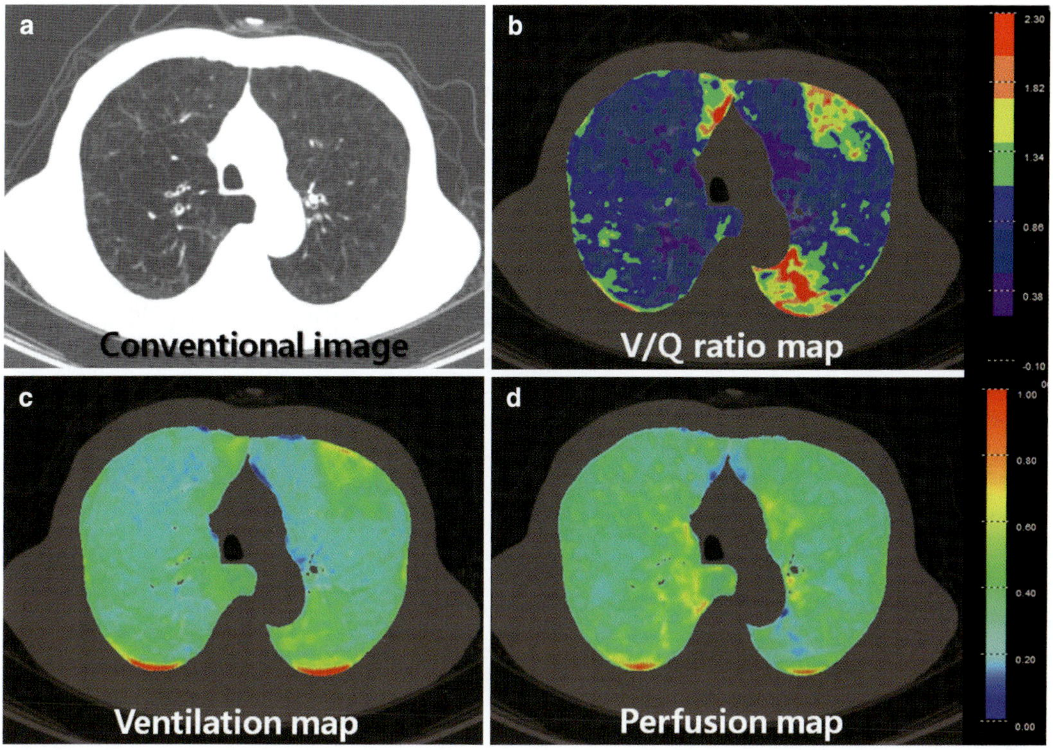

Fig. 8.23 Combined ventilation and perfusion assessment with dual-energy CT. From combined xenon ventilation and iodine perfusion CT using dual-energy CT, the conventional virtual non-contrast CT image (**a**), xenon ventilation/iodine perfusion map (**b**), ventilation map (**c**) and perfusion map (**d**) are generated. Lung parenchymal ventilation, perfusion and ventilation-perfusion imbalance with high-resolution anatomic CT information can be simultaneously evaluated with combined ventilation and perfusion dual-energy CT

SPECT-CT fusion image can better reflect the lung pathophysiology than the emphysema index on morphologic CT scan [164]. And there have been several intervention studies in COPD patients using perfusion scintigraphy and SPECT to predict and measure clinical success. As mentioned earlier, assessing the lung parenchymal perfusion has been particularly applicable in target lobe selection for lung volume reduction surgery or bronchoscopic lung volume reduction. Perfusion scintigraphy has been used in National Emphysema Treatment Trial with more than 1000 patients undergoing lung volume reduction surgery for selection of target lobe [149]. And perfusion scintigraphy was also useful for selection of target lobe for endobronchial valve therapy in advanced emphysema patients, and patients having heterogeneous emphysema with a low baseline target lobe perfusion benefited from endobronchial valve therapy [165]. Although scintigraphy and SPECT have constitutional problems, low spatial resolution and long image acquisition time, to date, they are widely applied due to their availability in many centers. Ventilation scintigraphy and SPECT use two types of inhalation radiotracers: gaseous radioisotopes or radiolabeled particulate aerosols. 81 m Kr and 133 Xe as gaseous radioisotopes have been used for ventilation scintigraphy and SPECT, and several studies with gaseous radioisotopes have demonstrated ventilation heterogeneity in COPD [166, 167]. And for radiolabeled particulate aerosol, Technegas (99 m Tc-labeled, aerosolized ultrafine carbon particle, approximately 200 nm diameter) is usually used in patients with COPD due to its small particle size [168], even in the presence of severe airflow obstruction [169]. With Technegas, the inhomogeneities in ventilation on scintigraphy and SPECT in COPD patients have been visualized and quantified [170, 171].

Ventilation/perfusion SPECT can also be applied for the evaluation of the imbalance between ventilation and perfusion in the patients with COPD. Jogi et al. have reported significant correlation between total reduction in lung function assessed with ventilation/perfusion SPECT and spirometric lung function and emphysema severity on CT in patients with COPD [172] (Fig. 8.24). Suga et al. have described that quantitative analysis of V/Q distribution by SPECT and the standard deviation and kurtosis of the V/Q profile could be adequate indicator for the severity of lung V-Q imbalance causing gas exchange impairment in patients with emphysema [173].

Positron Emission Tomography (PET)

Regional ventilation and perfusion also can be evaluated with PET using isotope $^{13}N_2$ gas dissolved in saline solution. Brudin et al. have reported that high V/Q tended to be more common in subjects with an emphysema dominant subtype, whereas low V/Q was more common in those with a bronchial inflammation dominant subtype. Spatial heterogeneity of lung perfusion also has been described with $^{13}N_2$ saline PET, and the regional heterogeneity in perfusion has been increased in patients with mild COPD compared to healthy controls, after adjusting for regional changes in lung tissue density and ventilation. [174]. These results suggest that regional perfusion changes may precede lung parenchymal destruction in COPD. Therefore, this imaging method may serve as an early biomarker for COPD.

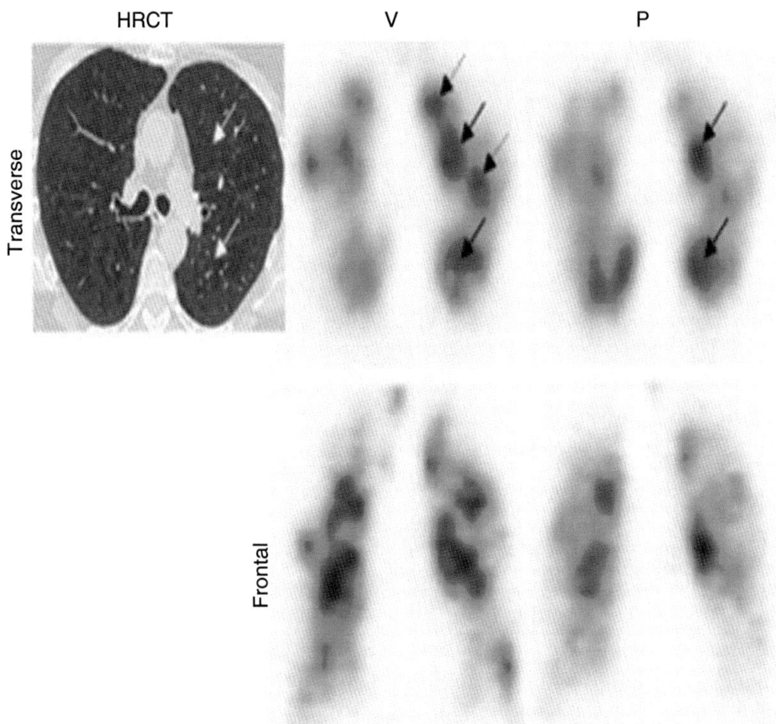

Fig. 8.24 Ventilation/perfusion SPECT. Patient with centrilobular emphysema on HRCT. Ventilation/perfusion SPECT shows uneven ventilation and perfusion. Extensive areas with reverse as well as matched ventilation/perfusion defects are found. Better perfused areas correspond to areas which are well ventilated (*black arrows*) and to better preserved parenchyma on HRCT (*white arrows*). Other areas appearing as hot spots on ventilation images are poorly perfused (*dotted arrows*). (Reprinted with permission, from reference 172)

Recent studies have been focused on systemic inflammation as a consequence of COPD, and patients with COPD are found to have higher levels of systemic biomarkers of inflammation and worse cardiovascular risk profile and prognosis [175–177]. Fluorine-18-fluorodeoxyglucose (^{18}F-FDG) is the most commonly used PET radioisotope, and it depicts increased glucose metabolism. In COPD patients, ^{18}F-FDG has been used to demonstrate both pulmonary and systemic inflammation. The pulmonary inflammation as ^{18}F-FDG uptake in COPD patients was significantly higher than in asthmatic and normal subjects [178]. Pulmonary ^{18}F-FDG uptake in usual (PiM phenotype) COPD patients was greater compared to patients with alpha-1 antitrypsin deficiency-associated emphysema (PiZ phenotype) and healthy controls, and it was correlated with FEV_1 [179]. Coulson et al. have evaluated the aortic inflammation as a measure of systemic inflammation using ^{18}F-FDG PET in seven COPD patients, five metabolic syndrome patients, and seven ex-smokers. Aortic inflammation in COPD patients was intermediate between ex-smokers and metabolic syndrome patients [180].

Optical Coherence Tomography (OCT)

OCT is an imaging method utilizing the refraction of light waves as it passes through tissues, and measures the lung structure with endobronchial approach. A fiberoptic probe with a near-infrared optical probe is introduced into the airways via a bronchoscope and the reflected light by the tissue is detected and reconstructed into an image. The spatial resolution of OCT is much higher than CT with the ability to resolve structures up to micrometers and distinguish between different tissue types within the airways. Thus, the main strength of OCT in COPD is the ability assessing small airway morphology in vivo. Coxson et al. have demonstrated an excellent correlation between airway lumen and wall area measured by OCT and by CT [181]. Furthermore, OCT airway dimensions measured at the fifth generation bronchi showed a stronger negative correlation with the subject's FEV_1 than CT, and had greater sensitivity in detecting changes in wall measurement than CT measurements. And OCT also provided data on airway wall morphology and subepithelial remodeling and collagen deposition. While OCT is not widely applicable to date, the novel ability on directly assessing small airway disease in COPD patients may allow increasing utilization of OCT in research and clinical practice.

References

1. Larke FJ, Kruger RL, Cagnon CH, Flynn MJ, McNitt-Gray MM, Wu X, et al. Estimated radiation dose associated with low-dose chest CT of average-size participants in the National Lung Screening Trial. AJR Am J Roentgenol. 2011;197(5):1165–9. doi:10.2214/AJR.11.6533.
2. Newell JD Jr, Sieren J, Hoffman EA. Development of quantitative computed tomography lung protocols. J Thorac Imaging. 2013;28(5):266–71. doi:10.1097/RTI.0b013e31829f6796.
3. Mayo JR. CT evaluation of diffuse infiltrative lung disease: dose considerations and optimal technique. J Thorac Imaging. 2009;24(4):252–9. doi:10.1097/RTI.0b013e3181c227b2.
4. Madani A, De Maertelaer V, Zanen J, Gevenois PA. Pulmonary emphysema: radiation dose and section thickness at multidetector CT quantification—comparison with macroscopic and microscopic morphometry. Radiology. 2007;243(1):250–7. doi:10.1148/radiol.2431060194.
5. Kemerink GJ, Kruize HH, Lamers RJ, van Engelshoven JM. CT lung densitometry: dependence of CT number histograms on sample volume and consequences for scan protocol comparability. J Comput Assist Tomogr. 1997;21(6):948–54.
6. Boedeker KL, McNitt-Gray MF, Rogers SR, Truong DA, Brown MS, Gjertson DW, et al. Emphysema: effect of reconstruction algorithm on CT imaging measures. Radiology. 2004;232(1):295–301. doi:10.1148/radiol.2321030383.
7. Choo JY, Goo JM, Lee CH, Park CM, Park SJ, Shim MS. Quantitative analysis of emphysema and airway measurements according to iterative reconstruction algorithms: comparison of filtered back projection, adaptive statistical iterative reconstruction and model-based iterative reconstruction. Eur Radiol. 2014;24(4):799–806. doi:10.1007/s00330-013-3078-5.
8. Mets OM, Willemink MJ, de Kort FP, Mol CP, Leiner T, Oudkerk M, et al. The effect of iterative reconstruction on computed tomography assessment

of emphysema, air trapping and airway dimensions. Eur Radiol. 2012;22(10):2103–9. doi:10.1007/s00330-012-2489-z.
9. Nishio M, Matsumoto S, Ohno Y, Sugihara N, Inokawa H, Yoshikawa T, et al. Emphysema quantification by low-dose CT: potential impact of adaptive iterative dose reduction using 3D processing. AJR Am J Roentgenol. 2012;199(3):595–601. doi:10.2214/AJR.11.8174.
10. Schroeder JD, McKenzie AS, Zach JA, Wilson CG, Curran-Everett D, Stinson DS, et al. Relationships between airflow obstruction and quantitative CT measurements of emphysema, air trapping, and airways in subjects with and without chronic obstructive pulmonary disease. AJR Am J Roentgenol. 2013;201(3):W460–70. doi:10.2214/AJR.12.10102.
11. Stockley RA, Mannino D, Barnes PJ. Burden and pathogenesis of chronic obstructive pulmonary disease. Proc Am Thorac Soc. 2009;6(6):524–6. doi:10.1513/pats.200904-016DS.
12. Roy K, Smith J, Kolsum U, Borrill Z, Vestbo J, Singh D. COPD phenotype description using principal components analysis. Respir Res. 2009;10:41. doi:10.1186/1465-9921-10-41.
13. Bergin C, Muller N, Nichols DM, Lillington G, Hogg JC, Mullen B, et al. The diagnosis of emphysema. A computed tomographic-pathologic correlation. Am Rev Respir Dis. 1986;133(4):541–6.
14. Bafadhel M, Umar I, Gupta S, Raj JV, Vara DD, Entwisle JJ, et al. The role of CT scanning in multidimensional phenotyping of COPD. Chest. 2011;140(3):634–42. doi:10.1378/chest.10-3007.
15. O'Brien C, Guest PJ, Hill SL, Stockley RA. Physiological and radiological characterisation of patients diagnosed with chronic obstructive pulmonary disease in primary care. Thorax. 2000;55(8):635–42.
16. McDonough JE, Yuan R, Suzuki M, Seyednejad N, Elliott WM, Sanchez PG, et al. Small-airway obstruction and emphysema in chronic obstructive pulmonary disease. N Engl J Med. 2011;365(17):1567–75. doi:10.1056/NEJMoa1106955.
17. Lehouck A, Boonen S, Decramer M, Janssens W. COPD, bone metabolism, and osteoporosis. Chest. 2011;139(3):648–57. doi:10.1378/chest.10-1427.
18. Miller RR, Muller NL, Vedal S, Morrison NJ, Staples CA. Limitations of computed tomography in the assessment of emphysema. Am Rev Respir Dis. 1989;139(4):980–3. doi:10.1164/ajrccm/139.4.980.
19. Kim SS, Seo JB, Lee HY, Nevrekar DV, Forssen AV, Crapo JD, et al. Chronic obstructive pulmonary disease: lobe-based visual assessment of volumetric CT by using standard images—comparison with quantitative CT and pulmonary function test in the COPDGene study. Radiology. 2013;266(2):626–35. doi:10.1148/radiol.12120385.
20. Cavigli E, Camiciottoli G, Diciotti S, Orlandi I, Spinelli C, Meoni E, et al. Whole-lung densitometry versus visual assessment of emphysema. Eur Radiol. 2009;19(7):1686–92. doi:10.1007/s00330-009-1320-y.
21. Bankier AA, De Maertelaer V, Keyzer C, Gevenois PA. Pulmonary emphysema: subjective visual grading versus objective quantification with macroscopic morphometry and thin-section CT densitometry. Radiology. 1999;211(3):851–8. doi:10.1148/radiology.211.3.r99jn05851.
22. Group COCW, Barr RG, Berkowitz EA, Bigazzi F, Bode F, Bon J, et al. A combined pulmonary-radiology workshop for visual evaluation of COPD: study design, chest CT findings and concordance with quantitative evaluation. COPD. 2012;9(2):151–9. doi:10.3109/15412555.2012.654923.
23. Hayhurst MD, MacNee W, Flenley DC, Wright D, McLean A, Lamb D, et al. Diagnosis of pulmonary emphysema by computerised tomography. Lancet. 1984;2(8398):320–2.
24. Muller NL, Staples CA, Miller RR, Abboud RT. "Density mask". An objective method to quantitate emphysema using computed tomography. Chest. 1988;94(4):782–7.
25. Madani A, Zanen J, de Maertelaer V, Gevenois PA. Pulmonary emphysema: objective quantification at multi-detector row CT—comparison with macroscopic and microscopic morphometry. Radiology. 2006;238(3):1036–43. doi:10.1148/radiol.2382042196.
26. Dirksen A, Friis M, Olesen KP, Skovgaard LT, Sorensen K. Progress of emphysema in severe alpha 1-antitrypsin deficiency as assessed by annual CT. Acta Radiol. 1997;38(5):826–32.
27. Dirksen A. Monitoring the progress of emphysema by repeat computed tomography scans with focus on noise reduction. Proc Am Thorac Soc. 2008;5(9):925–8. doi:10.1513/pats.200804-033QC.
28. Heussel CP, Herth FJ, Kappes J, Hantusch R, Hartlieb S, Weinheimer O, et al. Fully automatic quantitative assessment of emphysema in computed tomography: comparison with pulmonary function testing and normal values. Eur Radiol. 2009;19(10):2391–402. doi:10.1007/s00330-009-1437-z.
29. Stolk J, Dirksen A, van der Lugt AA, Hutsebaut J, Mathieu J, de Ree J, et al. Repeatability of lung density measurements with low-dose computed tomography in subjects with alpha-1-antitrypsin deficiency-associated emphysema. Investig Radiol. 2001;36(11):648–51.
30. Gietema HA, Muller NL, Fauerbach PV, Sharma S, Edwards LD, Camp PG, et al. Quantifying the extent of emphysema: factors associated with radiologists' estimations and quantitative indices of emphysema severity using the ECLIPSE cohort. Acad Radiol. 2011;18(6):661–71. doi:10.1016/j.acra.2011.01.011.
31. Parr DG, Stoel BC, Stolk J, Stockley RA. Pattern of emphysema distribution in alpha1-antitrypsin deficiency influences lung function impairment.

Am J Respir Crit Care Med. 2004;170(11):1172–8. doi:10.1164/rccm.200406-761OC.
32. Nakano Y, Sakai H, Muro S, Hirai T, Oku Y, Nishimura K, et al. Comparison of low attenuation areas on computed tomographic scans between inner and outer segments of the lung in patients with chronic obstructive pulmonary disease: incidence and contribution to lung function. Thorax. 1999;54(5):384–9.
33. Chae EJ, Seo JB, Song JW, Kim N, Park BW, Lee YK, et al. Slope of emphysema index: an objective descriptor of regional heterogeneity of emphysema and an independent determinant of pulmonary function. AJR Am J Roentgenol. 2010;194(3):W248–55. doi:10.2214/AJR.09.2672.
34. Nakano Y, Coxson HO, Bosan S, Rogers RM, Sciurba FC, Keenan RJ, et al. Core to rind distribution of severe emphysema predicts outcome of lung volume reduction surgery. Am J Respir Crit Care Med. 2001;164(12):2195–9. doi:10.1164/ajrccm.164.12.2012140.
35. Martinez-Garcia MA, Soler-Cataluna JJ, Donat Sanz Y, Catalan Serra P, Agramunt Lerma M, Ballestin Vicente J, et al. Factors associated with bronchiectasis in patients with COPD. Chest. 2011;140(5):1130–7. doi:10.1378/chest.10-1758.
36. Grydeland TB, Thorsen E, Dirksen A, Jensen R, Coxson HO, Pillai SG, et al. Quantitative CT measures of emphysema and airway wall thickness are related to D(L)CO. Respir Med. 2011;105(3):343–51. doi:10.1016/j.rmed.2010.10.018.
37. Nakano Y, Muro S, Sakai H, Hirai T, Chin K, Tsukino M, et al. Computed tomographic measurements of airway dimensions and emphysema in smokers. Correlation with lung function. Am J Respir Crit Care Med. 2000;162(3 Pt 1):1102–8. doi:10.1164/ajrccm.162.3.9907120.
38. Washko GR, Dransfield MT, Estepar RS, Diaz A, Matsuoka S, Yamashiro T, et al. Airway wall attenuation: a biomarker of airway disease in subjects with COPD. J Appl Physiol. 2009;107(1):185–91. doi:10.1152/japplphysiol.00216.2009.
39. Nakano Y, Wong JC, de Jong PA, Buzatu L, Nagao T, Coxson HO, et al. The prediction of small airway dimensions using computed tomography. Am J Respir Crit Care Med. 2005;171(2):142–6. doi:10.1164/rccm.200407-874OC.
40. Achenbach T, Weinheimer O, Biedermann A, Schmitt S, Freudenstein D, Goutham E, et al. MDCT assessment of airway wall thickness in COPD patients using a new method: correlations with pulmonary function tests. Eur Radiol. 2008;18(12):2731–8. doi:10.1007/s00330-008-1089-4.
41. Han MK, Kazerooni EA, Lynch DA, Liu LX, Murray S, Curtis JL, et al. Chronic obstructive pulmonary disease exacerbations in the COPDGene study: associated radiologic phenotypes. Radiology. 2011;261(1):274–82. doi:10.1148/radiol.11110173.
42. Lee HJ, Seo JB, Chae EJ, Kim N, Lee CW, Oh YM, et al. Tracheal morphology and collapse in COPD: correlation with CT indices and pulmonary function test. Eur J Radiol. 2011;80(3):e531–5. doi:10.1016/j.ejrad.2010.12.062.
43. Boiselle PM, Litmanovich DE, Michaud G, Roberts DH, Loring SH, Womble HM, et al. Dynamic expiratory tracheal collapse in morbidly obese COPD patients. COPD. 2013;10(5):604–10. doi:10.3109/15412555.2013.781149.
44. Regan EA, Hokanson JE, Murphy JR, Make B, Lynch DA, Beaty TH, et al. Genetic epidemiology of COPD (COPDGene) study design. COPD. 2010;7(1):32–43. doi:10.3109/15412550903499522.
45. Matsuoka S, Kurihara Y, Yagihashi K, Nakajima Y. Quantitative assessment of peripheral airway obstruction on paired expiratory/inspiratory thin-section computed tomography in chronic obstructive pulmonary disease with emphysema. J Comput Assist Tomogr. 2007;31(3):384–9. doi:10.1097/01.rct.0000243457.00437.10.
46. Matsuoka S, Kurihara Y, Yagihashi K, Hoshino M, Watanabe N, Nakajima Y. Quantitative assessment of air trapping in chronic obstructive pulmonary disease using inspiratory and expiratory volumetric MDCT. AJR Am J Roentgenol. 2008;190(3):762–9. doi:10.2214/AJR.07.2820.
47. Yamashiro T, Matsuoka S, Bartholmai BJ, San Jose Estepar R, Ross JC, Diaz A, et al. Collapsibility of lung volume by paired inspiratory and expiratory CT scans: correlations with lung function and mean lung density. Acad Radiol. 2010;17(4):489–95. doi:10.1016/j.acra.2009.11.004.
48. Lee YK, Oh YM, Lee JH, Kim EK, Lee JH, Kim N, et al. Quantitative assessment of emphysema, air trapping, and airway thickening on computed tomography. Lung. 2008;186(3):157–65. doi:10.1007/s00408-008-9071-0.
49. Galban CJ, Han MK, Boes JL, Chughtai KA, Meyer CR, Johnson TD, et al. Computed tomography-based biomarker provides unique signature for diagnosis of COPD phenotypes and disease progression. Nat Med. 2012;18(11):1711–5. doi:10.1038/nm.2971.
50. Barbosa EM Jr, Song G, Tustison N, Kreider M, Gee JC, Gefter WB, et al. Computational analysis of thoracic multidetector row HRCT for segmentation and quantification of small airway air trapping and emphysema in obstructive pulmonary disease. Acad Radiol. 2011;18(10):1258–69. doi:10.1016/j.acra.2011.06.004.
51. Ginsburg SB, Lynch DA, Bowler RP, Schroeder JD. Automated texture-based quantification of centrilobular nodularity and centrilobular emphysema in chest CT images. Acad Radiol. 2012;19(10):1241–51. doi:10.1016/j.acra.2012.04.020.
52. Park YS, Seo JB, Kim N, Chae EJ, Oh YM, Lee SD, et al. Texture-based quantification of pulmonary emphysema on high-resolution computed tomography: comparison with density-based quantification and correlation with pulmonary function test.

Investig Radiol. 2008;43(6):395–402. doi:10.1097/RLI.0b013e31816901c7.
53. Barr RG, Mesia-Vela S, Austin JH, Basner RC, Keller BM, Reeves AP, et al. Impaired flow-mediated dilation is associated with low pulmonary function and emphysema in ex-smokers: the emphysema and cancer action project (EMCAP) study. Am J Respir Crit Care Med. 2007;176(12):1200–7. doi:10.1164/rccm.200707-980OC.
54. Ross JC, Estepar RS, Diaz A, Westin CF, Kikinis R, Silverman EK, et al. Lung extraction, lobe segmentation and hierarchical region assessment for quantitative analysis on high resolution computed tomography images. Med Image Comput Comput Assist Interv. 2009;12(Pt 2):690–8.
55. Xiao C, Staring M, Shamonin D, Reiber JH, Stolk J, Stoel BC. A strain energy filter for 3D vessel enhancement with application to pulmonary CT images. Med Image Anal. 2011;15(1):112–24. doi:10.1016/j.media.2010.08.003.
56. Matsuoka S, Washko GR, Dransfield MT, Yamashiro T, San Jose Estepar R, Diaz A, et al. Quantitative CT measurement of cross-sectional area of small pulmonary vessel in COPD: correlations with emphysema and airflow limitation. Acad Radiol. 2010;17(1):93–9. doi:10.1016/j.acra.2009.07.022.
57. Harrison RA, Siminoski K, Vethanayagam D, Majumdar SR. Osteoporosis-related kyphosis and impairments in pulmonary function: a systematic review. J Bone Miner Res Off J Am Soc Bone Miner Res. 2007;22(3):447–57. doi:10.1359/jbmr.061202.
58. Ohara T, Hirai T, Muro S, Haruna A, Terada K, Kinose D, et al. Relationship between pulmonary emphysema and osteoporosis assessed by CT in patients with COPD. Chest. 2008;134(6):1244–9. doi:10.1378/chest.07-3054.
59. Kiyokawa H, Muro S, Oguma T, Sato S, Tanabe N, Takahashi T, et al. Impact of COPD exacerbations on osteoporosis assessed by chest CT scan. COPD. 2012;9(3):235–42. doi:10.3109/15412555.2011.650243.
60. Marquis K, Debigare R, Lacasse Y, LeBlanc P, Jobin J, Carrier G, et al. Midthigh muscle cross-sectional area is a better predictor of mortality than body mass index in patients with chronic obstructive pulmonary disease. Am J Respir Crit Care Med. 2002;166(6):809–13. doi:10.1164/rccm.2107031.
61. Soler-Cataluna JJ, Sanchez-Sanchez L, Martinez-Garcia MA, Sanchez PR, Salcedo E, Navarro M. Mid-arm muscle area is a better predictor of mortality than body mass index in COPD. Chest. 2005;128(4):2108–15. doi:10.1378/chest.128.4.2108.
62. Park MJ, Cho JM, Jeon KN, Bae KS, Kim HC, Choi DS, et al. Mass and fat infiltration of intercostal muscles measured by CT histogram analysis and their correlations with COPD severity. Acad Radiol. 2014;21(6):711–7. doi:10.1016/j.acra.2014.02.003.
63. Sin DD, Wu L, Man SF. The relationship between reduced lung function and cardiovascular mortality: a population-based study and a systematic review of the literature. Chest. 2005;127(6):1952–9. doi:10.1378/chest.127.6.1952.
64. Sin DD, Man SF. Chronic obstructive pulmonary disease as a risk factor for cardiovascular morbidity and mortality. Proc Am Thorac Soc. 2005;2(1):8–11. doi:10.1513/pats.200404-032MS.
65. Chae EJ, Seo JB, Oh YM, Lee JS, Jung Y, Lee SD. Severity of systemic calcified atherosclerosis is associated with airflow limitation and emphysema. J Comput Assist Tomogr. 2013;37(5):743–9. doi:10.1097/RCT.0b013e318299f9e7.
66. Ayres SM, Griesbach SJ, Reimold F, Evans RG. Bronchial component in chronic obstructive lung disease. Am J Med. 1974;57(2):183–91.
67. Pare PD, Lawson LM, Brooks LA. Patterns of response to inhaled bronchodilators in asthmatics. Am Rev Respir Dis. 1983;127(6):680–5.
68. Lee JS, Huh JW, Chae EJ, Seo JB, Ra SW, Lee JH, et al. Response patterns to bronchodilator and quantitative computed tomography in chronic obstructive pulmonary disease. Clin Physiol Funct Imaging. 2012;32(1):12–8. doi:10.1111/j.1475-097X.2011.01046.x.
69. Dirksen A, Piitulainen E, Parr DG, Deng C, Wencker M, Shaker SB, et al. Exploring the role of CT densitometry: a randomised study of augmentation therapy in alpha1-antitrypsin deficiency. Eur Respir J. 2009;33(6):1345–53. doi:10.1183/09031936.00159408.
70. Kim SS, Seo JB, Kim N, Chae EJ, Lee YK, Oh YM, et al. Improved correlation between CT emphysema quantification and pulmonary function test by density correction of volumetric CT data based on air and aortic density. Eur J Radiol. 2014;83(1):57–63. doi:10.1016/j.ejrad.2012.02.021.
71. Parr DG, Stoel BC, Stolk J, Nightingale PG, Stockley RA. Influence of calibration on densitometric studies of emphysema progression using computed tomography. Am J Respir Crit Care Med. 2004;170(8):883–90. doi:10.1164/rccm.200403-326OC.
72. Madani A, Van Muylem A, Gevenois PA. Pulmonary emphysema: effect of lung volume on objective quantification at thin-section CT. Radiology. 2010;257(1):260–8. doi:10.1148/radiol.10091446.
73. Grydeland TB, Dirksen A, Coxson HO, Pillai SG, Sharma S, Eide GE, et al. Quantitative computed tomography: emphysema and airway wall thickness by sex, age and smoking. Eur Respir J. 2009;34(4):858–65. doi:10.1183/09031936.00167908.
74. Camiciottoli G, Cavigli E, Grassi L, Diciotti S, Orlandi I, Zappa M, et al. Prevalence and correlates of pulmonary emphysema in smokers and former smokers. A densitometric study of participants in the ITALUNG trial. Eur Radiol. 2009;19(1):58–66. doi:10.1007/s00330-008-1131-6.
75. Ley-Zaporozhan J, Ley S, Kauczor HU. Morphological and functional imaging in COPD with CT and MRI: present and future. Eur Radiol. 2008;18(3):510–21. doi:10.1007/s00330-007-0772-1.

76. Bankier AA, O'Donnell CR, Mai VM, Storey P, De Maertelaer V, Edelman RR, et al. Impact of lung volume on MR signal intensity changes of the lung parenchyma. J Magn Reson Imaging. 2004;20(6):961–6. doi:10.1002/jmri.20198.
77. Rajaram S, Swift AJ, Capener D, Telfer A, Davies C, Hill C, et al. Lung morphology assessment with balanced steady-state free precession MR imaging compared with CT. Radiology. 2012;263(2):569–77. doi:10.1148/radiol.12110990.
78. Ley-Zaporozhan J, Ley S, Eberhardt R, Kauczor HU, Heussel CP. Visualization of morphological parenchymal changes in emphysema: comparison of different MRI sequences to 3D-HRCT. Eur J Radiol. 2010;73(1):43–9. doi:10.1016/j.ejrad.2008.09.029.
79. Ley-Zaporozhan J, Ley S, Kauczor HU. Proton MRI in COPD. COPD. 2007;4(1):55–65. doi:10.1080/15412550701198719.
80. Vogel-Claussen J, Renne J, Hinrichs J, Schonfeld C, Gutberlet M, Schaumann F, et al. Quantification of pulmonary inflammation after segmental allergen challenge using turbo-inversion recovery-magnitude magnetic resonance imaging. Am J Respir Crit Care Med. 2014;189(6):650–7. doi:10.1164/rccm.201310-1825OC.
81. Iwasawa T, Takahashi H, Ogura T, Asakura A, Gotoh T, Kagei S, et al. Correlation of lung parenchymal MR signal intensity with pulmonary function tests and quantitative computed tomography (CT) evaluation: a pilot study. J Magn Reson Imaging. 2007;26(6):1530–6. doi:10.1002/jmri.21183.
82. Mayo JR, MacKay A, Muller NL. MR imaging of the lungs: value of short TE spin-echo pulse sequences. AJR Am J Roentgenol. 1992;159(5):951–6. doi:10.2214/ajr.159.5.1414805.
83. Bergin CJ, Pauly JM, Macovski A. Lung parenchyma: projection reconstruction MR imaging. Radiology. 1991;179(3):777–81. doi:10.1148/radiology.179.3.2027991.
84. Ohno Y, Koyama H, Yoshikawa T, Matsumoto K, Takahashi M, Van Cauteren M, et al. T2* measurements of 3-T MRI with ultrashort TEs: capabilities of pulmonary function assessment and clinical stage classification in smokers. AJR Am J Roentgenol. 2011;197(2):W279–85. doi:10.2214/AJR.10.5350.
85. Takahashi M, Togao O, Obara M, van Cauteren M, Ohno Y, Doi S, et al. Ultra-short echo time (UTE) MR imaging of the lung: comparison between normal and emphysematous lungs in mutant mice. J Magn Reson Imaging. 2010;32(2):326–33. doi:10.1002/jmri.22267.
86. Johnson KM, Fain SB, Schiebler ML, Nagle S. Optimized 3D ultrashort echo time pulmonary MRI. Magn Reson Med. 2013;70(5):1241–50. doi:10.1002/mrm.24570.
87. Bianchi A, Ozier A, Ousova O, Raffard G, Cremillieux Y. Ultrashort-TE MRI longitudinal study and characterization of a chronic model of asthma in mice: inflammation and bronchial remodeling assessment. NMR Biomed. 2013;26(11):1451–9. doi:10.1002/nbm.2975.
88. Puderbach M, Eichinger M, Gahr J, Ley S, Tuengerthal S, Schmahl A, et al. Proton MRI appearance of cystic fibrosis: comparison to CT. Eur Radiol. 2007;17(3):716–24. doi:10.1007/s00330-006-0373-4.
89. Biederer J, Both M, Graessner J, Liess C, Jakob P, Reuter M, et al. Lung morphology: fast MR imaging assessment with a volumetric interpolated breath-hold technique: initial experience with patients. Radiology. 2003;226(1):242–9. doi:10.1148/radiol.2261011974.
90. Beckmann N, Cannet C, Zurbruegg S, Rudin M, Tigani B. Proton MRI of lung parenchyma reflects allergen-induced airway remodeling and endotoxin-aroused hyporesponsiveness: a step toward ventilation studies in spontaneously breathing rats. Magn Reson Med. 2004;52(2):258–68. doi:10.1002/mrm.20127.
91. Ogasawara N, Suga K, Zaki M, Okada M, Kawakami Y, Matsunaga N. Assessment of lung perfusion impairment in patients with pulmonary artery-occlusive and chronic obstructive pulmonary diseases with noncontrast electrocardiogram-gated fast-spin-echo perfusion MR imaging. J Magn Reson Imaging. 2004;20(4):601–11. doi:10.1002/jmri.20150.
92. Suga K, Ogasawara N, Okada M, Hara A, Matsunaga N. Potential of noncontrast electrocardiogram-gated half-fourier fast-spin-echo magnetic resonance imaging to monitor dynamically altered perfusion in regional lung. Investig Radiol. 2002;37(11):615–25. doi:10.1097/01.RLI.0000031079.78361.7D.
93. Hatabu H, Tadamura E, Levin DL, Chen Q, Li W, Kim D, et al. Quantitative assessment of pulmonary perfusion with dynamic contrast-enhanced MRI. Magn Reson Med. 1999;42(6):1033–8.
94. Levin DL, Chen Q, Zhang M, Edelman RR, Hatabu H. Evaluation of regional pulmonary perfusion using ultrafast magnetic resonance imaging. Magn Reson Med. 2001;46(1):166–71.
95. Keilholz SD, Mai VM, Berr SS, Fujiwara N, Hagspiel KD. Comparison of first-pass Gd-DOTA and FAIRER MR perfusion imaging in a rabbit model of pulmonary embolism. J Magn Reson Imaging. 2002;16(2):168–71. doi:10.1002/jmri.10138.
96. Korosec FR, Frayne R, Grist TM, Mistretta CA. Time-resolved contrast-enhanced 3D MR angiography. Magn Reson Med. 1996;36(3):345–51.
97. Fink C, Ley S, Kroeker R, Requardt M, Kauczor HU, Bock M. Time-resolved contrast-enhanced three-dimensional magnetic resonance angiography of the chest: combination of parallel imaging with view sharing (TREAT). Investig Radiol. 2005;40(1):40–8.
98. Fink C, Ley S, Risse F, Eichinger M, Zaporozhan J, Buhmann R, et al. Effect of inspiratory and expiratory breathhold on pulmonary perfusion: assessment by pulmonary perfusion magnetic resonance imaging. Investig Radiol. 2005;40(2):72–9.

99. Dehnert C, Risse F, Ley S, Kuder TA, Buhmann R, Puderbach M, et al. Magnetic resonance imaging of uneven pulmonary perfusion in hypoxia in humans. Am J Respir Crit Care Med. 2006;174(10):1132–8. doi:10.1164/rccm.200606-780OC.
100. Sergiacomi G, Sodani G, Fabiano S, Manenti G, Spinelli A, Konda D, et al. MRI lung perfusion 2D dynamic breath-hold technique in patients with severe emphysema. In Vivo. 2003;17(4):319–24.
101. Molinari F, Fink C, Risse F, Tuengerthal S, Bonomo L, Kauczor HU. Assessment of differential pulmonary blood flow using perfusion magnetic resonance imaging: comparison with radionuclide perfusion scintigraphy. Investig Radiol. 2006;41(8):624–30. doi:10.1097/01.rli.0000225399.65609.45.
102. Morino S, Toba T, Araki M, Azuma T, Tsutsumi S, Tao H, et al. Noninvasive assessment of pulmonary emphysema using dynamic contrast-enhanced magnetic resonance imaging. Exp Lung Res. 2006;32(1–2):55–67. doi:10.1080/01902140600691548.
103. Ley-Zaporozhan J, Ley S, Eberhardt R, Weinheimer O, Fink C, Puderbach M, et al. Assessment of the relationship between lung parenchymal destruction and impaired pulmonary perfusion on a lobar level in patients with emphysema. Eur J Radiol. 2007;63(1):76–83. doi:10.1016/j.ejrad.2007.01.020.
104. Jang YM, Oh YM, Seo JB, Kim N, Chae EJ, Lee YK, et al. Quantitatively assessed dynamic contrast-enhanced magnetic resonance imaging in patients with chronic obstructive pulmonary disease: correlation of perfusion parameters with pulmonary function test and quantitative computed tomography. Investig Radiol. 2008;43(6):403–10. doi:10.1097/RLI.0b013e31816901ab.
105. Ohno Y, Hatabu H, Murase K, Higashino T, Kawamitsu H, Watanabe H, et al. Quantitative assessment of regional pulmonary perfusion in the entire lung using three-dimensional ultrafast dynamic contrast-enhanced magnetic resonance imaging: preliminary experience in 40 subjects. J Magn Reson Imaging. 2004;20(3):353–65. doi:10.1002/jmri.20137.
106. Tadamura E, Hatabu H, Li W, Prasad PV, Edelman RR. Effect of oxygen inhalation on relaxation times in various tissues. J Magn Reson Imaging. 1997;7(1):220–5.
107. Brooks RA, Di Chiro G. Magnetic resonance imaging of stationary blood: a review. Med Phys. 1987;14(6):903–13.
108. Thulborn KR, Waterton JC, Matthews PM, Radda GK. Oxygenation dependence of the transverse relaxation time of water protons in whole blood at high field. Biochim Biophys Acta. 1982;714(2):265–70.
109. Ohno Y, Chen Q, Hatabu H. Oxygen-enhanced magnetic resonance ventilation imaging of lung. Eur J Radiol. 2001;37(3):164–71.
110. Bauman G, Eichinger M. Ventilation and perfusion magnetic resonance imaging of the lung. Pol J Radiol. 2012;77(1):37–46.
111. Ohno Y, Hatabu H. Basics concepts and clinical applications of oxygen-enhanced MR imaging. Eur J Radiol. 2007;64(3):320–8. doi:10.1016/j.ejrad.2007.08.006.
112. Ohno Y, Hatabu H, Takenaka D, Van Cauteren M, Fujii M, Sugimura K. Dynamic oxygen-enhanced MRI reflects diffusing capacity of the lung. Magn Reson Med. 2002;47(6):1139–44. doi:10.1002/mrm.10168.
113. Ohno Y, Hatabu H, Takenaka D, Adachi S, Van Cauteren M, Sugimura K. Oxygen-enhanced MR ventilation imaging of the lung: preliminary clinical experience in 25 subjects. AJR Am J Roentgenol. 2001;177(1):185–94. doi:10.2214/ajr.177.1.1770185.
114. Kirby M, Mathew L, Wheatley A, Santyr GE, McCormack DG, Parraga G. Chronic obstructive pulmonary disease: longitudinal hyperpolarized (3) He MR imaging. Radiology. 2010;256(1):280–9. doi:10.1148/radiol.10091937.
115. Kaushik SS, Cleveland ZI, Cofer GP, Metz G, Beaver D, Nouls J, et al. Diffusion-weighted hyperpolarized 129Xe MRI in healthy volunteers and subjects with chronic obstructive pulmonary disease. Magn Reson Med. 2011;65(4):1154–65. doi:10.1002/mrm.22697.
116. Altes TA, Salerno M. Hyperpolarized gas MR imaging of the lung. J Thorac Imaging. 2004;19(4):250–8.
117. de Lange EE, Altes TA, Patrie JT, Gaare JD, Knake JJ, Mugler JP III, et al. Evaluation of asthma with hyperpolarized helium-3 MRI: correlation with clinical severity and spirometry. Chest. 2006;130(4):1055–62. doi:10.1378/chest.130.4.1055.
118. van Beek EJ, Wild JM, Kauczor HU, Schreiber W, Mugler JP III, de Lange EE. Functional MRI of the lung using hyperpolarized 3-helium gas. J Magn Reson Imaging. 2004;20(4):540–54. doi:10.1002/jmri.20154.
119. Frahm J, Haase A, Matthaei D. Rapid NMR imaging of dynamic processes using the FLASH technique. Magn Reson Med. 1986;3(2):321–7.
120. Bock M. Simultaneous T2* and diffusion measurements with 3He. Magn Reson Med. 1997;38(6):890–5.
121. Salerno M, Altes TA, Brookeman JR, de Lange EE, Mugler JP III. Dynamic spiral MRI of pulmonary gas flow using hyperpolarized (3)He: preliminary studies in healthy and diseased lungs. Magn Reson Med. 2001;46(4):667–77.
122. Deninger AJ, Eberle B, Ebert M, Grossmann T, Heil W, Kauczor H, et al. Quantification of regional intrapulmonary oxygen partial pressure evolution during apnea by (3)He MRI. J Magn Reson. 1999;141(2):207–16. doi:10.1006/jmre.1999.1902.
123. Deninger AJ, Eberle B, Bermuth J, Escat B, Markstaller K, Schmiedeskamp J, et al. Assessment of a single-acquisition imaging sequence for oxygen-sensitive (3)He-MRI. Magn Reson Med. 2002;47(1):105–14.
124. van Beek EJ, Dahmen AM, Stavngaard T, Gast KK, Heussel CP, Krummenauer F, et al. Hyperpolarised 3He MRI versus HRCT in COPD and normal volunteers: PHIL trial. Eur Respir J. 2009;34(6):1311–21. doi:10.1183/09031936.00138508.

125. Kirby M, Svenningsen S, Owrangi A, Wheatley A, Farag A, Ouriadov A, et al. Hyperpolarized 3He and 129Xe MR imaging in healthy volunteers and patients with chronic obstructive pulmonary disease. Radiology. 2012;265(2):600–10. doi:10.1148/radiol.12120485.
126. Swift AJ, Wild JM, Fichele S, Woodhouse N, Fleming S, Waterhouse J, et al. Emphysematous changes and normal variation in smokers and COPD patients using diffusion 3He MRI. Eur J Radiol. 2005;54(3):352–8. doi:10.1016/j.ejrad.2004.08.002.
127. Salerno M, de Lange EE, Altes TA, Truwit JD, Brookeman JR, Mugler JP III. Emphysema: hyperpolarized helium 3 diffusion MR imaging of the lungs compared with spirometric indexes—initial experience. Radiology. 2002;222(1):252–60. doi:10.1148/radiol.2221001834.
128. Hermosillo G, Chefd'Hotel C, Faugeras O. Variational methods for multimodal image matching. Int J Comput Vision. 2002;50(3):329–43. doi:10.1023/A:1020830525823.
129. Bauman G, Puderbach M, Deimling M, Jellus V, Chefd'hotel C, Dinkel J, et al. Non-contrast-enhanced perfusion and ventilation assessment of the human lung by means of fourier decomposition in proton MRI. Magn Reson Med. 2009;62(3):656–64. doi:10.1002/mrm.22031.
130. Suga K, Ogasawara N, Okada M, Tsukuda T, Matsunaga N, Miyazaki M. Lung perfusion impairments in pulmonary embolic and airway obstruction with noncontrast MR imaging. J Appl Physiol. 2002;92(6):2439–51. doi:10.1152/japplphysiol.00900.2001.
131. Bauman G, Lutzen U, Ullrich M, Gaass T, Dinkel J, Elke G, et al. Pulmonary functional imaging: qualitative comparison of Fourier decomposition MR imaging with SPECT/CT in porcine lung. Radiology. 2011;260(2):551–9. doi:10.1148/radiol.11102313.
132. Gierada DS, Curtin JJ, Erickson SJ, Prost RW, Strandt JA, Goodman LR. Diaphragmatic motion: fast gradient-recalled-echo MR imaging in healthy subjects. Radiology. 1995;194(3):879–84. doi:10.1148/radiology.194.3.7862995.
133. Suga K, Tsukuda T, Awaya H, Takano K, Koike S, Matsunaga N, et al. Impaired respiratory mechanics in pulmonary emphysema: evaluation with dynamic breathing MRI. J Magn Reson Imaging. 1999;10(4):510–20.
134. Iwasawa T, Takahashi H, Ogura T, Asakura A, Gotoh T, Shibata H, et al. Influence of the distribution of emphysema on diaphragmatic motion in patients with chronic obstructive pulmonary disease. Jpn J Radiol. 2011;29(4):256–64. doi:10.1007/s11604-010-0552-8.
135. Iwasawa T, Yoshiike Y, Saito K, Kagei S, Gotoh T, Matsubara S. Paradoxical motion of the hemidiaphragm in patients with emphysema. J Thorac Imaging. 2000;15(3):191–5.
136. Millner MR, McDavid WD, Waggener RG, Dennis MJ, Payne WH, Sank VJ. Extraction of information from CT scans at different energies. Med Phys. 1979;6(1):70–1.
137. Rutherford RA, Pullan BR, Isherwood I. X-ray energies for effective atomic number determination. Neuroradiology. 1976;11(1):23–8.
138. Barbera JA, Riverola A, Roca J, Ramirez J, Wagner PD, Ros D, et al. Pulmonary vascular abnormalities and ventilation-perfusion relationships in mild chronic obstructive pulmonary disease. Am J Respir Crit Care Med. 1994;149(2 Pt 1):423–9. doi:10.1164/ajrccm.149.2.8306040.
139. Hale KA, Niewoehner DE, Cosio MG. Morphologic changes in the muscular pulmonary arteries: relationship to cigarette smoking, airway disease, and emphysema. Am Rev Respir Dis. 1980;122(2):273–8.
140. Peinado VI, Barbera JA, Ramirez J, Gomez FP, Roca J, Jover L, et al. Endothelial dysfunction in pulmonary arteries of patients with mild COPD. Am J Phys. 1998;274(6 Pt 1):L908–13.
141. Barbera JA, Roca J, Ferrer A, Felez MA, Diaz O, Roger N, et al. Mechanisms of worsening gas exchange during acute exacerbations of chronic obstructive pulmonary disease. Eur Respir J. 1997;10(6):1285–91.
142. Sandek K, Bratel T, Hellstrom G, Lagerstrand L. Ventilation-perfusion inequality and carbon dioxide sensitivity in hypoxaemic chronic obstructive pulmonary disease (COPD) and effects of 6 months of long-term oxygen treatment (LTOT). Clin Physiol. 2001;21(5):584–93.
143. Fuld MK, Halaweish AF, Haynes SE, Divekar AA, Guo J, Hoffman EA. Pulmonary perfused blood volume with dual-energy CT as surrogate for pulmonary perfusion assessed with dynamic multidetector CT. Radiology. 2013;267(3):747–56. doi:10.1148/radiol.12112789.
144. Barbera JA, Peinado VI, Santos S. Pulmonary hypertension in chronic obstructive pulmonary disease. Eur Respir J. 2003;21(5):892–905.
145. Ley S, Puderbach M, Fink C, Eichinger M, Plathow C, Teiner S, et al. Assessment of hemodynamic changes in the systemic and pulmonary arterial circulation in patients with cystic fibrosis using phase-contrast MRI. Eur Radiol. 2005;15(8):1575–80. doi:10.1007/s00330-005-2721-1.
146. Alford SK, van Beek EJ, McLennan G, Hoffman EA. Heterogeneity of pulmonary perfusion as a mechanistic image-based phenotype in emphysema susceptible smokers. Proc Natl Acad Sci U S A. 2010;107(16):7485–90. doi:10.1073/pnas.0913880107.
147. Pansini V, Remy-Jardin M, Faivre JB, Schmidt B, Dejardin-Bothelo A, Perez T, et al. Assessment of lobar perfusion in smokers according to the presence and severity of emphysema: preliminary experience with dual-energy CT angiography. Eur Radiol. 2009;19(12):2834–43. doi:10.1007/s00330-009-1475-6.

148. Lee CW, Seo JB, Lee Y, Chae EJ, Kim N, Lee HJ, et al. A pilot trial on pulmonary emphysema quantification and perfusion mapping in a single-step using contrast-enhanced dual-energy computed tomography. Investig Radiol. 2012;47(1):92–7. doi:10.1097/RLI.0b013e318228359a.
149. Chandra D, Lipson DA, Hoffman EA, Hansen-Flaschen J, Sciurba FC, Decamp MM, et al. Perfusion scintigraphy and patient selection for lung volume reduction surgery. Am J Respir Crit Care Med. 2010;182(7):937–46. doi:10.1164/rccm.201001-0043OC.
150. Park TS, Hong Y, Lee JS, Lee SM, Seo JB, Oh YM, et al. Efficacy of bronchoscopic lung volume reduction by endobronchial valves in patients with heterogeneous emphysema: report on the first Asian cases. J Korean Med Sci. 2014;29(10):1404–10. doi:10.3346/jkms.2014.29.10.1404.
151. Gur D, Drayer BP, Borovetz HS, Griffith BP, Hardesty RL, Wolfson SK. Dynamic computed tomography of the lung: regional ventilation measurements. J Comput Assist Tomogr. 1979;3(6):749–53.
152. Herbert DL, Gur D, Shabason L, Good WF, Rinaldo JE, Snyder JV, et al. Mapping of human local pulmonary ventilation by xenon enhanced computed tomography. J Comput Assist Tomogr. 1982;6(6):1088–93.
153. Chae EJ, Seo JB, Goo HW, Kim N, Song KS, Lee SD, et al. Xenon ventilation CT with a dual-energy technique of dual-source CT: initial experience. Radiology. 2008;248(2):615–24. doi:10.1148/radiol.2482071482.
154. Park EA, Goo JM, Park SJ, Lee HJ, Lee CH, Park CM, et al. Chronic obstructive pulmonary disease: quantitative and visual ventilation pattern analysis at xenon ventilation CT performed by using a dual-energy technique. Radiology. 2010;256(3):985–97. doi:10.1148/radiol.10091502.
155. Chae EJ, Seo JB, Lee J, Kim N, Goo HW, Lee HJ, et al. Xenon ventilation imaging using dual-energy computed tomography in asthmatics: initial experience. Investig Radiol. 2010;45(6):354–61. doi:10.1097/RLI.0b013e3181dfdae0.
156. Goo HW, Yu J. Redistributed regional ventilation after the administration of a bronchodilator demonstrated on xenon-inhaled dual-energy CT in a patient with asthma. Korean J Radiol. 2011;12(3):386–9. doi:10.3348/kjr.2011.12.3.386.
157. Kim WW, Lee CH, Goo JM, Park SJ, Kim JH, Park EA, et al. Xenon-enhanced dual-energy CT of patients with asthma: dynamic ventilation changes after methacholine and salbutamol inhalation. AJR Am J Roentgenol. 2012;199(5):975–81. doi:10.2214/AJR.11.7624.
158. Park SJ, Lee CH, Goo JM, Kim JH, Park EA, Jung JW, et al. Quantitative analysis of dynamic airway changes after methacholine and salbutamol inhalation on xenon-enhanced chest CT. Eur Radiol. 2012;22(11):2441–50. doi:10.1007/s00330-012-2516-0.
159. Hachulla AL, Pontana F, Wemeau-Stervinou L, Khung S, Faivre JB, Wallaert B, et al. Krypton ventilation imaging using dual-energy CT in chronic obstructive pulmonary disease patients: initial experience. Radiology. 2012;263(1):253–9. doi:10.1148/radiol.12111211.
160. Honda N, Osada H, Watanabe W, Nakayama M, Nishimura K, Krauss B, et al. Imaging of ventilation with dual-energy CT during breath hold after single vital-capacity inspiration of stable xenon. Radiology. 2012;262(1):262–8. doi:10.1148/radiol.11110569.
161. Thieme SF, Hoegl S, Nikolaou K, Fisahn J, Irlbeck M, Maxien D, et al. Pulmonary ventilation and perfusion imaging with dual-energy CT. Eur Radiol. 2010;20(12):2882–9. doi:10.1007/s00330-010-1866-8.
162. Zhang LJ, Zhou CS, Schoepf UJ, Sheng HX, Wu SY, Krazinski AW, et al. Dual-energy CT lung ventilation/perfusion imaging for diagnosing pulmonary embolism. Eur Radiol. 2013;23(10):2666–75. doi:10.1007/s00330-013-2907-x.
163. Noma S, Moskowitz GW, Herman PG, Khan A, Rojas KA. Pulmonary scintigraphy in elastase-induced emphysema in pigs. Correlation with high-resolution computed tomography and histology. Investig Radiol. 1992;27(6):429–35.
164. Suga K, Kawakami Y, Iwanaga H, Hayashi N, Seto A, Matsunaga N. Assessment of anatomic relation between pulmonary perfusion and morphology in pulmonary emphysema with breath-hold SPECT-CT fusion images. Ann Nucl Med. 2008;22(5):339–47. doi:10.1007/s12149-007-0137-5.
165. Argula RG, Strange C, Ramakrishnan V, Goldin J. Baseline regional perfusion impacts exercise response to endobronchial valve therapy in advanced pulmonary emphysema. Chest. 2013;144(5):1578–86. doi:10.1378/chest.12-2826.
166. Stavngaard T, Sogaard LV, Mortensen J, Hanson LG, Schmiedeskamp J, Berthelsen AK, et al. Hyperpolarized 3He MRI and 81mKr SPECT in chronic obstructive pulmonary disease. Eur J Nucl Med Mol Imaging. 2005;32(4):448–57. doi:10.1007/s00259-004-1691-x.
167. Suga K, Nishigauchi K, Kume N, Koike S, Takano K, Tokuda O, et al. Dynamic pulmonary SPECT of xenon-133 gas washout. J Nucl Med. 1996;37(5):807–14.
168. Amis TC, Crawford AB, Davison A, Engel LA. Distribution of inhaled 99mtechnetium labelled ultrafine carbon particle aerosol (Technegas) in human lungs. Eur Respir J. 1990;3(6):679–85.
169. Crawford AB, Davison A, Amis TC, Engel LA. Intrapulmonary distribution of 99mtechnetium labelled ultrafine carbon aerosol (Technegas) in severe airflow obstruction. Eur Respir J. 1990;3(6):686–92.
170. Cukic V, Begic A. Potential role of lung ventilation scintigraphy in the assessment of COPD. Acta Inform Med. 2014;22(3):170–3. doi:10.5455/aim.2014.22.170-173.

171. Xu J, Moonen M, Johansson A, Gustafsson A, Bake B. Quantitative analysis of inhomogeneity in ventilation SPET. Eur J Nucl Med. 2001;28(12):1795–800. doi:10.1007/s002590100649.
172. Jogi J, Ekberg M, Jonson B, Bozovic G, Bajc M. Ventilation/perfusion SPECT in chronic obstructive pulmonary disease: an evaluation by reference to symptoms, spirometric lung function and emphysema, as assessed with HRCT. Eur J Nucl Med Mol Imaging. 2011;38(7):1344–52. doi:10.1007/s00259-011-1757-5.
173. Suga K, Kawakami Y, Koike H, Iwanaga H, Tokuda O, Okada M, et al. Lung ventilation-perfusion imbalance in pulmonary emphysema: assessment with automated V/Q quotient SPECT. Ann Nucl Med. 2010;24(4):269–77. doi:10.1007/s12149-010-0369-7.
174. Vidal Melo MF, Winkler T, Harris RS, Musch G, Greene RE, Venegas JG. Spatial heterogeneity of lung perfusion assessed with (13)N PET as a vascular biomarker in chronic obstructive pulmonary disease. J Nucl Med. 2010;51(1):57–65. doi:10.2967/jnumed.109.065185.
175. Gan WQ, Man SF, Senthilselvan A, Sin DD. Association between chronic obstructive pulmonary disease and systemic inflammation: a systematic review and a meta-analysis. Thorax. 2004;59(7):574–80.
176. Karadag F, Karul AB, Cildag O, Yilmaz M, Ozcan H. Biomarkers of systemic inflammation in stable and exacerbation phases of COPD. Lung. 2008;186(6):403–9. doi:10.1007/s00408-008-9106-6.
177. Sinden NJ, Stockley RA. Systemic inflammation and comorbidity in COPD: a result of 'overspill' of inflammatory mediators from the lungs? Review of the evidence. Thorax. 2010;65(10):930–6. doi:10.1136/thx.2009.130260.
178. Jones HA, Marino PS, Shakur BH, Morrell NW. In vivo assessment of lung inflammatory cell activity in patients with COPD and asthma. Eur Respir J. 2003;21(4):567–73.
179. Subramanian DR, Jenkins L, Edgar R, Quraishi N, Stockley RA, Parr DG. Assessment of pulmonary neutrophilic inflammation in emphysema by quantitative positron emission tomography. Am J Respir Crit Care Med. 2012;186(11):1125–32. doi:10.1164/rccm.201201-0051OC.
180. Coulson JM, Rudd JH, Duckers JM, Rees JI, Shale DJ, Bolton CE, et al. Excessive aortic inflammation in chronic obstructive pulmonary disease: an 18F-FDG PET pilot study. J Nucl Med. 2010;51(9):1357–60. doi:10.2967/jnumed.110.075903.
181. Coxson HO, Quiney B, Sin DD, Xing L, McWilliams AM, Mayo JR, et al. Airway wall thickness assessed using computed tomography and optical coherence tomography. Am J Respir Crit Care Med. 2008;177(11):1201–6. doi:10.1164/rccm.200712-1776OC.

Biomarkers of COPD

9

Ho Il Yoon

Introduction

Chronic obstructive pulmonary disease (COPD) is a major health burden across the world. Globally, more than 300 million people suffer from COPD [1] and nearly three million die each year from this disease [2]. COPD mortality continues to climb at an alarming rate, such that by 2030, nearly nine million people will die annually from COPD [3]. The economic burden of COPD is also enormous. In the United States alone, COPD accounted for $20.9 billion USD in direct and $7.4 billion USD in indirect costs in 2004 [4]. Regrettably, the pipeline for new drugs for COPD is relatively dry compared to other major causes of mortality such as HIV/AIDs, cancer, and diabetes [5]. One major barrier to drug discovery in COPD is the paucity of well-accepted and well-validated biomarkers. Currently, the only "marker" that is widely accepted by regulatory agencies for new drug approval in COPD is FEV_1 (forced expiratory volume in 1 s), which is a robust measure of lung function. However, COPD is defined operationally as a chronic respiratory condition that results in airflow limitation which is progressive and not fully reversible [6]. In other words, COPD is defined by limited reversibility of FEV_1, making this endpoint unsuitable for drug discovery in COPD. The discovery of a validated, reliable, robust, and reproducible blood biomarker would provide a major boost to the development of novel compounds because it would allow investigators (and companies) to demonstrate the therapeutic promise of a drug in small (usually phase II) trials before proceeding to a much more expensive and logistically difficult phase III trials. Without such data, pharmaceutical companies are hesitant to invest millions of dollars on large phase III studies to bring compounds to market. For this reason, some international companies have recently abandoned COPD drug development altogether, while many others have scaled back their efforts significantly. The purpose of this chapter is to review potential biomarkers of COPD, especially those that could be used in predicting treatment responses.

Sources of Biomarkers

Biomarkers can originate from any organ. However, because COPD is predominantly a lung disease, the airways are the most logical source for identifying novel biomarkers in COPD. There are three major sources of airway samples. They include sputum (spontaneous or induced), exhaled gases or condensates, or bronchial washes or brushes. The latter source requires bronchoscopy, which is invasive. Thus, repeated measurements are usually not feasible. Furthermore, bronchial

HI. Yoon
Seoul National University Bundang Hospital,
Seongnam, South Korea
e-mail: dextro@snubh.org

S.-D. Lee (ed.), *COPD*, DOI 10.1007/978-3-662-47178-4_9

sampling is limited to one or two airways, which may result in sampling error because the human lung contains more than 40,000 terminal bronchioles [7]. For these and other reasons, bronchoscopic samples have not been used for biomarker discovery in COPD and will not be discussed any further in this chapter.

Both spontaneous and induced sputum and exhaled gases and condensates also have methodological challenges that limit their utility as a source of biomarker discovery. For example, induced sputum is hard to process and may contain contaminants such as saliva that makes it difficult to relate sputum findings to the pathophysiological processes that are occurring in the lungs [8]. Exhaled gases and more recently condensates have been used to identify novel biomarkers in COPD. However, the data to date have been variable and inconsistent, owing to lack of standardization of methods and heterogeneity in the techniques employed for sample collection and analysis [9] and the fact that most proteins are unpredictable or below the lower limit of quantification [10]. Nevertheless, these sources are commonly used for biomarker discovery in COPD because they are readily accessible and noninvasive.

Other than its sources, different criteria can be used to classify biomarkers of COPD. These can be by the biological process where they are modified, by purposes of which they can be used in the clinical field, and sometimes by the association with tobacco smoke. In effect, the respiratory biomarkers could be classified to five categories in relation to their association with exposure to tobacco smoke and/or with COPD [11]: (1) biomarkers of response to tobacco smoke exposure, associated with COPD activity, which are expressed at higher levels in healthy smokers than in non-smokers and at higher levels in COPD than in healthy smokers; (2) biomarkers of COPD inflammation whose expression level is not associated with tobacco smoke exposure, as it is higher in COPD patients than in controls, with no significant differences between healthy smokers and non-smokers; (3) biomarkers of response to tobacco smoke exposure, not associated with COPD activity; (4) biomarkers negatively associated with COPD and/or tobacco smoke exposure; and (5) molecules variably associated with COPD and/or tobacco smoke.

In addition, it would be crucial to differentiate biomarkers in terms of their reproducibility within and across laboratories and platforms to identify its relevance despite technical differences [12].

Sputum Neutrophils

By far, induced sputum has been the most popular source of biomarker discovery in COPD. Sputum contains a mixture of mucins (approximately 2–4% of the total weight), salts, tissue plasma, lipids, and inflammatory cells from tissue and airway lumen, microbial products, cellular debris, and inhaled particles from the environment [8]. The predominant mucins in sputum are MUC5B and MUC5AC [8]. Induced sputum is an attractive source of biomarker discovery because it is relatively noninvasive to obtain even in subjects who do not spontaneously expectorate and may reflect the inflammatory process in the airways. However, there are several challenges in identifying possible biomarkers in sputum. These include (1) the use of liquefaction agents such as DTT (dithiothreitol) or NAC (N-acetylcysteine), which may disturb or interfere with protein measurements in sputum; (2) the lack of consistent marker that can be used to normalize sputum data. This makes it difficult to compare results across subjects and across studies; (3) contamination of sputum by saliva, which may obscure biomarkers in sputum samples (largely by dilution); and (4) lack of standardization in the collection and processing of samples and in data analysis. Furthermore, the source of the induced sputum is likely the large (central) airways and not the small peripheral airways, which are thought to be the major site of disease in COPD [7]. The use of spontaneous sputum has similar issues but is more likely to reflect increased inflammation and can be sampled on a sequential basis reducing variability [13].

Notwithstanding these limitations, sputums have been used for biomarker discovery because they can be procured noninvasively and some components of sputum may reflect the active inflammatory process in the airways of COPD patients. One such biomarker is the neutrophil count in induced sputum. It is an attractive biomarker in COPD because neutrophils are thought to play an important role in the pathogenesis of COPD [14, 15], secreting various cytokines that provoke and perpetuate lung inflammation [16, 17]. Furthermore, neutrophils are easily measurable in sputum of COPD patients [18]. With smoking and with COPD progression, the sputum contains increasing percentages of neutrophils [19]. Interestingly, once COPD is firmly established, neutrophil count remains elevated even following smoking cessation [20]. Most importantly, elevated expression of sputum neutrophils has been associated with rapid decline in FEV_1, highlighting the importance of neutrophils in COPD pathogenesis [21]. However, the relationship between the neutrophil count and percent neutrophils is exponential and absolute count may therefore be more relevant.

Neutrophil counts in sputum have also been used as a biomarker to evaluate well-established COPD drugs. For instance, in the study by Barnes et al., sputum neutrophil count was used as a co-primary endpoint to evaluate the possible efficacy of fluticasone/salmeterol combination in the treatment of COPD [22]. Over 3 months, they did not find a significant change in sputum neutrophil count between fluticasone/salmeterol combination and placebo [22]. This was surprising as fluticasone/salmeterol combination has been shown to reduce the rate of COPD progression (albeit marginally) in patients with established COPD [23] suggesting the study may have been underpowered [13]. Similarly, Laperre et al. evaluated the effects of fluticasone alone and in combination with salmeterol on a variety of different outcomes included sputum neutrophil count. They showed that at 30 months of therapy, the group that received fluticasone had significantly lower sputum neutrophil count than did the placebo group [24]. On the other hand, salmeterol by itself had no significant effect on sputum neutrophilia [24]. These data are consistent with a meta-analysis published in 2005, showing that inhaled corticosteroid therapy for at least 6 weeks results in a significant reduction in sputum neutrophil count in patients with stable COPD [25]. Together, these studies validate the concept of using sputum neutrophilia as a biomarker to evaluate "neutrophilic" airway inflammation in patients with COPD.

Recently, several investigators have applied this biomarker to evaluate emerging (new) therapies in COPD. For instance, He and colleagues used sputum neutrophil count to assess the possible beneficial effects of erythromycin on airway inflammation [10]. In this randomized controlled trial, they found that erythromycin (at 125 mg three times per day) significantly reduced sputum neutrophilia by 3 months and interestingly also reduced the risk of exacerbations suggesting anti-inflammatory and/or antibacterial effects [10]. Ford and colleagues used sputum neutrophils to assess the possible benefits of low-dose theophylline in the management of COPD patients. Thirty patients with COPD were treated with placebo theophylline capsules plus either inhaled fluticasone propionate (500 microg bid) or inhaled placebo for 4 weeks in a double-dummy, randomized, double-blind, parallel study. Then following a two-week-washout period, patients were given active theophylline. However, contrary to expectations, they found that combination treatment with fluticasone and theophylline did not reduce total sputum neutrophils [13]. However, in another study, 8 weeks of low-dose theophylline therapy was associated with reduced sputum neutrophil count [26]. Sputum neutrophil count has also been used as a primary endpoint in clinical studies evaluating promising but not yet approved COPD drugs. For example, Gronke et al. used sputum neutrophils as a proof of concept that leukotriene B4 receptor antagonist, which in vitro and in animal studies decreased neutrophil recruitment to the lungs, unfortunately the study proved negative in COPD [27].

Although neutrophil counts in sputum have been widely used to assess possible therapeutic benefits of drugs for COPD, it has not been fully validated as a biomarker in COPD because sputum neutrophil measurements are only weakly associated with FEV_1 or with health status [28] and there have been no large-scale studies that have demonstrated its utility in predicting important health outcomes in COPD such as exacerbation or mortality [28]. Furthermore, despite the implication of neutrophils in the pathogenesis of emphysema, sputum neutrophils do not appear to correlate with the extent of emphysema in COPD patients [28] which seems to be natural because sputum neutrophil mainly reflects conditions of large airways not of lung parenchyma.

Other Sputum Biomarkers

There are other cellular elements in induced sputum that have been used as possible biomarkers in COPD. These include total cell count and sputum eosinophil and lymphocyte counts [25, 29]. The long-term use of inhaled corticosteroids has been shown to reduce total cell and lymphocyte counts, and eosinophilia in induced sputum [25]. However, as with sputum neutrophilia, none of these measurements has been consistently shown to predict important health outcomes in COPD. As such, their usefulness as biomarkers in COPD remains uncertain.

Some investigators have used supernatants from induced sputum to measure levels of inflammatory and oxidative molecules, which have been implicated in COPD pathogenesis. These include interleukin (IL)-8, IL-6, myeloperoxidase, and matrix metalloproteinases (MMP)-9. However, as with cellular components of induced sputum, the relationship of these inflammatory and oxidative stress molecules in sputum to health outcomes such as COPD progression and mortality has not been well established.

Fraction of Exhaled Nitric Oxide (FENO)

Given these limitations of induced sputum, there has been growing enthusiasm for developing exhaled gases as biomarkers in COPD [30]. Of these, the best studied has been FENO [31]. In general, FENO shows good specificity as a diagnostic marker in asthma [32] and a useful biomarker in assessing severity and control [33] and in evaluating treatment responses, especially to inhaled corticosteroids [34, 35]. The data in COPD are more scarce and generally less impressive. Levels of FENO are usually normal or only modestly elevated in COPD, except during exacerbations [36–38] and have not been demonstrated to predict important health outcomes in COPD. Thus, FENO is not a promising biomarker in COPD. However, with recent innovations in FENO measurements, there is renewed optimism of using FENO as a biomarker in COPD. One such modification is multiple exhalation flow technique (MEFT), which allows separate measurement of NO derived from small airways and alveoli (called corrected alveolar nitric oxide (CALV)) from those of larger airways. The subdivision of FENO into small and large airway compartments is very attractive in COPD as COPD is thought to involve largely the small airways and lung parenchyma. A recent study showed that CALV was elevated in COPD patients but disappointingly, it was not associated with COPD severity or smoking status of the patients [39]. Furthermore, CALV was not affected by inhaled corticosteroid treatment [39]. Additional work will be needed to understand the value, if any, that FENO has in COPD.

Other Exhaled Biomarkers

There are a number of other potential biomarkers from exhaled breath condensate (EBC). EBC pH is an acidification marker and was reported to be lower in smokers and COPD than in control nonsmokers. But it failed to differentiate COPD from smokers without COPD, to relate to disease severity, and to reflect response to corticosteroids [40]. Concentrations of leukotriene B4 (LTB4) and 8-isoprostane, markers of inflammation and oxidative stress, respectively, were known to increase in COPD exacerbations and decrease after antibiotic treatment [41]. LTB4 was further reported to contribute to neutrophil chemotactic activity [42]. Another oxidative stress marker, hydrogen peroxide, reflected level of oxidative stress in patients with COPD after exercise, but its performance in terms of therapeutic response biomarker is unknown yet [43].

Desmosine/Isodesmosine

While the pathogenesis of COPD is complex and poorly understood, there is some agreement that excess breakdown and turnover of extracellular matrix in the lungs is likely to be very important for the emphysema phenotype of COPD [44]. The extracellular matrix in the lungs acts as a three-dimensional scaffold, providing strength and support for the alveolar units. The extracellular matrix consists mostly of collagens (type 1 and 3), which provide tensile strength, elastin, which confers flexibility to the lung tissues and glycosaminoglycans [45]. In the normal lungs, the collagen fibers tightly wrap around elastic bands in an orderly manner. However, in COPD, this structure is disrupted, leading to a "random" distribution of collagen and elastic fibers [46]. Furthermore, with COPD disease progression, the ratio of collagen to elastin surrounding the alveolar units becomes distorted, owing largely to a severe loss in elastin [46]. The functional consequence is a loss in elastic recoil pressure and "floppy" airways. Consistent with these observations, deletion of the elastin gene in mice results in emphysematous changes in the lungs and mutations in the elastin gene in humans (e.g., cutix laxa) have been associated with severe early onset emphysema [47, 48].

Based on these and other findings, there has been some interest in using markers of elastin turnover as possible biomarkers in COPD. Of these, the best studied have been desmosine and isodesmosine [49]. Because these proteins are present only in mature elastin, it is thought that their expression in blood, urine, or sputum mostly reflects elastin degradation [50]. Consistent with this theory, injection of pancreatic elastase into animals leads to an acute loss of elastin and emphysematous changes in the lungs. Degradation of elastic fibers in the lungs in turn can be detected in the urine in the form of desmosine [51]. These changes have also been noted in mice exposed to acute cigarette smoke [52]. Interestingly, mice which are deficient in TNF-α or its receptors are protected against elastic fiber degradation and their urinary desmosine excretion is relatively normal in the presence of cigarette smoke. These mice are also relatively protected against smoking-induced emphysematous changes in the lungs [52, 53].

Blood desmosine levels were reported to be elevated in stable COPD patients compared to healthy control and asthma patients. It was found to be in negative relation with lung diffusing capacity. Moreover, urinary desmosine levels were reported to be elevated in exacerbations. [54] Human data, recently reviewed by Luisetti et al. [49], have been more mixed and less optimistic with some study showing a significant relationship of urinary (or plasma) desmosine/isodesmosine to COPD, while others failing to demonstrate this relationship. The heterogeneity in the human data reflects in part major differences in the modalities of measurement (e.g., immunoassays versus high-performance liquid chromatography), the biological source of assays (e.g., urine versus plasma), and the underlying clinical characteristics of the patients across the studies. Furthermore, most of the human studies to date have been relatively small in scope and did not consider the large variations in the phenotypes of the patients. Recently, ECLIPSE (Evaluation of COPD Longitudinally to Identify Predictive Surrogate Endpoints) investigators reported association between serum desmosine level and cardiovascular mortality in COPD, not emphysema progression [55]. Notwithstanding these limitations, the totality of data suggests that desmosine or isodesmosine is elevated in the urine of COPD patients [56–58].

Very few studies have evaluated these markers in therapeutic trials, demonstrating mixed results. For instance, a study by Stone and colleagues showed that short-term treatment with alpha-1-antrypsin replacement therapy led to significant reductions in urinary excretion of desmosine in two patients with severe COPD secondary to alpha-1-antitrypsin deficiency [59]. However, in another study, the use of alpha-1-antitrypsin replacement therapy did not modify urinary excretion of desmosine in these patients [60]. Ma and colleagues evaluated plasma, urine, and sputum expression of desmosine and isodesmosine related to the use of tiotropium, which is a long-acting muscarinic bronchodilator, and found that after 2 months of therapy, their expression decreased in COPD patients [61]. However, all of these studies contained very small sample sizes, which reduces the reliability of these reports. Thus, the possible role of desmosine or isodesmosine as biomarkers in COPD remains obscure. In a phase II trial, oral matrix metalloproteinase (MMP)-9 and -12 inhibitor has been shown to reduce urinary desmosine excretion [62]

PGP (Proline-Glycine-Proline), N-α-PGP

It is increasingly recognized that breakdown products of collagen in the lungs may be pro-inflammatory and exacerbate the inflammatory process in COPD, creating a vicious cycle. One such molecule produced by collagen metabolism is PGP. PGP shares structural homology with alpha chemokines and similarly to these chemokines induces the recruitment of neutrophils into lungs by stimulating CXCR-1 and most importantly, CXCR-2 receptors [63], which in turn augment the inflammatory cascade in the COPD lungs [64–66]. In mouse models, instillation of N-acetyl-Proline-Glycine-Proline (N-α-PGP) into the lungs of mice causes a marked recruitment of neutrophils to the airways and chronic airway exposure causes COPD-like pathology in the lungs characterized by alveolar enlargement and right ventricular hypertrophy [63]. Blockage of PGP using monoclonal antibody, on the other hand, suppresses both the in vitro chemotactic activity and in vivo recruitment of inflammatory cells into the lungs related to cigarette smoke [63, 67]. Additionally, treatment of these mice with a complementary peptide, L-arginine-threonine-arginine (RTR), which binds to PGP sequences, inhibits neutrophil infiltration and prevents development of pulmonary emphysema [68].

Could PGP or N-α-PGP be a useful biomarker in COPD? On the affirmative side, PGP is detectable in bronchoalveolar lavage samples of patients with COPD but not in control individuals [63]. Similarly, these markers are detectable in sputum samples of COPD patients but not in those of control subjects [69]. In serum, PGP levels are also significantly higher in COPD patients than in controls [69]. Interestingly, patients with cystic fibrosis also have increased PGP expression in sputum as in COPD, likely related to the intense neutrophilic inflammation observed in these conditions [64]. However, to date, PGP or N-α-PGP has not been associated with important health outcomes in COPD, and they have not been used in therapeutic trials. Thus, their possible role in evaluating new products in COPD is uncertain. In one study, levels of PGP in sputum were highest during exacerbation and azithromycin treatment lowered its levels [70]. Similarly, roflumilast has been reported to reduce sputum AcPGP by more than 50% in COPD patients with chronic bronchitis [71].

Leukotriene A4 Hydrolase (LTA4H)

Leukotriene A4 hydrolase (LTA4H) is an enzyme released from neutrophils and epithelial cells that generates leukotriene A4 (LTA4) via its hydrolase activity in the cytosol. LTA4 is a potent chemoattractant for neutrophils. LTA4H also has a peptidase activity. In the extracellular milieu, it degrades PGP or N-α-PGP, which, in turn, down-regulates neutrophilic inflammation. Interestingly, cigarette smoking inhibits the peptidase but not the hydrolase activity of LTA4H, thus up-regulating neutrophilic inflammation [72]. The balance between these two enzymatic activities of LTA4H may be important in determining the extent and duration of neutrophilic inflammation in the lungs of COPD patients.

Markers of Systemic Inflammation

Although biomarkers can be obtained from any organ, the most successful ones are from blood because blood is easy to obtain and its measurements can be standardized. Furthermore, with modern techniques, high throughput (and relatively inexpensive) assays can be developed for blood-based protein measurements. In COPD, there are no such blood biomarkers currently approved for use. Moreover, because blood samples are usually obtained in peripheral veins (e.g., antecubital fossa) and not from pulmonary veins or arteries, there is concern that blood biomarkers in COPD may not adequately reflect the disease activity (or severity) in the lungs, which are the primary sites of disease in COPD. Nevertheless, there is increasing evidence that the inflammatory process in the lungs "spill-over" into the systemic circulation, which may result in an "inflammatory signature" in blood related to COPD [73].

C-reactive Protein (CRP)

It is now well accepted that lung inflammation is an important component in the pathogenesis of COPD, and this inflammatory process carries over into the systemic circulation [73]. Accordingly, many groups of investigators are endeavoring to identify plasma proteins that are specific to the inflammatory process in COPD and relate these biomarkers to salient clinical health outcomes such as exacerbations and mortality. Of these, the best studied to date is C-reactive protein (CRP). CRP is a sensitive but not a specific marker of systemic inflammation and tissue damage. It has been extensively studied in patients with ischemic heart disease and other cardiovascular diseases (CVD) [74, 75] and has been shown to predict CVD morbidity and mortality. Importantly, CRP has also been shown to be a useful biomarker in guiding statin therapy for patients who do not have raised serum cholesterols [76].

CRP may also be useful in COPD [77]. Serum levels of CRP are associated with health status of COPD patients [78] and with all-cause, cardiovascular, and cancer-specific mortality [79]. Elevated levels are also associated with increased risk for hospitalization, comorbidity, and mortality from COPD [80, 81]. During acute exacerbations, CRP levels rise [82]. Oral glucocorticoid therapy (e.g., prednisone at 30 mg/d for 2 weeks) reduces serum CRP levels [83]. However, serum CRP is relatively insensitive to the effects of inhaled glucocorticoids [84, 85]. Thus, the role of CRP as a biomarker for therapeutic drugs in COPD remains uncertain.

Fibrinogen

Fibrinogen is another widely used biomarker of systemic inflammation. Plasma fibrinogen levels strongly associate with coronary heart disease (CHD), stroke, other vascular mortality, and nonvascular mortality [86]. They also predict future risk of moderate and severe exacerbations [87] and hospitalizations from COPD [88]. Moreover, serum levels of fibrinogen have been found to be related to mortality in COPD patients [89, 90]. However, plasma fibrinogen levels are not easily modifiable with medications [91, 92].

IL-6

The main up-stream regulator of CRP, fibrinogen, and other acute phase proteins such as serum amyloid A is interleukin (IL)-6 (93). IL-6, along with other primary inflammatory cytokines like TNF-α and IL-1β, responds to an acute insult by orchestrating and unleashing a cocktail of inflammatory mediators from the liver and other organs to contain the insult and protect the body from harm [93]. In the lungs, IL-6 is synthesized predominantly by alveolar macrophages and bronchial epithelial cells and is released in response to environmental triggers such as cigarette smoke and air pollution particles [94]. IL-6 in turn is accompanied by inflammatory cells including neutrophils into the lungs and limits the effects of the environment trigger. The mechanism of neutrophil recruitment of lung mediated by IL-6 is not fully elucidated, but there are data suggesting transcriptional activation of local chemokines such as IL-8 through signal transducer and activator of transcription-3 (STAT3). However, in certain circumstances, the IL-6 response can become dysregulated and spill into the systemic circulation, causing acute deleterious effects in the vascular system [95] and contribute to cardiovascular dysfunction related to acute lung injury [95].

Given these properties of IL-6, IL-6 has been investigated as a possible biomarker in COPD. COPD patients in general have higher serum IL-6 levels than those without COPD [96, 97]. Serum levels of IL-6 were significantly related to mortality in COPD patients [98]. However, serum IL-6 as a biomarker is limited in that it is not lung specific and is widely expressed throughout the body. Thus, serum IL-6 levels are poorly responsive to COPD medications and as such are less than ideal biomarker in COPD.

Serum Amyloid Protein A (SAA)

Serum amyloid protein A (SAA) is another promising biomarker of COPD exacerbation. This protein is known to be elevated in patients with exacerbation and decrease over time with recovery [99, 100].

Lung Predominant Proteins

To enhance the specificity of biomarkers, recent investigations have focused on proteins that are mostly synthesized in the lungs. These include surfactant proteins and Clara cell protein-16 (CC-16).

Surfactant Protein D

Surfactant proteins are produced predominantly by type II pneumocytes. Together with phospholipids they form pulmonary surfactants which act to reduce surface tension of alveoli preventing atelectasis. There are four kinds of surfactant proteins, A, B, C, and D. Of these, surfactant protein D (SP-D) has been the most widely explored biomarker in COPD because, dissimilar to other surfactant proteins, it is hydrophilic and is well expressed in plasma [101].

Although it has some minor role in regulating surface tension of alveoli, SP-D's main function is to modulate innate immunity [102, 103]. SP-D is a large multimeric calcium-dependent, collagenous glycoprotein that is part of the collectin family of carbohydrate-binding proteins [104]. SP-D is composed of three polypeptide chains of 43 kDa monomers, which aggregate to form a stable helical trimeric structure. Each trimeric structure contains four major domains: a cysteine-containing cross-linking domain, a carbohydrate recognition domain, a collagenous domain, and a peptide linking domain [105]. The main collagens in the trimeric complex are hydroxylysine and hydroxylysyl glycosides. In most cases, the trimeric structures are further modified into a complex quaternary cruciate structure, consisting of four trimeric subunits that undergo disulfide cross-linking within their amino-terminal domain, which results in a dodecamer. Under oxidizing conditions (e.g., in the presence of cigarette smoke), cysteine residues in the N-terminus can become nitrosylated, leading to the disruption of the multimeric structure into smaller trimers or monomers [106], which unlike the dodecamers are thought to be pro-inflammatory and are more likely to pass into the systemic circulation.

SP-D translocates from the lung into systemic circulation, which is dependent on several factors including rate of synthesis and the permeability of the alveolar-capillary barrier (i.e., lung permeability) [103]. With cigarette smoking, lung permeability increases. Thus, in smokers, the serum level of SP-D is elevated compared to nonsmokers but the concentration in the bronchoalveolar lavage (BAL) fluid is reduced [107, 108]. Similarly, with COPD, lung permeability increases independent of cigarette smoking [109]. Thus, with COPD progression, lung expression of SP-D decreases but the ratio of plasma SP-D to BAL SP-D increases [110]. Importantly, treatment of COPD patients with inhaled glucocorticoids with or without long-acting beta-2 agonists or oral glucocorticoids for 4 weeks significantly decreased measurable serum SP-D levels [109], which in turn is associated with improved health status of these patients. Serum SP-D levels may also identify patients at high risk of recurrent exacerbations [111, 112]. Together, these data suggest that SP-D is a promising modifiable biomarker in COPD.

Clara Cell-Derived Protein (CC-16)

Clara cell secretory protein-16 (CCSP, cc-16, cc-10, uteroglobin) is a member of the secretoglobin family of secreted disulfide-bridged dimeric proteins [113]. It is produced almost exclusively by non-ciliated Clara cells [114, 115], and its main function is to protect the lungs against oxidative stress and carcinogenesis [114]. Serum levels of CC-16 become elevated after acute exposure to various environmental triggers such as cigarette smoke, chlorine, and lipopolysaccharides [116]. They can also rise after ozone exposure and can be suppressed by inhaled glucocorticoids [117]. Interestingly, serum CC-16 levels are relatively low in obliterative bronchiolitis, asthma, and in healthy smokers [118–120]. In patients with COPD, serum CC-16 levels are lower compared to smokers without COPD [121, 122]. It is uncertain, however, whether in COPD, serum CC-16 levels are modifiable.

Pulmonary and Activation-Regulated Chemokine (PARC/CCL-18)

PARC/CCL-18 is protein that is mostly produced by monocytes, macrophages, and dendritic cells in lungs [123]. Serum levels of PARC/CCL-18 are elevated in acute coronary syndrome and idiopathic pulmonary fibrosis [124–126]. Serum PARC/CCL-18 levels are also significantly elevated in COPD and associated with the risk of cardiovascular hospitalization and mortality in mild-to-moderate disease and with total mortality in more advanced diseases [127]. Importantly, short-term uses of oral but not inhaled corticosteroids can down-regulated systemic expression of PARC/CCL-18 levels in COPD [127, 128].

Multiple Biomarkers

Finally, it seems very likely that multiple biomarkers, compared to individual ones, can reflect pathogenesis, natural course and prognosis, and response to the therapy more precisely. This is especially true when thinking about the enormous complexity of COPD in its pathogenesis and phenotype; the success of BODE index where multiple clinical factors were combined to predict its prognosis further raises this possibility [129]. In a recent study, selected panel of 24 biomarkers correlated with some clinical markers of COPD [130]. But there is no report with regard to validity of multiple biomarkers in evaluating drug response in this field as yet.

Molecular Biomarkers

Finally, there is a growing effort to find useful biomarker using gene expression profile. This approach has already been successful in some other fields of medicine [131, 132]. In a recent publication, a set of 220 biomarkers was identified and predicted disease in an independent data set with 97% accuracy [133]. The ability to identify COPD-related molecular processes in gene expression raises the possibility of serving as biomarkers of therapeutic response for novel and existing COPD therapies [134].

Future research effort and regulatory approval should include (1) the whole-OMIC high throughput technique to identify and validate useful biomarkers and (2) the evaluation of assays in validation of biomarkers in various cells/tissues/samples and evaluation of bioinformatics tools as suggested by Cazzola [12].

Conclusion

To date, there is no universally accepted biomarker in COPD. However, with the assembly of large cohorts and infusion of capital from various sources including government agencies and industry, there is renewed hope of finding a modifiable biomarker that will be useful in the discovery of novel compounds to treat COPD. Since COPD is a heterogeneous disorder with multiple different (but related) phenotypes, it is essential that future endeavors in biomarker discovery consider these phenotypes. Although biomarkers can originate from

Table 9.1 Summary of serum/plasma biomarkers of COPD

Biomarkers	Lung function	Exacerbation	Mortality	Modified by drug (s)
C-reactive protein (CRP)	Yes [135]	Yes [82]	Yes [79, 80]	Yes [83]
Interleukin 6 (IL-6)	Yes [129]	Yes [130]	Not known	Yes [136]
Fibrinogen	Yes [129, 137]	Yes [138]	Not known	Not known
Tumor necrosis factor receptor 1	Not known	Yes [82]	Not known	Not known
Eotaxin 2	Not known	Yes [82]	Not known	Not known
Serum amyloid A	Not known	Yes [99]	Not known	Yes [99]
Interleukin 1 (IL-1)	Not known	Yes [82]	Not known	Not known
Surfactant protein D (SP-D)	Yes [139]	Yes [109, 111]	Not known	Yes [85, 109]
Clara cell protein (cc16)	Not known	Not known	Not known	Yes [117]
Pulmonary and activation-regulated chemokine (PARC)	Yes [140]	Yes [82]	Yes [127]	Yes [127]

any source, sputum and blood are the most readily available sources and hence appear to be the most promising sites for large-scale biomarker discovery in COPD. However, clearer understanding of the pathophysiological role of the putative biomarkers, their variability, and importantly their relationship to disease progression are crucial defining factors (Table 9.1).

References

1. Buist AS, McBurnie MA, Vollmer WM, Gillespie S, Burney P, Mannino DM, et al. International variation in the prevalence of COPD (the BOLD study): a population-based prevalence study. Lancet. 2007;370(9589):741–50.
2. Murray CJ, Lopez AD. Alternative projections of mortality and disability by cause 1990-2020: global burden of disease study. Lancet. 1997;349(9064):1498–504.
3. Mathers CD, Loncar D. Projections of global mortality and burden of disease from 2002 to 2030. PLoS Med. 2006;3(11):e442.
4. National Heart L, and Blood Institute. Morbidity and mortality: chartbook on cardiovascular, lung, and blood diseases. In: US Department of Health and Human Services PHS, editor. National Institutes of Health; 2004.
5. Sin DD, Man SF. Steroids in COPD: still up in the air? Eur Respir J. 2010;35(5):949–51.
6. Rabe KF, Hurd S, Anzueto A, Barnes PJ, Buist SA, Calverley P, et al. Global strategy for the diagnosis, management, and prevention of chronic obstructive pulmonary disease: GOLD executive summary. Am J Respir Crit Care Med. 2007;176(6):532–55.
7. Hogg JC. Pathophysiology of airflow limitation in chronic obstructive pulmonary disease. Lancet. 2004;364(9435):709–21.
8. Dragonieri S, Tongoussouva O, Zanini A, Imperatori A, Spanevello A. Markers of airway inflammation in pulmonary diseases assessed by induced sputum. Monaldi Arch Chest Dis. 2009;71(3):119–26.
9. Borrill ZL, Roy K, Singh D. Exhaled breath condensate biomarkers in COPD. Eur Respir J. 2008;32(2):472–86.
10. He ZY, Ou LM, Zhang JQ, Bai J, Liu GN, Li MH, et al. Effect of 6 months of erythromycin treatment on inflammatory cells in induced sputum and exacerbations in chronic obstructive pulmonary disease. Respiration. 2010;80(6):445–52.
11. Comandini A, Rogliani P, Nunziata A, Cazzola M, Curradi G, Saltini C. Biomarkers of lung damage associated with tobacco smoke in induced sputum. Respir Med. 2009;103(11):1592–613.
12. Cazzola M, Novelli G. Biomarkers in COPD. Pulm Pharmacol Ther. 23(6):493–500.
13. Ford PA, Durham AL, Russell RE, Gordon F, Adcock IM, Barnes PJ. Treatment effects of low-dose theophylline combined with an inhaled corticosteroid in COPD. Chest. 2010;137(6):1338–44.
14. Sharafkhaneh A, Hanania NA, Kim V. Pathogenesis of emphysema: from the bench to the bedside. Proc Am Thorac Soc. 2008;5(4):475–7.
15. Cowburn AS, Condliffe AM, Farahi N, Summers C, Chilvers ER. Advances in neutrophil biology. Chest. 2008;134(3):606–12.
16. O'Donnell RA, Peebles C, Ward JA, Daraker A, Angco G, Broberg P, et al. Relationship between peripheral airway dysfunction, airway obstruction, and neutrophilic inflammation in COPD. Thorax. 2004;59(10):837–42.
17. Keatings VM, Collins PD, Scott DM, Barnes PJ. Differences in interleukin-8 and tumor necrosis factor-alpha in induced sputum from patients with chronic obstructive pulmonary disease or asthma. Am J Respir Crit Care Med. 1996;153(2):530–4.

18. Williams TJ, Jose PJ. Neutrophils in chronic obstructive pulmonary disease. Novartis Found Symp. 2001;234:136–41, discussion 41–8.
19. Perng DW, Huang HY, Chen HM, Lee YC, Perng RP. Characteristics of airway inflammation and bronchodilator reversibility in COPD: a potential guide to treatment. Chest. 2004;126(2):375–81.
20. Willemse BW, ten Hacken NH, Rutgers B, Lesman-Leegte IG, Postma DS, Timens W. Effect of 1-year smoking cessation on airway inflammation in COPD and asymptomatic smokers. Eur Respir J. 2005;26(5):835–45.
21. Stanescu D, Sanna A, Veriter C, Kostianev S, Calcagni PG, Fabbri LM, et al. Airways obstruction, chronic expectoration, and rapid decline of FEV1 in smokers are associated with increased levels of sputum neutrophils. Thorax. 1996;51(3):267–71.
22. Barnes NC, Qiu YS, Pavord ID, Parker D, Davis PA, Zhu J, et al. Antiinflammatory effects of salmeterol/fluticasone propionate in chronic obstructive lung disease. Am J Respir Crit Care Med. 2006;173(7):736–43.
23. Celli BR, Thomas NE, Anderson JA, Ferguson GT, Jenkins CR, Jones PW, et al. Effect of pharmacotherapy on rate of decline of lung function in chronic obstructive pulmonary disease: results from the TORCH study. Am J Respir Crit Care Med. 2008;178(4):332–8.
24. Lapperre TS, Snoeck-Stroband JB, Gosman MM, Jansen DF, van Schadewijk A, Thiadens HA, et al. Effect of fluticasone with and without salmeterol on pulmonary outcomes in chronic obstructive pulmonary disease: a randomized trial. Ann Intern Med. 2009;151(8):517–27.
25. Gan WQ, Man SF, Sin DD. Effects of inhaled corticosteroids on sputum cell counts in stable chronic obstructive pulmonary disease: a systematic review and a meta-analysis. BMC Pulm Med. 2005;5:3.
26. Kanehara M, Yokoyama A, Tomoda Y, Shiota N, Iwamoto H, Ishikawa N, et al. Anti-inflammatory effects and clinical efficacy of theophylline and tulobuterol in mild-to-moderate chronic obstructive pulmonary disease. Pulm Pharmacol Ther. 2008;21(6):874–8.
27. Gronke L, Beeh KM, Cameron R, Kornmann O, Beier J, Shaw M, et al. Effect of the oral leukotriene B4 receptor antagonist LTB019 on inflammatory sputum markers in patients with chronic obstructive pulmonary disease. Pulm Pharmacol Ther. 2008;21(2):409–17.
28. Singh D, Edwards L, Tal-Singer R, Rennard S. Sputum neutrophils as a biomarker in COPD: findings from the ECLIPSE study. Respir Res. 11(1):77.
29. Boorsma M, Lutter R, van de Pol MA, Out TA, Jansen HM, Jonkers RE. Long-term effects of budesonide on inflammatory status in COPD. COPD. 2008;5(2):97–104.
30. Kharitonov SA, Barnes PJ. Exhaled biomarkers. Chest. 2006;130(5):1541–6.
31. Barnes PJ, Dweik RA, Gelb AF, Gibson PG, George SC, Grasemann H, et al. Exhaled nitric oxide in pulmonary diseases: a comprehensive review. Chest. 2010;138(3):682–92.
32. Dupont LJ, Demedts MG, Verleden GM. Prospective evaluation of the validity of exhaled nitric oxide for the diagnosis of asthma*. Chest. 2003;123(3):751–6.
33. Van Den Toorn LM, Overbeek SE, De Jongste JC, Leman K, Hoogsteden HC, Prins J-B. Airway inflammation is present during clinical remission of atopic asthma. Am J Respir Crit Care Med. 2001;164(11):2107–13.
34. Kharitonov SA, Donnelly LE, Montuschi P, Corradi M, Collins JV, Barnes PJ. Dose-dependent onset and cessation of action of inhaled budesonide on exhaled nitric oxide and symptoms in mild asthma. Thorax. 2002;57(10):889–96.
35. Jones SL, Kittelson J, Cowan JO, Flannery EM, Hancox RJ, McLachlan CR, et al. The predictive value of exhaled nitric oxide measurements in assessing changes in asthma control. Am J Respir Crit Care Med. 2001;164(5):738–43.
36. Kharitonov SA, Barnes PJ. Exhaled markers of pulmonary disease. Am J Respir Crit Care Med. 2001;163(7):1693–722.
37. Verleden GM, Dupont LJ, Verpeut AC, Demedts MG. The effect of cigarette smoking on exhaled nitric oxide in mild steroid-naive asthmatics*. Chest. 1999;116(1):59–64.
38. Kharitonov SA, Robbins RA, Yates D, Keatings V, Barnes PJ. Acute and chronic effects of cigarette smoking on exhaled nitric oxide. Am J Respir Crit Care Med. 1995;152(2):609–12.
39. Brindicci C, Ito K, Resta O, Pride NB, Barnes PJ, Kharitonov SA. Exhaled nitric oxide from lung periphery is increased in COPD. Eur Respir J. 2005;26(1):52–9.
40. MacNee W, Rennard SI, Hunt JF, Edwards LD, Miller BE, Locantore NW, et al. Evaluation of exhaled breath condensate pH as a biomarker for COPD. Respir Med. 2011;105(7):1037–45.
41. Biernacki WA, Kharitonov SA, Barnes PJ. Increased leukotriene B4 and 8-isoprostane in exhaled breath condensate of patients with exacerbations of COPD. Thorax. 2003;58(4):294–8.
42. Corhay J-L, Henket M, Nguyen D, Duysinx B, Sele J, Louis R. Leukotriene B4 contributes to exhaled breath condensate and sputum neutrophil Chemotaxis in COPD. Chest. 2009;136(4):1047–54.
43. Mercken EM, Gosker HR, Rutten EP, Wouters EF, Bast A, Hageman GJ, et al. Systemic and pulmonary oxidative stress after single-leg exercise in COPD. Chest. 2009;136(5):1291–300.
44. Shifren A, Mecham RP. The stumbling block in lung repair of emphysema: elastic fiber assembly. Proc Am Thorac Soc. 2006;3(5):428–33.
45. Pelosi P, Rocco PR. Effects of mechanical ventilation on the extracellular matrix. Intensive Care Med. 2008;34(4):631–9.
46. Abraham T, Hogg J. Extracellular matrix remodeling of lung alveolar walls in three dimensional space identified using second harmonic generation and multiphoton excitation fluorescence. J Struct Biol. 2010;171(2):189–96.
47. Kelleher CM, Silverman EK, Broekelmann T, Litonjua AA, Hernandez M, Sylvia JS, et al. A functional

mutation in the terminal exon of elastin in severe, early-onset chronic obstructive pulmonary disease. Am J Respir Cell Mol Biol. 2005;33(4):355–62.
48. Wendel DP, Taylor DG, Albertine KH, Keating MT, Li DY. Impaired distal airway development in mice lacking elastin. Am J Respir Cell Mol Biol. 2000;23(3):320–6.
49. Luisetti M, Ma S, Iadarola P, Stone PJ, Viglio S, Casado B, et al. Desmosine as a biomarker of elastin degradation in COPD: current status and future directions. Eur Respir J. 2008;32(5):1146–57.
50. Rosenbloom J. Biochemical/immunologic markers of emphysema. Ann N Y Acad Sci. 1991;624:7–12.
51. Goldstein RA, Starcher BC. Urinary excretion of elastin peptides containing desmosin after intratracheal injection of elastase in hamsters. J Clin Invest. 1978;61(5):1286–90.
52. Churg A, Dai J, Tai H, Xie C, Wright JL. Tumor necrosis factor-alpha is central to acute cigarette smoke-induced inflammation and connective tissue breakdown. Am J Respir Crit Care Med. 2002;166(6):849–54.
53. Churg A, Wang RD, Tai H, Wang X, Xie C, Wright JL. Tumor necrosis factor-alpha drives 70% of cigarette smoke-induced emphysema in the mouse. Am J Respir Crit Care Med. 2004;170(5):492–8.
54. Huang JT-J, Chaudhuri R, Albarbarawi O, Barton A, Grierson C, Rauchhaus P, et al. Clinical validity of plasma and urinary desmosine as biomarkers for chronic obstructive pulmonary disease. Thorax. 2012;67(6):502–8.
55. Rabinovich RA, Miller BE, Wrobel K, Ranjit K, Williams MC, Drost E, et al. Circulating desmosine levels do not predict emphysema progression but are associated with cardiovascular risk and mortality in COPD. Eur Respir J. 2016;47(5):1365–73.
56. Fiorenza D, Viglio S, Lupi A, Baccheschi J, Tinelli C, Trisolini R, et al. Urinary desmosine excretion in acute exacerbations of COPD: a preliminary report. Respir Med. 2002;96(2):110–4.
57. Ma S, Lin YY, Turino GM. Measurements of desmosine and isodesmosine by mass spectrometry in COPD*. Chest. 2007;131(5):1363–71.
58. Cocci F, Miniati M, Monti S, Cavarra E, Gambelli F, Battolla L, et al. Urinary desmosine excretion is inversely correlated with the extent of emphysema in patients with chronic obstructive pulmonary disease. Int J Biochem Cell Biol. 2002;34(6):594–604.
59. Stone PJ, Morris TA 3rd, Franzblau C, Snider GL. Preliminary evidence that augmentation therapy diminishes degradation of cross-linked elastin in alpha-1-antitrypsin-deficient humans. Respiration. 1995;62(2):76–9.
60. Gottlieb DJ, Luisetti M, Stone PJ, Allegra L, Cantey-Kiser JM, Grassi C, et al. Short-term supplementation therapy does not affect elastin degradation in severe alpha(1)-antitrypsin deficiency. The American-Italian AATD study group. Am J Respir Crit Care Med. 2000;162(6):2069–72.
61. Ma S, Lin Y, Tartell L, Turino G. The effect of tiotropium therapy on markers of elastin degradation in COPD. Respir Res. 2009;10(1):12.
62. Dahl R, Titlestad I, Lindqvist A, Wielders P, Wray H, Wang M, et al. Effects of an oral MMP-9 and -12 inhibitor, AZD1236, on biomarkers in moderate/severe COPD: a randomised controlled trial. Pulm Pharmacol Ther. 2012;25(2):169–77.
63. Weathington NM, van Houwelingen AH, Noerager BD, Jackson PL, Kraneveld AD, Galin FS, et al. A novel peptide CXCR ligand derived from extracellular matrix degradation during airway inflammation. Nat Med. 2006;12(3):317–23.
64. Gaggar A, Jackson PL, Noerager BD, O'Reilly PJ, McQuaid DB, Rowe SM, et al. A novel proteolytic cascade generates an extracellular matrix-derived chemoattractant in chronic neutrophilic inflammation. J Immunol. 2008;180(8):5662–9.
65. Laskin DL, Kimura T, Sakakibara S, Riley DJ, Berg RA. Chemotactic activity of collagen-like polypeptides for human peripheral blood neutrophils. J Leukoc Biol. 1986;39(3):255–66.
66. Postlethwaite AE, Kang AH. Collagen-and collagen peptide-induced chemotaxis of human blood monocytes. J Exp Med. 1976;143(6):1299–307.
67. Houghton AM, Quintero PA, Perkins DL, Kobayashi DK, Kelley DG, Marconcini LA, et al. Elastin fragments drive disease progression in a murine model of emphysema. J Clin Invest. 2006;116(3):753–9.
68. van Houwelingen AH, Weathington NM, Verweij V, Blalock JE, Nijkamp FP, Folkerts G. Induction of lung emphysema is prevented by L-arginine-threonine-arginine. FASEB J. 2008;22(9):3403–8.
69. O'Reilly P, Jackson PL, Noerager B, Parker S, Dransfield M, Gaggar A, et al. N-alpha-PGP and PGP, potential biomarkers and therapeutic targets for COPD. Respir Res. 2009;10:38.
70. O'Reilly PJ, Jackson PL, Wells JM, Dransfield MT, Scanlon PD, Blalock JE. Sputum PGP is reduced by azithromycin treatment in patients with COPD and correlates with exacerbations. BMJ Open. 2013;3(12):e004140.
71. Wells JM, Jackson PL, Viera L, Bhatt SP, Gautney J, Handley G, et al. A randomized, placebo-controlled trial of Roflumilast. Effect on proline-glycine-proline and neutrophilic inflammation in chronic obstructive pulmonary disease. Am J Respir Crit Care Med. 2015;192(8):934–42.
72. Snelgrove RJ, Jackson PL, Hardison MT, Noerager BD, Kinloch A, Gaggar A, et al. A critical role for LTA4H in limiting chronic pulmonary neutrophilic inflammation. Science. 330(6000):90–4.
73. van Eeden SF, Sin DD. Chronic obstructive pulmonary disease: a chronic systemic inflammatory disease. Respiration. 2008;75(2):224–38.
74. Danesh J, Collins R, Appleby P, Peto R. Association of fibrinogen, C-reactive protein, albumin, or leukocyte count with coronary heart disease: meta-analyses of prospective studies. JAMA. 1998;279(18):1477–82.

75. Kaptoge S, Di Angelantonio E, Lowe G, Pepys MB, Thompson SG, Collins R, et al. C-reactive protein concentration and risk of coronary heart disease, stroke, and mortality: an individual participant meta-analysis. Lancet. 2010;375(9709):132–40.
76. Ridker PM, Danielson E, Fonseca FA, Genest J, Gotto AM Jr, Kastelein JJ, et al. Rosuvastatin to prevent vascular events in men and women with elevated C-reactive protein. N Engl J Med. 2008;359(21):2195–207.
77. Karadag F, Kirdar S, Karul AB, Ceylan E. The value of C-reactive protein as a marker of systemic inflammation in stable chronic obstructive pulmonary disease. Eur J Intern Med. 2008;19(2):104–8.
78. Garrod R, Marshall J, Barley E, Fredericks S, Hagan G. The relationship between inflammatory markers and disability in chronic obstructive pulmonary disease (COPD). Prim Care Respir J. 2007;16(4):236–40.
79. Man SFP, Connett JE, Anthonisen NR, Wise RA, Tashkin DP, Sin DD. C-reactive protein and mortality in mild to moderate chronic obstructive pulmonary disease. Thorax. 2006;61(10):849–53.
80. Dahl M, Vestbo J, Lange P, Bojesen SE, Tybjaerg-Hansen A, Nordestgaard BG. C-reactive protein as a predictor of prognosis in chronic obstructive pulmonary disease. Am J Respir Crit Care Med. 2007;175(3):250–5.
81. Thomsen M, Dahl M, Lange P, Vestbo J, Nordestgaard BG. Inflammatory biomarkers and comorbidities in chronic obstructive pulmonary disease. Am J Respir Crit Care Med. 2012;186(10):982–8.
82. Hurst JR, Donaldson GC, Perera WR, Wilkinson TMA, Bilello JA, Hagan GW, et al. Use of plasma biomarkers at exacerbation of chronic obstructive pulmonary disease. Am J Respir Crit Care Med. 2006;174(8):867–74.
83. Sin DD, Lacy P, York E, Man SFP. Effects of fluticasone on systemic markers of inflammation in chronic obstructive pulmonary disease. Am J Respir Crit Care Med. 2004;170(7):760–5.
84. Perng DW, Tao CW, Su KC, Tsai CC, Liu LY, Lee YC. Anti-inflammatory effects of salmeterol/fluticasone, tiotropium/fluticasone or tiotropium in COPD. Eur Respir J. 2009;33(4):778–84.
85. Sin DD, Man SF, Marciniuk DD, Ford G, FitzGerald M, Wong E, et al. The effects of fluticasone with or without salmeterol on systemic biomarkers of inflammation in chronic obstructive pulmonary disease. Am J Respir Crit Care Med. 2008;177(11):1207–14.
86. Fibrinogen SC. Plasma fibrinogen level and the risk of major cardiovascular diseases and nonvascular mortality. JAMA. 2005;294(14):1799–809.
87. Groenewegen KH, Postma DS, Hop WCJ, Wielders PLML, Schölsser NJ, Wouters EF. Increased systemic inflammation is a risk factor for COPD exacerbations*. Chest. 2008;133(2):350–7.
88. Engstrom G, Segelstorm N, Ekberg-Aronsson M, Nilsson PM, Lindgarde F, Lofdahl CG. Plasma markers of inflammation and incidence of hospitalisations for COPD: results from a population-based cohort study. Thorax. 2009;64(3):211–5.
89. Duvoix A, Dickens J, Haq I, Mannino D, Miller B, Tal-Singer R, et al. Blood fibrinogen as a biomarker of chronic obstructive pulmonary disease. Thorax. 2013;68(7):670–6.
90. Valvi D, Mannino DM, Müllerova H, Tal-Singer R. Fibrinogen, chronic obstructive pulmonary disease (COPD) and outcomes in two United States cohorts. Int J COPD. 2012;7:173–82.
91. Dentener MA, Creutzberg EC, Pennings HJ, Rijkers GT, Mercken E, Wouters EF. Effect of infliximab on local and systemic inflammation in chronic obstructive pulmonary disease: a pilot study. Respiration. 2008;76(3):275–82.
92. Kaczmarek P, Sladek K, Skucha W, Rzeszutko M, Iwaniec T, Dziedzina S, et al. The influence of simvastatin on selected inflammatory markers in patients with chronic obstructive pulmonary disease. Pol Arch Med Wewn. 2010;120(1–2):11–7.
93. Kishimoto T. IL-6: from its discovery to clinical applications. Int Immunol. 2010;22(5):347–52.
94. Ishii H, Hayashi S, Hogg JC, Fujii T, Goto Y, Sakamoto N, et al. Alveolar macrophage-epithelial cell interaction following exposure to atmospheric particles induces the release of mediators involved in monocyte mobilization and recruitment. Respir Res. 2005;6:87.
95. Kido T, Tamagawa E, Bai N, Suda K, Yang HH, Li Y, et al. Particulate matter induces translocation of IL-6 from the lung to the systemic circulation. Am J Respir Cell Mol Biol. 2011;44(2):197–204.
96. Thorleifsson SJ, Margretardottir OB, Gudmundsson G, Olafsson I, Benediktsdottir B, Janson C, et al. Chronic airflow obstruction and markers of systemic inflammation: results from the BOLD study in Iceland. Respir Med. 2009;103(10):1548–53.
97. Walter RE, Wilk JB, Larson MG, Vasan RS, Keaney JF Jr, Lipinska I, et al. Systemic inflammation and COPD: the Framingham heart study. Chest. 2008;133(1):19–25.
98. Celli BR, Locantore N, Yates J, Tal-Singer R, Miller BE, Bakke P, et al. Inflammatory biomarkers improve clinical prediction of mortality in chronic obstructive pulmonary disease. Am J Respir Crit Care Med. 2012;185(10):1065–72.
99. Bozinovski S, Hutchinson A, Thompson M, MacGregor L, Black J, Giannakis E, et al. Serum amyloid a is a biomarker of acute exacerbations of chronic obstructive pulmonary disease. Am J Respir Crit Care Med. 2008;177(3):269–78.
100. Koutsokera A, Kiropoulos TS, Nikoulis DJ, Daniil ZD, Tsolaki V, Tanou K, et al. Clinical, functional and biochemical changes during recovery from COPD exacerbations. Respir Med. 2009;103(6):919–26.
101. Cole FS. Surfactant protein B: unambiguously necessary for adult pulmonary function. Am J Physiol Lung Cell Mol Physiol. 2003;285(3):L540–L2.

102. Hartl D, Griese M. Surfactant protein D in human lung diseases. Eur J Clin Invest. 2006;36(6):423–35.
103. Sin DD, Pahlavan PS, Man SFP. Review: surfactant protein D: a lung specific biomarker in COPD? Ther Adv Respir Dis. 2008;2(2):65–74.
104. Kishore U, Greenhough TJ, Waters P, Shrive AK, Ghai R, Kamran MF, et al. Surfactant proteins SP-A and SP-D: structure, function and receptors. Mol Immunol. 2006;43(9):1293–315.
105. Crouch EC. Surfactant protein-D and pulmonary host defense. Respir Res. 2000;1(2):93–108.
106. Guo CJ, Atochina-Vasserman EN, Abramova E, Foley JP, Zaman A, Crouch E, et al. S-nitrosylation of surfactant protein-D controls inflammatory function. PLoS Biol. 2008;6(11):e266.
107. More JM, Voelker DR, Silveira LJ, Edwards MG, Chan ED, Bowler RP. Smoking reduces surfactant protein D and phospholipids in patients with and without chronic obstructive pulmonary disease. BMC Pulm Med. 2010;10:53.
108. Honda Y, Takahashi H, Kuroki Y, Akino T, Abe S. Decreased contents of surfactant proteins a and D in BAL fluids of healthy smokers. Chest. 1996;109(4):1006–9.
109. Lomas DA, Silverman EK, Edwards LD, Locantore NW, Miller BE, Horstman DH, et al. Serum surfactant protein D is steroid sensitive and associated with exacerbations of COPD. Eur Respir J. 2009;34(1):95–102.
110. Tkacova R, McWilliams A, Lam S, Sin DD. Integrating lung and plasma expression of pneumo-proteins in developing biomarkers in COPD: a case study of surfactant protein D. Med Sci Monit. 2010;16(11):CR540–4.
111. Shakoori TA, Sin DD, Ghafoor F, Bashir S, Bokhari SN. Serum surfactant protein D during acute exacerbations of chronic obstructive pulmonary disease. Dis Markers. 2009;27(6):287–94.
112. Hurst JR, Vestbo J, Anzueto A, Locantore N, Mullerova H, Tal-Singer R, et al. Susceptibility to exacerbation in chronic obstructive pulmonary disease. N Engl J Med. 2010;363(12):1128–38.
113. Umland TC, Swaminathan S, Singh G, Warty V, Furey W, Pletcher J, et al. Structure of a human Clara cell phospholipid-binding protein-ligand complex at 1.9 A resolution. Nat Struct Biol. 1994;1(8):538–45.
114. Broeckaert F, Bernard A. Clara cell secretory protein (CC16): characteristics and perspectives as lung peripheral biomarker. Clin Exp Allergy. 2000;30(4):469–75.
115. Yoneda K. Ultrastructural localization of phospholipases in the Clara cell of the rat bronchiole. Am J Pathol. 1978;93(3):745–52.
116. Lakind JS, Holgate ST, Ownby DR, Mansur AH, Helms PJ, Pyatt D, et al. A critical review of the use of Clara cell secretory protein (CC16) as a biomarker of acute or chronic pulmonary effects. Biomarkers. 2007;12(5):445–67.
117. Alexis NE, Lay JC, Haczku A, Gong H, Linn W, Hazucha MJ, et al. Fluticasone propionate protects against ozone-induced airway inflammation and modified immune cell activation markers in healthy volunteers. Environ Health Perspect. 2008;116(6):799–805.
118. Shijubo N, Itoh Y, Yamaguchi T, Shibuya Y, Morita Y, Hirasawa M, et al. Serum and BAL Clara cell 10 kDa protein (CC10) levels and CC10-positive bronchiolar cells are decreased in smokers. Eur Respir J. 1997;10(5):1108–14.
119. Shijubo N, Itoh Y, Yamaguchi T, Imada A, Hirasawa M, Yamada T, et al. Clara cell protein-positive epithelial cells are reduced in small airways of asthmatics. Am J Respir Crit Care Med. 1999;160(3):930–3.
120. Mattsson J, Remberger M, Andersson O, Sundberg B, Nord M. Decreased serum levels of clara cell secretory protein (CC16) are associated with bronchiolitis obliterans and may permit early diagnosis in patients after allogeneic stem-cell transplantation. Transplantation. 2005;79(10):1411–6.
121. Tsoumakidou M, Bouloukaki I, Thimaki K, Tzanakis N, Siafakas NM. Innate immunity proteins in chronic obstructive pulmonary disease and idiopathic pulmonary fibrosis. Exp Lung Res. 2010;36(6):373–80.
122. Lomas DA, Silverman EK, Edwards LD, Miller BE, Coxson HO, Tal-Singer R, et al. Evaluation of serum CC-16 as a biomarker for COPD in the ECLIPSE cohort. Thorax. 2008;63(12):1058–63.
123. Günther C, Bello-Fernandez C, Kopp T, Kund J, Carballido-Perrig N, Hinteregger S, et al. CCL18 is expressed in atopic dermatitis and mediates skin homing of human memory T cells. J Immunol. 2005;174(3):1723–8.
124. Prasse A, Probst C, Bargagli E, Zissel G, Toews GB, Flaherty KR, et al. Serum CC-chemokine ligand 18 concentration predicts outcome in idiopathic pulmonary fibrosis. Am J Respir Crit Care Med. 2009;179(8):717–23.
125. Prasse A, Pechkovsky DV, Toews GB, Schäfer M, Eggeling S, Ludwig C, et al. CCL18 as an indicator of pulmonary fibrotic activity in idiopathic interstitial pneumonias and systemic sclerosis. Arthritis Rheum. 2007;56(5):1685–93.
126. Kraaijeveld AO, de Jager SCA, de Jager WJ, Prakken BJ, McColl SR, Haspels I, et al. CC chemokine ligand-5 (CCL5/RANTES) and CC chemokine ligand-18 (CCL18/PARC) are specific markers of refractory unstable angina pectoris and are transiently raised during severe ischemic symptoms. Circulation. 2007;116(17):1931–41.
127. Sin DD, Miller B, Duvoix A, Man SFP, Zhang X, Silverman EK, et al. Serum PARC/CCL-18 concentrations and health outcomes in chronic obstructive pulmonary disease. Am J Respir Crit Care Med. 2011;183(9):1187–92.
128. Man SF, Xuekui Z, Vessey R, Walker T, Lee K, Park D, et al. The effects of inhaled and oral corticosteroids on serum inflammatory biomarkers in COPD: an exploratory study. Ther Adv Respir Dis. 2009;3(2):73–80.

129. Donaldson GC, Seemungal TAR, Patel IS, Bhowmik A, Wilkinson TMA, Hurst JR, et al. Airway and systemic inflammation and decline in lung function in patients with COPD*. Chest. 2005;128(4):1995–2004.
130. Karadag F, Karul A, Cildag O, Yilmaz M, Ozcan H. Biomarkers of systemic inflammation in stable and exacerbation phases of COPD. Lung. 2008;186(6):403–9.
131. Toedter G, Li K, Marano C, Ma K, Sague S, Huang CC, et al. Gene expression profiling and response signatures associated with differential responses to infliximab treatment in ulcerative colitis. Am J Gastroenterol. 2011;106(7):1272–80.
132. Elashoff MR, Wingrove JA, Beineke P, Daniels SE, Tingley WG, Rosenberg S, et al. Development of a blood-based gene expression algorithm for assessment of obstructive coronary artery disease in nondiabetic patients. BMC Med Genet. 2011;4(1):26.
133. Bhattacharya S, Srisuma S, DeMeo DL, Shapiro SD, Bueno R, Silverman EK, et al. Molecular biomarkers for quantitative and discrete COPD phenotypes. Am J Respir Cell Mol Biol. 2009;40(3):359–67.
134. Silverman EK, Spira A, Pare PD. Genetics and genomics of chronic obstructive pulmonary disease. Proc Am Thorac Soc. 2009;6(6):539–42.
135. Aronson D, Roterman I, Yigla M, Kerner A, Avizohar O, Sella R, et al. Inverse association between pulmonary function and C-reactive protein in apparently healthy subjects. Am J Respir Crit Care Med. 2006;174(6):626–32.
136. Cosio BG, Iglesias A, Rios A, Noguera A, Sala E, Ito K, et al. Low-dose theophylline enhances the anti-inflammatory effects of steroids during exacerbations of COPD. Thorax. 2009;64(5):424–9.
137. Dahl M, Tybjoerg-Hansen A, Vestbo J, Lange P, Nordestgaard BG. Elevated plasma fibrinogen associated with reduced pulmonary function and increased risk of chronic obstructive pulmonary disease. Am J Respir Crit Care Med. 2001;164(6):1008–11.
138. Wedzicha JA, Seemungal TA, MacCallum PK, Paul EA, Donaldson GC, Bhowmik A, et al. Acute exacerbations of chronic obstructive pulmonary disease are accompanied by elevations of plasma fibrinogen and serum IL-6 levels. Thromb Haemost. 2000;84(2):210–5.
139. Tkacova R, McWilliams A, Lam S, Sin DD. Integrating lung and plasma expression of pneumo-proteins in developing biomarkers in COPD: a case study of surfactant protein D. Med Sci Monit. 16(11):CR540–4.
140. Pinto-Plata V, Toso J, Lee K, Park D, Bilello J, Mullerova H, et al. Profiling serum biomarkers in patients with COPD: associations with clinical parameters. Thorax. 2007;62(7):595–601.

Part III

Heterogeneity

Phenotypes of COPD

10

Jamie Sheth and MeiLan Han

Introduction

Significant heterogeneity exists in chronic obstructive pulmonary disease (COPD) patients with respect to clinical presentation, physiology, imaging characteristics, response to therapy, disease progression, and ultimately survival [1]. While FEV_1 correlates to many outcomes of interest, no single measure adequately reflects this disease complexity. The goal of phenotyping is to identify patient subgroups with unique characteristics with the ultimate goal of altering clinically meaningful outcomes through targeted therapeutic approaches. While various definitions have been described, a consensus definition that was recently proposed defines a phenotype as, "a single or combination of disease attributes that describe differences between individuals with COPD as they relate to clinically meaningful outcomes (symptoms, exacerbations, response to therapy, rate of disease progression or death)" [1]. In many cases, the discovery and validation of phenotypes occurs through a multi-step process (Fig. 10.1) where for instance a unique group of patients may initially be identified through a biological or molecular signature and validated by demonstrating a similar response to therapy [2].

What follows in this chapter is a discussion of the "current state" for putative COPD phenotypes and data to support a relationship between proposed phenotypes and clinically meaningful metrics including prognosis, symptoms, and outcomes in COPD.

J. Sheth, M.D. (✉) • M. Han, M.D., M.S.
Division of Pulmonary and Critical Care,
University of Michigan, Ann Arbor, MI, USA
e-mail: jvotava@med.umich.edu;
mrking@med.umich.edu

S.-D. Lee (ed.), *COPD*, DOI 10.1007/978-3-662-47178-4_10

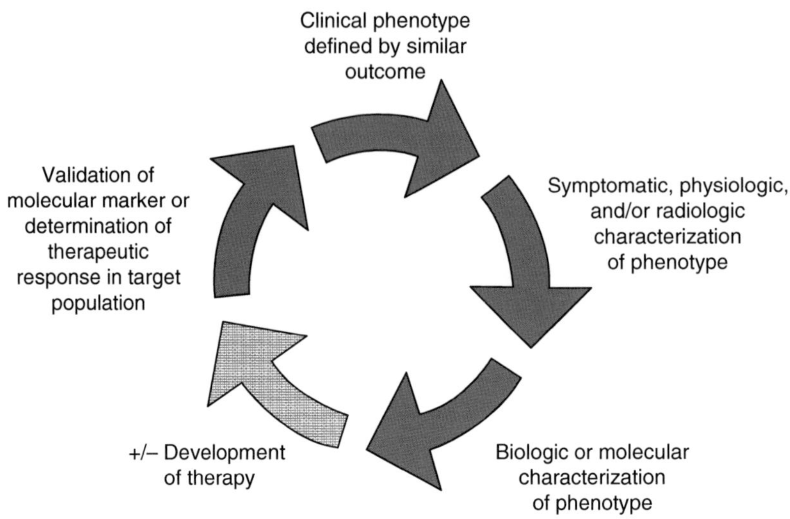

Fig. 10.1 Ideal phenotyping construct wherein candidate phenotypes are validated once their relevance to clinical outcomes is established. There are multiple potential points of entry into this iterative process of phenotype identification. For instance, similar clinical outcomes may define a subpopulation that leads to the identification of a biologic target and focused therapy. Alternatively, the process might begin with the differentiation of subgroups based on a biologic marker that is then validated by similar clinical response within subgroups [1]

Clinically Defined Phenotypes

Tobacco Smoke-Associated, Biomass Smoke-Associated, and Non-smoking COPD

Based on the GOLD definition, COPD is characterized by persistent airflow limitation that is usually progressive and associated with an enhanced chronic inflammatory response in the airways and the lung thought to be the result of exposure to noxious particles or gases [3]. Tobacco is the principal risk factor and environmental toxin responsible for disease in most patients with COPD. The prevalence of COPD in smokers is approximately 20% as compared to approximately 4% in nonsmokers [4]. Tobacco smoke exposure leads to decreases in expiratory flow through two distinct pathophysiological processes: the emphysematous destruction of the lung parenchyma and/or narrowing and obliteration of the small peripheral airways [5]. The Lung Health Study (an interventional smoking cessation study in smokers with COPD with a mild degree of airflow obstruction) demonstrated that the rate of FEV_1 (forced expiratory volume in one second) decline was greatest in patients who smoked the most and least in those who achieved sustained smoking cessation [6] with smokers losing lung function in a dose-dependent manner [7].

Compared to nonsmokers, COPD in smokers has been associated with greater amounts of emphysema, impaired gas exchange and greater amounts of chronic sputum production [8]. Classically, cigarette smoke-related COPD is manifest by upper lobe predominant centrilobular emphysema though a variety of subtypes have been described. As an example, the COPDGene study has identified four subtypes of smokers with distinct patterns of airway disease and emphysema that are strongly associated with COPD-related clinical characteristics including exacerbations and dyspnea [9]. The first cluster is the "relatively resistant smoker" characterized by heavy smoking exposure with no or minimal airflow obstruction. Second is "mild upper zone-predominant emphysema" characterized by mild airflow obstruction and mild emphysema which was also found to have a strong genetic association with single-nucleotide polymorphism (SNP) rs 1980057 near the *HHIP* gene. Cluster 3 represents "airway-predominant disease" characterized by thicker airway walls, lowest average emphysema of all clusters and high BMI. Cluster 4, "severe emphysema," is characterized by high emphysema, gas trapping, and severe airflow obstruction. It is associated with the lowest BMI, highest lifetime pack-years exposure, and oldest average age. A strong genetic association is seen with SNP rs8034191 in the chromosome 15q locus that includes the nicotinic receptor genes [9]. Clearly, tobacco cessation should be a predominant focus of treatment plan in all patients although we do not know whether the smoking cessation approach should be tailored to a patient's genetic variation in SNPs associated with nicotine dependence. One problem with this type of approach is that it can be difficult to separate differences due to differences exposure, disease severity, and disease biology.

A substantial proportion of COPD cases cannot be explained by smoking, especially among younger persons, females, and residents of developing countries [10]. In multiple population-based studies, approximately 30% of all cases of COPD occur in never-smokers [8]. Factors independently associated with COPD in nonsmokers include increasing age, a diagnosis of asthma, and severe childhood respiratory disease. Secondhand (also known as environmental) and biomass smoke exposure are additional gender-specific risk factors for women in non-smoking-related COPD [8]. For women in the developing world, where fuels such as coal and biomass are used for indoor cooking and heating, several studies have reported an association between exposure to biomass smoke and COPD [11]. Alternative risk factors for COPD include genetic factors, outdoor air pollution, secondhand smoke exposure, occupational exposures, diet, and tuberculosis [10]. Respiratory symptoms such as chronic cough, chronic phlegm, wheeze, and exertional dyspnea are features of COPD regardless of smoking status though are more frequent in ever-smokers [8]. However, the burden of COPD exacerbations has been shown to be equally prevalent, occurring in approximately 30% of ever-smokers and never-smokers with COPD [8]. While nonsmokers exhibit a similar respiratory symptoms profile to that seen in smokers, they demonstrate different radiologic and physiologic presentations.

In studies comparing radiologic phenotypes between tobacco smoked-exposed and biomass smoke-exposed patients matched for lung function, biomass-exposed individuals demonstrate more air trapping, peri-bronchial thickening and less emphysema than the tobacco-exposed group, suggesting an airway-predominant phenotype [12–14]. The early exposure and repeated respiratory infections associated with biomass smoke exposure may alter the structure and function of the airway walls and may predispose biomass smoke-exposed individuals to a different COPD phenotype as adults compared to tobacco smokers who may begin smoking at an older age.

Chemical composition, age of exposure, and inhalation pattern have all been suggested as factors that contribute to variable phenotypes between tobacco smoke- and biomass smoke-related COPD [12]. Compared to tobacco smoke COPD, those with disease related to biomass smoke exposure have more cough, sputum, and air trapping on CT scan.

Alpha-1 Antitrypsin Deficiency

Severe alpha-1 antitrypsin deficiency (AATD) is a well-established genetic risk factor for COPD in both smokers and nonsmokers. Alpha-1 antitrypsin (AAT) is a protease that inactivates neutrophil elastase. High-risk genotypes include S, Z, and null alleles. It has been estimated to be responsible for approximately 2–3% of cases of COPD [15]. The classic clinical phenotype is a young COPD patient, often a smoker, with lower lobe predominant emphysema and a family history of emphysema. Chest imaging frequently demonstrates a predominantly lower lobe distribution of emphysema with a panacinar pattern, different than the more common centriacinar pattern. In subjects homozygous for the AAT Z allele, cigarette smoking leads to a markedly increased risk of COPD and reduced survival. Non-smoking PI Z subjects are also at increased risk for developing COPD although to a lesser degree [16–19]. While the classic homozygous Z phenotype is associated with early-onset lower lung predominant, the heterozygous SZ patients are less susceptible to tobacco smoke and may have a clinical phenotype more consistent with "usual" COPD demonstrating upper lobe predominant emphysema [20]. Currently, treatment for AATD incorporates not only bronchodilator therapy but also a mechanism-directed treatment approach using clinical presentation in addition to serum AAT concentration, AAT protein phenotyping, and AAT genotyping to guide decision-making for treatment with AAT replacement therapy [21].

Chronic Bronchitis

Chronic bronchitis in the COPD population has been estimated to be between approximately 7 and 40%, depending on how it is defined. The most well-recognized definition for chronic bronchitis is the presence of chronic cough and sputum production for 3 months a year, for 2 consecutive years [22]. Chronic bronchitis is also present in the non-COPD population with cigarette smoking as a well-established shared risk factor for both obstructed and non-obstructed individuals [23]. Table 10.1 summarizes studies examining prevalence of chronic bronchitis in both the COPD and non-COPD patient populations.

Table 10.1 Summary of studies estimating the prevalence of chronic bronchitis [33]

Study	Patients	Findings
Lange et al., 1989 [34]	General population, Copenhagen; 12,698 adults	Bronchial hypersecretion: 10.1%
Sobradillo et al., 1999 [35]	General population, Spain; 4035 adults aged 40–69 years	Cough: 13.5% Expectoration 10.7% Chronic bronchitis 4.8%
Pallasaho et al., 1999 [36]	Random sample, Finland; 8000 patients aged 20–69 years	Productive cough: 27%
Von Hertzen et al., 2000 [37]	Random patients, Finland; 7217 patients aged >30 years	Chronic bronchitis and/or emphysema: 22% in men, 7% in women
Cerveri et al., 2001 [38]	General population, Europe; 17,966 patients aged 20–44 years	Chronic bronchitis: 2.6% (range 0.7–9.7% across countries)
Janson et al., 2001 [39]	Multinational; 18,277 patients aged 20–48 years	Productive cough: 10.2%
Huchon et al., 2002 [40]	General population, France; 14,076 patients	Chronic bronchitis: 4.1% Chronic cough and/or expectoration: 11.7%
Lundback et al., 2003 [41]	5892 patients from OLIN study cohort	Chronic productive cough: 60% in COPD patients
Miravitlles et al., 2006 [42]	General population, Spain; 6758 adults aged >40 years	Cough: 5% in never-smokers, 11% in smokers or ex-smokers Expectoration: 4% in never-smokers, 11% in smokers and ex-smokers
Pelkonen et al., 2006 [43]	Finnish cohort of 1711 adult men aged 40–59 years	Incidence of chronic productive cough: 42% current smokers, 26% past smokers, 22% never-smokers
De Marco et al., 2007 [44]	International cohort of 5002 patients aged 20–44 years with normal lung function	Chronic cough/phlegm production: 9.2%
Miravitlles et al., 2009 [45]	Population-based sample, Spain; 4274 adults aged 40–80 years	Chronic cough: 3.4% Chronic sputum production: 11.7%
Harmsen et al., 2010 [46]	Danish cohort of 29,180 (in 1994) and 21,130 (in 2004) twins aged 12–41 years	Cumulative prevalence of chronic mucus secretion over 10 years of study, 10.7% in women and 8.7% in men
Kim et al., 2011 [47]	US cohort of 1061 adults current or former smokers with COPD	Chronic bronchitis: 27.3%
Martinez et al., 2014 [48]	US cohort of 5858 adults past or previous smokers without airflow obstruction	Chronic bronchitis: 34.6%

Biomass smoke exposure may also contribute [12–14]. Genetic factors are likely at play as genome studies have identified a single-nucleotide polymorphism associated with chronic mucus hypersecretion on chromosome 3 [24]. Radiographically, chronic bronchitis is associated with greater airway disease manifest by higher bronchial wall thickness-to-diameter ratios [25].

In the COPDGene cohort, in addition to current smoking, allergic rhinitis, acute bronchitis, asthma, male gender, and Caucasian race (as opposed to African American race) were also associated with clinical phenotype of chronic bronchitis [26]. In this analysis, COPD subjects with chronic bronchitis were also more likely to have allergic nasal and ocular symptoms, higher exacerbation frequency, worse health-related quality of life, and lower 6-minute walk distance as compared to COPD patients without chronic bronchitis [26]. Most importantly, identification of the chronic bronchitis phenotype has important therapeutic implications.

Roflumilast, an oral phosphodiesterase-4 inhibitor, has been found to be most effective in patients with a chronic bronchitis phenotype and a history of repeated exacerbations [27, 28]. PDE-4 inhibitors such as roflumilast are believed to reduce airway inflammation through a variety of mechanisms [29–32]. While initial clinical trials showed inconsistent effects of PDE-4 inhibitors on clinically relevant outcomes such as frequency of acute exacerbation in all-comers with COPD, follow-up studies have demonstrated improved lung function and reduction in frequency of exacerbations in patients specifically with chronic bronchitis symptoms and severe airflow obstruction [27]. Use of roflumilast in this patient population results in reduced frequency of exacerbation, modest improvements in FEV_1, and improved dyspnea scores [27].

Asthma COPD Overlap Syndrome (ACOS)

Asthma COPD overlap syndrome (ACOS) is becoming increasingly recognized as a unique clinical subgroup but definitive criteria for identifying these patients are still evolving. Proposed definitions vary in complexity from "airflow obstruction that is not completely reversible, accompanied by symptoms or signs of increased obstruction reversibility" [49] to the presence of discrete major and minor criteria [50]. Clinically, patients with ACOS tend to be younger than those with COPD but older than those with "pure" asthma and have less smoking history than typically seen in traditional COPD [51]. They often demonstrate features associated with asthma including wheezing, atopy, elevated total immunoglobulin (Ig) E levels, and allergic problems such as allergic rhinitis and hay fever [52, 53]. Airway inflammation tends to be more eosinophilic than the usual neutrophilic inflammation described in COPD patients [54]. Pulmonary function testing also reveals a higher carbon monoxide diffusing capacity (DLCO) and more pronounced acute bronchodilator response [54, 55]. On HRCT, patients clinically identified with ACOS have more air trapping, less emphysema, and greater bronchial wall thickening [52, 56].

Part of the difficulty in creating criteria to identify these overlap patients is the heterogeneity that already exists within both asthma and COPD. For instance, not all asthmatics fit the typical eosinophilic, steroid-responsive profile [51]. Smoking asthmatics may fit a profile more consistent with traditional COPD including minimal lung function improvement with inhaled corticosteroids (ICS) [57–59]. However, in general, ACOS represents a group of COPD patients who are more likely to receive greater benefit from ICS, regardless of FEV_1 severity and exacerbation history, due to it ascribed features (eosinophila, bronchodilator responsiveness) [51].

Gender

Gender has been linked to disease susceptibility, symptoms, exacerbations, rate of progression, extent and distribution of airway abnormalities, and mortality in COPD. Several studies have demonstrated that women suffer more severe airflow limitation than men for a given tobacco exposure and are disproportionately represented among COPD patients without a history of significant smoking [60, 61]. The physiologic changes of COPD may also affect women and men differently in terms of symptoms and quality of life [11]. For a similar degree of physiologic impairment, several studies suggest women experience more severe dyspnea and worse health-related quality of life than men [62–64]. Additionally, the experience of symptoms may be further modified by gender-associated COPD comorbidities, with women for instance experiencing higher rates of anxiety and depression [11]. Female gender and the presence of anxiety and depression have both been independently linked to hospital readmissions for COPD exacerbations [11, 65]. Several studies have also demonstrated an increased frequency of exacerbation in women; however, it remains unclear if this is related to disease biology or difference in reporting patterns [66, 67]. From a physiologic perspective, data from the National Emphysema Trial suggest that men and women may respond differently in the type and location of lung damage due to tobacco exposure. In a population of patients with severe emphysema, women demonstrated less severe overall emphysema though on histologic examination had significantly thicker bronchiole airway walls. Work needs to be done to understand the therapeutic implications of these data. We do know that the effects of smoking cessation, the most impactful intervention for patients with COPD, vary by on gender. Smoking cessation benefits women more in regard to lung function (improvement in FEV_1) though men have greater improvement in symptoms. Unfortunately, multiple studies suggest women have greater difficulty in sustaining long-term abstinence from tobacco use but it may be more important [68].

Comorbidities

Accumulating data suggest that comorbidities must be included in the assessment of COPD with conditions such as cardiovascular disease and osteoporosis that are more prevalent in the COPD population and conditions such as obstructive sleep apnea (OSA) that may modify the disease course.

Cardiovascular Disease

Ischemic cardiovascular disease continues to be a leading cause of death in COPD [69]. While tobacco use is a shared risk factor, epidemiologic evidence suggests that impaired lung function itself is an independent risk factor for cardiovascular mortality, even when adjusted for smoking status [70]. Data from the National Health and Nutrition Examination Survey demonstrated that patients in the lowest FEV_1 quintile had the highest risk of cardiovascular mortality (RR 3.36), even after adjustment for smoking status, blood pressure, BMI, and presence of diabetes [70]. In patients with COPD, FEV_1 predicts the presence of atherosclerosis [71] as well as cardiovascular mortality [72, 73]. COPD is also a risk factor for hospitalization due to cardiovascular events [74]. The characterization of atherosclerosis as a disease of systemic inflammation helps may explain the connection to COPD [75]. Elevated C-reactive protein (CRP) levels correlate not only with the presence of COPD but also with the presence of exacerbations, severity of lung function, and risk for hospitalization and death [76]. Cardioselective beta-blockers, frequently used in patients with cardiovascular disease, have traditionally been used with caution in patients with COPD due to the theoretical risk of worsening bronchospasm. However, more recent data has suggested that beta-blockers may actually reduce all-cause mortality in COPD [77–79]. The use of other cardiovascular disease medications including statins alone or in combination with angiotensin-converting inhibitor or angiotensin receptor blockers has also been shown to improve overall mortality and reduce hospitalizations in several COPD cohort studies [80, 81].

Musculoskeletal Disease

Cachexia defined as a loss of fat and muscle tissues can be seen in severe COPD, with a reported prevalence of 5–15% [82]. Weight loss and muscular wasting play a role in low exercise capacity seen in COPD [83]. Additionally, low BMI is an important independent predictor of increased mortality in patients with COPD [84]. The prognostic effect of BMI is further supported by its inclusion in the BMI, airflow obstruction, dyspnea, and exercise capacity (BODE) index, which is one of the best mortality prediction indices in COPD [85]. Several studies have also correlated low BMI with greater extent of emphysema on HRCT, confirming its association with the classic pink puffer phenotype [86]. Conversely higher BMI has been associated with the presence of chronic bronchitis and HRCT indicators of airway disease [47]. Body composition is important in the assessment of COPD patients as the negative effect of low body weight on survival can be reversed by appropriate therapy in some COPD patients [87]. A relationship between increased mortality and low fat-free mass index (FFMI) has also been demonstrated, even in subjects with a normal BMI [88]. In fact, patients with low FFMI are often more severely disabled than COPD patients with low BMI and normal FFMI [89]. FFMI has been shown to be a strong predictor of peripheral skeletal muscle weakness, exercise capacity, and reduced health status [90–94]. In regard to exercise capacity, FFMI has been shown to correlate more specifically with 6-minute walk distance [95, 96]. Greater FFMI has also been inversely associated with emphysema extent on HRCT [86]. Assessment of FFM is important in patients referred to pulmonary rehabilitation, as exercise training results in a significant gain in FFM in normal-weight COPD patients [97].

As with low BMI, osteoporosis and low bone mineral density seems to be more strongly related to the presence and severity of emphysema, but not related to the severity of chronic bronchitis or airway wall thickness as assessed by HRCT [98]. A clear association has been shown between osteoporosis and COPD with studies suggesting a two- to five-fold increase in prevalence of osteoporosis in patients with COPD compared with age-matched controls [99, 100]. There are multiple shared risk factors between COPD and osteoporosis that likely influence this association including oral and inhaled steroid use, smoking, low body mass index (BMI), and physical inactivity [101]. However, low bone mineral density has also been shown in patients with COPD even in the absence of systemic steroids [101]. Pulmonary rehabilitation improves the functional status of patients with COPD and may diminish fracture risk by decreasing the risk of falls, but has not been shown to increase bone mineral density directly [102].

Diabetes

Diabetes is another comorbidity with increased prevalence in COPD. Lung function impairment has been associated with the coexistence of metabolic syndrome, insulin resistance, and the development of diabetes [103–105]. This association remains even after adjustment for BMI and smoking. The exact cause of this association is not known, but data implicates inhaled corticosteroids (ICS). While some studies have suggested a dose-dependent association between inhaled corticosteroid use and diabetes control and new onset diabetes, [106] a retrospective analysis of eight COPD trials and 26 asthma trials found no association between ICS and hyperglycemia [107]. A higher prevalence of diabetes has been seen with airway-disease-predominant COPD phenotype compared with emphysema-predominant phenotype [108]. Patients with airway-predominant disease also demonstrated a higher BMI and less frequent osteoporosis. Certain inflammatory mediators such as interleukin 6 (IL-6) and tumor necrosis factor-alpha (TNF-α) have been implicated in both bronchial inflammation and insulin resistance [2]. While data supports a relationship between certain metabolic pathways and COPD phenotypes, the exact pathways and therapeutic implications are currently unknown.

Gastroesophageal Reflux Disease

The association between gastroesophageal reflux disease (GERD) and COPD is also recognized. The presence of heartburn, regurgitation, and dysphagia has been found with higher frequency in patients with COPD compared with controls [109, 110]. Studies including esophageal pH monitoring have demonstrated that the actual proportion of GERD in the COPD population is higher than estimates based on symptoms alone. Both cross-section and longitudinal studies have reported associations between the presence of reflux and poor quality of life in COPD [111]. GERD has also been identified as a risk factor for COPD exacerbations [66, 112] and is specifically associated with the chronic bronchitic phenotype discussed previously. The presence of GERD is associated with increased symptoms, poorer quality of life, and increased frequency of exacerbations; associations which are maintained after controlling for PPI use [113]. Unfortunately, only limited data suggest that treatment of GERD may reduce the risk of exacerbations [114].

Obstructive Sleep Apnea (OSA)

In patients with COPD, the prevalence of obstructive sleep apnea has been estimated to be 16% [115], compared to an estimated 9% in women and 24% in men in the general population [116]. However, poor sleep quality, decreased sleep efficiency, and difficulties in initiating and maintaining sleep have been reported in more than 40% of patients with COPD [117]. In general, COPD patients with OSA are more severely hypercapnic, demonstrate more profound and frequent nocturnal oxygen desaturation, and have a higher risk of pulmonary hypertension [118]. Untreated OSA is also a risk factor for poor quality of live, acute exacerbations, and increased all-cause mortality [119, 120]. Diagnosis of OSA in COPD is important as initiation of continuous positive airway pressure therapy for patients with overlap has been associated with both decreased frisk of death and decreased incidence of severe exacerbations [119].

Depression and Anxiety

Coexistent depression and anxiety are seen in at least 10% of the general COPD population [121, 122]; however, with significantly higher estimated in patients with severe COPD [123]. Risk factors for depression in COPD include disease severity, limited mobility, low BMI, comorbid conditions, the need for supplemental oxygen, and female gender [124, 125]. COPD patients with comorbid anxiety are at risk for COPD exacerbations and higher morality [126], while depressive symptoms are associated with increased risk of death [127, 128]. While specific therapies for anxiety and depression have not been shown to improve COPD outcomes, pulmonary rehab has been shown to improve anxiety and depression in addition to overall quality of life and functional capacity [129].

Two general patterns of clinical features and comorbidities have been proposed which may represent unique phenotypes: [1] emphysema, low BMI and osteoporosis and [2] chronic bronchitis, airway disease, high BMI, OSA, and diabetes [2]. However, it is still unclear if these associations are related to specific mechanistic pathways that could lead to development of targeted therapies.

Physiologically Defined Phenotypes

Spirometric indices, including FEV_1, FVC, and their ratio, are used to define the presence and severity of disease. While pulmonary function explains less than 10–25% of disease impact on symptoms, quality of life, and exercise performance [130–132], FEV_1 remains an important outcome measure in COPD. Moreover, rapid physiologic progression as indicated by a change in FEV_1 may indicate a distinct phenotype. A more rapid decline in FEV_1 has been associated with morbidity, mortality, and hospitalization rates in COPD [133] and also has been linked to distinct plasma biomarker signatures [134]. The rate of FEV_1 decline has been associated with airway reactivity, exacerbations, and possibly a chronic inflammatory state [135–139]. There has been conflicting data regarding the role of inhaled corticosteroids in reducing decline in FEV_1 [140, 141]. Some genetic associations have also been seen, particularly with accelerated decline in FEV_1 in smokers with alpha-1 antitrypsin deficiency [142]. Additionally, a single nuclear polymorphism has been identified in the A disintegrin and metalloprotease 33 (ADAM33) gene, a susceptibility gene for asthma, that is associated with decline in FEV_1 in COPD [143]. While smoking cessation remains the best treatment for preventing FEV1 loss [133], it is unclear whether other currently available medications are effective in slowing lung function decline although several studies suggest bronchodilators and inhaled bronchodilator/corticosteroid combinations may be effective, particularly in moderate disease [144, 145].

GOLD defines an exacerbation as an event characterized by a change in the patient's baseline dyspnea, cough, and/or sputum production that is beyond normal day-to-day variation, is acute in onset, and may warrant a change in regular medication in a patient with underlying COPD [146]. In literature, exacerbations are often defined functionally (and not biologically) as "health care utilization" events requiring treatment with antibiotics, systemic corticosteroids, or both [147]. The natural history of COPD is punctuated by exacerbations that appear to be associated with accelerated decline in lung function [136, 137], reduced physical activity, poorer quality of life, increased health care utilization, and increased risk of death [148–151]. The Evaluation of COPD Longitudinally to Identify Predictive Surrogate Endpoints (ECLIPSE) cohort study demonstrated that while increased exacerbations occur as lung function declines, certain individuals demonstrate a relatively stable susceptibility phenotype irrespective of lung function [66]. Other factors identified as being associated with increased exacerbation frequency included a history of GERD, poorer quality of life, and elevated white blood cell count [66]. Controlled trials have shown that pharmacotherapy can reduce exacerbations [144, 152], which should be applied to all patients with the frequent exacerbation phenotype across all disease severities.

While COPD has been characterized as a disorder with airflow obstruction that is not fully reversible [146, 153], the presence of bronchodilator reversibility has been confirmed in patients clinically diagnosed with non-asthmatic COPD and may be clinically relevant [154–156]. There are various spirometric criteria for bronchoreversibility. The American Thoracic Society (ATS)/European Respiratory Society (ERS) defines bronchoreversibility as an increase in FEV_1 greater than or equal to 200 mL and greater than or equal to 12% absolute volume [157]. Alternate physiological criteria include a greater increase in FEV_1 or FVC (greater than or equal to 400 mL) and a 12% increase in either variable [147]. While bronchodilator reversibility defined as change in FEV_1 may be less common with an emphysema-dominant phenotype [147, 158], there is a small subgroup of patients with severe emphysema that meets ATS/ERS criteria for bronchoreversibility. However, the quantity of emphysema determined by HRCT is a negative predictor of meeting volume-guided bronchoreversibility criteria [147]. In the severe emphysema population, bronchoreversibility as defined by a change in FEV_1 is infrequent, varies over time, and is more common in males and those with less severe emphysema. The proportion of patients meeting bronchoreversibility criteria varies by the physiological criteria used to define a positive response, with a propensity for an increase in FVC in patients with emphysema [147].

The true impact of bronchoreversibility on clinically meaningful outcomes such as lung function decline and exacerbation frequency is controversial. The ISOLDE (Inhaled Steroids in Obstructive Lung Disease in Europe) and Lung Health Study data suggest that bronchoreversibility is not associated with accelerated decline in pulmonary function [159] or the number of exacerbations [154]. However, in patients with alpha 1 antitrypsin deficiency, bronchoreversibility has been associated with a greater rate of decline in FEV_1 [160]. Studies in relatives of COPD patients have shown familial clustering of spirometric and bronchodilators responsiveness phenotypes [161–166] and a genome-wide linkage analysis has suggested that bronchoreversibility can be linked to a specific COPD genotype [167], which increases its utility as meaningful phenotype.

In addition to the above, several other physiologic parameters have been identified that predict clinically meaningful outcomes. Airway hyperresponsiveness has been associated with more rapid longitudinal decline in lung function [147, 158], while hyperinflation has been related to mortality and functional impairments [168, 169]. Diffusing capacity impairment is an independent predictor of the extent of radiologic emphysema

[170], the presence of resting hypoxemia, exercise-induced arterial oxygen desaturation [171], and functional impairment [172]. Whether these parameters are truly reflective of a unique biologic processes is unclear and represent possibilities for unique therapeutic interventions is unknown [173, 174].

Radiographically Defined Phenotypes

Chest radiography and computed tomography (CT) are the two imaging modalities most commonly used in COPD. Chest radiography is neither sensitive nor specific for the diagnosis of COPD, but can reveal some characteristic features including radiolucency, diaphragmatic flattening, and hyperinflation. Chest CT allows for better detection and quantification of emphysema and can reveal thickened airways indicative of bronchial thickening. CT has also been used as a noninvasive tool to investigate the heterogeneous manifestations of COPD as they correlate to the clinical phenotypes discussed above.

Lung hyperinflation in COPD impairs chest wall and respiratory muscle mechanics, increases breathlessness, impairs weaning from mechanical ventilation, decreases exercise performance, and increases mortality [175]. This led to the development of techniques aimed at decreasing the markedly increased lung volumes seen in emphysema and ultimately lung volume reduction surgery (LVRS) [176–181]. The National Emphysema Treatment Trial (NETT) was a multicenter prospective randomized controlled trial that compared optimal medical treatment, including pulmonary rehabilitation, with optimal medical treatment plus LVRS in patients with severe emphysema [158, 182]. NETT demonstrated how physiological and radiographic phenotypes can predict patient survival as well as response to treatment. In COPD patients with upper lobe predominant emphysema and a low exercise capacity post-rehabilitation, LVRS improved survival and quality of life, as compared to those with upper lobe disease and high exercise capacity or COPD patients with non-upper lobe predominant disease regardless of exercise capacity [183]. CT imaging is required to assess emphysema extent and distribution for the purposes of lung volume reduction surgery [158].

Several studies have demonstrated a strong relationship between emphysema and both lung function decline [184, 185] and mortality [186, 187] (Table 10.2). Bronchial thickening seen on CT also has a strong correlation with symptoms [188]. Visually identified bronchiectasis may be associated with an increased risk of death compared to COPD patients without bronchiectasis [189].

Table 10.2 Summary of studies examining the relationship between emphysema and mortality

	Population	Risk factor	Hazard ratio	Outcome
Zulueta et al., [186]	Smokers $n = 9046$	Presence/absence visually scored emphysema	9.3[a]	Death from COPD
			1.7[a]	Death from lung cancer
Haruna et al., [187]	COPD $n = 251$	Emphysema ≥32%	1.52[b] ($p < 0.001$)	All-cause mortality
		Upper lobe emphysema ≥42%	1.55 ($p < 0.001$)	
		FEV1% 10–35%	1.25 ($p = 0.08$)	
Johannessen et al., [190]	Ever-smokers $n = 974$ (49% with COPD)	Emphysema 3–10%	56 months less survival ($p < 0.05$)	All-cause mortality[c], respiratory[c], cardiovascular[c], cancer and lung cancer
		Emphysema >10%	67 months less survival ($p < 0.05$)	

Table from "Clinical correlations of CT Imaging in COPD" [191]

[a]Adjusted for age and smoking history

[b]In multivariate models including age, emphysema, BMI, FEV1, RV/TLC, and DLCO/VA, only age and %LAA (low areas of attenuation) were significant predictors of mortality from respiratory disease. In models examining all-cause mortality, BMI, age, LAA% were all predictive

[c]Significant also in models adjusted for sex, interaction between sex and %LAA, COPD status, post-bronchodilator FEV! %predicted, age, smoking status, and inflation level for emphysema <10% group only

Different radiographic features have been utilized to define different physiologic parameters, which are associated with a variety of clinical outcomes. It is the airways less than 2 mm in diameter, that are thought to be the site of airflow obstruction in COPD [192], which unfortunately is below the limit of resolution for CT imaging. COPD's effects on small airways can be quantified indirectly through the measurement of air trapping using both inspiratory and expiratory images on chest CT [193–195]. One of these methods, the ratio of expiratory to inspiratory mean lung density has been found to correlate with spirometric measure of air trapping (ratio of residual volume to total lung capacity) [196] and has been shown to correlate with clinical outcomes including six-minute walk distance, dyspnea, and BODE score [197].

Pulmonary vascular disease has classically been described as a phenomenon of severe COPD. The total cross-sectional area of small pulmonary vessels assessed with CT has significant correlation with pulmonary artery pressures assess via right heart catheterization [198]. Pulmonary vascular abnormalities may also occur earlier in COPD and have clinical significance. In fact, CT detected pulmonary artery enlargement, defined as ratio of the diameter of the pulmonary artery to the diameter of the aorta, has been shown to identify patients at risk of COPD exacerbation [199].

Biologically Defined Phenotypes

While the term phenotype encompasses the clinically relevant properties of the disease, it does not necessarily defined a distinct to disease etiology or pathophysiology. Alternatively, endotypes describe subtypes of a disease defined by an intrinsically distinct pathogenetic mechanism [200]. Endotypes can then be utilized to identify biomarkers and potential novel therapeutic approaches [200]. Linking of endotypes to clinical phenotypes and to endotype-specific biomarkers will be crucial because phenotypes and biomarkers are more accessible to clinicians than endotypes [201] (Fig. 10.2).

Endotype identification in COPD is still in its relative infancy, but several possible endotypes have been identified. As previously discussed, the asthma-COPD overlap phenotype is a clinically apparent entity. A specific airway epithelial gene expression pattern that has previously been noted in Th2 inflammation in asthma has also been noted in COPD to correlate with decreased lung function, increased airway eosinophil counts, greater blood eosinophil percentage, bronchodilator reversibility, and improvement in hyperinflation with corticosteroid treatment [203]. Interestingly, the presence of Th2-associated signature is not predicted by a clinical history of asthma.

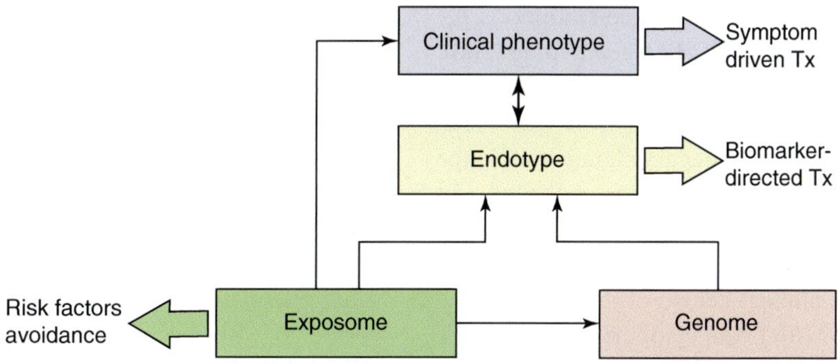

Fig. 10.2 Interrelations between exposome, genome, endotype, and clinical phenotype of COPD—Diagram of the interrelations (*thin black arrows*) between the exposome (the totality of human environmental exposures, from conception onwards [202]), genome (the genetic background of the individual), the endotype (biological networks that enable and restrict reactions), and the clinical phenotype (final clinical expression of the disease, e.g., symptoms, exacerbations, response to treatment, rate of disease progression, or death). *Large arrows* represent different treatment strategies. *COPD* chronic obstructive pulmonary disease, *Tx* treatment [200]

Related to this concept, previous studies in patients with COPD have also shown that eosinophilic airway inflammation is associated with acute exacerbations of COPD [204, 205] and can also predict a beneficial response to treatment with corticosteroids [206–209]. Eosinophilic airway inflammation can be seen in 10–20% of patients with COPD during both stable periods and acute exacerbations [204, 205, 207, 210, 211]. The use of corticosteroid therapy to reduce concentrations of airway eosinophils decreases frequency of severe acute exacerbation [205]. Benralizumab, an anti-interleukin-5 receptor (alpha) monoclonal antibody, depletes blood and sputum eosinophils [212, 213] and has been investigated as a therapeutic to decrease the frequency of acute exacerbation in COPD. Similar to roflumilast, a recent Phase II study of benralizumab compared to placebo did not reduce the rate of acute exacerbations; however, subgroup analysis support further investigation in patients with COPD and eosinophilia, which may represent a future target for directed therapy [214]. These data suggest several biomarkers related to inflammatory patterns seen in asthma have the potential to identify individuals with COPD who may be candidates for directed therapies.

Alpha-1 antitrypsin deficiency, as described above also meets criteria for an endotype of COPD. It has known genetic foundation, distinct clinical characteristics, characteristic histopathology, distinct epidemiology, and a mechanism-directed treatment approach that is guided by biomarkers, serum a1AT concentration, a1AT protein phenotyping, and a1AT genotyping [200].

Other possible endotypes in COPD are also under current investigation. COPD has been associated with signs of local inflammation in the airways involving neutrophils, macrophages, and T-cells [215]. Additionally, signs of systemic inflammation involving neutrophils have been linked to the clinical course of smoking-related COPD [215, 216]. Local cytokine signaling by T helper (Th)17 cells via Interleukin (IL)-17 is important for antibacterial host defense in the airways. In smokers with COPD including chronic bronchitis, systemic cytokine signaling via IL-17 appears to be impaired, and this alteration may be linked to colonization by opportunistic pathogens in the airways [217]. Further studies are needed to validate and evaluate potential therapeutic implications.

The six inflammatory biomarkers most studied in COPD include white blood cell (WBC) count, C-reactive protein (CRP), interleukins 6 (IL-6) and 8 (IL-8), fibrinogen, and tumor necrosis factor-alpha (TNF-α) [218]. A subgroup of COPD patients has been identified with persistently elevated inflammatory biomarker levels that, despite relatively similar lung function impairment, had significantly increased all-cause mortality and exacerbation frequency [219]. While the severity of airflow limitation has been largely used as the most important criteria to guide therapy in COPD [146], identification of this phenotype demonstrates that patients with similar levels of airflow limitation may have different outcomes depending on the presence or absence of persistent systemic inflammation. The treatment implications of these findings will require further investigation.

Conclusions

To date the majority of large trials investigating COPD therapies have not targeted-specific phenotypes. Nor have they been designed to clearly identify either predictors of response or harm, but development of a "personalized medicine" approach is a critical goal for the future of COPD treatment approaches. Future studies in COPD will be increasingly phenotype or ideally endotype driven. In order to achieve that goal, identification and validation of phenotypes in COPD will require analysis of longitudinal data in carefully characterized patient populations [1]. Multiple large observational and cohort studies, some of which have been mentioned above, have already begun this process by systematically gathering clinical, physiologic, radiologic, biologic, and genetic data on a wide spectrum of COPD patients. Representative studies include ECLIPSE, COPDGene, Subpopulations and Intermediate Outcome Measures in COPD (SPIROMICS), Canadian cohort obstructive lung disease (CanCOLD), and the Korean Obstructive Lung Disease (KOLD) cohort. Advanced statistical techniques incorporating systems biology and network medicine may also provide additional frameworks for understanding this disease's complexities [220–222] and aid in the identification of clinically meaningful groups [223–226].

References

1. Han MK, Agusti A, Calverley PM, Celli BR, Criner G, Curtis JL, Fabbri LM, Goldin JG, Jones PW, Macnee W, Make BJ, Rabe KF, Rennard SI, Sciurba FC, Silverman EK, Vestbo J, Washko GR, Wouters EF, Martinez FJ. Chronic obstructive pulmonary disease phenotypes: the future of COPD. Am J Respir Crit Care Med. 2010;182:598–604.
2. Martinez CH, Han MK. Contribution of the environment and comorbidities to chronic obstructive pulmonary disease phenotypes. Med Clin North Am. 2012;96:713–27.
3. Vestbo J, Hurd SS, Agusti AG, Jones PW, Vogelmeier C, Anzueto A, Barnes PJ, Fabbri LM, Martinez FJ, Nishimura M, Stockley RA, Sin DD, Rodriguez-Roisin R. Global strategy for the diagnosis, management, and prevention of chronic obstructive pulmonary disease: GOLD executive summary. Am J Respir Crit Care Med. 2013;187:347–65.
4. Lokke A, Lange P, Scharling H, Fabricius P, Vestbo J. Developing COPD: a 25 year follow up study of the general population. Thorax. 2006;61:935–9.
5. McDonough JE, Yuan R, Suzuki M, Seyednejad N, Elliott WM, Sanchez PG, Wright AC, Gefter WB, Litzky L, Coxson HO, Pare PD, Sin DD, Pierce RA, Woods JC, McWilliams AM, Mayo JR, Lam SC, Cooper JD, Hogg JC. Small-airway obstruction and emphysema in chronic obstructive pulmonary disease. N Engl J Med. 2011;365:1567–75.
6. Anthonisen NR, Connett JE, Kiley JP, Altose MD, Bailey WC, Buist AS, Conway WA Jr, Enright PL, Kanner RE, O'Hara P, et al. Effects of smoking intervention and the use of an inhaled anticholinergic bronchodilator on the rate of decline of FEV1. The Lung Health Study. JAMA. 1994;272:1497–505.
7. Shavelle RM, Paculdo DR, Kush SJ, Mannino DM, Strauss DJ. Life expectancy and years of life lost in chronic obstructive pulmonary disease: findings from the NHANES III follow-up study. Int J Chron Obstruct Pulmon Dis. 2009;4:137–48.
8. Tan WC, Sin DD, Bourbeau J, Hernandez P, Chapman KR, Cowie R, FitzGerald JM, Marciniuk DD, Maltais F, Buist AS, Road J, Hogg JC, Kirby M, Coxson H, Hague C, Leipsic J, O'Donnell DE, Aaron SD, Can CCRG. Characteristics of COPD in never-smokers and ever-smokers in the general population: results from the CanCOLD study. Thorax. 2015;70(9):822–9.
9. Castaldi PJ, Dy J, Ross J, Chang Y, Washko GR, Curran-Everett D, Williams A, Lynch DA, Make BJ, Crapo JD, Bowler RP, Regan EA, Hokanson JE, Kinney GL, Han MK, Soler X, Ramsdell JW, Barr RG, Foreman M, van Beek E, Casaburi R, Criner GJ, Lutz SM, Rennard SI, Santorico S, Sciurba FC, DeMeo DL, Hersh CP, Silverman EK, Cho MH. Cluster analysis in the COPDGene study identifies subtypes of smokers with distinct patterns of airway disease and emphysema. Thorax. 2014;69:415–22.
10. Eisner MD, Anthonisen N, Coultas D, Kuenzli N, Perez-Padilla R, Postma D, Romieu I, Silverman EK, Balmes JR, Committee on Nonsmoking Copd E, Occupational Health A. An official American Thoracic Society public policy statement: novel risk factors and the global burden of chronic obstructive pulmonary disease. Am J Respir Crit Care Med. 2010;182:693–718.
11. Han MK, Postma D, Mannino DM, Giardino ND, Buist S, Curtis JL, Martinez FJ. Gender and chronic obstructive pulmonary disease: why it matters. Am J Respir Crit Care Med. 2007;176:1179–84.
12. Camp PG, Ramirez-Venegas A, Sansores RH, Alva LF, McDougall JE, Sin DD, Pare PD, Muller NL, Silva CI, Rojas CE, Coxson HO. COPD phenotypes in biomass smoke- versus tobacco smoke-exposed Mexican women. Eur Respir J. 2014;43:725–34.
13. Gonzalez-Garcia M, Maldonado Gomez D, Torres-Duque CA, Barrero M, Jaramillo Villegas C, Perez JM, Varon H. Tomographic and functional findings in severe COPD: comparison between the wood smoke-related and smoking-related disease. J Bras Pneumol. 2013;39:147–54.
14. Moreira MA, Barbosa MA, Queiroz MC, Teixeira KI, Torres PP, Santana Junior PJ, Montadon Junior ME, Jardim JR. Pulmonary changes on HRCT scans in nonsmoking females with COPD due to wood smoke exposure. J Bras Pneumol. 2013;39:155–63.
15. Lieberman J, Winter B, Sastre A. Alpha 1-antitrypsin Pi-types in 965 COPD patients. Chest. 1986;89:370–3.
16. Tobin MJ, Cook PJ, Hutchison DC. Alpha 1 antitrypsin deficiency: the clinical and physiological features of pulmonary emphysema in subjects homozygous for Pi type Z. A survey by the British Thoracic Association. Br J Dis Chest. 1983;77:14–27.
17. Larsson C. Natural history and life expectancy in severe alpha1-antitrypsin deficiency, Pi Z. Acta Med Scand. 1978;204:345–51.
18. Janus ED, Phillips NT, Carrell RW. Smoking, lung function, and alpha 1-antitrypsin deficiency. Lancet. 1985;1:152–4.
19. Black LF, Kueppers F. Alpha1-antitrypsin deficiency in nonsmokers. Am Rev Respir Dis. 1978;117:421–8.
20. Green CE, Vayalapra S, Hampson JA, Mukherjee D, Stockley RA, Turner AM. PiSZ alpha-1 antitrypsin deficiency (AATD): pulmonary phenotype and prognosis relative to PiZZ AATD and PiMM COPD. Thorax. 2015;70(10):939–45.
21. Stockley RA, Turner AM. Alpha-1-antitrypsin deficiency: clinical variability, assessment, and treatment. Trends Mol Med. 2014;20:105–15.

22. Ferris BG. Epidemiology standardization project (American Thoracic Society). Am Rev Respir Dis. 1978;118:1–120.
23. Forey BA, Thornton AJ, Lee PN. Systematic review with meta-analysis of the epidemiological evidence relating smoking to COPD, chronic bronchitis and emphysema. BMC Pulm Med. 2011;11:36.
24. Dijkstra AE, Smolonska J, van den Berge M, Wijmenga C, Zanen P, Luinge MA, Platteel M, Lammers JW, Dahlback M, Tosh K, Hiemstra PS, Sterk PJ, Spira A, Vestbo J, Nordestgaard BG, Benn M, Nielsen SF, Dahl M, Verschuren WM, Picavet HS, Smit HA, Owsijewitsch M, Kauczor HU, de Koning HJ, Nizankowska-Mogilnicka E, Mejza F, Nastalek P, van Diemen CC, Cho MH, Silverman EK, Crapo JD, Beaty TH, Lomas DA, Bakke P, Gulsvik A, Bosse Y, Obeidat MA, Loth DW, Lahousse L, Rivadeneira F, Uitterlinden AG, Hofman A, Stricker BH, Brusselle GG, van Duijn CM, Brouwer U, Koppelman GH, Vonk JM, Nawijn MC, Groen HJ, Timens W, Boezen HM, Postma DS, LifeLines Cohort s. Susceptibility to chronic mucus hypersecretion, a genome wide association study. PLoS One. 2014;9:e91621.
25. Orlandi I, Moroni C, Camiciottoli G, Bartolucci M, Pistolesi M, Villari N, Mascalchi M. Chronic obstructive pulmonary disease: thin-section CT measurement of airway wall thickness and lung attenuation. Radiology. 2005;234:604–10.
26. Kim V, Davey A, Comellas AP, Han MK, Washko G, Martinez CH, Lynch D, Lee JH, Silverman EK, Crapo JD, Make BJ, Criner GJ, Investigators CO. Clinical and computed tomographic predictors of chronic bronchitis in COPD: a cross sectional analysis of the COPDGene study. Respir Res. 2014;15:52.
27. Calverley PM, Rabe KF, Goehring UM, Kristiansen S, Fabbri LM, Martinez FJ, M, groups Ms. Roflumilast in symptomatic chronic obstructive pulmonary disease: two randomised clinical trials. Lancet. 2009;374:685–94.
28. Rennard SI, Calverley PM, Goehring UM, Bredenbroker D, Martinez FJ. Reduction of exacerbations by the PDE4 inhibitor roflumilast—the importance of defining different subsets of patients with COPD. Respir Res. 2011;12:18.
29. Grootendorst DC, Gauw SA, Verhoosel RM, Sterk PJ, Hospers JJ, Bredenbroker D, Bethke TD, Hiemstra PS, Rabe KF. Reduction in sputum neutrophil and eosinophil numbers by the PDE4 inhibitor roflumilast in patients with COPD. Thorax. 2007;62:1081–7.
30. Spina D. PDE4 inhibitors: current status. Br J Pharmacol. 2008;155:308–15.
31. Bundschuh DS, Eltze M, Barsig J, Wollin L, Hatzelmann A, Beume R. In vivo efficacy in airway disease models of roflumilast, a novel orally active PDE4 inhibitor. J Pharmacol Exp Ther. 2001;297:280–90.
32. Hatzelmann A, Schudt C. Anti-inflammatory and immunomodulatory potential of the novel PDE4 inhibitor roflumilast in vitro. J Pharmacol Exp Ther. 2001;297:267–79.
33. Miravitlles M. Cough and sputum production as risk factors for poor outcomes in patients with COPD. Respir Med. 2011;105:1118–28.
34. Lange P, Groth S, Nyboe J, Appleyard M, Mortensen J, Jensen G, Schnohr P. Chronic obstructive lung disease in Copenhagen: cross-sectional epidemiological aspects. J Intern Med. 1989;226:25–32.
35. Sobradillo V, Miravitlles M, Jimenez CA, Gabriel R, Viejo JL, Masa JF, Fernandez-Fau L, Villasante C. Epidemiological study of chronic obstructive pulmonary disease in Spain (IBERPOC): prevalence of chronic respiratory symptoms and airflow limitation. Arch Bronconeumol. 1999;35:159–66.
36. Pallasaho P, Lundback B, Laspa SL, Jonsson E, Kotaniemi J, Sovijarvi AR, Laitinen LA. Increasing prevalence of asthma but not of chronic bronchitis in Finland? Report from the FinEsS-Helsinki Study. Respir Med. 1999;93:798–809.
37. von Hertzen L, Reunanen A, Impivaara O, Malkia E, Aromaa A. Airway obstruction in relation to symptoms in chronic respiratory disease—a nationally representative population study. Respir Med. 2000;94:356–63.
38. Cerveri I, Accordini S, Verlato G, Corsico A, Zoia MC, Casali L, Burney P, de Marco R, European Community Respiratory Health Survey Study G. Variations in the prevalence across countries of chronic bronchitis and smoking habits in young adults. Eur Respir J. 2001;18:85–92.
39. Janson C, Chinn S, Jarvis D, Burney P. Determinants of cough in young adults participating in the European Community Respiratory Health Survey. Eur Respir J. 2001;18:647–54.
40. Huchon GJ, Vergnenegre A, Neukirch F, Brami G, Roche N, Preux PM. Chronic bronchitis among French adults: high prevalence and underdiagnosis. Eur Respir J. 2002;20:806–12.
41. Lundback B, Lindberg A, Lindstrom M, Ronmark E, Jonsson AC, Jonsson E, Larsson LG, Andersson S, Sandstrom T, Larsson K, Obstructive lung disease in Northern Sweden S. Not 15 but 50% of smokers develop COPD?—report from the obstructive lung disease in Northern Sweden studies. Respir Med. 2003;97:115–22.
42. Miravitlles M, de la Roza C, Morera J, Montemayor T, Gobartt E, Martin A, Alvarez-Sala JL. Chronic respiratory symptoms, spirometry and knowledge of COPD among general population. Respir Med. 2006;100:1973–80.
43. Pelkonen M, Notkola IL, Nissinen A, Tukiainen H, Koskela H. Thirty-year cumulative incidence of chronic bronchitis and COPD in relation to 30-year pulmonary function and 40-year mortality: a follow-up in middle-aged rural men. Chest. 2006;130:1129–37.

44. de Marco R, Accordini S, Cerveri I, Corsico A, Anto JM, Kunzli N, Janson C, Sunyer J, Jarvis D, Chinn S, Vermeire P, Svanes C, Ackermann-Liebrich U, Gislason T, Heinrich J, Leynaert B, Neukirch F, Schouten JP, Wjst M, Burney P. Incidence of chronic obstructive pulmonary disease in a cohort of young adults according to the presence of chronic cough and phlegm. Am J Respir Crit Care Med. 2007;175:32–9.
45. Miravitlles M, Soriano JB, Garcia-Rio F, Munoz L, Duran-Tauleria E, Sanchez G, Sobradillo V, Ancochea J. Prevalence of COPD in Spain: impact of undiagnosed COPD on quality of life and daily life activities. Thorax. 2009;64:863–8.
46. Harmsen L, Thomsen SF, Ingebrigtsen T, Steffensen IE, Skadhauge LR, Kyvik KO, Backer V. Chronic mucus hypersecretion: prevalence and risk factors in younger individuals. Int J Tuberc Lung Dis. 2010;14:1052–8.
47. Kim V, Han MK, Vance GB, Make BJ, Newell JD, Hokanson JE, Hersh CP, Stinson D, Silverman EK, Criner GJ, Investigators CO. The chronic bronchitic phenotype of COPD: an analysis of the COPDGene study. Chest. 2011;140:626–33.
48. Martinez CH, Kim V, Chen Y, Kazerooni EA, Murray S, Criner GJ, Curtis JL, Regan EA, Wan E, Hersh CP, Silverman EK, Crapo JD, Martinez FJ, Han MK, Investigators CO. The clinical impact of non-obstructive chronic bronchitis in current and former smokers. Respir Med. 2014;108:491–9.
49. Miravitlles M, Calle M, Soler-Cataluna JJ. Clinical phenotypes of COPD: identification, definition and implications for guidelines. Arch Bronconeumol. 2012;48:86–98.
50. Soler-Cataluna JJ, Cosio B, Izquierdo JL, Lopez-Campos JL, Marin JM, Aguero R, Baloira A, Carrizo S, Esteban C, Galdiz JB, Gonzalez MC, Miravitlles M, Monso E, Montemayor T, Morera J, Ortega F, Peces-Barba G, Puente L, Rodriguez JM, Sala E, Sauleda J, Soriano JB, Viejo JL. Consensus document on the overlap phenotype COPD-asthma in COPD. Arch Bronconeumol. 2012;48:331–7.
51. Bujarski S, Parulekar AD, Sharafkhaneh A, Hanania NA. The asthma COPD overlap syndrome (ACOS). Curr Allergy Asthma Rep. 2015;15:509.
52. Hardin M, Silverman EK, Barr RG, Hansel NN, Schroeder JD, Make BJ, Crapo JD, Hersh CP, Investigators CO. The clinical features of the overlap between COPD and asthma. Respir Res. 2011;12:127.
53. Zeki AA, Schivo M, Chan A, Albertson TE, Louie S. The Asthma-COPD overlap syndrome: a common clinical problem in the elderly. J Allergy. 2011;2011:861926.
54. Kitaguchi Y, Komatsu Y, Fujimoto K, Hanaoka M, Kubo K. Sputum eosinophilia can predict responsiveness to inhaled corticosteroid treatment in patients with overlap syndrome of COPD and asthma. Int J Chron Obstruct Pulmon Dis. 2012;7:283–9.
55. Menezes AM, Montes de Oca M, Perez-Padilla R, Nadeau G, Wehrmeister FC, Lopez-Varela MV, Muino A, Jardim JR, Valdivia G, Talamo C, Team P. Increased risk of exacerbation and hospitalization in subjects with an overlap phenotype: COPD-asthma. Chest. 2014;145:297–304.
56. Kitaguchi Y, Fujimoto K, Kubo K, Honda T. Characteristics of COPD phenotypes classified according to the findings of HRCT. Respir Med. 2006;100:1742–52.
57. Chaudhuri R, Livingston E, McMahon AD, Thomson L, Borland W, Thomson NC. Cigarette smoking impairs the therapeutic response to oral corticosteroids in chronic asthma. Am J Respir Crit Care Med. 2003;168:1308–11.
58. Chalmers GW, MacLeod KJ, Thomson L, Little SA, McSharry C, Thomson NC. Smoking and airway inflammation in patients with mild asthma. Chest. 2001;120:1917–22.
59. Boulet LP, Lemiere C, Archambault F, Carrier G, Descary MC, Deschesnes F. Smoking and asthma: clinical and radiologic features, lung function, and airway inflammation. Chest. 2006;129:661–8.
60. Chapman KR. Chronic obstructive pulmonary disease: are women more susceptible than men? Clin Chest Med. 2004;25:331–41.
61. Birring SS, Brightling CE, Bradding P, Entwisle JJ, Vara DD, Grigg J, Wardlaw AJ, Pavord ID. Clinical, radiologic, and induced sputum features of chronic obstructive pulmonary disease in nonsmokers: a descriptive study. Am J Respir Crit Care Med. 2002;166:1078–83.
62. Watson L, Vestbo J, Postma DS, Decramer M, Rennard S, Kiri VA, Vermeire PA, Soriano JB. Gender differences in the management and experience of chronic obstructive pulmonary disease. Respir Med. 2004;98:1207–13.
63. de Torres JP, Casanova C, Hernandez C, Abreu J, Aguirre-Jaime A, Celli BR. Gender and COPD in patients attending a pulmonary clinic. Chest. 2005;128:2012–6.
64. Martinez FJ, Curtis JL, Sciurba F, Mumford J, Giardino ND, Weinmann G, Kazerooni E, Murray S, Criner GJ, Sin DD, Hogg J, Ries AL, Han M, Fishman AP, Make B, Hoffman EA, Mohsenifar Z, Wise R, National Emphysema Treatment Trial Research G. Sex differences in severe pulmonary emphysema. Am J Respir Crit Care Med. 2007;176:243–52.
65. Jennings JH, Digiovine B, Obeid D, Frank C. The association between depressive symptoms and acute exacerbations of COPD. Lung. 2009;187:128–35.
66. Hurst JR, Vestbo J, Anzueto A, Locantore N, Mullerova H, Tal-Singer R, Miller B, Lomas DA, Agusti A, Macnee W, Calverley P, Rennard S, Wouters EF, Wedzicha JA, Evaluation of CLtIPSEI. Susceptibility to exacerbation in chronic obstructive pulmonary disease. N Engl J Med. 2010;363:1128–38.

67. Tashkin D, Celli B, Kesten S, Lystig T, Decramer M. Effect of tiotropium in men and women with COPD: results of the 4-year UPLIFT trial. Respir Med. 2010;104:1495–504.
68. Varkey AB. Chronic obstructive pulmonary disease in women: exploring gender differences. Curr Opin Pulm Med. 2004;10:98–103.
69. Hansell AL, Walk JA, Soriano JB. What do chronic obstructive pulmonary disease patients die from? A multiple cause coding analysis. Eur Respir J. 2003;22:809–14.
70. Sin DD, Wu L, Man SF. The relationship between reduced lung function and cardiovascular mortality: a population-based study and a systematic review of the literature. Chest. 2005;127:1952–9.
71. Beaty TH, Newill CA, Cohen BH, Tockman MS, Bryant SH, Spurgeon HA. Effects of pulmonary function on mortality. J Chronic Dis. 1985;38:703–10.
72. Speizer FE, Fay ME, Dockery DW, Ferris BG Jr. Chronic obstructive pulmonary disease mortality in six U.S. cities. Am Rev Respir Dis. 1989;140:S49–55.
73. Hospers JJ, Postma DS, Rijcken B, Weiss ST, Schouten JP. Histamine airway hyper-responsiveness and mortality from chronic obstructive pulmonary disease: a cohort study. Lancet. 2000;356:1313–7.
74. Anthonisen NR, Connett JE, Enright PL, Manfreda J, Lung Health Study Research G. Hospitalizations and mortality in the lung health study. Am J Respir Crit Care Med. 2002;166:333–9.
75. Ross R. Atherosclerosis—an inflammatory disease. N Engl J Med. 1999;340:115–26.
76. Han MK, McLaughlin VV, Criner GJ, Martinez FJ. Pulmonary diseases and the heart. Circulation. 2007;116:2992–3005.
77. Short PM, Lipworth SI, Elder DH, Schembri S, Lipworth BJ. Effect of beta blockers in treatment of chronic obstructive pulmonary disease: a retrospective cohort study. BMJ. 2011;342:d2549.
78. Dransfield MT, Rowe SM, Johnson JE, Bailey WC, Gerald LB. Use of beta blockers and the risk of death in hospitalised patients with acute exacerbations of COPD. Thorax. 2008;63:301–5.
79. Rutten FH, Zuithoff NP, Hak E, Grobbee DE, Hoes AW. Beta-blockers may reduce mortality and risk of exacerbations in patients with chronic obstructive pulmonary disease. Arch Intern Med. 2010;170:880–7.
80. Soyseth V, Brekke PH, Smith P, Omland T. Statin use is associated with reduced mortality in COPD. Eur Respir J. 2007;29:279–83.
81. Mancini GB, Etminan M, Zhang B, Levesque LE, FitzGerald JM, Brophy JM. Reduction of morbidity and mortality by statins, angiotensin-converting enzyme inhibitors, and angiotensin receptor blockers in patients with chronic obstructive pulmonary disease. J Am Coll Cardiol. 2006;47:2554–60.
82. von Haehling S, Anker SD. Cachexia as a major underestimated and unmet medical need: facts and numbers. J Cachex Sarcopenia Muscle. 2010;1:1–5.
83. Gologanu D, Ionita D, Gartonea T, Stanescu C, Bogdan MA. Body composition in patients with chronic obstructive pulmonary disease. Maedica. 2014;9:25–32.
84. Landbo C, Prescott E, Lange P, Vestbo J, Almdal TP. Prognostic value of nutritional status in chronic obstructive pulmonary disease. Am J Respir Crit Care Med. 1999;160:1856–61.
85. Nishimura K, Izumi T, Tsukino M, Oga T. Dyspnea is a better predictor of 5-year survival than airway obstruction in patients with COPD. Chest. 2002;121:1434–40.
86. Marquez-Martin E, Ramos PC, Lopez-Campos JL, Serrano Gotarredona Mdel P, Herrero SN, Aguilar RT, Cortes EB, Ruiz FO. Components of physical capacity in patients with chronic obstructive pulmonary disease: relationship with phenotypic expression. Int J Chron Obstruct Pulmon Dis. 2011;6:105–12.
87. Schols AM, Slangen J, Volovics L, Wouters EF. Weight loss is a reversible factor in the prognosis of chronic obstructive pulmonary disease. Am J Respir Crit Care Med. 1998;157:1791–7.
88. Vestbo J, Prescott E, Almdal T, Dahl M, Nordestgaard BG, Andersen T, Sorensen TI, Lange P. Body mass, fat-free body mass, and prognosis in patients with chronic obstructive pulmonary disease from a random population sample: findings from the Copenhagen City heart study. Am J Respir Crit Care Med. 2006;173:79–83.
89. Schols AM. Pulmonary cachexia. Int J Cardiol. 2002;85:101–10.
90. Engelen MP, Schols AM, Does JD, Wouters EF. Skeletal muscle weakness is associated with wasting of extremity fat-free mass but not with airflow obstruction in patients with chronic obstructive pulmonary disease. Am J Clin Nutr. 2000;71:733–8.
91. Mostert R, Goris A, Weling-Scheepers C, Wouters EF, Schols AM. Tissue depletion and health related quality of life in patients with chronic obstructive pulmonary disease. Respir Med. 2000;94:859–67.
92. Baarends EM, Schols AM, Mostert R, Wouters EF. Peak exercise response in relation to tissue depletion in patients with chronic obstructive pulmonary disease. Eur Respir J. 1997;10:2807–13.
93. Schols AM, Mostert R, Soeters PB, Wouters EF. Body composition and exercise performance in patients with chronic obstructive pulmonary disease. Thorax. 1991;46:695–9.
94. Sabino PG, Silva BM, Brunetto AF. Nutritional status is related to fat-free mass, exercise capacity and inspiratory strength in severe chronic obstructive pulmonary disease patients. Clinics (Sao Paulo). 2010;65:599–605.
95. Budweiser S, Meyer K, Jorres RA, Heinemann F, Wild PJ, Pfeifer M. Nutritional depletion and its relationship to respiratory impairment in patients with chronic respiratory failure due to COPD or restrictive thoracic diseases. Eur J Clin Nutr. 2008;62:436–43.

96. Ischaki E, Papatheodorou G, Gaki E, Papa I, Koulouris N, Loukides S. Body mass and fat-free mass indices in COPD: relation with variables expressing disease severity. Chest. 2007;132:164–9.
97. Franssen FM, Broekhuizen R, Janssen PP, Wouters EF, Schols AM. Effects of whole-body exercise training on body composition and functional capacity in normal-weight patients with COPD. Chest. 2004;125:2021–8.
98. Bon J, Fuhrman CR, Weissfeld JL, Duncan SR, Branch RA, Chang CC, Zhang Y, Leader JK, Gur D, Greenspan SL, Sciurba FC. Radiographic emphysema predicts low bone mineral density in a tobacco-exposed cohort. Am J Respir Crit Care Med. 2011;183:885–90.
99. Bolton CE, Ionescu AA, Shiels KM, Pettit RJ, Edwards PH, Stone MD, Nixon LS, Evans WD, Griffiths TL, Shale DJ. Associated loss of fat-free mass and bone mineral density in chronic obstructive pulmonary disease. Am J Respir Crit Care Med. 2004;170:1286–93.
100. Nuti R, Siviero P, Maggi S, Guglielmi G, Caffarelli C, Crepaldi G, Gonnelli S. Vertebral fractures in patients with chronic obstructive pulmonary disease: the EOLO study. Osteoporos Int. 2009;20:989–98.
101. Dam TT, Harrison S, Fink HA, Ramsdell J, Barrett-Connor E. Osteoporotic fractures in men research G. Bone mineral density and fractures in older men with chronic obstructive pulmonary disease or asthma. Osteoporos Int. 2010;21:1341–9.
102. Beauchamp MK, O'Hoski S, Goldstein RS, Brooks D. Effect of pulmonary rehabilitation on balance in persons with chronic obstructive pulmonary disease. Arch Phys Med Rehabil. 2010;91:1460–5.
103. Leone N, Courbon D, Thomas F, Bean K, Jego B, Leynaert B, Guize L, Zureik M. Lung function impairment and metabolic syndrome: the critical role of abdominal obesity. Am J Respir Crit Care Med. 2009;179:509–16.
104. Song Y, Klevak A, Manson JE, Buring JE, Liu S. Asthma, chronic obstructive pulmonary disease, and type 2 diabetes in the Women's health study. Diabetes Res Clin Pract. 2010;90:365–71.
105. Lazarus R, Sparrow D, Weiss ST. Baseline ventilatory function predicts the development of higher levels of fasting insulin and fasting insulin resistance index: the normative aging study. Eur Respir J. 1998;12:641–5.
106. Suissa S, Kezouh A, Ernst P. Inhaled corticosteroids and the risks of diabetes onset and progression. Am J Med. 2010;123:1001–6.
107. O'Byrne PM, Rennard S, Gerstein H, Radner F, Peterson S, Lindberg B, Carlsson LG, Sin DD. Risk of new onset diabetes mellitus in patients with asthma or COPD taking inhaled corticosteroids. Respir Med. 2012;106:1487–93.
108. Han MK, Kazerooni EA, Lynch DA, Liu LX, Murray S, Curtis JL, Criner GJ, Kim V, Bowler RP, Hanania NA, Anzueto AR, Make BJ, Hokanson JE, Crapo JD, Silverman EK, Martinez FJ, Washko GR, Investigators CO. Chronic obstructive pulmonary disease exacerbations in the COPDGene study: associated radiologic phenotypes. Radiology. 2011;261:274–82.
109. Mokhlesi B, Morris AL, Huang CF, Curcio AJ, Barrett TA, Kamp DW. Increased prevalence of gastroesophageal reflux symptoms in patients with COPD. Chest. 2001;119:1043–8.
110. Terada K, Muro S, Sato S, Ohara T, Haruna A, Marumo S, Kinose D, Ogawa E, Hoshino Y, Niimi A, Terada T, Mishima M. Impact of gastro-oesophageal reflux disease symptoms on COPD exacerbation. Thorax. 2008;63:951–5.
111. Rascon-Aguilar IE, Pamer M, Wludyka P, Cury J, Vega KJ. Poorly treated or unrecognized GERD reduces quality of life in patients with COPD. Dig Dis Sci. 2011;56:1976–80.
112. Rascon-Aguilar IE, Pamer M, Wludyka P, Cury J, Coultas D, Lambiase LR, Nahman NS, Vega KJ. Role of gastroesophageal reflux symptoms in exacerbations of COPD. Chest. 2006;130:1096–101.
113. Martinez CH, Okajima Y, Murray S, Washko GR, Martinez FJ, Silverman EK, Lee JH, Regan EA, Crapo JD, Curtis JL, Hatabu H, Han MK, Investigators CO. Impact of self-reported gastroesophageal reflux disease in subjects from COPDGene cohort. Respir Res. 2014;15:62.
114. Sasaki T, Nakayama K, Yasuda H, Yoshida M, Asamura T, Ohrui T, Arai H, Araya J, Kuwano K, Yamaya M. A randomized, single-blind study of lansoprazole for the prevention of exacerbations of chronic obstructive pulmonary disease in older patients. J Am Geriatr Soc. 2009;57:1453–7.
115. Simon-Tuval T, Scharf SM, Maimon N, Bernhard-Scharf BJ, Reuveni H, Tarasiuk A. Determinants of elevated healthcare utilization in patients with COPD. Respir Res. 2011;12:7.
116. Young T, Palta M, Dempsey J, Skatrud J, Weber S, Badr S. The occurrence of sleep-disordered breathing among middle-aged adults. N Engl J Med. 1993;328:1230–5.
117. Kinsman RA, Yaroush RA, Fernandez E, Dirks JF, Schocket M, Fukuhara J. Symptoms and experiences in chronic bronchitis and emphysema. Chest. 1983;83:755–61.
118. Weitzenblum E, Chaouat A, Kessler R, Canuet M. Overlap syndrome: obstructive sleep apnea in patients with chronic obstructive pulmonary disease. Proc Am Thorac Soc. 2008;5:237–41.
119. Marin JM, Soriano JB, Carrizo SJ, Boldova A, Celli BR. Outcomes in patients with chronic obstructive pulmonary disease and obstructive sleep apnea: the overlap syndrome. Am J Respir Crit Care Med. 2010;182:325–31.
120. Mermigkis C, Kopanakis A, Foldvary-Schaefer N, Golish J, Polychronopoulos V, Schiza S, Amfilochiou A, Siafakas N, Bouros D. Health-related quality of life in patients with obstructive sleep apnoea and

chronic obstructive pulmonary disease (overlap syndrome). Int J Clin Pract. 2007;61:207–11.
121. Kunik ME, Roundy K, Veazey C, Souchek J, Richardson P, Wray NP, Stanley MA. Surprisingly high prevalence of anxiety and depression in chronic breathing disorders. Chest. 2005;127:1205–11.
122. Yohannes AM, Willgoss TG, Baldwin RC, Connolly MJ. Depression and anxiety in chronic heart failure and chronic obstructive pulmonary disease: prevalence, relevance, clinical implications and management principles. Int J Geriatr Psychiatry. 2010;25:1209–21.
123. Solano JP, Gomes B, Higginson IJ. A comparison of symptom prevalence in far advanced cancer, AIDS, heart disease, chronic obstructive pulmonary disease and renal disease. J Pain Symptom Manag. 2006;31:58–69.
124. Laurin C, Lavoie KL, Bacon SL, Dupuis G, Lacoste G, Cartier A, Labrecque M. Sex differences in the prevalence of psychiatric disorders and psychological distress in patients with COPD. Chest. 2007;132:148–55.
125. Hanania NA, Mullerova H, Locantore NW, Vestbo J, Watkins ML, Wouters EF, Rennard SI, Sharafkhaneh A, Evaluation of CLtIPSEsi. Determinants of depression in the ECLIPSE chronic obstructive pulmonary disease cohort. Am J Respir Crit Care Med. 2011;183:604–11.
126. Eisner MD, Blanc PD, Yelin EH, Katz PP, Sanchez G, Iribarren C, Omachi TA. Influence of anxiety on health outcomes in COPD. Thorax. 2010;65:229–34.
127. Fan VS, Ramsey SD, Giardino ND, Make BJ, Emery CF, Diaz PT, Benditt JO, Mosenifar Z, McKenna R Jr, Curtis JL, Fishman AP, Martinez FJ, National Emphysema Treatment Trial Research G. Sex, depression, and risk of hospitalization and mortality in chronic obstructive pulmonary disease. Arch Intern Med. 2007;167:2345–53.
128. de Voogd JN, Wempe JB, Koeter GH, Postema K, van Sonderen E, Ranchor AV, Coyne JC, Sanderman R. Depressive symptoms as predictors of mortality in patients with COPD. Chest. 2009;135:619–25.
129. von Leupoldt A, Taube K, Lehmann K, Fritzsche A, Magnussen H. The impact of anxiety and depression on outcomes of pulmonary rehabilitation in patients with COPD. Chest. 2011;140:730–6.
130. Mahler DA, Ward J, Fierro-Carrion G, Waterman LA, Lentine TF, Mejia-Alfaro R, Baird JC. Development of self-administered versions of modified baseline and transition dyspnea indexes in COPD. COPD. 2004;1:165–72.
131. Jones PW. Health status measurement in chronic obstructive pulmonary disease. Thorax. 2001;56:880–7.
132. Brown CD, Benditt JO, Sciurba FC, Lee SM, Criner GJ, Mosenifar Z, Shade DM, Slivka WA, Wise RA, National emphysema Treatment Trial Research G. Exercise testing in severe emphysema: association with quality of life and lung function. COPD. 2008;5:117–24.
133. Wise RA. The value of forced expiratory volume in 1 second decline in the assessment of chronic obstructive pulmonary disease progression. Am J Med. 2006;119:4–11.
134. Devanarayan V, Scholand MB, Hoidal J, Leppert MF, Crackower MA, O'Neill GP, Gervais FG. Identification of distinct plasma biomarker signatures in patients with rapid and slow declining forms of COPD. COPD. 2010;7:51–8.
135. Tashkin DP, Altose MD, Connett JE, Kanner RE, Lee WW, Wise RA. Methacholine reactivity predicts changes in lung function over time in smokers with early chronic obstructive pulmonary disease. The Lung Health Study Research Group. Am J Respir Crit Care Med. 1996;153:1802–11.
136. Donaldson GC, Seemungal TA, Bhowmik A, Wedzicha JA. Relationship between exacerbation frequency and lung function decline in chronic obstructive pulmonary disease. Thorax. 2002;57:847–52.
137. Kanner RE, Anthonisen NR, Connett JE, Lung Health Study Research G. Lower respiratory illnesses promote FEV(1) decline in current smokers but not ex-smokers with mild chronic obstructive pulmonary disease: results from the lung health study. Am J Respir Crit Care Med. 2001;164:358–64.
138. Kanazawa H, Hirata K, Yoshikawa J. Accelerated decline of lung function in COPD patients with chronic hepatitis C virus infection: a preliminary study based on small numbers of patients. Chest. 2003;123:596–9.
139. Vergnenegre A, Pugnere N, Antonini MT, Arnaud M, Melloni B, Treves R, Bonnaud F. Airway obstruction and rheumatoid arthritis. Eur Respir J. 1997;10:1072–8.
140. Highland KB, Strange C, Heffner JE. Long-term effects of inhaled corticosteroids on FEV1 in patients with chronic obstructive pulmonary disease. A meta-analysis. Ann Intern Med. 2003;138:969–73.
141. Sutherland ER, Allmers H, Ayas NT, Venn AJ, Martin RJ. Inhaled corticosteroids reduce the progression of airflow limitation in chronic obstructive pulmonary disease: a meta-analysis. Thorax. 2003;58:937–41.
142. Sandford AJ, Silverman EK. Chronic obstructive pulmonary disease. 1: susceptibility factors for COPD the genotype-environment interaction. Thorax. 2002;57:736–41.
143. van Diemen CC, Postma DS, Vonk JM, Bruinenberg M, Schouten JP, Boezen HM. A disintegrin and metalloprotease 33 polymorphisms and lung function decline in the general population. Am J Respir Crit Care Med. 2005;172:329–33.
144. Tashkin DP, Celli B, Senn S, Burkhart D, Kesten S, Menjoge S, Decramer M, Investigators US. A 4-year trial of tiotropium in chronic obstructive pulmonary disease. N Engl J Med. 2008;359:1543–54.
145. Celli BR, Thomas NE, Anderson JA, Ferguson GT, Jenkins CR, Jones PW, Vestbo J, Knobil K, Yates JC, Calverley PM. Effect of pharmacotherapy on rate of decline of lung function in chronic obstructive pul-

monary disease: results from the TORCH study. Am J Respir Crit Care Med. 2008;178:332–8.
146. Rabe KF, Hurd S, Anzueto A, Barnes PJ, Buist SA, Calverley P, Fukuchi Y, Jenkins C, Rodriguez-Roisin R, van Weel C, Zielinski J, Global Initiative for Chronic Obstructive Lung D. Global strategy for the diagnosis, management, and prevention of chronic obstructive pulmonary disease: GOLD executive summary. Am J Respir Crit Care Med. 2007;176:532–55.
147. Han MK, Wise R, Mumford J, Sciurba F, Criner GJ, Curtis JL, Murray S, Sternberg A, Weinman G, Kazerooni E, Fishman AP, Make B, Hoffman EA, Mosenifar Z, Martinez FJ, Group NR. Prevalence and clinical correlates of bronchoreversibility in severe emphysema. Eur Respir J. 2010;35:1048–56.
148. Soler-Cataluna JJ, Martinez-Garcia MA, Roman Sanchez P, Salcedo E, Navarro M, Ochando R. Severe acute exacerbations and mortality in patients with chronic obstructive pulmonary disease. Thorax. 2005;60:925–31.
149. Donaldson GC, Wilkinson TM, Hurst JR, Perera WR, Wedzicha JA. Exacerbations and time spent outdoors in chronic obstructive pulmonary disease. Am J Respir Crit Care Med. 2005;171:446–52.
150. Seemungal TA, Donaldson GC, Paul EA, Bestall JC, Jeffries DJ, Wedzicha JA. Effect of exacerbation on quality of life in patients with chronic obstructive pulmonary disease. Am J Respir Crit Care Med. 1998;157:1418–22.
151. Sullivan SD, Ramsey SD, Lee TA. The economic burden of COPD. Chest. 2000;117:5S–9S.
152. Calverley PM, Anderson JA, Celli B, Ferguson GT, Jenkins C, Jones PW, Yates JC, Vestbo J, investigators T. Salmeterol and fluticasone propionate and survival in chronic obstructive pulmonary disease. N Engl J Med. 2007;356:775–89.
153. Celli BR, MacNee W, Force AET. Standards for the diagnosis and treatment of patients with COPD: a summary of the ATS/ERS position paper. Eur Respir J. 2004;23:932–46.
154. Calverley PM, Burge PS, Spencer S, Anderson JA, Jones PW. Bronchodilator reversibility testing in chronic obstructive pulmonary disease. Thorax. 2003;58:659–64.
155. Tashkin DP, Celli B, Decramer M, Liu D, Burkhart D, Cassino C, Kesten S. Bronchodilator responsiveness in patients with COPD. Eur Respir J. 2008;31:742–50.
156. Anthonisen NR, Wright EC. Bronchodilator response in chronic obstructive pulmonary disease. Am Rev Respir Dis. 1986;133:814–9.
157. Pellegrino R, Viegi G, Brusasco V, Crapo RO, Burgos F, Casaburi R, Coates A, van der Grinten CP, Gustafsson P, Hankinson J, Jensen R, Johnson DC, MacIntyre N, McKay R, Miller MR, Navajas D, Pedersen OF, Wanger J. Interpretative strategies for lung function tests. Eur Respir J. 2005;26:948–68.
158. Fishman A, Martinez F, Naunheim K, Piantadosi S, Wise R, Ries A, Weinmann G, Wood DE, National Emphysema Treatment Trial Research G. A randomized trial comparing lung-volume-reduction surgery with medical therapy for severe emphysema. N Engl J Med. 2003;348:2059–73.
159. Anthonisen NR, Lindgren PG, Tashkin DP, Kanner RE, Scanlon PD, Connett JE, Lung Health Study Research G. Bronchodilator response in the lung health study over 11 yrs. Eur Respir J. 2005;26:45–51.
160. Dowson LJ, Guest PJ, Stockley RA. Longitudinal changes in physiological, radiological, and health status measurements in alpha(1)-antitrypsin deficiency and factors associated with decline. Am J Respir Crit Care Med. 2001;164:1805–9.
161. Kueppers F, Miller RD, Gordon H, Hepper NG, Offord K. Familial prevalence of chronic obstructive pulmonary disease in a matched pair study. Am J Med. 1977;63:336–42.
162. Beaty TH, Liang KY, Seerey S, Cohen BH. Robust inference for variance components models in families ascertained through probands: II. Analysis of spirometric measures. Genet Epidemiol. 1987;4:211–21.
163. Cohen BH, Ball WC Jr, Brashears S, Diamond EL, Kreiss P, Levy DA, Menkes HA, Permutt S, Tockman MS. Risk factors in chronic obstructive pulmonary disease (COPD). Am J Epidemiol. 1977;105:223–32.
164. Cohen BH. Chronic obstructive pulmonary disease: a challenge in genetic epidemiology. Am J Epidemiol. 1980;112:274–88.
165. Celedon JC, Speizer FE, Drazen JM, Weiss ST, Campbell EJ, Carey VJ, Reilly JJ, Ginns L, Silverman EK. Bronchodilator responsiveness and serum total IgE levels in families of probands with severe early-onset COPD. Eur Respir J. 1999;14:1009–14.
166. Silverman EK, Chapman HA, Drazen JM, Weiss ST, Rosner B, Campbell EJ, O'Donnell WJ, Reilly JJ, Ginns L, Mentzer S, Wain J, Speizer FE. Genetic epidemiology of severe, early-onset chronic obstructive pulmonary disease. Risk to relatives for airflow obstruction and chronic bronchitis. Am J Respir Crit Care Med. 1998;157:1770–8.
167. Palmer LJ, Celedon JC, Chapman HA, Speizer FE, Weiss ST, Silverman EK. Genome-wide linkage analysis of bronchodilator responsiveness and post-bronchodilator spirometric phenotypes in chronic obstructive pulmonary disease. Hum Mol Genet. 2003;12:1199–210.
168. Casanova C, Cote C, de Torres JP, Aguirre-Jaime A, Marin JM, Pinto-Plata V, Celli BR. Inspiratory-to-total lung capacity ratio predicts mortality in patients with chronic obstructive pulmonary disease. Am J Respir Crit Care Med. 2005;171:591–7.
169. O'Donnell DE, Lam M, Webb KA. Spirometric correlates of improvement in exercise performance after anticholinergic therapy in chronic obstructive pulmonary disease. Am J Respir Crit Care Med. 1999;160:542–9.
170. Gelb AF, Hogg JC, Muller NL, Schein MJ, Kuei J, Tashkin DP, Epstein JD, Kollin J, Green RH,

Zamel N, Elliott WM, Hadjiaghai L. Contribution of emphysema and small airways in COPD. Chest. 1996;109:353–9.
171. Owens GR, Rogers RM, Pennock BE, Levin D. The diffusing capacity as a predictor of arterial oxygen desaturation during exercise in patients with chronic obstructive pulmonary disease. N Engl J Med. 1984;310:1218–21.
172. Dillard TA, Piantadosi S, Rajagopal KR. Determinants of maximum exercise capacity in patients with chronic airflow obstruction. Chest. 1989;96:267–71.
173. Pinto-Plata V, Toso J, Lee K, Park D, Bilello J, Mullerova H, De Souza MM, Vessey R, Celli B. Profiling serum biomarkers in patients with COPD: associations with clinical parameters. Thorax. 2007;62:595–601.
174. Hersh CP, Demeo DL, Lazarus R, Celedon JC, Raby BA, Benditt JO, Criner G, Make B, Martinez FJ, Scanlon PD, Sciurba FC, Utz JP, Reilly JJ, Silverman EK. Genetic association analysis of functional impairment in chronic obstructive pulmonary disease. Am J Respir Crit Care Med. 2006;173:977–84.
175. Criner GJ, Cordova F, Sternberg AL, Martinez FJ. The National Emphysema Treatment Trial (NETT): part I: lessons learned about emphysema. Am J Respir Crit Care Med. 2011;184:763–70.
176. Cooper JD, Trulock EP, Triantafillou AN, Patterson GA, Pohl MS, Deloney PA, Sundaresan RS, Roper CL. Bilateral pneumectomy (volume reduction) for chronic obstructive pulmonary disease. J Thorac Cardiovasc Surg. 1995;109:106–16. discussion 116-109
177. Keenan RJ, Landreneau RJ, Sciurba FC, Ferson PF, Holbert JM, Brown ML, Fetterman LS, Bowers CM. Unilateral thoracoscopic surgical approach for diffuse emphysema. J Thorac Cardiovasc Surg. 1996;111:308–15. discussion 315-306
178. McKenna RJ Jr, Brenner M, Gelb AF, Mullin M, Singh N, Peters H, Panzera J, Calmese J, Schein MJ. A randomized, prospective trial of stapled lung reduction versus laser bullectomy for diffuse emphysema. J Thorac Cardiovasc Surg. 1996;111:317–21. discussion 322
179. Sciurba FC, Rogers RM, Keenan RJ, Slivka WA, Gorcsan J 3rd, Ferson PF, Holbert JM, Brown ML, Landreneau RJ. Improvement in pulmonary function and elastic recoil after lung-reduction surgery for diffuse emphysema. N Engl J Med. 1996;334:1095–9.
180. Gelb AF, Zamel N, McKenna RJ Jr, Brenner M. Mechanism of short-term improvement in lung function after emphysema resection. Am J Respir Crit Care Med. 1996;154:945–51.
181. Dantzker DR, Scharf SM. Surgery to reduce lung volume. N Engl J Med. 1996;334:1128–9.
182. Weinmann GG, Chiang YP, Sheingold S. The National Emphysema Treatment Trial (NETT): a study in agency collaboration. Proc Am Thorac Soc. 2008;5:381–4.
183. Naunheim KS, Wood DE, Mohsenifar Z, Sternberg AL, Criner GJ, DeCamp MM, Deschamps CC, Martinez FJ, Sciurba FC, Tonascia J, Fishman AP, National Emphysema Treatment Trial Research G. Long-term follow-up of patients receiving lung-volume-reduction surgery versus medical therapy for severe emphysema by the National Emphysema Treatment Trial Research Group. Ann Thorac Surg. 2006;82:431–43.
184. Vestbo J, Edwards LD, Scanlon PD, Yates JC, Agusti A, Bakke P, Calverley PM, Celli B, Coxson HO, Crim C, Lomas DA, MacNee W, Miller BE, Silverman EK, Tal-Singer R, Wouters E, Rennard SI, Investigators E. Changes in forced expiratory volume in 1 second over time in COPD. N Engl J Med. 2011;365:1184–92.
185. Nishimura M, Makita H, Nagai K, Konno S, Nasuhara Y, Hasegawa M, Shimizu K, Betsuyaku T, Ito YM, Fuke S, Igarashi T, Akiyama Y, Ogura S, Hokkaido CCSI. Annual change in pulmonary function and clinical phenotype in chronic obstructive pulmonary disease. Am J Respir Crit Care Med. 2012;185:44–52.
186. Zulueta JJ, Wisnivesky JP, Henschke CI, Yip R, Farooqi AO, McCauley DI, Chen M, Libby DM, Smith JP, Pasmantier MW, Yankelevitz DF. Emphysema scores predict death from COPD and lung cancer. Chest. 2012;141:1216–23.
187. Haruna A, Muro S, Nakano Y, Ohara T, Hoshino Y, Ogawa E, Hirai T, Niimi A, Nishimura K, Chin K, Mishima M. CT scan findings of emphysema predict mortality in COPD. Chest. 2010;138:635–40.
188. Grydeland TB, Dirksen A, Coxson HO, Eagan TM, Thorsen E, Pillai SG, Sharma S, Eide GE, Gulsvik A, Bakke PS. Quantitative computed tomography measures of emphysema and airway wall thickness are related to respiratory symptoms. Am J Respir Crit Care Med. 2010;181:353–9.
189. Martinez-Garcia MA, de la Rosa CD, Soler-Cataluna JJ, Donat-Sanz Y, Serra PC, Lerma MA, Ballestin J, Sanchez IV, Selma Ferrer MJ, Dalfo AR, Valdecillos MB. Prognostic value of bronchiectasis in patients with moderate-to-severe chronic obstructive pulmonary disease. Am J Respir Crit Care Med. 2013;187:823–31.
190. Johannessen A, Skorge TD, Bottai M, Grydeland TB, Nilsen RM, Coxson H, Dirksen A, Omenaas E, Gulsvik A, Bakke P. Mortality by level of emphysema and airway wall thickness. Am J Respir Crit Care Med. 2013;187:602–8.
191. Han MK. Clinical correlations of computed tomography imaging in chronic obstructive pulmonary disease. Ann Am Thorac Soc. 2013;10(Suppl):S131–7.
192. Hogg JC. Pathophysiology of airflow limitation in chronic obstructive pulmonary disease. Lancet. 2004;364:709–21.
193. Jain N, Covar RA, Gleason MC, Newell JD Jr, Gelfand EW, Spahn JD. Quantitative computed tomography detects peripheral airway disease in asthmatic children. Pediatr Pulmonol. 2005;40:211–8.
194. Matsuoka S, Kurihara Y, Yagihashi K, Hoshino M, Watanabe N, Nakajima Y. Quantitative assessment of air trapping in chronic obstructive pulmonary

disease using inspiratory and expiratory volumetric MDCT. AJR Am J Roentgenol. 2008;190:762–9.
195. O'Donnell RA, Peebles C, Ward JA, Daraker A, Angco G, Broberg P, Pierrou S, Lund J, Holgate ST, Davies DE, Delany DJ, Wilson SJ, Djukanovic R. Relationship between peripheral airway dysfunction, airway obstruction, and neutrophilic inflammation in COPD. Thorax. 2004;59:837–42.
196. Mets OM, Zanen P, Lammers JW, Isgum I, Gietema HA, van Ginneken B, Prokop M, de Jong PA. Early identification of small airways disease on lung cancer screening CT: comparison of current air trapping measures. Lung. 2012;190:629–33.
197. Lee YK, Oh YM, Lee JH, Kim EK, Lee JH, Kim N, Seo JB, Lee SD, Group KS. Quantitative assessment of emphysema, air trapping, and airway thickening on computed tomography. Lung. 2008;186:157–65.
198. Matsuoka S, Washko GR, Yamashiro T, Estepar RS, Diaz A, Silverman EK, Hoffman E, Fessler HE, Criner GJ, Marchetti N, Scharf SM, Martinez FJ, Reilly JJ, Hatabu H, National Emphysema Treatment Trial Research G. Pulmonary hypertension and computed tomography measurement of small pulmonary vessels in severe emphysema. Am J Respir Crit Care Med. 2010;181:218–25.
199. Wells JM, Washko GR, Han MK, Abbas N, Nath H, Mamary AJ, Regan E, Bailey WC, Martinez FJ, Westfall E, Beaty TH, Curran-Everett D, Curtis JL, Hokanson JE, Lynch DA, Make BJ, Crapo JD, Silverman EK, Bowler RP, Dransfield MT, Investigators CO, Investigators ES. Pulmonary arterial enlargement and acute exacerbations of COPD. N Engl J Med. 2012;367:913–21.
200. Woodruff PG, Agusti A, Roche N, Singh D, Martinez FJ. Current concepts in targeting chronic obstructive pulmonary disease pharmacotherapy: making progress towards personalised management. Lancet. 2015;385:1789–98.
201. Lotvall J, Akdis CA, Bacharier LB, Bjermer L, Casale TB, Custovic A, Lemanske RF Jr, Wardlaw AJ, Wenzel SE, Greenberger PA. Asthma endotypes: a new approach to classification of disease entities within the asthma syndrome. J Allergy Clin Immunol. 2011;127:355–60.
202. Vrijheid M. The exposome: a new paradigm to study the impact of environment on health. Thorax. 2014;69:876–8.
203. Christenson SA, Steiling K, van den Berge M, Hijazi K, Hiemstra PS, Postma DS, Lenburg ME, Spira A, Woodruff PG. Asthma-COPD overlap. Clinical relevance of genomic signatures of type 2 inflammation in chronic obstructive pulmonary disease. Am J Respir Crit Care Med. 2015;191:758–66.
204. Bafadhel M, McKenna S, Terry S, Mistry V, Reid C, Haldar P, McCormick M, Haldar K, Kebadze T, Duvoix A, Lindblad K, Patel H, Rugman P, Dodson P, Jenkins M, Saunders M, Newbold P, Green RH, Venge P, Lomas DA, Barer MR, Johnston SL, Pavord ID, Brightling CE. Acute exacerbations of chronic obstructive pulmonary disease: identification of biologic clusters and their biomarkers. Am J Respir Crit Care Med. 2011;184:662–71.
205. Siva R, Green RH, Brightling CE, Shelley M, Hargadon B, McKenna S, Monteiro W, Berry M, Parker D, Wardlaw AJ, Pavord ID. Eosinophilic airway inflammation and exacerbations of COPD: a randomised controlled trial. Eur Respir J. 2007;29:906–13.
206. Brightling CE, McKenna S, Hargadon B, Birring S, Green R, Siva R, Berry M, Parker D, Monteiro W, Pavord ID, Bradding P. Sputum eosinophilia and the short term response to inhaled mometasone in chronic obstructive pulmonary disease. Thorax. 2005;60:193–8.
207. Brightling CE, Monteiro W, Ward R, Parker D, Morgan MD, Wardlaw AJ, Pavord ID. Sputum eosinophilia and short-term response to prednisolone in chronic obstructive pulmonary disease: a randomised controlled trial. Lancet. 2000;356:1480–5.
208. Leigh R, Pizzichini MM, Morris MM, Maltais F, Hargreave FE, Pizzichini E. Stable COPD: predicting benefit from high-dose inhaled corticosteroid treatment. Eur Respir J. 2006;27:964–71.
209. Pizzichini E, Pizzichini MM, Gibson P, Parameswaran K, Gleich GJ, Berman L, Dolovich J, Hargreave FE. Sputum eosinophilia predicts benefit from prednisone in smokers with chronic obstructive bronchitis. Am J Respir Crit Care Med. 1998;158:1511–7.
210. Barker BL, Brightling CE. Phenotyping the heterogeneity of chronic obstructive pulmonary disease. Clin Sci (Lond). 2013;124:371–87.
211. Singh D, Kolsum U, Brightling CE, Locantore N, Agusti A, Tal-Singer R, investigators E. Eosinophilic inflammation in COPD: prevalence and clinical characteristics. Eur Respir J. 2014;44:1697–700.
212. Busse WW, Katial R, Gossage D, Sari S, Wang B, Kolbeck R, Coyle AJ, Koike M, Spitalny GL, Kiener PA, Geba GP, Molfino NA. Safety profile, pharmacokinetics, and biologic activity of MEDI-563, an anti-IL-5 receptor alpha antibody, in a phase I study of subjects with mild asthma. J Allergy Clin Immunol. 2010;125:1237–44. e1232
213. Laviolette M, Gossage DL, Gauvreau G, Leigh R, Olivenstein R, Katial R, Busse WW, Wenzel S, Wu Y, Datta V, Kolbeck R, Molfino NA. Effects of benralizumab on airway eosinophils in asthmatic patients with sputum eosinophilia. J Allergy Clin Immunol. 2013;132:1086–96. e1085
214. Brightling CE, Bleecker ER, Panettieri RA Jr, Bafadhel M, She D, Ward CK, Xu X, Birrell C, van der Merwe R. Benralizumab for chronic obstructive pulmonary disease and sputum eosinophilia: a randomised, double-blind, placebo-controlled, phase 2a study. Lancet Respir Med. 2014;2:891–901.
215. Barbu C, Iordache M, Man MG. Inflammation in COPD: pathogenesis, local and systemic effects. Rom J Morphol Embryol. 2011;52:21–7.

216. Nussbaumer-Ochsner Y, Rabe KF. Systemic manifestations of COPD. Chest. 2011;139:165–73.
217. Andelid K, Tengvall S, Andersson A, Levanen B, Christenson K, Jirholt P, Ahren C, Qvarfordt I, Ekberg-Jansson A, Linden A. Systemic cytokine signaling via IL-17 in smokers with obstructive pulmonary disease: a link to bacterial colonization? Int J Chron Obstruct Pulmon Dis. 2015;10:689–702.
218. Gan WQ, Man SF, Senthilselvan A, Sin DD. Association between chronic obstructive pulmonary disease and systemic inflammation: a systematic review and a meta-analysis. Thorax. 2004;59:574–80.
219. Agusti A, Edwards LD, Rennard SI, MacNee W, Tal-Singer R, Miller BE, Vestbo J, Lomas DA, Calverley PM, Wouters E, Crim C, Yates JC, Silverman EK, Coxson HO, Bakke P, Mayer RJ, Celli B, Evaluation of CLtIPSEI. Persistent systemic inflammation is associated with poor clinical outcomes in COPD: a novel phenotype. PLoS One. 2012;7:e37483.
220. Agusti A, Anto JM, Auffray C, Barbe F, Barreiro E, Dorca J, Escarrabill J, Faner R, Furlong LI, Garcia-Aymerich J, Gea J, Lindmark B, Monso E, Plaza V, Puhan MA, Roca J, Ruiz-Manzano J, Sampietro-Colom L, Sanz F, Serrano L, Sharpe J, Sibila O, Silverman EK, Sterk PJ, Sznajder JI. Personalized respiratory medicine: exploring the horizon, addressing the issues. Summary of a BRN-AJRCCM workshop held in Barcelona on June 12, 2014. Am J Respir Crit Care Med. 2015;191:391–401.
221. Vanfleteren LE, Kocks JW, Stone IS, Breyer-Kohansal R, Greulich T, Lacedonia D, Buhl R, Fabbri LM, Pavord ID, Barnes N, Wouters EF, Agusti A. Moving from the Oslerian paradigm to the post-genomic era: are asthma and COPD outdated terms? Thorax. 2014;69:72–9.
222. Loscalzo J, Kohane I, Barabasi AL. Human disease classification in the postgenomic era: a complex systems approach to human pathobiology. Mol Syst Biol. 2007;3:124.
223. Burgel PR, Paillasseur JL, Caillaud D, Tillie-Leblond I, Chanez P, Escamilla R, Court-Fortune I, Perez T, Carre P, Roche N, Initiatives BSC. Clinical COPD phenotypes: a novel approach using principal component and cluster analyses. Eur Respir J. 2010;36:531–9.
224. Weatherall M, Travers J, Shirtcliffe PM, Marsh SE, Williams MV, Nowitz MR, Aldington S, Beasley R. Distinct clinical phenotypes of airways disease defined by cluster analysis. Eur Respir J. 2009;34:812–8.
225. Paoletti M, Camiciottoli G, Meoni E, Bigazzi F, Cestelli L, Pistolesi M, Marchesi C. Explorative data analysis techniques and unsupervised clustering methods to support clinical assessment of Chronic Obstructive Pulmonary Disease (COPD) phenotypes. J Biomed Inform. 2009;42:1013–21.
226. Cho MH, Washko GR, Hoffmann TJ, Criner GJ, Hoffman EA, Martinez FJ, Laird N, Reilly JJ, Silverman EK. Cluster analysis in severe emphysema subjects using phenotype and genotype data: an exploratory investigation. Respir Res. 2010;11:30.

Genetics of COPD

11

Woo Jin Kim

Introduction

Although environmental factors, including cigarette smoking and biomass smoke exposure, are major risk factors of COPD, genetic risk factors are also important [1]. In addition, an interaction between genetics and environment is believed to drive the development of COPD.

Pathways that play a role in COPD pathogenesis include the response to oxidative stress, the protease–antiprotease imbalance, cell death, and inflammation [2–5]. Genetic studies have been performed to identify genetic risk factors and to understand the pathogenesis of COPD. Family-based studies and candidate gene association studies have found associations for many genes and loci. However, alpha-1 antitrypsin deficiency caused by mutations in *SERPINA1* is the only established genetically driven cause of COPD that has a potential intervention so far [6].

Future research is needed to characterize the effect of genetic variants, validate gene function in humans and model systems, and elucidate the genes' transcriptional and post-transcriptional regulatory mechanisms [7].

W.J. Kim
Department of Internal Medicine and Environmental Health Center, Kangwon National University, Chuncheon, South Korea
e-mail: pulmo2@kangwon.ac.kr

History of Genetic Studies for COPD

Family studies have supported genetic factors to play an important role in the development of COPD [8]. Twin studies have reported heritability of lung function between 30 and 50% [9]. Recently, heritability of COPD was estimated 35–40% in population-based study [10].

Genome-wide linkage analysis using Boston early onset COPD identified several loci that were associated with lung function that is the most important phenotype of COPD [11].

Candidate gene strategies were used to test hypothesis of genetic associations with COPD. However, there were few genetic associations that were consistently significant, and this strategy has limitation in identifying novel mechanisms of COPD.

Genome-Wide Association Study

Although whole-genome and exome sequencing may be the next tools used for the genetic study of COPD, genome-wide association study (GWAS) is currently the most widely used method for the discovery of candidate genes [12]. Several GWASs have discovered novel genes and pathways that are associated with COPD susceptibility. Even more genes have been found to be significantly associated with lung function in the general population. Some of these lung function genes are also associated with COPD susceptibility. The genetic basis of different

S.-D. Lee (ed.), *COPD*, DOI 10.1007/978-3-662-47178-4_11

COPD-related phenotypes, including emphysema and chronic bronchitis, also overlaps with that of COPD susceptibility. After being implicated in disease pathogenesis, these genes can be used as potential drug targets or as biomarkers that can influence diagnosis and personalized treatment.

Currently, the most well-known candidate genes for COPD are *CHRNA3/5* (cholinergic nicotine receptor alpha 3/5), *IREB2* (iron regulatory binding protein 2), *HHIP* (hedgehog-interacting protein), *FAM13A* (family with sequence similarity 13, member A), and *AGER* (advanced glycosylation end product-specific receptor). They have been replicated in multiple populations. None of them are targeted by treatments for COPD yet, and the mechanisms by which they alter COPD risk are still largely unknown. There is some emerging evidence that they may be good targets for treatments or useful as biomarkers. However, more study is required to understand the functional roles of these candidate genes.

CHRNA3, *CHRNA5*, and *IREB2*

There are several genes at chromosome 15q25 that have been identified by GWAS for affecting COPD risk, including *CHRNA3*, *CHRNA5*, and *IREB2* [13–15]. The COPD cohorts investigated were the Norway case/control cohort (GenKOLS), the family-based ICGN cohort, the NETT (National Emphysema Treatment Trial)/NAS (normative aging study) cohorts, the Boston early onset COPD cohort, and the COPDGene study cohort. The association between *CHRNA3/5* and COPD has been replicated in multiple ethnic populations by direct genotyping [16–18]. The *CHRNA3/5* region is also associated with lung cancer and nicotine addiction. It has been debated whether this common susceptibility region is the result of a common pathogenic pathway for lung cancer and COPD, or if it is simply associated with nicotine addiction, a risk factor for both diseases. In addition, the causal variant within the *CHRNA3/5* locus may be different in lung cancer than in COPD. There is some evidence that this locus has independent roles in the pathogenesis of COPD and smoking behavior [19].

CHRNA3/5 and CHRNB4 are subunits of the nicotine cholinergic receptor, and the cholinergic system is active not only in cholinergic neuronal cells, but also in bronchial epithelial cells and airway inflammatory cells. The proteins are responsive to nicotine and are upregulated during chronic tobacco exposure. A recent study integrating GWAS results with expression quantitative trait loci (eQTL) study results found that SNPs in the 15q25 region were associated with the expression of *IREB2* and *CHRNA3* in blood and sputum samples [20]. CHRNA3/5 and IREB2 may play different roles in the pathogenesis of COPD.

IREB2 was first identified by characterizing the differential gene expression in lung tissue between COPD patients and controls, and genotyping the SNPs within the candidate regions [21]. IREB2 is a protein that binds iron-responsive elements (IREs), maintains cellular iron metabolism, and is regulated in response to oxygen and iron supply. *IREB2* expression is higher in the lung tissue of COPD cases. The *Ireb2* knockout mouse has abnormal iron metabolism in the brain, which causes cellular dysfunction [22]. However, the role of *IREB2* in COPD pathogenesis is still not known. A GWAS of the pulmonary artery measurement obtained by computed tomography (CT) in cohorts from the COPDGene Study and the Evaluation of COPD Longitudinally to Identify Predictive Surrogate Endpoints (ECLIPSE) study found a genome-wide significant association to *IREB2* [23]. This suggests a role for IREB2 in the pathogenesis of pulmonary hypertension in COPD, particularly in the vascular subtype.

HHIP

Many recently identified COPD-associated variants are located at chromosome 4q31, upstream of *HHIP*. This intergenic region has associated with COPD susceptibility in several GWASs [13, 14, 24], and has consistently replicated in multiple ethnicities [25–28]. This region is also associated with lung function in the general population [29–31]. *HHIP* is also associated with adult height in the general population [32]. Considering that the FEV_1 prediction is determined by height, there may be genetic factors that control both phenotypes. Using the candidate gene strategy, it was found that the *HHIP* gene interacted with environmental tobacco smoke in utero, suggesting that this gene is involved in the lung response to smoke exposure in early life [33].

HHIP encodes a membrane glycoprotein that is an endogenous antagonist for the Hedgehog pathway. Hedgehog signaling is important for the morphogenesis of the lung and other organs [34]. Although the role of HHIP in COPD is not fully understood, several studies have validated the function of this gene in COPD pathogenesis. The associated SNPs are located upstream of *HHIP*, suggesting that they may affect promoter activity. A lung eQTL study revealed that SNPs associated with COPD affect the expression of *HHIP*, and the risk allele of rs1828591 decreases expression [35]. Zhou et al. reported that *HHIP* expression is reduced in COPD lung tissues and the genomic region upstream of *HHIP* interacts with the *HHIP* promoter. The risk allele of a variant in the *HHIP* enhancer region reduces promoter activity via a differential binding affinity to transcription factors [36].

These studies suggest that the genetic variation of the *HHIP* region affects the risk of COPD by affecting *HHIP* expression in lung tissues. HHIP silencing in an airway epithelial cell line leads to a change in gene expression, and these differentially expressed genes are enriched in pathways related to the extracellular matrix and cell growth, which are processes relevant to COPD pathogenesis [37]. Recently, Lao et al. found that Hhip-haploinsufficient mice have increased airspace size after cigarette smoke exposure, increased lung compliance, and increased numbers of lymphoid aggregates. The functions of the genes with altered expression in $Hhip^{+/-}$ mice exposed to cigarette smoke were enriched in the pathway of lymphocyte activation [38]. They used haploinsufficient mice because $Hhip^{-/-}$ mice die shortly after birth due to lung branching morphogenesis failure.

HHIP was also found to be associated with lung cancer by a candidate gene study [39]. The Hedgehog pathway is a critical mediator of cigarette smoke-induced lung cancer, and it may act as a common pathway for the development of COPD and lung cancer [40].

FAM13A

A GWAS using three COPD cohorts, GenKOLS, NETT/NAS, and the ECLIPSE study, identified variants at chromosome 4q22 in the gene *FAM13A* [41]. These are some of the most highly associated SNPs in COPD and are located in an intron. These associations have replicated in a subset of the patients in the COPDGene Study and the cohort of the International COPD Genetics Network. They also replicated in Asian populations, assayed using the candidate gene strategy [42, 43]. *FAM13A* was first found to associate with lung function in a GWAS using the general population [29], and it is associated with lung function in asthmatic subjects [44]. Of note, *FAM13A* is also associated with idiopathic pulmonary disease (IPF) [45], but the expression of *FAM13A* in lung tissues does not differ by case/control status or by genotype.

FAM13A was originally identified in cattle near a quantitative trait locus affecting milk production, and is expressed in the kidney, pancreas, lung, and thymus [46]. Although the function of FAM13A has not been extensively studied, its RhoGAP domain may be related to COPD. Rho GTPases are key regulators of cytoskeletal dynamics, are involved in the pulmonary endothelial barrier, and are dysregulated in several lung diseases [47]. A lung eQTL study suggested that the expression of *FAM13A* may be associated with particular SNPs [35]. In the case of COPD, the *FAM13A* risk allele is associated with increased *FAM13A* expression in the lung although expression does not differ in lung tissues between COPD cases and controls [42]. A recent study by Jin et al. found that FAM13A activates Wnt signaling by increasing the stability of β-catenin [48]. Although depletion of FAM13A in a lung cancer cell line reduces Wnt signaling activity, *FAM13A* knockout mice are viable and *FAM13A*-mutant lungs are morphologically indistinguishable from wild-type lungs, and Wnt signaling remains normal in

Fam13a-knockout lungs. They also found that Akt regulates the phosphorylation of FAM13A, which can lead to cytoplasmic sequestration of FAM13A. Considering that Akt has a role in the pathogenesis of COPD [49], FAM13A may contribute to lung disease through aberrant Akt signaling. Further work is needed to validate the functional role of FAM13A in the pathogenesis of COPD.

AGER

GWASs of lung function in the general population have found that chromosome 6p21 is associated with FEV_1/FVC and FEV_1, which are important physiologic parameters of COPD [31, 29, 50]. This association was investigated in COPD patients identified from the population cohort using spirometry criteria, and the study found a suggestive association between COPD risk and *AGER*, although it was not statistically significant [51]. A candidate gene study in NETT/NAS, GenKOLS, ECLIPSE, and a subset of the COPDGene Study cohort found that it is associated with COPD susceptibility although a subsequent GWAS did not find a significant association [52]. On the other hand, an association has been found in multiple ethnic populations [53].

Chromosome 6p21 region that showed significant association with COPD includes many genes: *TNXB*, *PPT2*, *AGER*, and *NOTCH4*. However, *AGER* has a potential functional variant, rs2070600, and has been studied the most in the pathogenesis of COPD. A GWAS of percent emphysema determined by CT using the Multi-Ethnic Study of Atherosclerosis cohort identified a significant association with the *AGER*/*PPT* region [54]. This region did associate with emphysema severity and gas trapping in a GWAS using cohorts from the COPDGene, ECLIPSE, NETT, and GenKOLS studies [55].

The protein product of *AGER*, the receptor for advanced glycan end-products (RAGE), is a multi-ligand receptor of the immunoglobulin superfamily and interacts with molecules implicated in homeostatic function, inflammation, and development [56]. RAGE levels are increased in the airway and alveolar walls of COPD lungs [57]. RAGE expression in mice increases after cigarette smoke exposure, and cigarette smoking-induced inflammatory responses by alveolar macrophages are diminished in RAGE knockout mice [58]. Transgenic mice with upregulated RAGE have impaired alveolar morphogenesis during lung development, distal airspace enlargement, and increased alveolar cell apoptosis [59]. Another study using RAGE transgenic mice found incremental dilation of alveolar spaces, as well as pronounced inflammation in the peripheral lung and alveolar destabilization [60]. A promoter variant of *AGER* in cystic fibrosis patients is associated with poor lung function, and it increases expression in airway epithelial cell lines, suggesting that it is a modifier of lung disease severity [61].

The soluble isoform of RAGE (sRAGE) contains the RAGE extracellular domain and can bind to circulating proinflammatory ligands, preventing RAGE activation. Mice that are exposed to chronic hypoxia have down-regulated pulmonary RAGE protein and increased levels of sRAGE, which might be adaptive to and protective against chronic hypoxia [62]. Circulatory levels of sRAGE are reduced in COPD patients [63]. Reduced sRAGE levels are associated with increased emphysema in two COPD cohorts [64]. Decreased plasma sRAGE levels are also associated with the progression of airflow limitation over time [65]. In patients of the Treatment of Emphysema with a Selective Retinoid Agonist (TESRA) and ECLIPSE studies, sRAGE is associated with diffusing capacity, emphysema, and COPD disease status, and the variant rs2070600 is associated with circulating sRAGE levels [66]. The significant association between rs2070600 and plasma sRAGE levels was also found in Dutch diabetes mellitus and control subjects [67]. RAGE has been studied in metabolic diseases, and decreased levels of sRAGE are linked to vascular complications. RAGE contributes to the pathogenesis of COPD in the lung probably via the regulation of inflammation and apoptosis, and further study of the functions of this gene may lead to it being identified as a potential therapeutic target.

Other Candidate Genes

There have been several more regions identified in GWASs of COPD. A GWAS using subjects from the ECLIPSE, NETT/NAS, GenKOLS, and COPDGene studies identified chromosome 19q13 as being associated with COPD, along with the previously identified *HHIP*, *FAM13A*, and 15q25 regions [14]. Chromosome 19q13 contains *CYP2A6*, *RAB4B*, *MIA*, and *EGLN*, which could potentially be involved in COPD pathogenesis, and *EGLN2* was found to be dysregulated in the airway epithelium of smokers [68]. A GWAS using the full COPDGene cohort identified additional associations with *TGFB2*, *MMP12*, and *RIN3* [24]. *TGFB2* and *MMP12* have been previously studied in COPD or related phenotypes [69, 70], whereas *RIN3* has not been studied in COPD and needs to be investigated further. *SERPINE2* was identified using a linkage analysis of gene expression changes in lung tissue [71]. A recent GWAS of airway thickness identified rs734556 on chromosome 2q, which is associated with *SERPINE2* expression [72]. These associations require more replications and further fine-mapping studies are needed to find the causal variants of COPD, as well as studies to functionally validate the identified genes.

GWAS for Heterogeneity

CT phenotypes including emphysema severity and airway thickness quantitatively measured using standardized methods are useful in understanding heterogeneity of COPD by characterizing lung parenchyma and airways. Previous study using candidate gene approach reported that associations between *SERPINE2* and upper lobe dominance [73], *ADRB2* and airway lumen area [74]. Another study reported that *EPHX1, SERPINE2*, and *GSTP1* were associated with emphysema severity and *TGFB1, EPHX1, SERPINE2*, and *ADRB2* were associated with airway phenotypes [75].

After GWAS identified several COPD-associated genes, those identified genes were tested for CT phenotypes, and also GWAS was performed on CT phenotypes.

The *CHRNA3/5* locus is associated with emphysema and smoking intensity in COPD [76, 77].

HHIP is associated with various CT phenotypes in COPD including distinct patterns of emphysema [77] and the severity of emphysema [55]. *HHIP* is more associated with emphysema measurements than with airway phenotypes and has a more significant association in emphysema subgroups [78]. This difference may reflect a different pathogenic process driven by HHIP, or may be driven by correlations between COPD status and imaging measurements.

Genome-wide association studies using COPD cases with chronic bronchitis in the COPDGene Study, GenKOLS, and ECLIPSE cohorts identified a significant association with *FAM13A* [79], whereas several GWASs for emphysema did not identify a genome-wide association. The odds ratios of *FAM13A* SNPs for COPD with chronic bronchitis were significantly higher than those for non-chronic bronchitis COPD, suggesting that *FAM13A* is more related to the pathogenesis of the chronic bronchitis subtype.

GWAS in the presence of emphysema identified BICD as a susceptibility gene for emphysema [80]. GWAS of percent emphysema in the general population identified SNRPF and PPT2 [54]. GWAS on airway wall thickness *MAGI2* and *NT5C3B* were associated with airway wall thickness [72].

As pulmonary hypertension is a well-established complication and an important factor of prognosis, GWAS of pulmonary artery enlargement have found IREB2 and GALC associated with pulmonary artery enlargement defined as PA/A ratio more than 1 in COPD subjects [23].

BMI is important in prognosis of COPD. The *HHIP* locus is associated with fat-free mass and exacerbations in COPD subjects [76]. GWAS on BMI in COPD identified *FTO* was associated with BMI and fat-free mass index [81].

Pharmacogenetics

Recently, genotype variation can be used to individualized therapy. In COPD, the most studied subject is *ADRB2* polymorphisms of β2-adrenergic receptor on β2 agonist therapy [82, 83]. Another gene included *CRHR1* polymorphism [84]. Warfarin is a good example of individual variation in pharmacokinetics; however, drug used in COPD are not known for gene influencing drug metabolism.

Previous study reported that COPD candidate genes may influence bronchodilator responsiveness [85]. Considering that treatment with PDE4 inhibitor is effective only for the chronic bronchitis subtype, there may be a mechanism that is unique to this subtype. Candidate genes can be used to determine personalized treatment because they may help identify a subtype-unique pathogenesis, as well as variation in a drug-action site, or variable drug metabolism [86].

Conclusion

Recently, several candidate genes associated with COPD risk have been identified using GWAS. Replication and functional validation studies may lead to clinical applications for these genes such as novel therapeutics, subtyping, and risk prediction for COPD. Also, phenotype heterogeneity can be investigated using association studies on various COPD-related phenotypes. More regions have been identified in GWASs on FEV_1 and FEV_1/FVC in the general population, probably because of the larger sample sizes than COPD case/control subjects. GWASs using a greater sample size of COPD subjects may find more candidate genes [87]. Another approach for finding more candidate genes is to identify rare variation using exome sequencing or arrays.

References

1. Postma DS, Bush A, van den Berge M. Risk factors and early origins of chronic obstructive pulmonary disease. Lancet. 2015;385:899–909.
2. Cosio MG, Saetta M, Agusti A. Immunologic aspects of chronic obstructive pulmonary disease. N Engl J Med. 2009;360:2445–54.
3. Tuder R, Petrache I. Pathogenesis of chronic obstructive pulmonary disease. J Clin Invest. 2012;122: 2749–55.
4. Kirkham PA, Barnes PJ. Oxidative stress in COPD. Chest. 2013;144:266–73.
5. Bagdonas E, Raudoniute J, Bruzauskaite I, et al. Novel aspects of pathogenesis and regeneration mechanisms in COPD. Int J Chron Obstruct Pulmon Dis. 2015;10:995–1013.
6. Silverman EK, Sandhaus RA. Alpha1-antitrypsin deficiency. N Engl J Med. 2009;360:2749–57.
7. Ober C, Butte AJ, Elias JA, et al. Getting from genes to function in lung disease. Am J Respir Crit Care Med. 2010;182:732–7.
8. Silverman EK, Chapman HA, Drazen JM, et al. Genetic epidemiology of severe, early-onset chronic obstructive pulmonary disease. Am J Respir Crit Care Med. 1998;157:1770–8.
9. Ingebrigtsen T, Thomsen S, van der Sluis S, et al. Genetic influences on pulmonary function: a large sample twin study. Lung. 2011;189:323–30.
10. Zhou JJ, Cho MH, Castaldi PJ, et al. Heritability of chronic obstructive pulmonary disease and related phenotypes in smokers. Am J Respir Crit Care Med. 2013;188:941–7.
11. Silverman EK, Palmer LJ, Mosley JD, et al. Genomewide linkage analysis of quantitative Spirometric phenotypes in severe early-onset chronic obstructive pulmonary disease. Am J Hum Genet. 2002;70:1229–39.
12. Todd JL, Goldstein DB, Ge D, et al. The state of genome-wide association studies in pulmonary disease. Am J Respir Crit Care Med. 2011;184:873–80.
13. Pillai SG, Ge D, Zhu G, et al. A genome-wide association study in chronic obstructive pulmonary disease (COPD): identification of two major susceptibility loci. PLoS Genet. 2009;5:e1000421.
14. Cho MH, Castaldi PJ, Wan ES, et al. A genome-wide association study of COPD identifies a susceptibility locus on chromosome 19q13. Hum Mol Genet. 2012;21:947–57.
15. Wilk JB, Shrine NR, Loehr LR, et al. Genome-wide association studies identify CHRNA5/3 and HTR4 in the development of airflow obstruction. Am J Respir Crit Care Med. 2012;186:622–32.
16. Hardin M, Zielinski J, Wan ES, et al. CHRNA3/5, IREB2, and ADCY2 are associated with severe chronic obstructive pulmonary disease in Poland. Am J Respir Cell Mol Biol. 2012;47:203–8.
17. Kim WJ, Oh YM, Kim TH, et al. ***CHRNA3*** variant for lung cancer is associated with chronic obstructive pulmonary disease in Korea. Respiration. 2013;86:117–22.
18. Yang L, Qiu F, Lu X, et al. Functional polymorphisms of CHRNA3 predict risks of chronic obstructive pulmonary disease and lung cancer in Chinese. PLoS One. 2012;7:e46071.
19. Siedlinski M, Tingley D, Lipman PJ, et al. Dissecting direct and indirect genetic effects on chronic obstructive pulmonary disease (COPD) susceptibility. Hum Genet. 2013;132:431–41.
20. Castaldi PJ, Cho MH, Zhou X, et al. Genetic control of gene expression at novel and established chronic

obstructive pulmonary disease loci. Hum Mol Genet. 2015;24:1200–10.
21. DeMeo DL, Mariani T, Bhattacharya S, et al. Integration of genomic and genetic approaches implicates IREB2 as a COPD susceptibility Gene. Am J Hum Genet. 2009;85:493–502.
22. Zumbrennen-Bullough KB, Becker L, Garrett L, et al. Abnormal brain iron metabolism in *Irp2* deficient mice is associated with mild neurological and behavioral impairments. PLoS One. 2014;9:e98072.
23. Lee JH, Cho MH, Hersh CP, et al. IREB2 and GALC are associated with pulmonary artery enlargement in chronic obstructive pulmonary disease. Am J Respir Cell Mol Biol. 2015;52:365–76.
24. Cho MH, McDonald ML, Zhou X, et al. Risk loci for chronic obstructive pulmonary disease: a genome-wide association study and meta-analysis. Lancet Respir Med. 2014;2:214–25.
25. Van Durme YM, Eijgelsheim M, Joos GF, et al. Hedgehog-interacting protein is a COPD susceptibility gene: the Rotterdam study. Eur Respir J. 2010;36:89–95.
26. Kim WJ, Oh YM, Lee JH, et al. Genetic variants in HHIP are associated with FEV1 in subjects with chronic obstructive pulmonary disease. Respirology. 2013;18:1202–9.
27. Xie J, Wu H, Xu Y, et al. Gene susceptibility identification in a longitudinal study confirms new loci in the development of chronic obstructive pulmonary disease and influences lung function decline. Respir Res. 2015;16:49.
28. Wang B, Zhou H, Yang J, et al. Association of HHIP polymorphisms with COPD and COPD-related phenotypes in a Chinese Han population. Gene. 2013;531:101–5.
29. Hancock DB, Eijgelsheim M, Wilk JB, et al. Meta-analyses of genome-wide association studies identify multiple loci associated with pulmonary function. Nat Genet. 2010;42:45–52.
30. Wilk JB, Chen TH, Gottlieb DJ, et al. A genome-wide association study of pulmonary function measures in the Framingham heart study. PLoS Genet. 2009;5:e1000429.
31. Repapi E, Sayers I, Wain LV, et al. Genome-wide association study identifies five loci associated with lung function. Nat Genet. 2010;42:36–44.
32. van der Valk RJP, Kreiner-Møller E, Kooijman MN, et al. A novel common variant in DCST2 is associated with length in early life and height in adulthood. Hum Mol Genet. 2015;24:1155–68.
33. Kerkhof M, Boezen HM, Granell R, et al. Transient early wheeze and lung function in early childhood associated with chronic obstructive pulmonary disease genes. J Allergy Clin Immunol. 2014;133:68–76.e64.
34. Chuang PT, Kawcak T, McMahon AP. Feedback control of mammalian hedgehog signaling by the hedgehog-binding protein, Hip1, modulates Fgf signaling during branching morphogenesis of the lung. Genes Dev. 2003;17:342–7.
35. Lamontagne M, Couture C, Postma DS, et al. Refining susceptibility loci of chronic obstructive pulmonary disease with lung eqtls. PLoS One. 2013;8:e70220.
36. Zhou X, Baron RM, Hardin M, et al. Identification of a chronic obstructive pulmonary disease genetic determinant that regulates HHIP. Hum Mol Genet. 2012;21:1325–35.
37. Zhou X, Qiu W, Sathirapongsasuti JF, et al. Gene expression analysis uncovers novel hedgehog interacting protein (HHIP) effects in human bronchial epithelial cells. Genomics. 2013;101:263–72.
38. Lao T, Glass K, Qiu W, et al. Haploinsufficiency of hedgehog interacting protein causes increased emphysema induced by cigarette smoke through network rewiring. Genome Med. 2015;7:12.
39. Young RP, Whittington CF, Hopkins RJ, et al. Chromosome 4q31 locus in COPD is also associated with lung cancer. Eur Respir J. 2010;36: 1375–82.
40. Lemjabbar-Alaoui H, Dasari V, Sidhu SS, et al. Wnt and hedgehog are critical mediators of cigarette smoke-induced lung cancer. PLoS One. 2006;1:e93.
41. Cho MH, Boutaoui N, Klanderman BJ, et al. Variants in FAM13A are associated with chronic obstructive pulmonary disease. Nat Genet. 2010;42:200–2.
42. Kim WJ, Lim MN, Hong Y, et al. Association of lung function genes with chronic obstructive pulmonary disease. Lung. 2014;192:473–80.
43. Guo Y, Lin H, Gao K, et al. Genetic analysis of IREB2, FAM13A and XRCC5 variants in Chinese Han patients with chronic obstructive pulmonary disease. Biochem Biophys Res Commun. 2011;415:284–7.
44. Li X, Hawkins GA, Ampleford EJ, et al. Genome-wide association study identifies TH1 pathway genes associated with lung function in asthmatic patients. J Allergy Clin Immunol. 2013;132:313–20, e315.
45. Fingerlin TE, Murphy E, Zhang W, et al. Genome-wide association study identifies multiple susceptibility loci for pulmonary fibrosis. Nat Genet. 2013;45:613–20.
46. Cohen M, Reichenstein M, Everts-van der Wind A, et al. Cloning and characterization of FAM13A1—a gene near a milk protein QTL on BTA6: evidence for population-wide linkage disequilibrium in Israeli Holsteins. Genomics. 2004;84:374–83.
47. Corvol H, Hodges CA, Drumm ML, et al. Moving beyond genetics: is FAM13A a major biological contributor in lung physiology and chronic lung diseases? J Med Genet. 2014;51:646–9.
48. Jin Z, Chung JW, Mei W, et al. Regulation of nuclear-cytoplasmic shuttling and function of family with sequence similarity 13, member a (Fam13a), by B56-containing PP2As and Akt. Mol Biol Cell. 2015;26:1160–73.
49. Bozinovski S, Vlahos R, Hansen M, et al. Akt in the pathogenesis of COPD. Int J Chron Obstruct Pulmon Dis. 2006;1:31–8.
50. Kim WJ, Lee MK, Shin C, et al. Genome-wide association studies identify locus on 6p21 influencing lung function in the Korean population. Respirology. 2014;19:360–8.
51. Soler Artigas M, Wain LV, Repapi E, et al. Effect of five genetic variants associated with lung function on the risk of chronic obstructive lung disease, and their

joint effects on lung function. Am J Respir Crit Care Med. 2011;184:786–95.
52. Castaldi PJ, Cho MH, Litonjua AA, et al. The association of genome-wide significant spirometric loci with chronic obstructive pulmonary disease susceptibility. Am J Respir Cell Mol Biol. 2011;45:1147–53.
53. Li Y, Yang C, Ma G, et al. Association of Polymorphisms of the receptor for advanced glycation end products Gene with COPD in the Chinese population. DNA Cell Biol. 2014;33:251–8.
54. Manichaikul A, Hoffman EA, Smolonska J, et al. Genome-wide study of percent emphysema on computed tomography in the general population. The multi-ethnic study of atherosclerosis lung/SNP health association resource study. Am J Respir Crit Care Med. 2014;189:408–18.
55. Cho MH, Castaldi PJ, Hersh CP, et al. A genome-wide association study of emphysema and airway quantitative imaging phenotypes. Am J Respir Crit Care Med. 2015;192(5):559–69.
56. Sorci G, Riuzzi F, Giambanco I, et al. RAGE in tissue homeostasis, repair and regeneration. Biochim Biophys Acta. 2013;1833:101–9.
57. Wu L, Ma L, Nicholson LFB, et al. Advanced glycation end products and its receptor (RAGE) are increased in patients with COPD. Respir Med. 2011;105:329–36.
58. Robinson AB, Johnson KD, Bennion BG, et al. RAGE signaling by alveolar macrophages influences tobacco smoke-induced inflammation. Am J Physiol Lung Cell Mol Physiol. 2012;302(11):L1192–9.
59. Fineschi S, De Cunto G, Facchinetti F, et al. Receptor for advanced glycation end products contributes to postnatal pulmonary development and adult lung maintenance program in mice. Am J Respir Cell Mol Biol. 2013;48:164–71.
60. Stogsdill MP, Stogsdill JA, Bodine BG, et al. Conditional overexpression of receptors for advanced glycation end-products in the adult murine lung causes airspace enlargement and induces inflammation. Am J Respir Cell Mol Biol. 2013;49:128–34.
61. Beucher J, Boëlle P-Y, Busson P-F, et al. *AGER*-429T/C is associated with an increased lung disease severity in cystic fibrosis. PLoS One. 2012;7:e41913.
62. Gopal P, Gosker HR, de Theije CC, et al. Effect of chronic hypoxia on RAGE and its soluble forms in lungs and plasma of mice. Biochim Biophys Acta 2015;1852:992–1000
63. Miniati M, Monti S, Basta G, et al. Soluble receptor for advanced glycation end products in COPD: relationship with emphysema and chronic cor pulmonale: a case-control study. Respir Res. 2011;12:37.
64. Carolan B, Hughes G, Morrow J, et al. The association of plasma biomarkers with computed tomography-assessed emphysema phenotypes. Respir Res. 2014;15:127.
65. Iwamoto H, Gao J, Pulkkinen V, et al. Soluble receptor for advanced glycation end-products and progression of airway disease. BMC Pulm Med. 2014;14:68.
66. Cheng DT, Kim DK, Cockayne DA, et al. Systemic soluble receptor for advanced glycation endproducts is a biomarker of emphysema and associated with AGER genetic variants in patients with chronic obstructive pulmonary disease. Am J Respir Crit Care Med. 2013;188: 948–57.
67. Gaens KHJ, Ferreira I, van der Kallen CJH, et al. Association of polymorphism in the receptor for advanced glycation end products (RAGE) Gene with circulating RAGE levels. J Clin Endocrinol Metabol. 2009;94:5174–80.
68. Ryan DM, Vincent TL, Salit J, et al. Smoking dysregulates the human airway basal cell transcriptome at COPD risk locus 19q13.2. PLoS One. 2014;9:e88051.
69. Hunninghake GM, Cho MH, Tesfaigzi Y, et al. MMP12, lung function, and COPD in high-risk populations. N Engl J Med. 2009;361:2599–608.
70. Artigas MS, Loth DW, Wain LV, et al. Genome-wide association and large-scale follow up identifies 16 new loci influencing lung function. Nat Genet. 2011;43:1082–90.
71. DeMeo DL, Mariani TJ, Lange C, et al. The SERPINE2 gene is associated with chronic obstructive pulmonary disease. Am J Hum Genet. 2006;78:253–64.
72. Dijkstra AE, Postma DS, van Ginneken B, et al. Novel genes for airway wall thickness identified with combined genome-wide association and expression analyses. Am J Respir Crit Care Med. 2014; 191:547–56.
73. DeMeo DL, Hersh CP, Hoffman EA, et al. Genetic determinants of emphysema distribution in the National Emphysema Treatment Trial. Am J Respir Crit Care Med. 2007;176:42–8.
74. Kim WJ, Oh Y-M, Sung J, et al. CT scanning-based phenotypes vary with ADRB2 polymorphisms in chronic obstructive pulmonary disease. Respir Med. 2009;103:98–103.
75. Kim WJ, Hoffman E, Reilly J, et al. Association of COPD candidate genes with computed tomography emphysema and airway phenotypes in severe COPD. Eur Respir J. 2011;37:39–43.
76. Pillai SG, Kong X, Edwards LD, et al. Loci identified by genome-wide association studies influence different disease-related phenotypes in chronic obstructive pulmonary disease. Am J Respir Crit Care Med. 2010;182:1498–505.
77. Castaldi PJ, Cho MH, San Jose Estepar R, et al. Genome-wide association identifies regulatory loci associated with distinct local histogram emphysema patterns. Am J Respir Crit Care Med. 2014;190:399–409.
78. Castaldi PJ, Dy J, Ross J, et al. Cluster analysis in the COPDGene study identifies subtypes of smokers with distinct patterns of airway disease and emphysema. Thorax. 2014;69:416–23.
79. Lee JH, Cho MH, Hersh CP, et al. Genetic susceptibility for chronic bronchitis in chronic obstructive pulmonary disease. Respir Res. 2014;15:113.
80. Kong X, Cho MH, Anderson W, et al. Genome-wide association study identifies BICD1 as a susceptibil-

ity gene for emphysema. Am J Respir Crit Care Med. 2011;183:43–9.
81. Wan ES, Cho MH, Boutaoui N, et al. Genome-wide association analysis of body mass in chronic obstructive pulmonary disease. Am J Respir Cell Mol Biol. 2011;45:304–10.
82. Kim W, Oh Y-M, Sung J, et al. Lung function response to 12-week treatment with combined inhalation of long-acting β2 agonist and glucocorticoid according to ADRB2 polymorphism in patients with chronic obstructive pulmonary disease. Lung. 2008;186:381–6.
83. Bleecker ER, Meyers DA, Bailey WC, et al. ADrb2 polymorphisms and budesonide/formoterol responses in COPD. Chest. 2012;142:320–8.
84. Kim WJ, Sheen SS, Kim T-H, et al. Association between CRHR1 polymorphism and improved lung function in response to inhaled corticosteroid in patients with COPD. Respirology. 2009;14:260–3.
85. Kim WJ, Hersh CP, DeMeo DL, et al. Genetic association analysis of COPD candidate genes with bronchodilator responsiveness. Respir Med. 2009;103:552–7.
86. Hersh CP. Pharmacogenetics of chronic obstructive pulmonary disease: challenges and opportunities. Pharmacogenomics. 2010;11:237–47.
87. Silverman EK, Vestbo J, Agusti A, et al. Opportunities and challenges in the genetics of COPD 2010: an international COPD genetics conference report. COPD. 2011;8:121–35.

Imaging Heterogeneity of COPD

12

Sang Min Lee and Joon Beom Seo

Overview

Although chronic obstructive pulmonary disease (COPD) is defined as persistent airflow limitation which is usually progressive and associated with an enhanced chronic inflammatory response [1], heterogeneity of COPD has been realized while our understanding of this agonizing disease has grown over the past two decades [2]. Patients with same or similar pulmonary function impairment show different symptoms, disease progression, and prognosis. As a result, the concept of COPD has been changing from an airflow limitation-centric view to a complex and heterogeneous condition, preferring multidimensional approaches and finding phenotypes. In this context, imaging features, especially quantitative analysis of CT, have garnered attention as they have been demonstrated to be of help in evaluating patients' status as well as predicting acute exacerbation and prognosis of patients. The two main components of COPD, emphysema and small airway disease, can be accurately and reliably assessed by quantitative CT analysis [3, 4]. In this chapter, we reviewed previous research on imaging in COPD patients briefly and addressed the current concept and future direction of imaging phenotyping.

CT: Airway vs. Emphysema Predominance

The concept that COPD phenotype can be divided according to varying combination and severity of emphysema and small airway disease on CT was firstly suggested by Nakano et al. [5]. Initially, Nakano et al. showed that CT could quantify airway abnormalities in 114 smokers [6]. They demonstrated the accuracy and reproducibility of quantitative airway measurement on CT and revealed that both quantitative analyses of airway and emphysema on CT were useful and complementary in the evaluation of patients with COPD [6]. This technical advance allows to evaluate structural change due to airway inflammation and remodeling in vivo. Nakano et al. finally suggested that COPD patients can be divided into groups who had predominant emphysema or thickening and narrowing of the apical segmental bronchus using quantitative assessment of relative area of low parenchymal attenuation and percent airway wall area. In Korean Obstructive Lung Disease (KOLD) Cohort study [7], 530 patients also demonstrate a similar distribution (Fig. 12.1).

S.M. Lee, M.D. • J.B. Seo, M.D., Ph.D. (✉)
Division of Cardiothoracic Radiology, Department of Radiology, Asan Medical Center, University of Ulsan College of Medicine, Ulsan, South Korea
e-mail: sangmin.lee.md@gmail.com; joonbeom.seo@gmail.com

S.-D. Lee (ed.), *COPD*, DOI 10.1007/978-3-662-47178-4_12

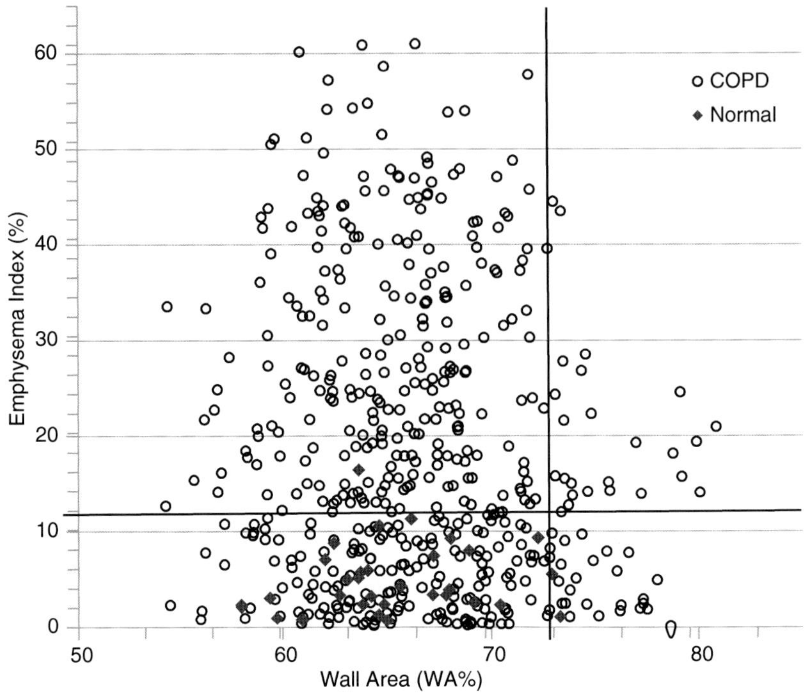

Fig. 12.1 Emphysema index and airway wall thickening in Korean Obstructive Lung Disease (KOLD) Cohort. This graph demonstrates the distribution of 497 COPD patients and 33 normal individuals according to emphysema index and airway wall thickening. *Horizontal line* indicates the mean + 2 standard deviation of emphysema index of the normal individuals (12.8%). *Vertical line* indicates the mean + 2 standard deviation of wall area of the normal individuals (73.0%). COPD patients can be categorized as different groups using these thresholds: airway-predominant, emphysema-predominant, and a mixed group. In KOLD cohort, the emphysema-predominant group comprises a large proportion of COPD patients

This concept of dividing patients based on CT imaging characteristics evolves and expands in recent article by Fleischner society [8]. They suggested seven different subtypes of COPD patients: five different patterns of emphysema-predominant subtype according to severity and location of emphysema (mild centrilobular emphysema, moderate centrilobular emphysema, confluent emphysema, advanced destructive emphysema, panlobular emphysema, and paraseptal emphysema) and two patterns of airway-predominant subtype according to level of involved airways (bronchial disease and small airway disease). The most important factor differentiating subtypes of COPD is quantitative amount of emphysema, that is, emphysema-predominant subgroup can be defined as more than 6% of pixels less than −950 HU at quantitative CT and airway-predominant subgroup can be defined as pixels less than 6% of −950 HU at quantitative CT. Although this classification is tentative and much area remains for future research, the key concept that two components of emphysema and airway disease mainly consist of COPD will be effective.

In addition, technical advances in imaging processing enable novel and detailed quantification of COPD and provide imaging-biomarkers for diagnosis of COPD phenotypes and disease progression. Galban et al. [3] demonstrated more clear separation of emphysema and functional small airway disease using non-rigid registration between inspiratory and expiratory CT images. Furthermore, Kim et al. [4] showed a new approach to quantifying air-trapping using a co-registration method which defined air-trapping as a volume with attenuation increase less than 50 HU between inspiration and expiration CT

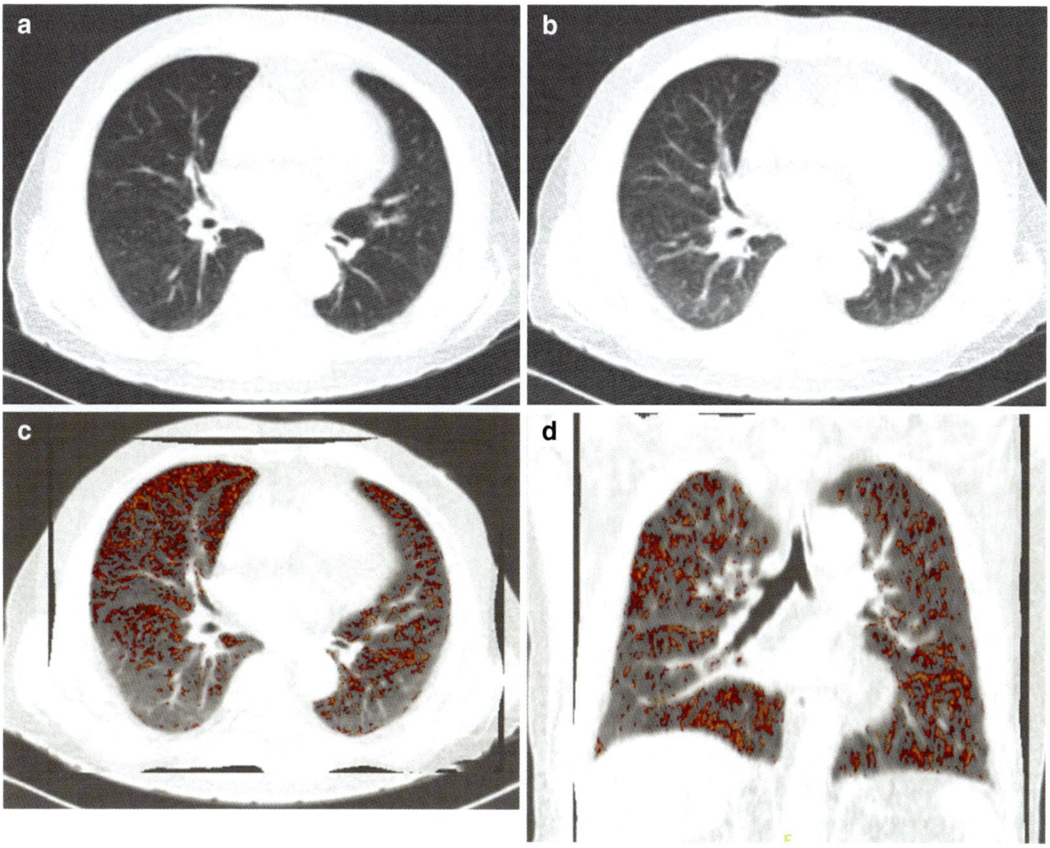

Fig. 12.2 Co-registration of inspiration and expiration CT scans for analysis on air-trapping. (**a**) Inspiration CT and (**b**) expiration CT were obtained in a 77-year-old male patient. Expiration CT was deformed and registered to the inspiration CT using a non-rigid registration method. Color mapping according to differences of voxel attenuation between inspiration and expiration CT was performed in co-registered images (**c**, **d**). These images allow to easily detect the areas of air-trapping with small attenuation change on respiration. *Red color* represents voxels with a difference of voxel attenuation between inspiration and expiration CT below a threshold of 50

(Fig. 12.2). Using this approach, respective contributions of different densities seen on inspiration CT to air-trapping could be assessed in detail. The previous two studies quantified air-trapping area rather than airway wall for evaluation of small airway disease as it is difficult to quantify small airway disease because there are limitations in the direct visualization of small airways (diameter < 2 mm) on CT.

Prediction of Treatment Response

One of important roles of CT phenotyping is to predict treatment response in COPD patients. In a study by Kitaguchi et al. [9], they subjectively classified into three phenotypes of 85 COPD patients according to components of emphysema and bronchial wall thickening on CT; airway-predominant, emphysema-dominant, and mixed airway and emphysema. They assessed area of emphysema and airway wall thickness visually. Interestingly, three CT phenotypes showed different characteristics in terms of body mass index, onset of dyspnea, proportion of never-smoker, and dependency of long-term oxygen therapy. This implies that CT phenotyping can explain clinical features. More importantly, CT phenotyping was significantly related to treatment response with inhaled ß$_2$-agonist and corticosteroid. Airway-predominant phenotype showed significantly greater reversibility with inhaled ß$_2$-agonist (change in FEV_1: airway-predominant, 253.3 mL; emphysema-predominant, 94.0 mL; mixed phenotype, 133.7 mL). Airway-predominant phenotype and mixed phenotype were significantly associated with improvement in FEV_1 when using inhaled corticosteroid (change in FEV_1: airway-predominant, 313.9 mL; emphysema-predominant, 116.2 mL; mixed phenotype, 247.9 mL). This result suggests that bronchial wall thickening on CT may be an indicator for predicting good response to treatment. However, semiquantitative evaluation has limitation due to requirement for expert radiologists and interobserver variation.

Similar study was performed using a quantitative method in KOLD cohort by Lee et al. [10]. They objectively categorized 165 patients into four subtypes using extent of emphysema on CT and FEV_1: emphysema-dominant, obstruction-dominant, mild-mixed subtype, and severe-mixed subtype. They also reported that obstruction-dominant and mixed subtypes showed significantly greater improvement in FEV_1 than emphysema-dominant group after 3 months of combined inhalation of long-acting beta-agonist and corticosteroid. Furthermore, obstruction-dominant subtype patients showed marked improvement of dyspnea compared with emphysema-dominant patients. Given the results of two studies, we can safely tell that bronchial wall thickening on CT should be assessed to predict treatment response before treatment.

Prediction of Acute Exacerbation

Acute exacerbation of COPD is defined as acute event characterized by a worsening of patients' respiratory symptoms that is beyond normal day-to-day variations and leads to a change in medication [1]. It is known that all-cause mortality 3 years after hospitalization due to acute exacerbation is as high as 49% [11]. Therefore, early detection and prompt treatment of acute exacerbations as well as prevention are crucial to reduce the burden of COPD [12]. Regarding acute exacerbation, Han et al. [13] performed a study to investigate a relationship between quantitative CT measures and COPD exacerbation frequency. According to their study, greater extent of emphysema and airway wall thickness was associated with COPD exacerbations, irrespective of the severity of airflow obstruction. Importantly, mean segmental bronchial wall thickness showed the highest odds ratio (1.84) among significant variables on multivariate analysis. This result corresponds well with essential role of airway inflammation and remodeling in development and progression of COPD [14, 15]. Based on Han et al.'s study, we can identify subgroups of patients who experience exacerbations more frequently and subsequently provide more personalized therapy.

Regional Heterogeneity of Emphysema

Emphysema can vary according to subtypes (centrilobular, paraseptal, and panlobular) and regional distribution. It is known that regional heterogeneity of emphysema in anterior-posterior and upper-lower direction was independent determinants of FEV_1 and FEV_1/FVC and the lower and posterior regional dominant emphysema is associated with a decrease in FEV_1 and FEV_1/FVC [16]. Basal distribution of emphysema is also associated with greater impairment of FEV_1 [17].

Such regional heterogeneity of emphysema has clinical relevance to the treatment of COPD. According to results of a randomized trial for lung volume reduction surgery (LVRS) [18], it has a survival gain for patients with both predominantly upper-lobe emphysema and low base-line exercise capacity even though upper-lobe predominance of emphysema was visually determined by each center's radiologist. Thus, assessment of regional heterogeneity of emphysema using CT is important and useful for selecting candidates for LVRS. In addition, even in endobronchial valves for advanced emphysema, heterogeneity of emphysema on CT is the criteria for selecting patients [19]. In Sciurba et al.'s study [19], the percentage of heterogeneity was defined as the difference in the quantitative emphysema score (the proportion of pixels of less than −910 Hounsfield units) between the targeted lobe and the ipsilateral adjacent nontargeted lobe. After that, this percentage was then converted to a Likert scale, with a score of 1 for 1–25%, 2 for 26–50%, 3 for 51–75%, and 4 for 76–100%. A 1-unit difference between treated and untreated lobes was required for inclusion in the effect analyses of endobronchial valve.

Other Issues in Imaging Heterogeneity

Silent Emphysema with Normal PFT Abnormality

COPD is basically diagnosed by spirometry. Patients with normal PFT, even though CT demonstrates pulmonary parenchyma abnormality, are not diagnosed as COPD. Therefore, there can be discrepancy between CT findings and PFT. As previous studies showed that emphysema severity on CT in COPD patients was significantly correlated with rapid decline in FEV_1 [20] and mortality [21], some patients with emphysema on CT can be underdiagnosed. Regarding this issue, Lutchmedial et al. [22] conducted a study including 274 patients with more than or equal to 5% of emphysema extent on CT with a threshold of −950 HU. According to their results, GOLD criteria missed 19 patients and lower limit of normal (LLN) criteria missed 38 patients who were diagnosed by clinical criteria for COPD. Although this study was not performed in screening population and we cannot estimate the prevalence of silent emphysema which affects no significant pulmonary function impairment in general population, about 6.9–13.9% patients with more than or equal to 5% of emphysema extent on CT may be underdiagnosed for COPD.

Vascular Subtype

Pulmonary vascular disease such as pulmonary hypertension is an independent predictor of morbidity and mortality in COPD patients [23]. The mechanisms for this process likely include inflammation or hypoxic vasoconstriction due to emphysematous destruction of the tissue. While the standard visual assessment of pulmonary vascular remodeling includes measurements of the diameter of the main pulmonary artery, the recent study has demonstrated that remodeling of the distal intraparenchymal pulmonary vasculature yields insights into the relation of vascular disease and emphysema and the effect of pulmonary vascular disease on pulmonary artery pressure [24]. In this context, Estepar et al. [25] showed that smoking-related chronic obstructive pulmonary disease is characterized by distal pruning of the small blood vessels ($<5\ mm^2$) and loss of tissue in excess of the vasculature. The magnitude of these changes predicts the clinical severity of disease [25]. Alford et al. [26] investigated whether early regional vascular dysfunction was correlated with emphysematous changes or not. They included 41 individuals (17 normal, 12 smokers with no emphysema and normal lung function, and 12 smokers with very mild emphysema). They demonstrated that functional lung-imaging measure that provides a more mechanistically oriented phenotype using perfusion imaging differentiates smokers with and without evidence of emphysema susceptibility.

GOLD U Group

When GOLD criteria are applied for diagnosis of COPD, about 8–14% of individuals with a normal FEV_1/FVC ratio and a reduced FEV_1 are detected [27–29]. These individuals are designated as GOLD-nonobstructed (GOLDU). Individuals with GOLDU were associated with increased BMI, reduced total lung capacity, and higher proportion of non-white individuals, and diabetes mellitus as well as increased bronchial wall thickness when compared with smoking control group [30]. Kim et al. [31] investigated more detailed analysis of CT findings and showed that chest wall abnormalities (diaphragmatic eventration) and parenchymal lung disease (emphysema, airway wall thickening, air-trapping), which contribute to restrictive physiologic impairment, are associated with GOLDU in cigarette smokers when compared with a control group of smokers with normal lung function. However, there remains uncertainty about a specific phenotype of GOLDU regarding disease progression or prognosis.

Asthma/COPD Overlap Syndrome (ACOS)

Asthma/COPD overlap syndrome is characterized by persistent airflow limitation with several features usually associated with asthma and COPD. ACOS is therefore identified by the features that it shares with both asthma and COPD [1]. Patients with ACOS are usually 40 or more years old, but overlap syndrome percentages are increased from mid to later life progressively [32]. Marco et al. showed that the frequency of ACOS was 1.6, 2.1, and 4.5% in the 20–44, 45–64, and 65–84 age groups, respectively [33]. Patients can have respiratory symptoms including exertional dyspnea. Exacerbations in patients with ACOS may be more common up to three times than patients with COPD [34, 35]. Overlap subjects had more severe and more frequent respiratory exacerbations, less emphysema, and greater airway wall thickness compared to subjects with COPD alone [36]. Kim et al. [37] also demonstrated that ACOS is associated with a higher risk of hospitalization due to respiratory problems than COPD alone in a retrospective study dealing with 2933 COPD patients. However, further study on imaging characteristics of AOCS is awaited.

Combined Emphysema and Pulmonary Fibrosis

Combined pulmonary fibrosis and emphysema (CPFE) is characterized by the presence of emphysema predominantly in the upper lobes, with diffuse interstitial opacities in the lower lobes [38, 39] (IPF). According to Cottin et al. [39], CPFE can be diagnosed based on radiologic findings: (1) the presence of emphysema with upper zone predominance on CT; (2) the presence of diffuse parenchymal lung disease with significant pulmonary fibrosis on CT, defined as reticular opacities, honeycombing, architectural distortion, and/or traction bronchiectasis with peripheral and basal predominance. It is now considered as a different phenotype of idiopathic pulmonary fibrosis. In terms of prevalence, 3.1% of asymptomatic smokers were diagnosed with CPFE using Cottin et al.'s criteria in Kim et al.'s study [40]. Ryerson et al. [41] reported 8.0% of CPFE in IPF patients when emphysema in CPFE was defined as 10% or more in extent. The prevalence of CPFE varies depending on study population and diagnostic criteria.

The main characteristic of CPFE is relative preservation of FVC even when the affected lung parenchyma increases in extent because of countereffect of emphysema and pulmonary fibrosis, that is, compensation of hyperinflation of emphysema for decreased lung volume due to pulmonary fibrosis. This implies that PFT cannot accurately assess disease status in CPFE patients. For this reason, CT has attracted clinical interest in evaluation of disease progression as well as diagnosis in CPFE patients. The prognosis of CPFE compared with IPF is not clearly determined. Mejia et al.'s study [42] showed that CPFE was associated with poorer prognosis compared with IPF due to higher incidence of pulmonary hypertension. However, Ryerson et al. [41] reported that there were no significant differences in survival between CPFE and IPF. Furthermore, Kurashima et al. [43] demonstrated that patients with UIP and emphysema had greater lung volumes and better survival compared with those with UIP alone. At present, prospective studies of CPFE are needed to clarify the natural course of CPFE including prognosis.

Imaging and Genetic Association Studies

Individual susceptibility to COPD and manifestation of COPD may vary according to genetic variation, and there have been several studies on the association between genetic variation and CT phenotype [44–49].

With respect to emphysema on CT, Ito et al. [44] reported that polymorphism of MMP-9 (C-1562T) was associated with upper lung-dominant emphysema in patients with COPD. Demeo et al. [46] suggested that polymorphisms in the xenobiotic enzymes, GSTP1 and EPHX1, are associated with apical-predominant emphysema and altered detoxification of cigarette smoke metabolites may contribute to emphysema distribution. Sakao et al. also reported that the TNF-alpha-308 allele 2 may be partly associated with the extent of emphysematous changes in patients with COPD. Cheng [47] demonstrated that systemic soluble receptor for advanced glycation end products is a biomarker of emphysema in COPD patients. Recently, Bowler et al. [48] showed that sphingomyelins are strongly associated with emphysema and glycosphingolipids are associated with COPD exacerbations.

In terms of airway disease, Kim et al. found that Gly16 variant in ADRB2 gene was associated with airway wall phenotypes measured using CT scanning in COPD patients [49]. Kim et al. also reported that single nucleotide polymorphisms in EPHX1, SERPINE2, TGFB1, and ADRB2 were associated with airway wall phenotypes [50]. Recently, Dijkstra et al. showed that three significant loci on chromosomes 2q (rs734556) and 10q (rs10794108 and rs7078439) were associated with AWT and confirmed in the meta-analysis in cohorts [51].

In summary, many researchers have made a lot of effort to uncover pathogenesis of COPD by investigating the relationship between genotype and phenotype of COPD (especially imaging phenotype). Although much things to do remain, these works may open the path to the personalized medicine.

References

1. Global initiative for chronic obstructive pulmonary disease. Global strategy for the diagnosis, management, and prevention of chronic obstructive pulmonary disease. 2015. Available via http://www.goldcopd.org/.
2. Agusti A, Sobradillo P, Celli B. Addressing the complexity of chronic obstructive pulmonary disease: from phenotypes and biomarkers to scale-free networks, systems biology, and P4 medicine. Am J Respir Crit Care Med. 2011;183(9):1129–37. doi:10.1164/rccm.201009-1414PP.
3. Galban CJ, Han MK, Boes JL, Chughtai KA, Meyer CR, Johnson TD, et al. Computed tomography-based biomarker provides unique signature for diagnosis of COPD phenotypes and disease progression. Nat Med. 2012;18(11):1711–5. doi:10.1038/nm.2971.
4. Kim EY, Seo JB, Lee HJ, Kim N, Lee E, Lee SM, et al. Detailed analysis of the density change on chest CT of COPD using non-rigid registration of inspiration/expiration CT scans. Eur Radiol. 2015;25(2):541–9. doi:10.1007/s00330-014-3418-0.
5. Nakano Y, Muller NL, King GG, Niimi A, Kalloger SE, Mishima M, et al. Quantitative assessment of airway remodeling using high-resolution CT. Chest. 2002;122(6 Suppl):271S–5S.
6. Nakano Y, Muro S, Sakai H, Hirai T, Chin K, Tsukino M, et al. Computed tomographic measurements of airway dimensions and emphysema in smokers. Correlation with lung function. Am J Respir Crit Care Med. 2000;162(3 Pt 1):1102–8. doi:10.1164/ajrccm.162.3.9907120.
7. Park TS, Lee JS, Seo JB, Hong Y, Yoo JW, Kang BJ, et al. Study design and outcomes of Korean obstructive lung disease (KOLD) cohort study. Tuberc Respir Dis. 2014;76(4):169–74. doi:10.4046/trd.2014.76.4.169.
8. Lynch DA, Austin JH, Hogg JC, Grenier PA, Kauczor HU, Bankier AA, et al. CT-definable subtypes of chronic obstructive pulmonary disease: a statement of the Fleischner society. Radiology. 2015;277(1):192–205. doi:10.1148/radiol.2015141579.
9. Kitaguchi Y, Fujimoto K, Kubo K, Honda T. Characteristics of COPD phenotypes classified according to the findings of HRCT. Respir Med. 2006;100(10):1742–52. doi:10.1016/j.rmed.2006.02.003.
10. Lee JH, Lee YK, Kim EK, Kim TH, Huh JW, Kim WJ, et al. Responses to inhaled long-acting beta-agonist and corticosteroid according to COPD subtype. Respir Med. 2010;104(4):542–9. doi:10.1016/j.rmed.2009.10.024.
11. Gunen H, Hacievliyagil SS, Kosar F, Mutlu LC, Gulbas G, Pehlivan E, et al. Factors affecting survival of hospitalised patients with COPD. Eur Respir J. 2005;26(2):234–41. doi:10.1183/09031936.05.00024804.
12. Wilkinson TM, Donaldson GC, Hurst JR, Seemungal TA, Wedzicha JA. Early therapy improves outcomes of exacerbations of chronic obstructive pulmonary disease. Am J Respir Crit Care Med. 2004;169(12):1298–303. doi:10.1164/rccm.200310-1443OC.
13. Han MK, Kazerooni EA, Lynch DA, Liu LX, Murray S, Curtis JL, et al. Chronic obstructive pulmonary disease exacerbations in the COPDGene study: associated radiologic phenotypes. Radiology. 2011;261(1):274–82. doi:10.1148/radiol.11110173.

14. Hogg JC, Chu F, Utokaparch S, Woods R, Elliott WM, Buzatu L, et al. The nature of small-airway obstruction in chronic obstructive pulmonary disease. N Engl J Med. 2004;350(26):2645–53. doi:10.1056/NEJMoa032158.
15. McDonough JE, Yuan R, Suzuki M, Seyednejad N, Elliott WM, Sanchez PG, et al. Small-airway obstruction and emphysema in chronic obstructive pulmonary disease. N Engl J Med. 2011;365(17):1567–75. doi:10.1056/NEJMoa1106955.
16. Chae EJ, Seo JB, Song JW, Kim N, Park BW, Lee YK, et al. Slope of emphysema index: an objective descriptor of regional heterogeneity of emphysema and an independent determinant of pulmonary function. AJR Am J Roentgenol. 2010;194(3):W248–55. doi:10.2214/AJR.09.2672.
17. Parr DG, Stoel BC, Stolk J, Stockley RA. Pattern of emphysema distribution in alpha1-antitrypsin deficiency influences lung function impairment. Am J Respir Crit Care Med. 2004;170(11):1172–8. doi:10.1164/rccm.200406-761OC.
18. Fishman A, Martinez F, Naunheim K, Piantadosi S, Wise R, Ries A, et al. A randomized trial comparing lung-volume-reduction surgery with medical therapy for severe emphysema. N Engl J Med. 2003;348(21):2059–73. doi:10.1056/NEJMoa030287.
19. Sciurba FC, Ernst A, Herth FJ, Strange C, Criner GJ, Marquette CH, et al. A randomized study of endobronchial valves for advanced emphysema. N Engl J Med. 2010;363(13):1233–44. doi:10.1056/NEJMoa0900928.
20. Nishimura M, Makita H, Nagai K, Konno S, Nasuhara Y, Hasegawa M, et al. Annual change in pulmonary function and clinical phenotype in chronic obstructive pulmonary disease. Am J Respir Crit Care Med. 2012;185(1):44–52. doi:10.1164/rccm.201106-0992OC.
21. Johannessen A, Skorge TD, Bottai M, Grydeland TB, Nilsen RM, Coxson H, et al. Mortality by level of emphysema and airway wall thickness. Am J Respir Crit Care Med. 2013;187(6):602–8. doi:10.1164/rccm.201209-1722OC.
22. Lutchmedial SM, Creed WG, Moore AJ, Walsh RR, Gentchos GE, Kaminsky DA. How common is airflow limitation in patients with emphysema on CT scan of the chest? Chest. 2015;148(1):176–84. doi:10.1378/chest.14-1556.
23. Chaouat A, Naeije R, Weitzenblum E. Pulmonary hypertension in COPD. Eur Respir J. 2008;32(5):1371–85. doi:10.1183/09031936.00015608.
24. Matsuoka S, Washko GR, Yamashiro T, Estepar RS, Diaz A, Silverman EK, et al. Pulmonary hypertension and computed tomography measurement of small pulmonary vessels in severe emphysema. Am J Respir Crit Care Med. 2010;181(3):218–25. doi:10.1164/rccm.200908-1189OC.
25. Estepar RS, Kinney GL, Black-Shinn JL, Bowler RP, Kindlmann GL, Ross JC, et al. Computed tomographic measures of pulmonary vascular morphology in smokers and their clinical implications. Am J Respir Crit Care Med. 2013;188(2):231–9. doi:10.1164/rccm.201301-0162OC.
26. Alford SK, van Beek EJ, McLennan G, Hoffman EA. Heterogeneity of pulmonary perfusion as a mechanistic image-based phenotype in emphysema susceptible smokers. Proc Natl Acad Sci U S A. 2010;107(16):7485–90. doi:10.1073/pnas.0913880107.
27. Kohler D, Fischer J, Raschke F, Schonhofer B. Usefulness of GOLD classification of COPD severity. Thorax. 2003;58(9):825.
28. Arne M, Lisspers K, Stallberg B, Boman G, Hedenstrom H, Janson C, et al. How often is diagnosis of COPD confirmed with spirometry? Respir Med. 2010;104(4):550–6. doi:10.1016/j.rmed.2009.10.023.
29. Zielinski J, Bednarek M, Gorecka D, Viegi G, Hurd SS, Fukuchi Y, et al. Increasing COPD awareness. Eur Respir J. 2006;27(4):833–52. doi:10.1183/09031936.06.00025905.
30. Wan ES, Hokanson JE, Murphy JR, Regan EA, Make BJ, Lynch DA, et al. Clinical and radiographic predictors of GOLD-unclassified smokers in the COPDGene study. Am J Respir Crit Care Med. 2011;184(1):57–63. doi:10.1164/rccm.201101-0021OC.
31. Kim SS, Yagihashi K, Stinson DS, Zach JA, McKenzie AS, Curran-Everett D, et al. Visual assessment of CT findings in smokers with nonobstructed spirometric abnormalities in the COPDGene Study. Chronic Obstr Pulm Dis (Miami). 2014;1(1):88–96. doi:10.15326/jcopdf.1.1.2013.0001#sthash.L0atdpjM.dpuf.
32. Soriano JB, Davis KJ, Coleman B, Visick G, Mannino D, Pride NB. The proportional Venn diagram of obstructive lung disease: two approximations from the United States and the United Kingdom. Chest. 2003;124(2):474–81.
33. de Marco R, Pesce G, Marcon A, Accordini S, Antonicelli L, Bugiani M, et al. The coexistence of asthma and chronic obstructive pulmonary disease (COPD): prevalence and risk factors in young, middle-aged and elderly people from the general population. PLoS One. 2013;8(5):e62985. doi:10.1371/journal.pone.0062985.
34. Soriano JB, Visick GT, Muellerova H, Payvandi N, Hansell AL. Patterns of comorbidities in newly diagnosed COPD and asthma in primary care. Chest. 2005;128(4):2099–107. doi:10.1378/chest.128.4.2099.
35. Hardin M, Silverman EK, Barr RG, Hansel NN, Schroeder JD, Make BJ, et al. The clinical features of the overlap between COPD and asthma. Respir Res. 2011;12:127. doi:10.1186/1465-9921-12-127.
36. Hardin M, Cho M, McDonald ML, Beaty T, Ramsdell J, Bhatt S, et al. The clinical and genetic features of COPD-asthma overlap syndrome. Eur Respir J. 2014;44(2):341–50. doi:10.1183/09031936.00216013.
37. Kim MA, Noh CS, Chang YJ, Hong YK, Lee JS, Lee SW, et al. Asthma and COPD overlap syndrome is associated with increased risk of hospitalisation. Int

J Tuberc Lung Dis. 2015;19(7):864–9. doi:10.5588/ijtld.14.0327.
38. Cottin V, Cordier JF. The syndrome of combined pulmonary fibrosis and emphysema. Chest. 2009;136(1):1–2. doi:10.1378/chest.09-0538.
39. Cottin V, Nunes H, Brillet PY, Delaval P, Devouassoux G, Tillie-Leblond I, et al. Combined pulmonary fibrosis and emphysema: a distinct underrecognised entity. Eur Respir J. 2005;26(4):586–93. doi:10.1183/09031936.05.00021005.
40. Chae KJ, Jin GY, Han YM, Kim YS, Chon SB, Lee YS, et al. Prevalence and progression of combined pulmonary fibrosis and emphysema in asymptomatic smokers: a case-control study. Eur Radiol. 2015;25(8):2326–34. doi:10.1007/s00330-015-3617-3.
41. Ryerson CJ, Hartman T, Elicker BM, Ley B, Lee JS, Abbritti M, et al. Clinical features and outcomes in combined pulmonary fibrosis and emphysema in idiopathic pulmonary fibrosis. Chest. 2013;144(1):234–40. doi:10.1378/chest.12-2403.
42. Mejia M, Carrillo G, Rojas-Serrano J, Estrada A, Suarez T, Alonso D, et al. Idiopathic pulmonary fibrosis and emphysema: decreased survival associated with severe pulmonary arterial hypertension. Chest. 2009;136(1):10–5. doi:10.1378/chest.08-2306.
43. Kurashima K, Takayanagi N, Tsuchiya N, Kanauchi T, Ueda M, Hoshi T, et al. The effect of emphysema on lung function and survival in patients with idiopathic pulmonary fibrosis. Respirology. 2010;15(5):843–8. doi:10.1111/j.1440-1843.2010.01778.x.
44. Ito I, Nagai S, Handa T, Muro S, Hirai T, Tsukino M, et al. Matrix metalloproteinase-9 promoter polymorphism associated with upper lung dominant emphysema. Am J Respir Crit Care Med. 2005;172(11):1378–82. doi:10.1164/rccm.200506-953OC.
45. Sakao S, Tatsumi K, Igari H, Watanabe R, Shino Y, Shirasawa H, et al. Association of tumor necrosis factor-alpha gene promoter polymorphism with low attenuation areas on high-resolution CT in patients with COPD. Chest. 2002;122(2):416–20.
46. DeMeo DL, Hersh CP, Hoffman EA, Litonjua AA, Lazarus R, Sparrow D, et al. Genetic determinants of emphysema distribution in the national emphysema treatment trial. Am J Respir Crit Care Med. 2007;176(1):42–8. doi:10.1164/rccm.200612-1797OC.
47. Cheng DT, Kim DK, Cockayne DA, Belousov A, Bitter H, Cho MH, et al. Systemic soluble receptor for advanced glycation endproducts is a biomarker of emphysema and associated with AGER genetic variants in patients with chronic obstructive pulmonary disease. Am J Respir Crit Care Med. 2013;188(8):948–57. doi:10.1164/rccm.201302-0247OC.
48. Bowler RP, Jacobson S, Cruickshank C, Hughes GJ, Siska C, Ory DS, et al. Plasma sphingolipids associated with chronic obstructive pulmonary disease phenotypes. Am J Respir Crit Care Med. 2015;191(3):275–84. doi:10.1164/rccm.201410-1771OC.
49. Kim WJ, Oh YM, Sung J, Lee YK, Seo JB, Kim N, et al. CT scanning-based phenotypes vary with ADRB2 polymorphisms in chronic obstructive pulmonary disease. Respir Med. 2009;103(1):98–103. doi:10.1016/j.rmed.2008.07.025.
50. Kim WJ, Hoffman E, Reilly J, Hersh C, Demeo D, Washko G, et al. Association of COPD candidate genes with computed tomography emphysema and airway phenotypes in severe COPD. Eur Respir J. 2011;37(1):39–43. doi:10.1183/09031936.00173009.
51. Dijkstra AE, Postma DS, van Ginneken B, Wielputz MO, Schmidt M, Becker N, et al. Novel genes for airway wall thickness identified with combined genome-wide association and expression analyses. Am J Respir Crit Care Med. 2015;191(5):547–56. doi:10.1164/rccm.201405-0840OC.

Asthma-COPD Overlap Syndrome 13

Chin Kook Rhee

Introduction

Although asthma and COPD are characterized by reversible airway obstruction and by persistent airway obstruction, respectively, these two features are not mutually exclusive. Thus, some patients may show both characteristics of asthma and COPD. For example, if a patient shows positive for bronchodilator test and post-bronchodilator FEV_1 (forced expiratory volume in 1 s)/FVC (forced vital capacity) < 0.7 at the same time, the patient meets both characteristics of asthma and COPD. Asthma is clinically characterized by respiratory symptoms such as wheeze, shortness of breath, chest tightness, and cough [1]. However, these clinical characteristics are also frequently observed in patients with COPD, too. Patients who showed overlapped feature of asthma and COPD have been always existed. However, these patients have been usually excluded in clinical trial of asthma or COPD. Many experts of each filed (asthma and COPD) sometimes denied the existence of these patients and considered them only as heterogeneity of each disease. However, since these patients definitely exist, the concept of asthma-COPD overlap syndrome (ACOS) has emerged recently.

Definition

Until now, firm definition of ACOS is not settled yet. However, there are some promising definitions regarding ACOS (Table 13.1). First, spirometric definition is very simple and easy to apply in clinical practice. The spirometric criteria for asthma is positive for bronchodilator test or provocation test. The spirometric criteria for COPD is post-bronchodilator FEV_1/FVC < 0.7. Gibson et al. [2] suggested ACOS as combination of these two spirometric definitions. One of the merits of this definition is very simple and clear-cut. However, the problem of this definition is that it is too broad a definition. According to this definition, too many patients of each disease (asthma or COPD) belong to ACOS. Pure asthma patients who simply showed fixed airway obstruction can be regarded as ACOS by definition. Also, pure COPD patients who simply showed reversibility can be regarded as ACOS. Second, ACOS can be defined as COPD patients who have history of diagnosis of asthma by physician before age 40 [3]. This definition is also very easy to apply in clinical practice. However, the limitation of this definition is inaccuracy of asthma diagnosis. Often, asthma is misdiagnosis by physician. Without firm evidence of

C.K. Rhee
Division of Pulmonary, Allergy and Critical Care Medicine, Department of Internal Medicine, Seoul St. Mary's Hospital, College of Medicine, The Catholic University of Korea, Seoul, South Korea
e-mail: chinkook@catholic.ac.kr

S.-D. Lee (ed.), *COPD*, DOI 10.1007/978-3-662-47178-4_13

Table 13.1 Definitions of ACOS

Definition 1
• Positive for bronchodilator response test (increase in FEV_1 of >12% and >200 mL from baseline, 10–15 min after 200–400 μg albuterol or equivalent)
OR
• Positive for provocation test (fall in FEV_1 from baseline of 20% with standard doses of methacholine or histamine, or 15% with standardized hyperventilation, hypertonic saline, or mannitol challenge)
AND
• Post-bronchodilator $FEV_1/FVC < 0.7$
Definition 2
• Diagnosis of asthma by physician before age 40
AND
• COPD (post-bronchodilator $FEV_1/FVC < 0.7$ and smoking ≥10 pack years)
Definition 3
• Positive for bronchodilator response test
OR
• Positive for provocation test
AND
• History of asthma before age of 40
OR
• Eosinophilic inflammation in lung (elevated sputum eosinophil or FENO)
OR
• History of allergic disease
AND
• Post-bronchodilator $FEV_1/FVC < 0.7$
AND
• Smoking ≥10 pack years

asthma (reversible airway obstruction by PFT), clinical trial by these definitions is not desirable. Third, ACOS can be defined as patients who meet both spirometric and clinical characteristics of both diseases [4]. This definition is ideal for clinical trial since ACOS patients by this definition are clearly compatible with both diseases. Limitation of this definition is that it is too narrow. Thus, many patients with overlapped feature may be excluded by this strict criteria. Until now, which definition is correct is not yet validated. Actually, these three definitions represent broad to narrow spectrum of chronic obstructive airway disease. Thus, researchers may choose appropriate definition according to the need. First or second definition may be suitable for epidemiologic or population-based study, while third definition is suitable for strict clinical trial.

Prevalence

Prevalence is different according to the definition of ACOS. However, there are substantial number of ACOS patients among asthma and COPD patients. According to database-based studies [5–7], prevalence of ACOS was 52–55% among COPD. However, the prevalence of ACOS was from 5.8 to 24.3% in clinical studies [3, 8–13]. In a meta-analysis, prevalence of ACOS among COPD was 27% (95% CI: 16–38%) [14]. Prevalence of ACOS among asthma patients is 38% over 40 according to very strict diagnostic criteria [15]. Interestingly, the proportion of ACOS was increased significantly according to the age [15, 16]. Prevalence of ACOS among chronic obstructive airway disease was 14% (asthma only: 38%, COPD only: 48%) [17].

Clinical Characteristics

Eosinophilic Inflammation

Serum IgE and blood eosinophil levels were significantly higher in ACOS compared with COPD only [18, 19]. Sputum eosinophil percentage in ACOS was significantly higher in ACOS than COPD only [19, 20]. Blood eosinophil levels were significantly higher in asthma only compared with ACOS [15]. Interestingly, total IgE level was significantly higher in ACOS patients compared with asthma only [15].

Respiratory Symptoms

According to the analysis of NHANES III and COPD cohort, chronic phlegm, nocturnal cough, and wheeze were significantly higher in allergic phenotype COPD patients [21]. According to population-based study, dyspnea and wheezing were significantly higher in ACOS than COPD only [10]. Also, according to another population-based study, ACOS patients had more symptoms of dyspnea, cough, phlegm, and wheezing [16]. According to the analysis of PLATINO study, ACOS was associated with more cough, phlegm, wheeze, and dyspnea [9].

Radiologic Finding

Compared with COPD only patients, ACOS patients showed less emphysema and more airway disease in CT [22].

Exacerbation

Compared with COPD only, ACOS patients exacerbate more frequently. According to the analysis of national health insurance data, the percentage of ER visit was three times higher in ACOS compared with COPD only. Hospitalization was two times higher and ICU admission was 2.5 times higher [5]. According to hospital-based analysis of COPD hospitalization for 10 years, odds ratio of ACOS was 2.183 (95% CI: 1.821–2.618) [23]. According to the analysis of PLATINO study, ACOS was associated with higher risks of exacerbations (prevalence ratio [PR]: 2.11; 95% CI: 1.08–4.12) and hospitalizations (PR: 4.11; 95% CI: 1.45–11.67) [9]. According to the analysis of NHANES III and COPD cohort, risk of ER visit or hospitalization was significantly higher in allergic phenotype COPD patients [21]. In a 9-year follow-up study, risk of hospital/ER admission compared with normal control was 3.76 in asthma only, 5.12 in ACOS, and 2.10 in COPD only [24].

Lung Function Decline

According to longitudinal study in young European adults, change of lung function (mL/yr) was −0.92 in asthma only, −4.84 in ACOS, and −13.83 in COPD only, respectively [24].

Survival

In an analysis of NHANES III data, ACOS patients had higher risk of death during follow-up. Hazard ratio (HR) were ACOS: 1.45 (95% CI: 1.06–1.98), COPD only: 1.28 (95% CI: 1.13–1.45), and asthma only: 1.04 (95% CI: 0.85–1.27).

Treatment

Generally, bronchodilator single therapy is not recommended in asthma patients and inhaled corticosteroid (ICS) single therapy is also not recommended in COPD patients. Thus, combined inhalation of ICS + bronchodilator treatment is a safe option for ACOS patients. There has been no well-designed clinical trial in patients with ACOS. However, several reports support the role of ICS + bronchodilator for ACOS. In a prospective study, response to ICS is much greater in ACOS patients compared with COPD only (372 mL vs. 120 mL) [19]. Christenson and colleagues [25] analyzed the T helper type 2 (Th2) signature (T2S) score, a gene expression metric induced in Th2-high asthma in COPD cohorts. Interestingly, higher T2S scores correlated with increased airway wall eosinophil counts ($P = 0.003$), blood eosinophil percentage ($P = 0.03$), bronchodilator reversibility ($P = 0.01$), and improvement in hyperinflation after ICS ± long-acting beta agonist (LABA) ($P = 0.019$). In a retrospective cohort study, among older adults with COPD, particularly those with asthma and those not receiving a long-acting muscarinic antagonist (LAMA), newly prescribed ICS + LABA combination therapy, compared with newly prescribed LABAs alone, was associated with a significantly lower risk of the composite outcome of death or COPD hospitalization [26]. In a study by Suzuki et al. [27], ACOS was characterized by an airway lesion-dominant phenotype, in contrast to COPD only. Compared to baseline, budesonide/formoterol treatment significantly increased the FEV_1 and decreased the degree of airway wall thickness (percentage of wall area) as well as pulmonary microvascular density in ACOS patients. Although there is limited evidence, other possible treatment for ACOS is listed in Table 13.2.

Future Direction

Since firm definition of ACOS has not been settled, consensus for the definition of ACOS is needed. Then, well-designed prospective clinical trial should be performed in patients with ACOS. Wide definition of ACOS can include variety of obstructive airway disease patients. Thus, in the future, phenotypical approach for patients with ACOS is mandatory [4, 28]. Since asthma and COPD are heterogeneous diseases, management of ACOS should also be based on phenotype and endotype of diseases.

Table 13.2 Possible treatment options for ACOS

ICS + LABA
Recommended for all ACOS patients
LAMA
COPD predominant patients Patients who have neutrophilic inflammation in sputum Add on therapy to ICS + LABA in asthma predominant patients
LTRA (recommend to add on therapy to ICS + LABA)
Smoker asthma Old age asthma ACOS patients combined with allergic rhinitis
PDE4 inhibitor
COPD predominant patients Asthma patients who have neutrophilic inflammation in sputum
LABA + LAMA
COPD predominant patients
Anti-IL5
ACOS patients who have eosinophilic inflammation in sputum

Summary

1. There are substantial number of ACOS patients among asthma and COPD patients.
2. Although definition of ACOS is not settled yet, combination of both asthma and COPD definition is needed for the definition of ACOS.
3. ACOS is characterized by more symptom, frequent exacerbation, frequent admission, higher mortality, and poor prognosis compared with asthma only or COPD only.
4. Although treatment for ACOS is not settled, ICS + bronchodilator is recommended.

References

1. Global strategy for asthma management and prevention. 2015; http://ginasthma.org/wp-content/uploads/2016/01/GINA_Report_2015_Aug11-1.pdf. Accessed October 15, 2016.
2. Gibson PG, Simpson JL. The overlap syndrome of asthma and COPD: what are its features and how important is it? Thorax. 2009;64(8):728–35.

3. Hardin M, Silverman EK, Barr RG, et al. The clinical features of the overlap between COPD and asthma. Respir Res. 2011;12:127.
4. Rhee CK. Phenotype of asthma-chronic obstructive pulmonary disease overlap syndrome. Korean J Intern Med. 2015;30(4):443–9.
5. Rhee CK, Yoon HK, Yoo KH, et al. Medical utilization and cost in patients with overlap syndrome of chronic obstructive pulmonary disease and asthma. COPD. 2014;11(2):163–70.
6. Soriano JB, Davis KJ, Coleman B, Visick G, Mannino D, Pride NB. The proportional Venn diagram of obstructive lung disease: two approximations from the United States and the United Kingdom. Chest. 2003;124(2):474–81.
7. Marsh SE, Travers J, Weatherall M, et al. Proportional classifications of COPD phenotypes. Thorax. 2008;63(9):761–7.
8. Louie S, Zeki AA, Schivo M, et al. The asthma-chronic obstructive pulmonary disease overlap syndrome: pharmacotherapeutic considerations. Expert Rev Clin Pharmacol. 2013;6(2):197–219.
9. Menezes AM, Montes de Oca M, Perez-Padilla R, et al. Increased risk of exacerbation and hospitalization in subjects with an overlap phenotype: COPD-asthma. Chest 2014;145(2):297–304.
10. Miravitlles M, Soriano JB, Ancochea J, et al. Characterisation of the overlap COPD-asthma phenotype. Focus on physical activity and health status. Respir Med. 2013;107(7):1053–60.
11. Miravitlles M, Huerta A, Fernandez-Villar JA, et al. Generic utilities in chronic obstructive pulmonary disease patients stratified according to different staging systems. Health Qual Life Outcomes. 2014;12:120.
12. Izquierdo-Alonso JL, Rodriguez-Gonzalezmoro JM, de Lucas-Ramos P, et al. Prevalence and characteristics of three clinical phenotypes of chronic obstructive pulmonary disease (COPD). Respir Med. 2013;107(5):724–31.
13. Golpe R, Sanjuan Lopez P, Cano Jimenez E, Castro Anon O, Perez de llano LA. Distribution of clinical phenotypes in patients with chronic obstructive pulmonary disease caused by biomass and tobacco smoke. Arch Bronconeumol. 2014;50(8):318–24.
14. Alshabanat A, Zafari Z, Albanyan O, Dairi M, FitzGerald JM. Asthma and COPD overlap syndrome (ACOS): a systematic review and meta analysis. PLoS One. 2015;10(9):e0136065.
15. Lee HY, Kang JY, Yoon HK, et al. Clinical characteristics of asthma combined with COPD feature. Yonsei Med J. 2014;55(4):980–6.
16. de Marco R, Pesce G, Marcon A, et al. The coexistence of asthma and chronic obstructive pulmonary disease (COPD): prevalence and risk factors in young, middle-aged and elderly people from the general population. PLoS One. 2013;8(5):e62985.
17. Chung JW, Kong KA, Lee JH, Lee SJ, Ryu YJ, Chang JH. Characteristics and self-rated health of overlap syndrome. Int J Chron Obstruct Pulmon Dis. 2014;9:795–804.
18. Cosio BG, Soriano JB, Lopez-Campos JL, et al. Defining the asthma-COPD overlap syndrome in a COPD cohort. Chest. 2015;149(1):45–52.
19. Kitaguchi Y, Komatsu Y, Fujimoto K, Hanaoka M, Kubo K. Sputum eosinophilia can predict responsiveness to inhaled corticosteroid treatment in patients with overlap syndrome of COPD and asthma. Int J Chron Obstruct Pulmon Dis. 2012;7:283–9.
20. Iwamoto H, Gao J, Koskela J, et al. Differences in plasma and sputum biomarkers between COPD and COPD-asthma overlap. Eur Respir J. 2014;43(2):421–9.
21. Jamieson DB, Matsui EC, Belli A, et al. Effects of allergic phenotype on respiratory symptoms and exacerbations in patients with chronic obstructive pulmonary disease. Am J Respir Crit Care Med. 2013;188(2):187–92.
22. Hardin M, Cho M, McDonald ML, et al. The clinical and genetic features of COPD-asthma overlap syndrome. Eur Respir J. 2014;44(2):341–50.
23. Kim MA, Noh CS, Chang YJ, et al. Asthma and COPD overlap syndrome is associated with increased risk of hospitalisation. Int J Tuberc Lung Dis. 2015;19(7):864–9.
24. de Marco R, Marcon A, Rossi A, et al. Asthma, COPD and overlap syndrome: a longitudinal study in young European adults. Eur Respir J. 2015;46(3):671–9.
25. Christenson SA, Steiling K, van den Berge M, et al. Asthma-COPD overlap. Clinical relevance of genomic signatures of type 2 inflammation in chronic obstructive pulmonary disease. Am J Respir Crit Care Med. 2015;191(7):758–66.
26. Gershon AS, Campitelli MA, Croxford R, et al. Combination long-acting beta-agonists and inhaled corticosteroids compared with long-acting beta-agonists alone in older adults with chronic obstructive pulmonary disease. JAMA. 2014;312(11):1114–21.
27. Suzuki T, Tada Y, Kawata N, et al. Clinical, physiological, and radiological features of asthma-chronic obstructive pulmonary disease overlap syndrome. Int J Chron Obstruct Pulmon Dis. 2015;10:947–54.
28. Bateman ED, Reddel HK, van Zyl-Smit RN, Agusti A. The asthma-COPD overlap syndrome: towards a revised taxonomy of chronic airways diseases? Lancet Respir Med. 2015;3(9):719–28.

The Spectrum of Pulmonary Disease in COPD

14

Norbert F. Voelkel, Shiro Mizuno, and Carlyne D. Cool

Introduction

The pulmonary vascular disease component in COPD/emphysema has initially been described by A. Liebow at the dawn of emphysema research [1], and radiologists pointed out that vessel loss on the routine chest X-ray films was the best indicator of emphysema. Benjamin Burrows published the first systematic hemodynamic evaluation of patients with COPD and illustrated the great variability of pulmonary hypertension at rest and during exercise in these patients [2]. Since these early investigations, there have been additional remarkable observations. J. Barbera and coworkers [3] demonstrated histologically the presence of vascular abnormalities in chronic smokers without evidence of pulmonary hypertension (PH); the group of E. Weitzenblum reported severe PH in a subgroup of COPD patients [4] and H.J. Bogaard et al. described a severe reduction in the DLCO in their Dutch cohort of cigarette-smoking patients with idiopathic PH [5]. Finally, it has been recognized that a subset of patients with COPD and with interstitial pulmonary fibrosis has significant PH [6]. It thus appears that chronic cigarette abuse is the common denominator, which can explain an element—or "the element"—of the vascular disease component in a large number of patients with PH, and also that there is a spectrum of severity of PH and of lung vessel pathology.

The lung vessel abnormalities include small vessel- and lung capillary loss, intima and media abnormalities, in situ thrombosis, pulmonary embolism, and bronchial artery thrombosis. Presently, we do not understand how the various vascular abnormalities relate to the severity of PH at rest and during exercise; the contributing role of chronic or intermittent nocturnal hypoxia remains also unresolved. Genetic determinants of PH in COPD/emphysema are by and large unknown. One recent study found an association between IREB2 (iron regulatory protein 2, an RNA binding protein) and GALC (encoding galactosylceramidase) and pulmonary artery enlargement in COPD patients [7].

The concept of a homeostatic lung structure maintenance "program" [8, 9] allows us to explain the loss of pulmonary vessels as a consequence of the action of endothelial cell toxic factors like acrolein [10], leukotriene B4 [11], and sphingolipids (ceramides) [12], and apoptosis

N.F. Voelkel (✉)
School of Pharmacy, Virginia Commonwealth University, Richmond, VA, USA
e-mail: nfvoelkel@gmail.com

S. Mizuno
Department of Respiratory Medicine, Kanazawa Medical University, Ishikawa, Japan
e-mail: shirotan@kanazawa-med.ac.jp

C.D. Cool
Department of Pathology and Pulmonary Division, University of Colorado School of Medicine, Aurora, CO, USA

Department of Pathology, National Jewish Health, Denver, CO, USA

S.-D. Lee (ed.), *COPD*, DOI 10.1007/978-3-662-47178-4_14

induced by loss of endothelial cell maintenance factors like VEGF [13].

Paradoxically, the expression of HIF 1 alpha, VEGF, and VEGF receptors is reduced [14]—however, one would expect rather an increased expression of HIF 1 alpha in the setting of hypoxia and chronic inflammation. Studies designed to phenotype and genotype COPD patients are required in order to understand why some patients develop PH and others do not [15]. There are major unresolved questions, like: Why does not every smoker develop PH? What are the root causes of "cor pulmonale" [15, 16]? Why do smokers with COPD develop a functional impairment of the left ventricle? These are just a few of the unanswered questions.

Therapy of patients with COPD/emphysema with PH-targeting drugs remains problematic because of the possibility of inducing V/Q mismatch, yet there may be still ill-characterized subgroups of COPD patients with PAH that can be treated with PH drugs.

In animal models of emphysema, it can be shown that loss of alveolar structures can be reversed. New, non-broncho/vaso/dilator drugs need to be developed which halt lung cell apoptosis and improve pulmonary vascular endothelial cell function [17].

Why Is There a Spectrum of Lung Vascular Abnormalities in COPD?

At present, there is no generally accepted explanation for the variability of pulmonary vascular abnormalities in COPD/emphysema and we resort to the hypothesis of a genetically and epigenetically controlled lung structure maintenance program which may be more or less effective in defending the lung vessels against the toxic effects of the multiple components of cigarette smoke [7]. Figure 14.1 depicts and puts in context the most commonly accepted elements of the pathophysiology of COPD, including pulmonary vasoconstriction and vessel loss. Although traditionally defined as a disease of airflow limitation, it is now apparent that all compartments of the lung (Fig. 14.2)—including the pleura (Fig. 14.3) can show histological abnormalities. A scale-free model of pathobiologically important disease components is shown in Fig. 14.4; some of these components may also explain why COPD is also a systemic disease

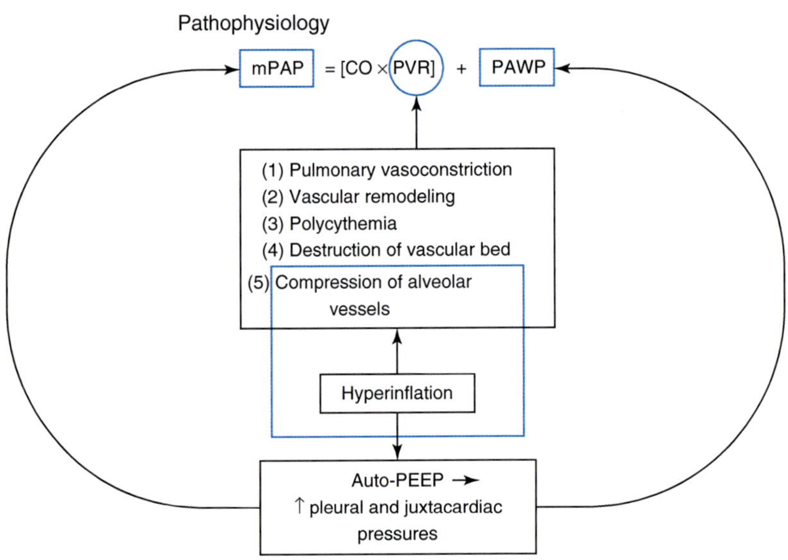

Fig. 14.1 A schematic depicting how different factors contribute to the development of PH in patients with COPD/emphysema. Note that "bad humor" and the contribution of "sick lung vessel" and their metabolic products are not included in this concept

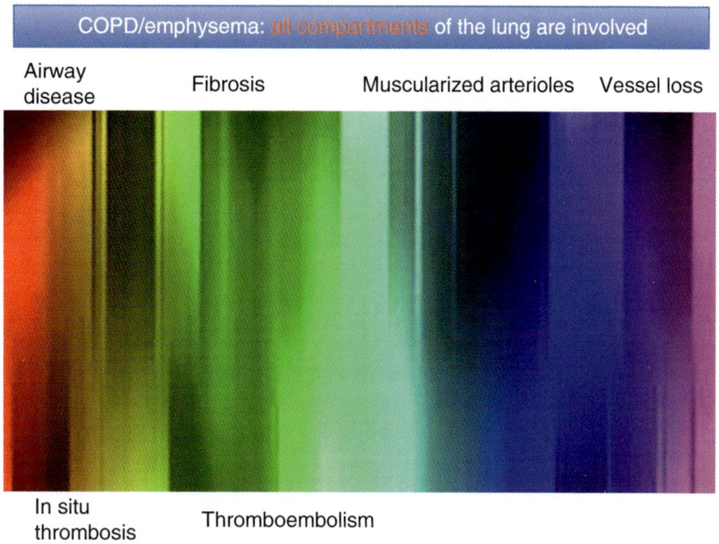

Fig. 14.2 COPD/emphysema patients represent a spectrum of lung pathologies. Which include airway, lung vessel and pleura and interstitial abnormalities. The lung encounters the impact of environmental insults in all of its cells and functional compartments

with multiple extrapulmonary disease manifestations. It is somewhat intuitive that inhaled tobacco smoke causes airway irritation and inflammation; however, the damage to the lung vascular endothelium by smoke continues to be a fact that is not immediately intuitive and difficult to accept by many investigators.

The striking accumulation of anthracotic pigment deposits in the perivascular space (Figs. 14.5 and 14.6) is proof of a particle contribution to the vascular injury and remodeling. Very likely these carbon and iron particles are being transported to the perivascular space via the lymphatics. In addition, inhaled tobacco smoke components gain access to the circulation and affect the function and fate of lung vessel endothelial cells. The best example is acrolein, a highly chemically aggressive aldehyde, which is measurably elevated in blood and excreted in the urine [10]. Cytokines like IL-6 are likewise circulating through the lung vessels and can damage the endothelium. Circulating microparticles can also damage the lung vessel endothelium [18]. The studies by Barbera's group, which documented endothelial cell abnormalities in normoxemic smokers without airflow limitation [3], leave no doubt about the toxicity of cigarette smoke components that can also be easily demonstrated by studies of cultured lung vascular endothelial cells [19]. Parajuli et al. [20] showed an impressive loss of lung vessels in chronically cigarette smoke-exposed mice—iNOS-deficient mice were protected; Misonou et al. [21] suggested that acrolein generates nitric oxide-dependent endothelial cell apoptosis. Thus, there is animal- and cell experimental evidence that categorically supports the notion of cigarette smoke-related lung endothelial cell damage. Yet, we are ill informed about the genetically and epigenetically controlled mechanisms that direct the protective forces of the lung and those that lead to severe PH with or without interstitial fibrosis. Mizuno et al. [22] reported that deficiency of p53 promotes lung vascular remodeling and development of PH and studies in COPD patients have revealed a polymorphism in the MDM2 gene; the MDM2 protein is involved in the breakdown of p53. A possible model of lung vessel loss due to cigarette smoking is shown in Fig. 14.7.

To summarize: the spectrum of lung vascular structural abnormalities is large, reaching from intima thickening in asymptomatic smokers to severe vascular pathology (Fig. 14.8) which can include plexiform lesions [23].

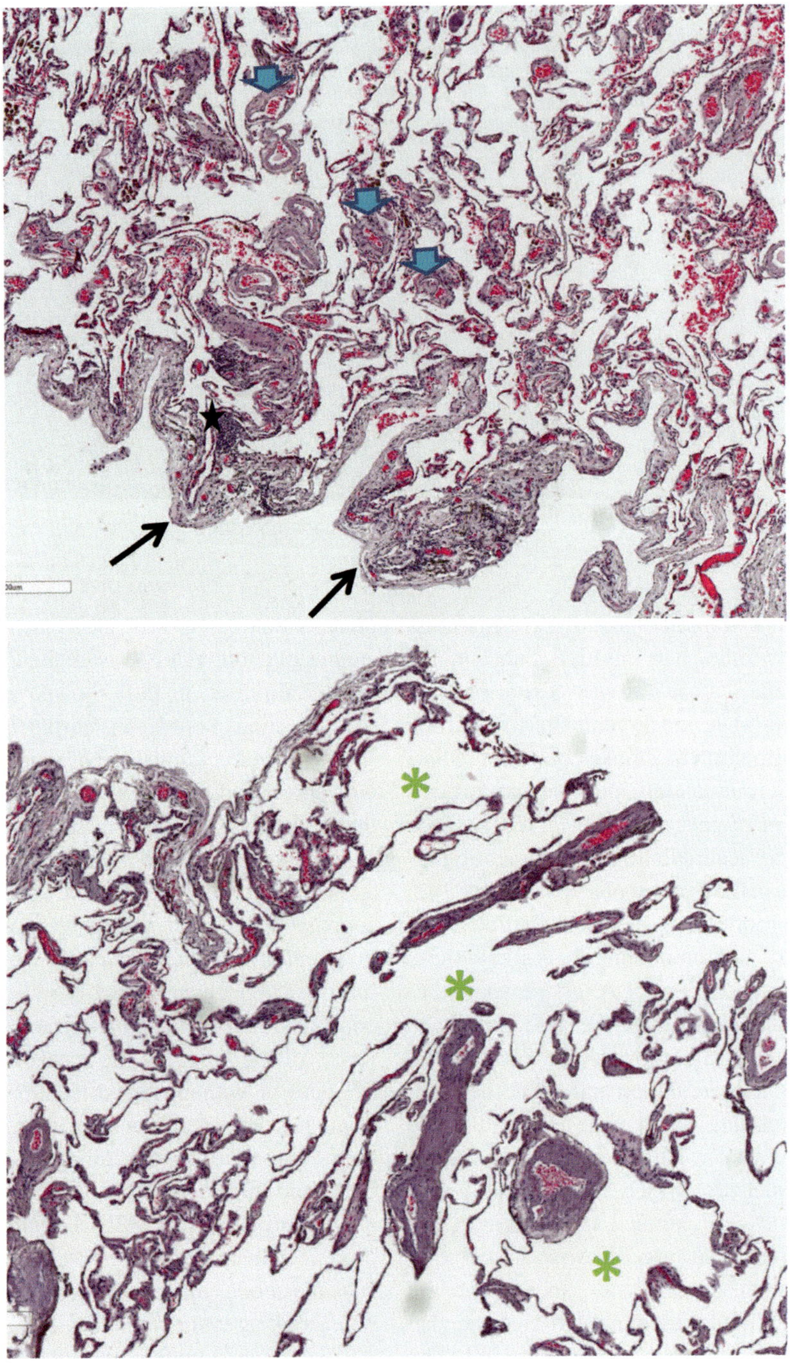

Fig. 14.3 (**a**) The pleura, highlighted by arrows, is mildly thickened and shows patchy lymphocyte clusters (*star*). Small vessel within the pleura are congested, filled with red blood cells. Although much of the septa are destroyed by emphysematous changes, the parenchymal small vessels (*block arrows*) stand out in stark relief to the airspaces. In contrast, small airways appear decreased in number. (**b**) This is an image from the same patient in which the small pulmonary arteries show medial hypertrophy; the arteries are unaccompanied by small airways. Marked emphysematous changes, characterized by enlarged airspaces (*asterisk*), are evident. There is congestion of the pleural vessels, highlighted by the intraluminal red blood cells

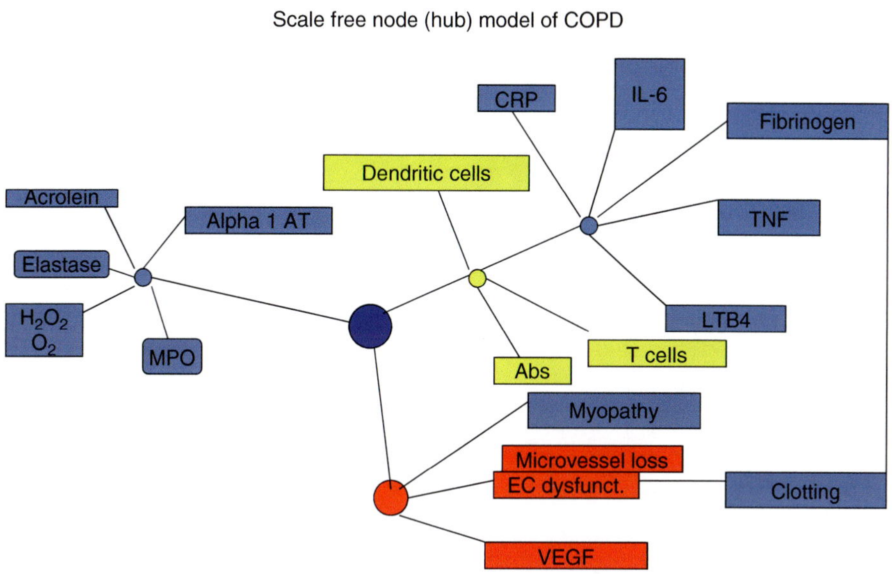

Fig. 14.4 A scale-free hub model of pulmonary and extrapulmonary disease components. The center (*blue circle*) is the adult lung structure maintenance program. Highlighted (*in yellow*) are immune and autoimmune mechanisms and (*in red*) vascular abnormalities both of which likely are also responsible for extrapulmonary disease components

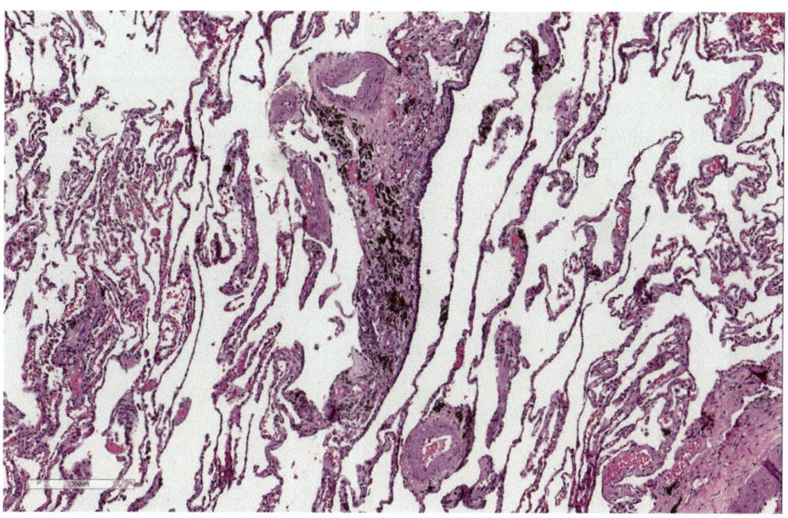

Fig. 14.5 A longitudinal view of a bronchiole line by ciliated, columnar to cuboidal epithelium. The underlying connective tissue demonstrates dense anthracosis. Additionally, the alveolar septa surrounding the bronchiole show clubbing of the tips and enlarged spaces, consistent with emphysematous changes

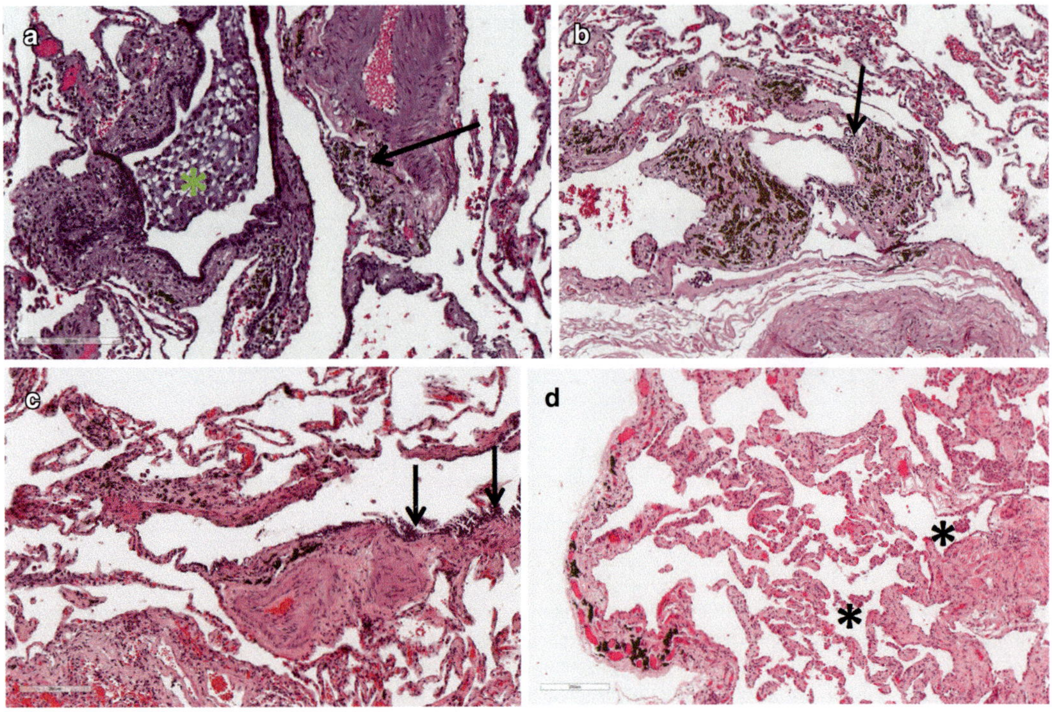

Fig. 14.6 (**a**) High power image of a bronchiole demonstrating dense anthracotic (carbon) pigment deposition (*arrow*) in peri-airway interstitium. The lumen of the bronchiole contains macrophages admixed with mucin (*asterisk*). The airspace macrophages extend into the adjacent lumens of the respiratory bronchioles and alveolar spaces. (**b**) Dense anthracotic pigment deposition in peri-airway distribution. There is mild lymphocytic inflammation in association with the anthracosis (*arrows*). The adjacent alveolar septa are thin and delicate. A portion of a pulmonary artery is visible at the bottom right. (**c**) Longitudinal view of an airway with anthracosis of the surrounding connective tissue. The bronchiolar epithelium is ciliated and columnar (*arrows*). The adjacent alveolar septa are thin and anthracosis is focally visible in the septal tissue. The pleura is highlighted by the dense anthracosis that accumulates along vascular channels within the pleura. The bronchial arteries within the pleura are ectatic and congested. The adjacent alveolar septa are mildly thickened, presumably as a response to repeated septal breaking and accompanying scarring. Alveolar macrophages (*asterisks*) accumulate within the airspaces

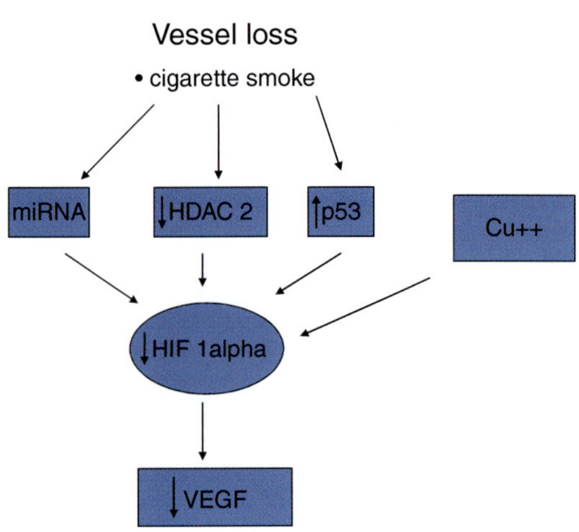

Fig. 14.7 A model of lung vessel loss. This model shows how several factors converge on the important transcription factor hypoxia-inducible factor 1 alpha which importantly controls the gene expression of vascular endothelial growth factor (VEGF). HDAC 2 = histone deacetylase 2

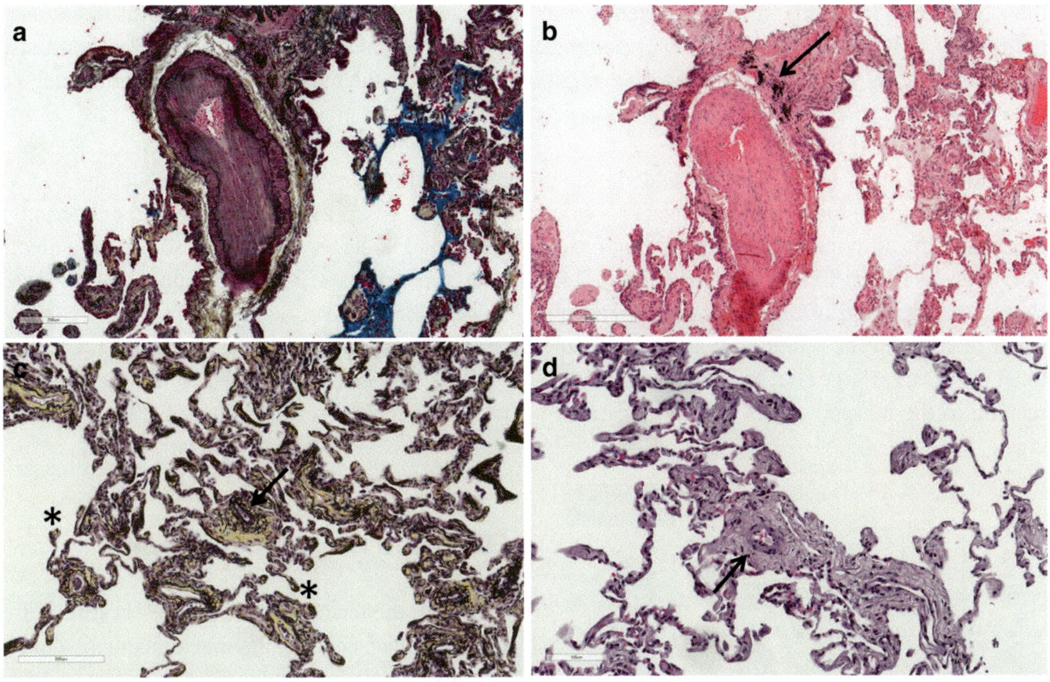

Fig. 14.8 (**a**) Pentachrome (Movat) stain of a small pulmonary artery. The intima, which is located between the internal elastic lamina (*black*) and the lumen (containing red blood cells), is thickened by fibroblastic tissue. The media (between internal and external elastic laminae) is of normal thickness. The adventitia (*yellow collagen*) is normal in thickness. Airspace mucin, visible to the right of the vessel, stains bright blue. (**b**) Corresponding H & E stained image to the pentachrome stain described above. Here, one can appreciate the thickened vessel wall, but the elastic layers are difficult to discern on H & E. In addition, the abundant mucin visible on the pentachrome stain is more subtle on the standard H & E. However, the peri-airway anthracosis (*arrow*) is easier to appreciate on this stain. (**c**) Arteriole within the alveolar parenchyma demonstrating thickening of the wall with prominent elastic laminae (elastic tissue highlighted by black on pentachrome/Movat stain, *arrow*). The airspaces are enlarged and clubbed septal tips are evident (*asterisks*). (**d**) H & E stained image corresponding to the pentachrome image above. The wall of the arteriole is thickened, indicating small vessel disease. There is increased perivascular collagen deposition (*arrow*), which is yellow on the corresponding pentachrome stain in (**c**)

A Spectrum of Vasoreactivity and Response to Exercise

As there are several histopathological pulmonary vascular manifestations, there is a spectrum of responses of the COPD patient's lung circulation to acute and chronic hypoxia and to exercise. Ideally, the testing of pulmonary vascular reactivity should include a hypoxic challenge of normoxemic patients and an attempt to normalize the hypoxemia in those patients that are hypoxemic and are using supplemental oxygen. To assess the degree of pulmonary vasoconstriction, a vasodilator drug like prostacyclin or acetylcholine should be administered [24] following the correction of the hypoxemia. In such a way, the hypoxic and non-hypoxic component of vasoconstriction can be separated. At present, right heart catheterization and pulmonary vasoreactivity testing are not standard procedures that are regularly performed during the workup of PH in patients with COPD/emphysema, perhaps because the degree of PH in most PH patients is mild—when evaluated at rest!

While the magnitude of the acute hypoxic pressure response appears to be greater in older men when compared with younger man [25], chronic intermittent nocturnal hypoxemia may be the condition missed most frequently in pulmonary hypertensive COPD patients. Supplementation of oxygen during the night, with or without CPAP is the treatment of choice for the PH of those patients.

Little new information can be added—since Benjamin Burrows pioneering studies [2]—when it comes to the description of the spectrum of exercise-induced PH in COPD patients. Figure 14.9 shows this spectrum of responses ranging from a small increase in the pulmonary arterial pressure to an impressive, large rise. In the absence of data relating to the morphology of the lung vessels in individual patients [26], the degree of pulmonary hyperinflation or air trapping (Fig. 14.1) is usually proposed as the mechanism explaining the degree of pulmonary pressure response [27, 28]. Some authors have found a mild correlation between resting pulmonary arterial pressure and the DLCO [29]. The group of Joan Albert Barbera recently conducted a large population study of patients with GOLD class 2–4 and found that exercise induced PH was very common in COPD patients (Fig. 14.10), for example, in GOLD Class 3 patients the mean pulmonary artery pressure increased from a resting value of 20 mmHg to a peak exercise value of 45 mmHg [30].

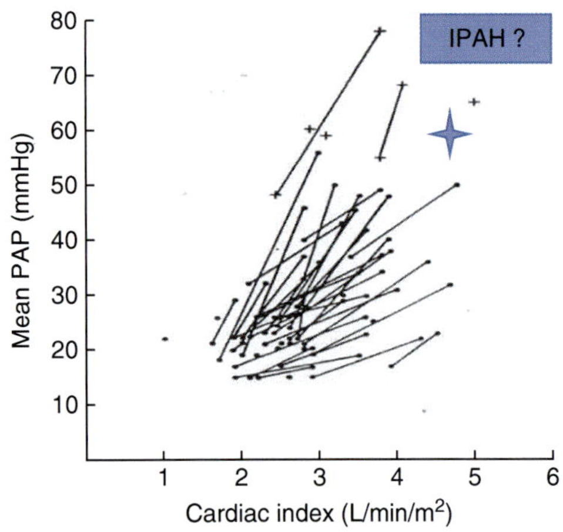

Fig. 14.9 The classical hemodynamic studies showing a spectrum of exercise-induced reponses (Burrows B et al., NEJM 1972; (Reference [2]))

COPD and Heart Involvement

Although the term "cor pulmonale" is still in use (for a review see [31], the mechanisms responsible for cardiac involvement remain largely obscure. It is now accepted that hypoxic pulmonary vasoconstriction or pulmonary hypertension are insufficient as a causal explanation for the development of "cor pulmonale"—in particular since right ventricular dysfunction has been described in COPD patients without resting pulmonary hypertension [32]. Apparently, there is a correlation between the degree of emphysematous tissue destruction and pulmonary hypertension [33]. There is also evidence for impaired left

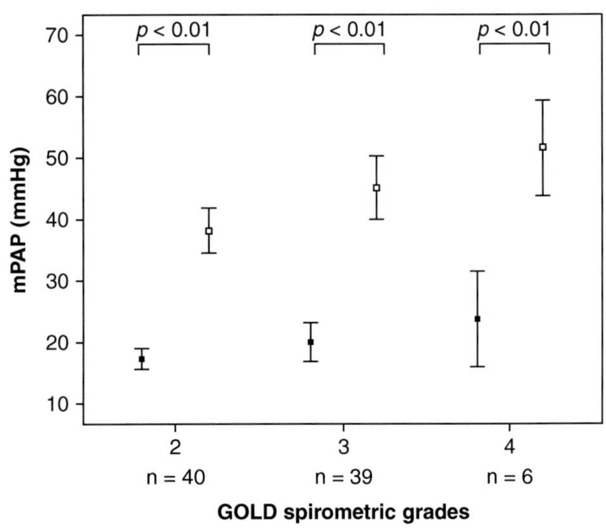

Fig. 14.10 Recent data showing the degree of exercise-induced PH in COPD patients in relationship to their GOLD classification. From Portillo K et al., Int J Chr Obstruct Pulm Disease 2015, (Reference [30])

ventricular function in COPD patients [34] and for these reasons it appears that the term "cor pulmonale" is neither timely nor accurate. Certainly, coronary artery disease is a comorbidity in patients with COPD [35], yet cardiac dysfunction can be documented also in patients where coronary artery disease has been ruled out by angiography. One hypothetical explanation or concept is the effect of a "sick" lung circulation on the myocardial microcirculation [26]. Briefly, functional and morphological alterations of the lung vessels—in particular of the small vessel endothelial cells—generate a "bad humor" which impacts on the cardiac microvessels. The bad humor contains inflammatory mediators, cytokines, microparticles, and vasoactive substances normally removed from the circulation during the passage of blood through the lung circulation. This loss of filter activity is a part of the well-documented pulmonary endothelial cell dysfunction in COPD [36]. It is now appreciated that microparticles contain RNA which could influence the gene expression pattern of myocardial capillary endothelium. To formally address this hypothesis assessment of the blood exiting the lung (arteriovenous gradient) will be necessary; the bioactivity of microparticle-enriched plasma can be examined using vascular rings or cultured endothelial cells.

Taken together, impaired cardiac performance in patients with COPD can occur with and without pulmonary hypertension and with and without coronary artery disease. Both a pulmonary vascular and a cardiac "secretome" may be participating in the pathogenesis of myocardial dysfunction in patients with COPD. As we are learning more about the specific components of lung inflammation and altered pulmonary immunity in COPD [37–39], we may also gain a better understanding of the details of lung–heart interactions in chronic lung diseases and the very opaque term "cor pulmonale" may eventually be understood mechanistically. We want to point out that to date there have been no studies that have used modern immunohistochemical methods or tools that allow the assessment of gene and protein expression in the hearts from patients with COPD. This is a large deficiency and partially explains why we have this knowledge gap. Thus, while we have some histological and molecular information that characterizes right ventricular hypertrophy and to a lesser extent right heart failure in patients with severe PH [40, 41], similar data in COPD are lacking.

Treatment of COPD-Associated Pulmonary Hypertension

The conventional wisdom has it that underlying causes of COPD should be strategically targeted-like inflammation, hypoxemia or polycythemia, and sleep apnea if present. For years now investigators and practitioners have asked whether drugs used for the treatment of patients with PAH (WHO Group 1) should also be used to treat patients with COPD-associated PH. This question is particularly directed towards the COPD patients with "out-of-proportion" PH [42–46]. Over the last three decades, many vasoactive drugs have been considered for the treatment of PH in patients with COPD [47–50]; usually, the study cohorts were small and the patients were not well phenotyped. Reports using calcium antagonist for the treatment of COPD-associated PH showed mixed results [48–50]. Acetylcholine infusion and inhaled NO have been tested, and it was shown that acetylcholine worsened gas exchange while inhaled NO induced pulmonary selective vasodilation [51, 52]. These studies were the precursor studies, which are now leading to clinical trials of sildenafil and riociguat [53–56]. Because prostacyclins are effective in the treatment of severe PAH a small number of patients with COPD-associated PH have been treated with epoprostenol or inhaled iloprost. Ishikawa et al. [57] treated a COPD patient with severe PH and a low cardiac output with infusion of epoprostenol and reported improved right heart function, and Hegewald and Eliott [58] reported a treatment effect that was sustained for 2 years in a COPD patient treated with inhaled iloprost who had a mean pulmonary artery pressure of 74 mmHg. The acutely inhaled iloprost was found to be safe in exercising patients with COPD-associated PH [59], yet Boeck et al. [60]

studied 16 patients with COPD-associated PH after acute iloprost inhalation and reported an unchanged 6-min walking distance. A preclinical study by Gomez-Arroyo et al. [61] demonstrated in a rat model of severe PAH reduction in right heart fibrosis and improved right heart function after 14 days of inhaled iloprost treatment. Taken together, these results may suggest that chronic prostacyclin treatment may improve right heart function in patients with severe PH.

Reed et al. [62] conducted a cross-sectional analysis of 112 COPD patients evaluated for lung transplantation and found that the 30% of these patients that been treated with a statin had a lower pulmonary artery pressure; a prospective study evaluating a potential effect of statin use on PH in COPD patients should be conducted. A small pilot study (eight patients with COPD-associated PH) evaluated the 3 months oral treatment with dehydroepiandrosterone (DHEA) and the authors [63] found a remarkable improvement of the diffusing capacity, pulmonary hemodynamics, and 6-min walking distance.

Summary and Conclusions

There are several manifestations of pulmonary vascular abnormalities in COPD patients and wide variations in the degree of pulmonary hypertension—ranging from mild during exercise to very severe at rest. We are still at the beginning of the work of phenotyping and genotyping this disease spectrum. We predict that a deeper understanding of the disease mechanisms that may have different importance for those patients with a genetically controlled disease susceptibility to the toxic effects of inhaled cigarette smoke will lead to individualized treatments. Cigarette smoke is directly toxic to the lung vessels [20], (Fig. 14.11), and pulmonary vascular remodeling in chronic smokers but may also involve the activation of a host of xenobiotic metabolism pathways, including cytochrome P450 enzyme catalyzed responses [64, 65]. Induced xenobiotic metabolites are also endothelial cell toxic—as is acrolein.

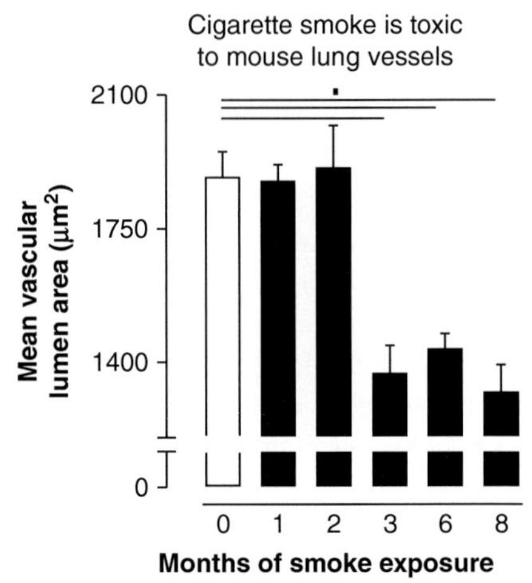

Fig. 14.11 In mice cigarette smoking causes time (and dose dependently), loss of lung vessels and pulmonary vascular remodeling. From Parajuli N et al. AJRCCM, 2015, (Reference [20])

Historically, chronic hypoxic vasoconstriction ranked premier as the mechanism of COPD-associated PH; surely, we now must consider inflammation, immune mechanisms, and the chronic toxic effects of cigarette smoke as pathobiologically important.

While investigators have traditionally been highly reluctant to recommend drug treatment for COPD-associated forms of PH, more recently we witness the process of an opinion shift: patients at the severe end of the PH spectrum should be evaluated for treatment with PAH-targeting drugs—in specialized PH centers.

A recent longitudinal smokers cohort study of the Lovelace Clinic identified approximately 32% of ever smokers as patients which demonstrated a rapid decline in postbronchodilator FEV1; of interest, use of angiotensin-converting enzyme (ACE) inhibitors protected against this rapid decline [66]. It remains to be seen whether ACE inhibitor use can likewise protect against the development of COPD-associated PH—or mitigate the severity of PH or the development of cardiac dysfunction. A recent publication by the MESA COPD study group [67] found that a reduction of microvascular blood flow in patients with mild COPD; this imaging study provides strong support for the concept of a microvascular pathogenesis of COPD/emphysema [8].

As pointed out above, we recommend to retire the diagnosis of "cor pulmonale" and replace the term with a more accurate diagnosis of right or left ventricular dysfunction.

While vasodilator drugs may be effective in the treatment of a few COPD patients with severe PH, perhaps most patients with COPD may benefit in the long run from treatment with drugs like statins or ACE inhibitors. Multicenter controlled clinical trials should follow small exploratory pilot trials of well-phenotyped COPD/PH patients. It appears that the time of treating PH in patients with COPD—and the prevention of PH and associated cardiac dysfunction—in this group of patients, has come. Much work is needed as illustrated by the recent ATS/EUR RESPIR SOCIETY research agenda for COPD statement, as unfortunately, PH was but a footnote [35].

In so many words: it is a great time for COPD-associated PH research [68–71].

References

1. Liebow A. Pulmonary emphysema with special emphasis to vascular changes. Am Rev Respir Dis. 1959;80:67–93.
2. Burrows B, Kettel LJ, Niden AH, Rabinowitz M, Diener CF. Patterns of cardiovascular dysfunction in chronic obstructive lung disease. N Engl J Med. 1972;286:912–8.
3. Santos S, Peinado VI, Ramirez J, Melgosa T, Roca J, Rodriguez-Roisin R, Barbera JA. Characterization of pulmonary vascular remodeling in smokers and patients with mild COPD. Eur Respir J. 2002;19:632–8.
4. Weitzenblum E, Chaouat A. Severe pulmonary hypertension in COPD: is it a distinct disease? Chest. 2005;127:1480–2.
5. Trip P, Nossent EJ, de Man FS, van den Berk IA, Boonstra A, Groepenhoff H, Leter EM, Westerhoff N, Gruenberg K, Bogaard HJ, Vonk-Noordegraaf A. Severly reduced diffudion capacity in idiopathic pulmonary arterial hypertension: patient characteristics and treatment responses. Eur Respir J. 2013;42:1575–85.
6. Tanabe N, Taniguchi H, Tsujino I, Sakamaki F, Emoto N, Kimura H, Takamura K, Hanaoka M, Nishimura M, Tatsumi K. Multi-institutional retrospective cohort study of patients with severe pulmonary hypertension associated with chronic lung diseases. Respirology. 2015;5:805–12.
7. Lee J-H, Cho MH, Hersh CP, McDonald M-L, Wells JM, et al. IREB2 and GALC are associated with pulmonary artery enlargement in chronic obstructive pulmonary disease. Am J Respir Cell Mol Biol. 2015;52:365–76.
8. Tuder RM, Voelkel NF. The pathobiology of chronic bronchitis and emphysema. In: Voelkel NF, MacNee W, editors. Chronic obstructive lung diseases. 1st ed. London: BC Decker; 2002. p. 90–113.
9. Barbera JA, Peinado VI. Disruption of the lung structure maintenance programme: a comprehensive view of emphysema development. Eur Respir J. 2011;37:752–4.
10. Kitaguchi Y, Taraseveciene-Stewart L, Hanaoka M, Natarajan R, Kraskauskas D, Voelkel NF. Acrolein induces endoplasmic reticulum stress and causes airspace enlargement. PLoS One. 2012;7(5):e38038.
11. Tian W, Jiang X, Tamosiuniene R, Sung YK, Quian J, Dhillon G, Gera L, Farkas L, Rabinovitch M, Zamanian RT, Inayathullah M, Fridlib M, Rajadas J, Peters-Golden M, Voelkel NF, Nicholls MR. Blocking macrophage leukotriene b4 prevents endothelial injury and reverses pulmonary hypertension. Sci Tranl Med. 2013;5(200):ra 117.
12. Petrache I, Petrusca DN. Involvement of sphingolipids in chronic obstructive lung diseases. Handb Exp Pharmacol. 2013;216:247–64.
13. Voelkel NF, Vandivier RW, Tuder RM. Vascular endothelial growth factor in the lung. Am J Physiol Lung Cell Mol Physiol. 2006;290(2):L209–21.
14. Yasuo M, Mizuno S, Kraskauskas D, Bogaard HJ, Natarajan R, Cool CD, Zamora M, Voelkel NF. Hypoxiainducible factor 1 alpha in human emphysema lung tissue. Eur Respir J. 2011;37:775–83.
15. MacNee W. The pathophysiology of cor pulmonale in chronic obstructive pulmonary disease. Part two. Am J Respir Crit Care Med. 1994;150:1158–68.
16. Weitzenblum E, Chaouat A. Cor pulmonale. Chron Respir Dis. 2009;6:177–85.
17. Saluja B, Li H, Desai UR, Voelkel NF, Sakagami M. Sulfated caffeic acid dehydropolymer attenuates elastase and cigarette smoke extract induced emphysema in rats: sustained activity and a need of pulmonary delivery. Lung. 2014;192:481–92.
18. Thomashow MA, Shimbo D, Parikh MA, Hoffman EA, Vogel-Clausen J, Hueper K, Fu J, Liu CY. Endothelial microparticles in mild chronic obstructive pulmonary disease and emphysema. The Mulyi-ethnic study of atherosclerosis chronic obstructive pulmonary disease study. Am J Respir Crit Care Med. 2013;188:60–8.
19. Nana-Sinkam SP, Lee JD, Sotto-Santiago S, Stearman RS, Keith RL, Choudhury Q, Cool CD, Parr J, Moore MD, et al. Prostacyclin prevents pulmonary endothelial cell apoptosis induced by cigarette smoke. Am J Respir Crit Care Med. 2007;175:676–85.
20. Weissmann N, Lobo B, Pichl A, Parajuli N, Seimetz M, Puig-Pey R, Ferrer E, Peinado VI, Dominguez-Fandos D, Fysikopoulos A et al. Stimulation of soluble guanylate cyclase prevents cigarette smoke-induced pulmonary hypertension and emphysema. Am J Respir Crit Care Med. 2014;189:1359–1373.

21. Misonou Y, et al. Acrolein produces nitric oxide through the elevation of intracellular calcium levels to induce apoptosis in human umbilical endothelial cell: implications for smoke angiopathy. Nitric Oxide. 2006;14:180–7.
22. Mizuno S, Bogaard HJ, Kraskauskas D, Alhusseini A, Gomez-Arroyo J, Voelkel NF, Ishizaki T. p53 gene deficiency promotes hypoxia-induced pulmonary hypertension and vascularremodeling in mice. Am J Physiol Lung Cell Mol Physiol. 2011;300:L753–61.
23. Carlsen J, Hasseriis Andersen K, Kjaergaard J, Mortensn J, et al. Prevalence, predictors and survival in pulmonary hypertension related to end-stage chronic obstructive disease. J Heart Lung Transplant. 2012;4:373–80.
24. Stevens D, Sharma K, Szidon P, Rich S, McLaughlin V, Kesten S. Severe pulmonary hypertension associated with COPD. Ann Transplant. 2000;5:8–12.
25. Balanos GM, Pugh K, Frise MC, Dorrington KL. Exaggerated pulmonary vascular response to acute hypoxia in older men. Exp Physiol. 2015;100(10):1187–98.
26. Voelkel NF, Gomez-Arroyo J, Mizuno S. COPD/emphysema: the vascular story. Pulm Circ. 2011;3:320–6.
27. Boerrigter BC, Bogaard HJ, Vonk-Noordegraaf A. Spirometry in chronic obstructive oulmonary hypertension. A hemodynamic roller coaster? Am J Respir Crit Care Med. 2012;186:e6–7.
28. Boerrigter BC, Bogaard HC, Trip P, Groepenhoff H, Rietema H, et al. Ventilatory and cardiocirculatory exercise profile in COPD: the role of pulmonary hypertension. Chest. 2012;142:1166–74.
29. Minai OA, Fessler H, Stoller JK, Criner GJ, Scharf SM, et al. Clinical characteristics and prediction of pulmonary hypertension in severe emphysema. Respir Med. 2014;108:482–90.
30. Portillo K, Torralba Y, Blanco I, Burgos F, et al. Pulmonary hemodynamic profile in chronic obstructive pulmonary disease. Int J Chr Obstruct Pulm Dis. 2015;10:1313–20.
31. Shujaat A, Minkin R, Eden E. Pulmonary hypertension and chronic cor pulmonale in COPD. Int J Chron Obstruct Pulmon Dis. 2007;2:273–82.
32. Hilde JM, Skjorten I, Grotta OJ, Hansteen V, Melsom MN, et al. Right ventricular dysfunction and remodeling in chronic obstructive pulmonary disease without pulmonary hypertension. J Am Coll Cardiol. 2013;62:1103–11.
33. Huang YS, Hsu HH, Chen JY, Tai MH, Jaw FS, Chang YC. Quantitative computed tomography of pulmonary emphysema and ventricular function in chronic obstructive pulmonary disease patients with pulmonary hypertension. Korean J Rad. 2014;15(6):871–7.
34. Funk GC, Lang I, Schenk P, Valipor A, Hartl S, Burghuber OC. Left ventricular diastolic dysfunction in patients with COPD in the presence and absence of elevated pulmonary arterial pressure. Chest. 2008;133:1354–9.
35. Celli BR, Decramer M, Wedzicha JA, Wilson KC, et al. An official American Thoracic Society/European Respiratory Society statement: research questions in chronic obstructive pulmonary disease. Am J Respir Crit Care Med. 2015;191:e4–e27.
36. Yang Q, Underwood MJ, Hsin MK, Liu XC, He GW. Dysfunction of the pulmonary vascular endothelium in chronic obstructive pulmonary disease: considerations for future drug development. Curr Drug Metab. 2008;9:661–7.
37. Peinado VI, Barbera JA, Abate P, et al. Inflammatory reaction in pulmonary muscular arteries of patients with mild chronic obstructive pulmonary disease. Am J Respir Crit Care Med. 1999;159:1605–12.
38. Gopi Kalathil S, Lugade AA, Pradhan V, Miller A, et al. T regulatory cells and programmed death 1 + T cells contribute to effector T cell dysfunction in patients with chronic obstructive pulmonary disease. Am J Respir Crit Care Med. 2013;190:40–50.
39. Roos AB, Sanden C, Mori M, Bjermer L, et al. IL-17A is elevated in end-stage chronic obstructive pulmonary disease and contributes to cigarette smoke-induced lymphoid neogenesis. Am J Respir Crit Care Med. 2015;191:1232–41.
40. Lowes BD, Minobe W, Abraham WT, Rizeq MN, et al. Changes in gene expression in the intact normal heart. Downregulation of alpha-myosin heavy chain in hypertrophied, failing ventricular myocardium. J Clin Invest. 1997;100:2315–24.
41. Di Salvo TG, Guo X, Su YR, Clark T, Brittain T, et al. Right ventricular long noncoding RNA expression in human heart failure. Pulm Circ. 2015;5:135–61.
42. Girard A, Jouneau S, Chabanne C, Khouatra C, Lannes M, et al. Severe pulmonary hypertension associated with COPD: hemodynamic improvement with specific therapy. Respiration. 2015;90(3):220–8.
43. Burger CD. Pulmonary hypertension in COPD: a review and consideration of the role of arterial vasodilators. COPD. 2009;6:137–44.
44. Barbera JA, Blanco I. Management of pulmonary hypertension in patients with chronic lung disease. Curr Hypertens Rep. 2015;8:62.
45. Zangiabadi A, De Pasquale CG, Sajkov D. Pulmonary hypertension and right heart dysfunction in chronic lung disease. Biomed Res Int. 2014;2014:739674.
46. Fossati L, Mueller-Mottet S, Haslaer E, Speich R, Bloch KE, Huber LC, Ulrich Somaini S. Long-term effect of vasodilator therapy in pulmonary hypertension secondary due to COPD: a retrospective analysis. Lung. 2014;192:987–95.
47. Gruetzmacher I, Schicht R, Schlaeger R, Sill V. Hemodynamics of pulmonary circulation in patients with chronic obstructive lung disease and pulmonary hypertension as dependent on the theophylline concentration of the serum. Prax Klin Pneumonol. 1984;38:19–25.
48. Saadjian AY, Philip-Joet FF, Vestri R, Arnaud AG. Long-term treatment of obstructive lung disease by nifedipine: an 18 month hemodynamic study. Eur Respir J. 1988;1:716–20.

49. Mookherjee S, Ashutosh K, Dunsky M, Hill N, Vardan S, et al. Nifedipine in chronic corpulmonale: acute and relatively long-term effects. Clin Pharmacol Ther. 1988;44:289–96.
50. Sajkov D, Wang T, Frith PA, Bune AJ, et al. A comparison of two long-acting calcium antagonists in pulmonary hypertension secondary to COPD. Chest. 1997;111:1622–30.
51. Adnot S, Kouyoumdjian C, Defouilloy C, Andrivet P, et al. Hemodynamic and gas exchange responses to infusion of acetylcholine and inhalation of nitric oxide in patients with chronic obstructive lung disease and pulmonary hypertension. Am Rev Respir Dis. 1993;148:310–6.
52. Roger N, Barbera JA, Roca J, Rovira J, Gomez FP, Rodriguez-Roison R. Nitric oxide inhalation during exercise in chronic obstructive pulmonary disease. Am J Respir Crit Care Med. 1997;156:800–6.
53. Holverda S, Rietema H, Bogaard HJ, Westerhof N, Postmus PE, et al. Acute effects of sildenafil on exercise pulmonary hemodynamics and capacity in patients with COPD. Pulm Pharmacol Ther. 2008;21:558–64.
54. Blanco I, Gimeno E, Munoz PA, Pizarro S, Gistau C, et al. Hemodynamic and gas exchange effects of sidenafil in patients with chronic obstructive pulmonary disease and pulmonary hypertension. Am J Respir Crit Care Med. 2010;181:270–8.
55. Maron BA, Goldstein RH, Rounds SI, Shapiro S, Jankowich M, et al. Study design and rationale for investigating phoshodiesterase 5 inhibition for the treatment of pulmonary hypertension due to chronic obstructive lung disease; the TAD-PHILD trial. Pulm Circ. 2013;3:889–97.
56. Ghofrani HA, Staehler G, Gruenig E, Halank M, Mitrovic V, Unger S, et al. Acute effects of riociguat I borderline or manifest pulmonary hypertension associated with chronic obstructive pulmonary disease. Pulm Circ. 2015;5:296–304.
57. Ishikawa S, Yano S, Wakabayashi K, Tokuda Y, Kobayashi K, et al. A case of severe pulmonary hypertension associated with COPD treated with epoprostenol. Nihon Kokyuki Gakkai Zasshi. 2008;46:660–06.
58. Hegewald M, Eliott CG. Sustained improvement with iloprost in a COPD patient with severe pulmonary hypertension. Chest. 2009;135:536–44.
59. Dernaika TA, Beavin M, Kinasewitz GT. Iloprost improves gas exchange and exercise tolerance in patients with pulmonary hypertension and chronic obstructive pulmonary disease. Respiration. 2010;79:377–82.
60. Boeck L, Tamm M, Grendelmeier P, Stolz D. Acute effects of aerosolized iloprost in COPD related pulmonary hypertension-a randomized controlled crossover trial. PLoS One. 2012;7:e52248.
61. Gomez-Arroyo J, Sakagami M, Syed AA, Farkas L, Van Tassel B, et al. Iloprost reverses established fibrosis in experimental right ventricular failure. Eur Respir J. 2015;45:449–62.
62. Reed RM, Iacono A, De Filippis A, Jones S, et al. Statin therapy is associated with decreased pulmonary vascular pressures in severe COPD. COPD. 2011;8:96–102.
63. Dumas de La Rogue E, Savineau JP, Metivier AV, et al. Dehydroepiandrosterone (DHEA) improves pulmonary hypertension in chronic obstructive pulmonary disease (COPD): a pilot study. Ann Endocrinol (Paris). 2012;73:20–5.
64. Budhi A, Hiyama K, Isobe T, Oshima Y, Hara H, et al. Genetic susceptibility for emphysematous changes of the lung in Japanese. Int J Mol Med. 2003;11:321–9.
65. Sacks PG, Zhao ZL, Kosinska W, Fleisher KE, Gordon T, Guttenplan JB. Concentration dependent effects of tobacco particulates from different types of cigarettes on expression of drug metabolizing proteins, and benzo(a)pyrene metabolism in primary oral human epithelial cells. Food Chem Toxicol. 2011;49:2348–55.
66. Petersen H, Sood A, Meek PM, Shen X, Cheng Y, Bellisky SA, et al. Rapid lung function decline in smokers is a risk factor for COPD and is attenuated by angiogensin-converting enzyme inhibitor use. Chest. 2014;145:695–703.
67. Hueper K, Vogel-Clausen J, Parikh MA, Austin JHM, Bluemke DA, et al. Pulmonary microvascular blood flow in mild chronic obstructive pulmonary disease and emphysema. Am J Respir Crit Care Med. 2015;192:570–80.
68. Weir-McCall JR, Struthers AD, Lipworth BJ, Houston JG. The role of pulmonary arterial stiffness in COPD. Respir Med. 2015;109(11):1381–90.
69. Dournes G, Laurent F, Coste F, Dromer C, Blanchard E, Picard F, et al. Computed tomographic measurement of airway remodeling and emphysema in advanced chronic obstructive pulmonary disease. Correlation with pulmonary hypertension. Am J Respir Crit Care Med. 2015;191:63–70.
70. Sakao S, Voelkel NF, Tatsumi K. The vascular bed in COPD: pulmonary hypertension and vascular alterations. Eur Respir Rev. 2014;133:350–5.
71. Hoffmann J, Wilhelm J, Marsh LM, Ghanim B, Klepetko W, Kovacs G, Olschewski H, Olschewski A, Kwapiszewska G. Distinct gene expression patterns in pulmonary arteries of patients with chronic obstructive pulmonary disease and idiopathic pulmonary fibrosis with pulmonary hypertension. Am J Respir Crit Care Med. 2014;190:98–111.

Part IV

Management

Prevention of COPD

15

HyoungKyu Yoon

Introduction

Chronic obstructive pulmonary disease (COPD), a common preventable and treatable disease, is characterized by persistent airflow limitation that is usually progressive and associated with an enhanced chronic inflammatory response in the airways and lungs to noxious particles or gases [1]. Chronic airway inflammation, which is a pathogenic mechanism of COPD, is caused by gene–environment interactions. Although the genetic factors contributing to gene–environment interactions cannot be controlled, COPD can be prevented if the environmental risk factors are eliminated. COPD prevention is more important than treatment because it is almost impossible to lung function normalization after airflow limitation occurs in COPD.

Rates of COPD have continuously increased worldwide, as people become increasingly exposed to COPD environmental risk factors, especially in developing countries. Until now, the majority of research and therapeutic interventions have focused on treating COPD after it develops. There has been limited focus on COPD prevention. Efforts to prevent COPD are lacking, particularly because they have not focused on primary prevention.

Strategies used to prevent any chronic disease can be divided into three stages: (1) primary prevention to suppress the occurrence of disease, (2) secondary prevention to diagnose and treat a disease in its early stages, and (3) tertiary prevention to treat a patient with a disease in progress so that he or she can resume a normal life.

In the case of COPD, primary prevention involves preventing healthy people from becoming exposed to COPD risk factors to prevent the development of COPD. Primary prevention is the most crucial aspect of COPD management. To make an effective COPD prevention strategy, it is necessary to clarify what a COPD risk factor is. Among several risk factors, smoking is the most important for COPD. Smoking prevention and smoking cessation are central aspects of epidemiological measurements to counteract COPD epidemics [2].

However, at least one-fourth of patients with COPD are nonsmokers, and the burden of COPD in nonsmokers is higher than previously believed [3]. Risk factors for COPD in nonsmokers include genetics, long-standing asthma, outdoor air pollution (from traffic and other sources), environmental smoke exposure, indoor air pollution such as biomass smoke, diet, recurrent respiratory infection in early childhood, tuberculosis, and exposure to toxic gas or dust in the workplace. Indoor pollution, which is caused by using biomass for heating and cooking in developing

HK. Yoon
Yeouido St. Mary's Hospital, The Catholic University of Korea, Seoul, South Korea
e-mail: cmcyhg@catholic.ac.kr

S.-D. Lee (ed.), *COPD*, DOI 10.1007/978-3-662-47178-4_15

countries, is a significant problem. Additional causes of COPD include old age, low socioeconomic status, chronic bronchitis, airway hypersensitivity, and infection.

Preventive strategies are also important in patients with established COPD. Continued exposure to noxious agents promotes a more rapid decline in lung function and increases the risk of repeated exacerbations, eventually leading to end-stage disease. Without major prevention efforts, there will be an increasing proportion of end-stage patients who can live longer through long-term oxygen therapy and assisted ventilation, but with increased suffering and costs. Therefore, secondary prevention, which involves diagnosing COPD in its early stages and preventing constant exposure to risk factors, is also very important. Indeed, preliminary research has shown that early intervention based on minimizing these risk factors might be a cost-effective way to prevent COPD.

The main point of tertiary prevention is to prevent death by COPD by controlling the rapid decrease of lung function through proper treatment and by preventing acute exacerbation.

This chapter primarily discusses the primary prevention of COPD and the use of spirometry related to early diagnosis during secondary prevention. Tertiary prevention is about controlling the progression of COPD and treatment related to the prevention of acute exacerbation.

Primary Prevention: COPD Risk Factors and Their Prevention

Interventions based on reducing exposure to COPD risk factors are critical to strategies aimed at preventing COPD. The most important way to prevent COPD is to avoid smoking and reduce exposure to toxic gases or dust in many ways, such as via occupational exposure.

Smoking

The major risk factor for the development of COPD is cigarette smoking, and 90% of deaths due to COPD are directly attributable to smoking. It is well known that cigarette smoking accounts for 80% of the total COPD burden. Therefore, smoking cessation is the most effective means of halting or slowing the progress of this disease.

Although previous studies suggested that 10–15% of smokers develop COPD, more recent studies indicate that some degree of airflow limitation is present in up to 50% of smokers, with clinically significant COPD being present in approximately 25% of smokers [4]. Smoking cessation is the most effective means of stopping the progression of COPD as well as increasing survival and reducing morbidity. This is why smoking cessation should be the top priority in the treatment of COPD [5]. Presently, quitting smoking and home oxygen therapy are the only ways to lower mortality rates among COPD patients.

Smoking cessation can lead to primary, secondary, and tertiary prevention, so it is the most important part of any COPD prevention strategy. Encouraging people to quit smoking in order to prevent further lung damage is the most important and valuable task and should be the most important goal of all doctors who treat COPD. Of course, this is true for all smokers, whether they are COPD patients or not. However, many COPD patients are unable to quit smoking. Smoking is very common among COPD patients; 54–77% of mild COPD patients and 38–51% of severe COPD patients smoke [5]. In order to achieve a reasonable quit rate, it is necessary to administer behavioral support (e.g., counseling) in combination with pharmacological drugs [6].

Preventing or limiting lung damage through smoking cessation should be the foremost goal of all physicians managing COPD. Of course, all smokers should be encouraged to stop smoking, whether they have COPD or not. Smoking cessation reduces the rate of FEV_1 decline and improves respiratory symptoms and health-related quality of life.

Even brief counseling can be effective. All doctors must ask their patients whether they smoke and determine if they want to quit smoking, and smokers should be encouraged to quit.

Of the various behavioral interventions available that can increase the likelihood of smoking cessation, one of the simplest and most effective strategies that physicians can use is to simply advise their patients to quit, particularly if this advice is combined with information about the patient's "lung age" [7].

However, doctors should consider drug treatment to induce more effective smoking cessation results. First-line pharmacological drugs used for smoking cessation include nicotine-replacement therapy (patches, gum, inhalers, nasal sprays, lozenge/tablets, and oral sprays), varenicline, and bupropion SR. These drugs have scientific, well-documented efficacy when used for 2–3 months [6, 8, 9]. All pharmacologic therapies must be combined with support and counseling for maximum efficacy [10]. Verified quit rates at 12 months of follow-up were 13.6 and 6.4% in the intervention and control groups, respectively. Thus, telling smokers their lung age based on spirometry results may increase the likelihood that they will quit smoking [11].

Exposure to Biomass Smoke

It is increasingly recognized that a significant proportion of patients with COPD are nonsmokers.

This proportion is generally higher in developing countries, where exposure to biomass smoke for heating and cooking is common (e.g., up to nearly 70% of people in India with COPD are nonsmokers) [3], but it is also significant in the developed world, with just under 40% of people with COPD in a recent New Zealand study being people who smoked and overall international figures ranging from 25 to 45% [12]. According to the World Health Organization, approximately 50% of all households and 90% of rural households utilize biomass or coal fuels for cooking and heating in the world. About three billion people worldwide are exposed to smoke produced from biomass or coal fuel burning [3].

According to the World Health Organization, approximately 50% of all families and 90% of families in rural areas use biomass or coal for cooking and heating in developing countries. About three billion people are affected by smoke from biomass or coal combustion.

There are several ways to reduce indoor air pollution exposure, such as by changing fuel type or using an improved vented coal stove. Most of all, recognition of indoor air pollution as a cause of COPD is a key element of prevention.

Outdoor Air Pollution

According to longitudinal cohort studies, outdoor air pollution is related to a decrease in lung function in children and adolescents [13, 14]. Therefore, the risk of COPD can be increased upon exposure to air pollution. This harmful effect of air pollution may be caused by lung development impairment during childhood. Several studies have indicated that particulate pollution and nitrogen dioxide (NO_2) are significantly associated with impaired lung development.

The two air pollutants that most commonly exceed standards are ozone and particulate matter. Ozone and particulate matter can harm anyone if levels are sufficiently elevated, but health risks from air pollution are greatest among vulnerable populations. Both ozone and particulate matter can cause pulmonary inflammation, decreased lung function, and exacerbation of asthma. Particulate matter is also strongly associated with increased cardiovascular morbidity and mortality. Children, older adults, and other vulnerable persons may be sensitive to lower levels of air pollution. For persons who are aware of local air pollution levels, the seriousness of air pollution (provided by a government agency) can be checked on the Internet in real time. For avoiding exposure to outdoor pollution, simple measures can be taken; these include limiting the exertion and time spent outdoors when air pollution levels are highest and reducing the infiltration of outdoor air pollutants into indoor spaces [15].

In adults, higher levels of particulate matter (<10 mm [PM10]) are negatively associated with FVC, FEV_1, and FEV_1/FVC. Higher PM10 levels are also correlated with an increased risk of COPD.

COPD acute exacerbation and symptoms become worse when outdoor air pollution is high. COPD patients should limit their outdoor activity, and younger people also needed to avoid exposure to outside when air pollution levels are high. The most effective solution is to reduce air pollution, which will require more effort across the country as well as international cooperation, as pollution is not limited to the country; it is produced in and also influences nearby countries.

Occupational Exposure

There is consistent evidence from population studies that a median of 10–15% of the total burden of COPD is associated with exposure to inhaled vapors, gases, dust, and fumes (VGDF) in the workplace [16]. The evidence supporting these risks varies. For example, the role of coal, cadmium, silica, and biomass in COPD is relatively well established, and the role of more generic exposure to potentially harmful inhaled substances in the workplace is supported by evidence from a number of studies.

The causes of inorganic dust exposure are welding, coal, coke, asphalt, silica, cement, tunnel work, cadmium, glass, bangle, and bleach. The causes of organic dust are cotton, flax, jute, farming, grain, and wood.

Control measures to prevent or reduce exposure to VGDF in the workplace are the most effective methods of reducing occupational COPD. However, it is also important to diagnose COPD at the early stage and in patients with rapidly decreasing lung function. These individuals can be identified at work by accurate annual assessments of lung function [16]. Lung function programs and health surveillance systems are needed for this purpose. Workers in high-COPD-risk workplaces should undergo regular examinations of lung function and surveys of pulmonary symptoms.

Nutrition

Many studies have reported that people who eat a diet high in antioxidants, such as vitamin C and vitamin E, have good lung function, but the reasons for this are not clear. Many studies report COPD "outbreaks" in obese patients although many other studies have opposite findings [17]. The relationship between nutrition and COPD prevention is not clear, but proper nutrition and maintaining a normal weight lead to a better prognosis in COPD patients.

Bronchial Asthma

Asthma is associated with accelerated lung function decline. This decline is greater in smoking asthmatics. Low baseline lung function (FEV_1% predicted), less reversibility to β2-agonists, more severe bronchial hyperresponsiveness, mucus production, male sex, and frequent exacerbations are associated with an excess decline in FEV_1 among persons with asthma. Most studies indicated that irreversible obstruction occurs in older patients with a longer duration of asthma; duration of asthma appears to be more important than chronological age. Whether interventions designed to control tissue remodeling in asthma can prevent the development of COPD is a question that needs to be addressed.

Several studies have shown that childhood asthma may be associated with abnormal lung function in adults. Optimal control of bronchial asthma, especially during childhood and adolescence, is important to prevent permanent impairment of lung function.

Risk Factors of Early Origin

There is growing evidence that COPD may begin very early in life. It may be associated with lung damage to the developing lung during the intrauterine period and the first few years of postnatal life, when lung growth and development are rapid. Early-life risk factors may include fetal and early infant growth patterns; preterm birth; maternal obesity, diet, and smoking; the child's diet; allergen exposure; respiratory tract infections; and genetic susceptibility [18]. The most important risk factor for chronic obstructive lung diseases in childhood is maternal tobacco smoking [19].

Recently, information about early-life risk factors has become more accessible, but people do not know how big this influence is, and there is no effective prevention. However, it will be very important to identify those individuals who are exposed to these risk factors early in life in order to begin proper observation and treatment. Furthermore, physicians need to recognize that lung disease is potentially associated with early-life insults and provide better education regarding diet, exercise, and the avoidance of smoking to preserve the precious reserves of lung function in susceptible adults [20].

Secondary Prevention

Early Detection: Spirometry

According to the Lung Health Study (LHS), lack of awareness and knowledge about COPD among healthcare providers is an important factor in misdiagnosis and/or delays in diagnosis. Major overhauls in both cultural and primary care settings are needed to achieve the goal of early COPD diagnosis. Extensive innovation and changes are needed in primary treatment to diagnose COPD in its early stages. Spirometry is a method commonly used to diagnose early-stage COPD. Medical personnel should be educated to perform spirometry when smokers older than 40 years show respiratory symptoms [21].

The LHS showed that spirometry can be successfully used to assess smoking cessation as a means to prevent COPD progression [22]. According to recent research, spirometry can effectively encourage patients to quit smoking, especially those whose spirometry results show respiratory obstruction [23]. However, in other studies, public spirometry not with high-risk groups did not effectively encourage people to quit smoking. However, there are limitations to these findings, as many young people were included as a target group in this research. There is no definite evidence showing that public spirometry in smokers older than 40 years increases the possibility that a person will quit smoking or identifies early-stage COPD patients.

Smoking Cessation in COPD Patients

The LHS, a 5-year early intervention study combining behavioral therapy and nicotine gum versus standard care in 3926 smokers with mild-to-moderate airflow limitation due to COPD, demonstrated that participants who quit smoking and remained abstinent had improved FEV_1 in the year after quitting smoking and demonstrated a subsequent age-related decline in FEV_1 that was half the rate of continuing smokers [24]. This benefit of sustained smoking cessation in slowing the rate of progressive lung function loss to a level comparable to that of never-smokers persisted for at least an additional 6 years among the quitters who remained abstinent [7].

Brief advice and spirometry are effective to support smoking cessation in COPD patients. In one study, subjects were made to underwent spirometry and were given smoking cessation advice by a nurse and a letter from a physician reinforcing the results of their spirometry annually for 3 years. After various exclusions, of those remaining in the study after 3 years, 25% of smokers with COPD at baseline had been smoke-free for 1 year compared to 7% of those smokers with normal lung function who received the same level of intervention [25]. In a separate analysis of data from the LHS, a reduction in the number of cigarettes smoked per day in the absence of complete cessation did not influence the rate of decline in lung function unless the percentage reduction was very marked (>85%), a degree that was achieved by only a small minority of subjects [26].

When COPD patients quit smoking, infection causing acute exacerbation and a decrease in lung function occurs at lower rates. Additionally, COPD patients who quit smoking consistently show reasonable decreases in all-cause mortality, cardiovascular disease, lung cancer, coronary heart disease, and death due to other factors [27].

Tertiary Prevention

Prevention of Disease Progression

COPD is a heterogeneous disease. As shown in the ECLIPSE study, the speed of decrease in lung function varies among patients, such that one patient can show almost no decrease in lung function while another patient shows a rapid decrease. Tertiary prevention of COPD involves controlling this decrease of lung function by finding the causes of the rapid decrease in lung function and providing active treatment that is designed for end-stage COPD. It is very important to discover biomarkers to help identify this rapid-decliner group early. To discover this biomarker, it is necessary to use diverse methods, such as spirometry and chest computed tomography scan and to assess airway hyperreactivity, health status, physical activity, and comorbidity. The proper treatment of COPD phenotypes has not been identified, but phenotypic-specific treatment will be a crucial aspect of COPD tertiary prevention in the future.

Smoking cessation is the most crucial and effective method to control the speed of lung function decline in COPD patients. Therefore, all COPD patients must not smoke, regardless of the severity of COPD.

Several large randomized controlled studies [22, 28, 29], suggest that disease progression can be slowed in established COPD. In the TORCH study, spirometry also showed significantly reduced progression with fluticasone propionate (13 mL/year), salmeterol (13 mL/year), and the combination (16 mL/year) compared with placebo although these differences are less than the generally accepted clinical target of 20 mL/year. The UPLIFT study reported no significant difference in lung function decline between patients given tiotropium and those given placebo. However, among individuals with moderate disease, the rate of FEV_1 loss among those given tiotropium was 6 mL less than that of controls. Although not tested for primary or secondary prevention, these findings suggest that, as with smoking cessation, pharmacological interventions could be more effective in early disease than in late disease [30].

Prevention of Acute Exacerbation

Acute exacerbation represents the biggest portion of the socioeconomic cost of COPD treatment. Additionally, acute exacerbations reduce quality of life and lung function and can even cause death. Therefore, prevention of COPD acute exacerbation is very important in tertiary prevention.

Influenza vaccine reduces approximately 37% of the total number of exacerbations per patient compared with placebo because vaccination prevents late exacerbation after 3–4 weeks [31]. However, 23 valent pneumococcal vaccines cannot prevent acute exacerbation and reduce the number of deaths due to COPD.

According to a large randomized controlled study, long-acting β agonist (LABA) or long-acting antimuscarinic (LAMA) bronchodilators and inhaled corticosteroid-LABA combinations prevent exacerbation. Triple therapy with inhaled corticosteroid-LABA plus LAMA shows an additional prevention effect. Antibiotics such as PDE4 inhibitors and azithromycin can also prevent exacerbation. Strong evidence indicates that daily variation in exposure to outdoor air pollution is correlated with acute exacerbations of COPD.

References

1. Vestbo J, Hurd SS, Agusti AG, Jones PW, Vogelmeier C, Anzueto A, et al. Global strategy for the diagnosis, management, and prevention of chronic obstructive pulmonary disease: GOLD executive summary. Am J Respir Crit Care Med. 2013;187(4):347–65.
2. Viegi G, Pistelli F, Sherrill DL, Maio S, Baldacci S, Carrozzi L. Definition, epidemiology and natural history of COPD. Eur Respir J. 2007;30(5):993–1013.
3. Zeng G, Sun B, Zhong N. Non-smoking-related chronic obstructive pulmonary disease: a neglected entity? Respirology. 2012;17(6):908–12.
4. Lundback B, Lindberg A, Lindstrom M, Ronmark E, Jonsson AC, Jonsson E, et al. Not 15 but 50% of smokers develop COPD?—report from the obstructive

lung disease in northern Sweden studies. Respir Med. 2003;97(2):115–22.
5. Tonnesen P. Smoking cessation and COPD. Eur Respir Rev. 2013;22(127):37–43.
6. Stead LF, Perera R, Bullen C, Mant D, Hartmann-Boyce J, Cahill K, et al. Nicotine replacement therapy for smoking cessation. Cochrane Database Syst Rev. 2012;11:CD000146.
7. Tashkin DP, Murray RP. Smoking cessation in chronic obstructive pulmonary disease. Respir Med. 2009;103(7):963–74.
8. Cahill K, Stead LF, Lancaster T. Nicotine receptor partial agonists for smoking cessation. Cochrane Database Syst Rev. 2012;4:CD006103.
9. Hughes JR, Stead LF, Lancaster T. Antidepressants for smoking cessation. Cochrane Database Syst Rev. 2007;1:CD000031.
10. McDonald CF, Khor Y. Advances in chronic obstructive pulmonary disease. Intern Med J. 2013;43(8):854–62.
11. Parkes G, Greenhalgh T, Griffin M, Dent R. Effect on smoking quit rate of telling patients their lung age: the Step2quit randomised controlled trial. BMJ. 2008;336(7644):598–600.
12. Salvi SS, Barnes PJ. Chronic obstructive pulmonary disease in non-smokers. Lancet. 2009;374(9691):733–43.
13. Rojas-Martinez R, Perez-Padilla R, Olaiz-Fernandez G, Mendoza-Alvarado L, Moreno-Macias H, Fortoul T, et al. Lung function growth in children with long-term exposure to air pollutants in Mexico City. Am J Respir Crit Care Med. 2007;176(4):377–84.
14. Gauderman WJ, Avol E, Gilliland F, Vora H, Thomas D, Berhane K, et al. The effect of air pollution on lung development from 10 to 18 years of age. N Engl J Med. 2004;351(11):1057–67.
15. Laumbach RJ. Outdoor air pollutants and patient health. Am Fam Physician. 2010;81(2):175–80.
16. Fishwick D, Sen D, Barber C, Bradshaw L, Robinson E, Sumner J, et al. Occupational chronic obstructive pulmonary disease: a standard of care. Occup Med (Lond). 2015;65(4):270–82.
17. Hanson C, Rutten EP, Wouters EF, Rennard S. Influence of diet and obesity on COPD development and outcomes. Int J Chron Obstruct Pulmon Dis. 2014;9:723–33.
18. Duijts L, Reiss IK, Brusselle G, de Jongste JC. Early origins of chronic obstructive lung diseases across the life course. Eur J Epidemiol. 2014;29(12):871–85.
19. Neuman A, Hohmann C, Orsini N, Pershagen G, Eller E, Kjaer HF, et al. Maternal smoking in pregnancy and asthma in preschool children: a pooled analysis of eight birth cohorts. Am J Respir Crit Care Med. 2012;186(10):1037–43.
20. Stocks J, Sonnappa S. Early life influences on the development of chronic obstructive pulmonary disease. Ther Adv Respir Dis. 2013;7(3):161–73.
21. Jagana R, Bartter T, Joshi M. Delay in diagnosis of chronic obstructive pulmonary disease: reasons and solutions. Curr Opin Pulm Med. 2015;21(2):121–6.
22. Anthonisen NR, Connett JE, Kiley JP, Altose MD, Bailey WC, Buist AS, et al. Effects of smoking intervention and the use of an inhaled anticholinergic bronchodilator on the rate of decline of FEV1. The Lung Health Study. JAMA. 1994;272(19):1497–505.
23. Bednarek M, Gorecka D, Wielgomas J, Czajkowska-Malinowska M, Regula J, Mieszko-Filipczyk G, et al. Smokers with airway obstruction are more likely to quit smoking. Thorax. 2006;61(10):869–73.
24. Scanlon PD, Connett JE, Waller LA, Altose MD, Bailey WC, Buist AS, et al. Smoking cessation and lung function in mild-to-moderate chronic obstructive pulmonary disease. The lung health study. Am J Respir Crit Care Med. 2000;161(2 Pt 1):381–90.
25. Stratelis G, Molstad S, Jakobsson P, Zetterstrom O. The impact of repeated spirometry and smoking cessation advice on smokers with mild COPD. Scand J Prim Health Care. 2006;24(3):133–9.
26. Simmons MS, Connett JE, Nides MA, Lindgren PG, Kleerup EC, Murray RP, et al. Smoking reduction and the rate of decline in FEV(1): results from the lung health study. Eur Respir J. 2005;25(6):1011–7.
27. Anthonisen NR, Skeans MA, Wise RA, Manfreda J, Kanner RE, Connett JE, et al. The effects of a smoking cessation intervention on 14.5-year mortality: a randomized clinical trial. Ann Intern Med. 2005;142(4):233–9.
28. Decramer M, Celli B, Kesten S, Lystig T, Mehra S, Tashkin DP, et al. Effect of tiotropium on outcomes in patients with moderate chronic obstructive pulmonary disease (UPLIFT): a prespecified subgroup analysis of a randomised controlled trial. Lancet. 2009;374(9696):1171–8.
29. Celli BR, Thomas NE, Anderson JA, Ferguson GT, Jenkins CR, Jones PW, et al. Effect of pharmacotherapy on rate of decline of lung function in chronic obstructive pulmonary disease: results from the TORCH study. Am J Respir Crit Care Med. 2008;178(4):332–8.
30. Rennard SI, Drummond MB. Early chronic obstructive pulmonary disease: definition, assessment, and prevention. Lancet. 2015;385(9979):1778–88.
31. Poole PJ, Chacko E, Wood-Baker RW, Cates CJ. Influenza vaccine for patients with chronic obstructive pulmonary disease. Cochrane Database Syst Rev. 2006;1:CD002733.

Pharmacologic Management 16

Seong Yong Lim

Inhaled Corticosteroids (ICS)

ICS are the cornerstone of anti-inflammatory agents in asthma, and are recommended as monotherapy or combination with long-acting β2-agonists (LABA) or leukotriene receptor antagonists. In contrast to the crucial role in asthma, evidence that ICS therapy is beneficial to patients with COPD is limited. ICS provide little benefit in COPD patients and are generally reserved for patients with severe COPD with frequent exacerbations or asthma-COPD overlap syndrome.

Molecular Mechanism

Corticosteroid-Induced Gene Transcription

Corticosteroids belong to the family of 21-carbon steroid nuclear hormones [1] and act by binding to and activating specific cytosolic glucocorticoid receptors (GRs). GRs are held in a resting state by a number of chaperone proteins, such as heat-shock protein 90 and FK-binding protein, which protect the GRs and prevent its nuclear localization by covering the receptor sites [2].

Dissociation of chaperone proteins occurred after corticosteroids bound to GRs, which resulted in rapid transport of the activated GR-corticosteroid complex into the nucleus where it induces the expression of a number of key anti-inflammatory gene transcription (trans-activation) following a direct association with DNA at specific sequences in the promoter region of corticosteroid-responsive genes known as glucocorticoid response elements (GREs) [1, 2].

Alternatively, corticosteroids may act by inhibiting the synthesis of multiple inflammatory gene transcription (trans-repression) including NF-κB and AP-1, which regulate the expression of genes that code for many inflammatory proteins, such as cytokines, inflammatory enzymes, adhesion molecules, and inflammatory receptors (Fig. 16.1) [3].

Effects on Histone Acetylation

GRs, after activation by corticosteroids, translocate to the nucleus and bind to coactivators in order to inhibit histone acetyltransferase (HAT) activity [4] directly and recruit histone deacetylase-2 (HDAC2), which reverses histone acetylation, leading to suppression of these activated inflammatory genes.

Cigarette smoke and reactive oxygen species (ROS) stress can prevent GR nuclear translocation or reduce the activity of HDAC2 reducing

S.Y. Lim, M.D., Ph.D.
Division of Pulmonary and Critical Care Medicine, Department of Medicine, Kangbuk Samsung Hospital, Sungkyunkwan University School of Medicine, 29, Saemunan-Ro, Jongno-Gu, Seoul 110-746, South Korea
e-mail: symd21.lim@gmail.com

S.-D. Lee (ed.), *COPD*, DOI 10.1007/978-3-662-47178-4_16

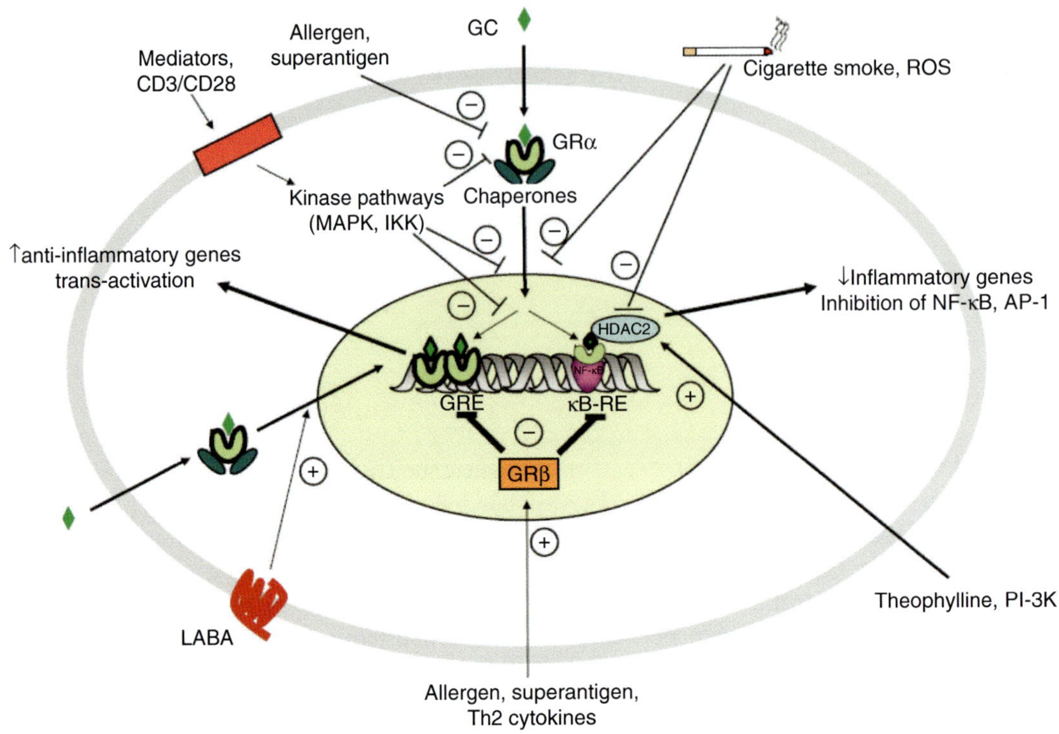

Fig. 16.1 Mechanism of corticosteroid action (from Adcock et al. [3], reproduced with kind permission). *GC* glucocorticoid, *GRE* glucocorticoid response element, *HDAC2* histone deacetylase-2, *IKK* inhibitor of NF-κB kinase, *LABA* long-acting β2-agonists, *MAPK* mitogen-activated protein kinase

the ability of GR to switch off inflammatory genes [3]. Theophylline is known to have the anti-inflammatory effects in patients with COPD mediated through the enhancement of HDAC2 activity that is independent of its bronchodilator actions [5].

Mechanism of Corticosteroid Resistance in COPD

The reduction in the corticosteroid responsiveness in patients with COPD has been variably ascribed to the reduced GR expression, altered affinity of the ligand for GRs, reduced ability of the GRs to bind to DNA, reduced expression and/or activity of corepressor proteins, or increased expression of inflammatory transcription factors, such as NF-kB and AP-1 [1, 3].

The enhanced inflammatory response and corticosteroid resistance may be explained by the reduced activity and expression of HDAC2 as a result of oxidative and nitrative stress in the lungs of patients with COPD. Cigarette smoke and pro-inflammatory stimuli activate p38MAPK, but attenuate HDAC2 expression and activity in patients with COPD. The reduction in GR-alpha expression, while GR-beta expression is enhanced, results in enhanced activation of NF-kB p65 and unresponsiveness to corticosteroid (Fig. 16.2) [6].

Specimens of lung tissue obtained from patients with increasing severity of COPD showed that mRNA expression of HDAC and expression of the HDAC2 protein were significantly lower with increasing COPD severity [7]. In addition, HDAC activity was decreased in patients with COPD, as compared with normal subjects. The reduction in HDAC2 expression is associated with increased acetylation of the GRs, which prevents it from inhibiting NF-kB-driven inflammation [8, 9].

Several promising therapeutic strategies have been investigated in order to reverse corticosteroid resistance by increasing the expression and activity of HDAC2 (Fig. 16.3) [8].

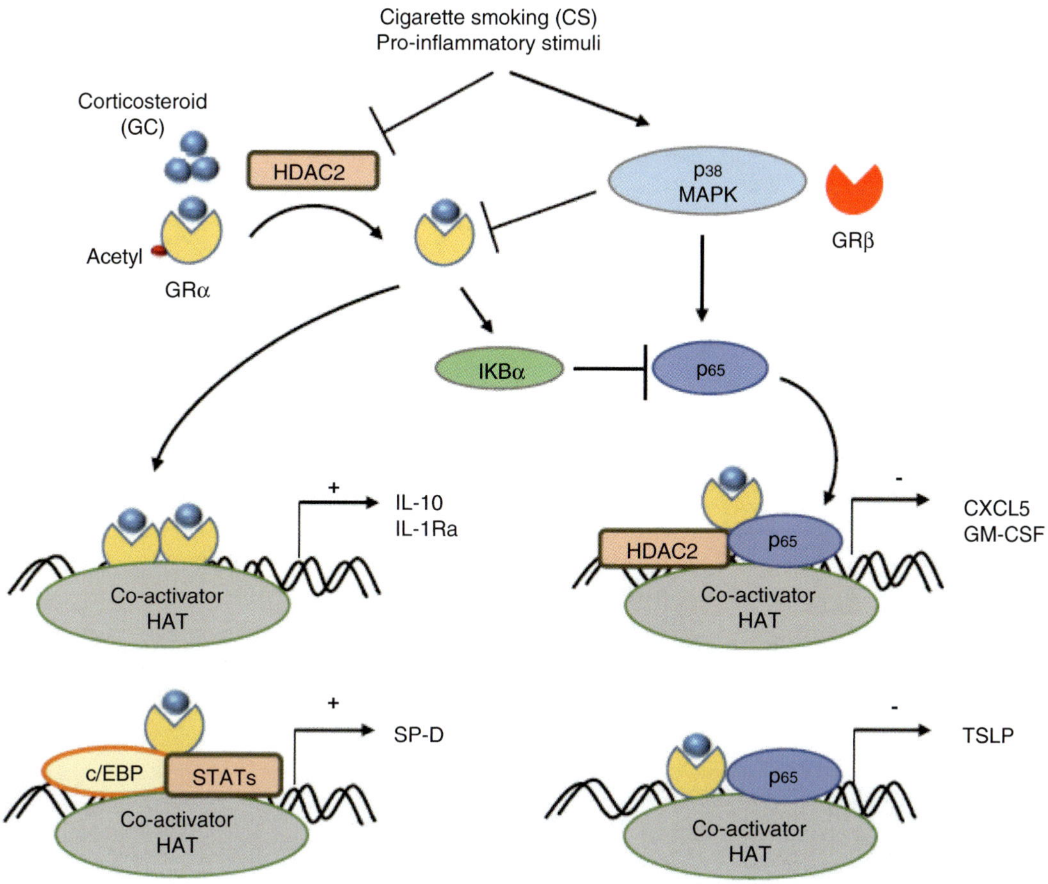

Fig. 16.2 Diagram of steroid resistance in patients with COPD and smokers (from Jiang et al. [6], reproduced with kind permission). *HAT* histone acetyltransferase, *MAPK* mitogen-activated kinase, *SP-D* surfactant protein D, *TSLP* thymic stromal lymphopoietin

Clinical Evidence on the Role of ICS in COPD

Although ICS has been widely prescribed for COPD, the effects of ICS in the treatment of stable COPD are still controversial. Numerous long-term studies regarding the impact of ICS on lung function, exacerbation, health-related quality of life, and mortality have been reported over the last two decades.

Effect of ICS on Lung Function

Whether treatment with ICS has favorable long-term effects by reducing the accelerated decline in FEV_1 remains unclear. Early trials of ICS therapy published in late 1990s in patients with mild-to-moderate COPD did not show the benefit on decline in FEV_1 [10, 11]. Vestbo and colleagues investigated the effects of budesonide 400 μg b.i.d. in 290 mild-to-moderate COPD (mean FEV_1, 86% of predicted) for 3 years [10]. They did not find any significant difference in the annual rate of FEV_1 decline with either budesonide (−46 mL/year) or placebo (−49 mL/year) ($P = 0.70$).

In the European Respiratory Society Study on Chronic Obstructive Pulmonary Disease (EUROSCOP) study, Pauwels and colleagues evaluated the effect of twice-daily budesonide 400 μg for 3 years in 1277 subjects with mild COPD (mean FEV_1, 77% of predicted) who continued smoking [11]. During the first 6 months of the study, the FEV_1 improved at the rate of 17 mL/year in the budesonide group, as compared

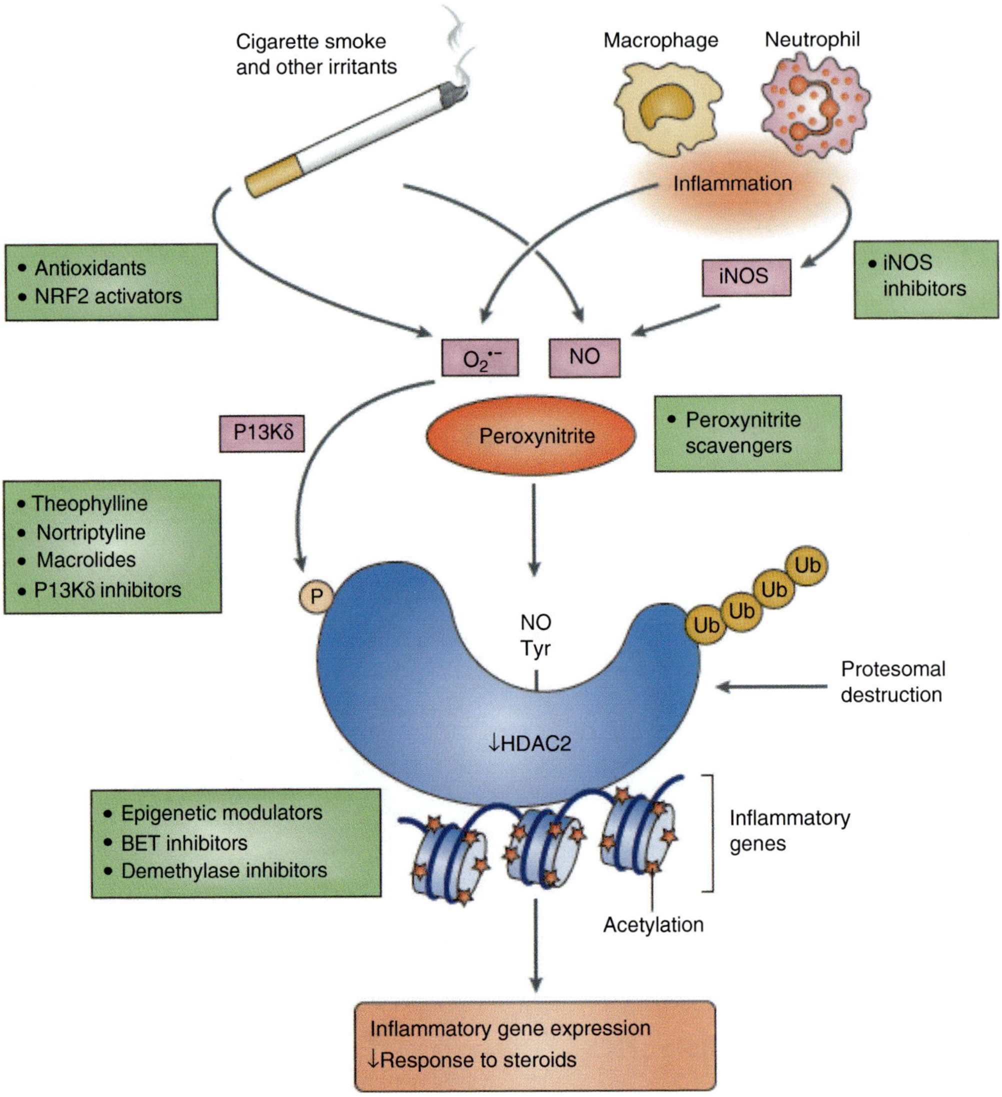

Fig. 16.3 Therapeutic strategies for reversing corticosteroid resistance in COPD. HDAC2 function may be restored by antioxidants (including NRF2 (nuclear factor erythroid 2-related factor 2) activators), iNOS inhibitors, or peroxynitrite scavengers. Theophylline, nortriptyline, or selective PI3Kδ inhibitors restore HDAC function through the inhibition of PI3Kδ (from Barnes [8], reproduced with kind permission)

with a decline of 81 mL/year in the placebo group ($P < 0.001$). However, decline in FEV_1 between 9-month and 3-year follow-up did not differ between budesonide and placebo group (−57 vs. −67 mL/year, respectively; $P = 0.39$).

In the Inhaled Steroids in Obstructive Lung Disease in Europe (ISOLDE) study, no significant difference in annual decline in FEV_1 was also observed between the fluticasone propionate (FP) 500 μg b.i.d. group (−50 mL/year) and the placebo group (−59 mL/year) [12]. The Lung Health Study (LHS) enrolled COPD patients with FEV_1 between 30 and 90% and found that FEV_1 decline was similar in the triamcinolone and placebo group (−44 vs. −47 mL/year, $P = 0.50$) [13].

Based on these study results, ICS therapy did not appear to be effective to slow down the natural course of COPD. Moreover, inconsistent conclusion was published in two subsequent

Table 16.1 Yearly rate of FEV_1 decline by treatment group in TORCH study [17]

	Placebo (n = 1261)	SAL (n = 1334)	FP (n = 1356)	SFC (n = 1392)
Adjusted rate of FEV_1 decline (SE), mL/year	−55.3 (3.2)	−42.3 (3.1)	−42.3 (3.1)	−39.0 (3.0)
Adjusted rate of FEV_1 decline (SE), %/year	−1.5 (0.1)	−1.0 (0.1)	−1.1 (0.1)	−0.9 (0.1)

FP fluticasone propionate, *SAL* salmeterol, *SFC* salmeterol/fluticasone propionate combination

Fig. 16.4 Rate of decline in FEV_1 by baseline post-bronchodilator FEV_1% predicted (reproduced from Jenkins et al. [18])

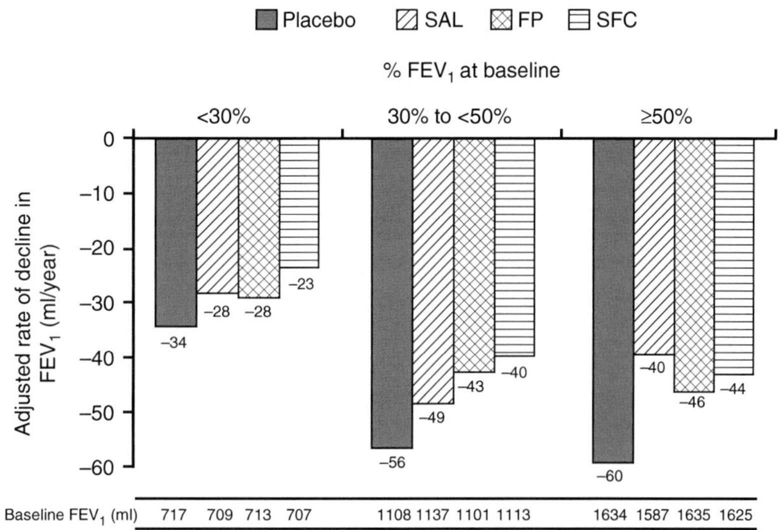

meta-analyses. One meta-analysis concluded that ICS could reduce FEV_1 decline by a small statistical mean rate of 7.7 mL/year [14]. However, another meta-analysis showed a nonsignificant statistical mean rate of 5.0 mL/year reduction [15]. Recently, a Cochrane review in 2012, that examined 55 studies with 15,154 subjects, concluded that long-term use of ICS (> 6 months) did not consistently modify FEV_1 decline in COPD patients [16].

However, in contrast with the results of these meta-analyses, in the 3-year Toward a Revolution in COPD Health (TORCH) study, which was a large landmark study that evaluated the effect of fluticasone, salmeterol, and their combination on mortality over 3 years in 6112 patients with COPD (mean FEV_1, 44% of predicted), FP showed a significant improvement in FEV_1 decline (−42 mL/year, −1.1%/year) compared to placebo (−55 mL/year, −1.5%/year) (Table 16.1) [17].

In a subgroup analysis of the TORCH study, the reduction in the rate of decline in FEV_1 with FP vs. placebo was 14 mL/year in GOLD grade II patients, 13 mL/year in GOLD grade III patients, and 6 mL/year in GOLD grade IV patients (Fig. 16.4) [18].

In addition, the Groningen Leiden Universities Corticosteroids in Obstructive Lung Disease (GLUCOLD) study evaluated the long-term effects of fluticasone with or without salmeterol in patients with COPD who had not used ICS for at least 6 months prior to inclusion [19]. Placebo, or first 6 months' FP treatment followed by 24-month placebo, experienced a considerable decline in FEV_1 of −87 and −65 mL/year over 2-year follow-up, respectively. Notably, treatment with FP improved not only the rate of decline in FEV_1, being close to zero, but also, at the same time, the bronchial hyperresponsiveness and inflammatory parameters.

The TORCH and GLUCOLD study demonstrated significant favorable effect of ICS treatment on the long-term decline in FEV_1, which is opposite conclusion compared to previous early ICS trials. Interpretation of less FEV_1 decline in TORCH study has been debated. The authors stated that the difference in FEV_1 decline compared with placebo group was diminished because of the greater dropout rate in the placebo group. However, some authors criticized that TORCH analysis of lung function decline was not a true intent-to-treat analysis since it was based on only 5343 out of the 6112 patients with randomized FEV_1 values. Moreover, nearly twice as many patients in the placebo group (18%) discontinued before the end of full follow-up measurement. Placebo patients who discontinued had a faster decline in FEV_1 (76 mL/year) than those completing the trial (54 mL/year). These missing results did not occur at random and exaggerate differences in FEV_1 decline between the placebo and treatment groups through the statistical phenomenon of regression to the mean [20].

Nonetheless, effect of ICS treatment on lung function decline in TORCH study was likely to have been observed since it was implemented with adequate sample size which increases the power to detect statistical differences. It should also be emphasized that majority of GLUCOLD patients demonstrated bronchial hyperresponsiveness as well as a modest reversibility of FEV_1 (6.9% of the predicted value), which are characteristics of asthma, and could be useful in identifying a subgroup of COPD with a favorable response to ICS treatment [21].

Effects of ICS on Quality of Life

In a number of previous studies the effects of ICS on health-related quality of life (HRQL) were evaluated. The St George's Respiratory Questionnaire (SGRQ) is a disease-specific HRQL questionnaire [22] and a difference of four units in the SGRQ score is considered the minimum clinically important difference (MCID) [23].

In the ISOLDE study, FP treatment significantly reduced the decline of HRQL compared to placebo (2.0 units/year vs. 3.2 units/year, respectively; $P = 0.004$) [12]. In the TORCH study, HRQL, measured by the SGRQ, also showed an improvement of 1.8 units in the fluticasone group compared to placebo (−1.8 units/year vs. 0.2 units/year; $P < 0.001$) [24]. Fluticasone treatment in the GLUCOLD study was also associated with an improvement in dyspnea, SGRQ activity score, and clinical COPD questionnaire (CCQ) compared to placebo [19]. However, ICS treatment with fluticasone in the TRISTAN study was not associated with significant improvement of SGRQ compared to placebo (−3.1 units/year vs. -2.3 units/year). In the review of the Cochrane Airways Group analyzing pooling of rate of change in SGRQ, it showed that ICS slowed the rate of decline in SGRQ. However, the magnitude of this benefit was relatively small (mean difference: −1.22 units/year; 95% CI: -1.83-0.60; 2507 participants) [16].

Although most studies demonstrated statistically favorable effect of ICS on HRQL, it is not clear whether this improvement may be attributed to other benefits such as reduced frequency of exacerbations. In addition, no studies have shown that significant clinical benefit exceeds the 4-point threshold of MCID. Moreover, there have been arguments against the use of ICS since it is associated with HRQL deterioration in some COPD patients, which could be linked to adverse events by prolonged use of ICS [25].

Effects of ICS on Exacerbation

Until late 1990s no studies were able to show a benefit on the reduction of exacerbation rate. Two positive studies including Lung Health Study [13] and ISOLDE study [12] were followed after year 2000. The ISOLDE study found that the fluticasone-treated group reported lower median yearly exacerbation rate (0.99/year) compared with the placebo (1.32/year), a reduction of 25% in those receiving fluticasone, and a subgroup analysis revealed that this was predominant in patients with more severe disease ($FEV_1 < 50\%$ predicted). The meta-analysis by Alsaeedi et al. [26] concluded that there was surprisingly 30% reduction in acute exacerbation of COPD receiving ICS (rate ratio (RR), 0.70; 95% CI: 0.58–0.84). However, these positive studies received criticism because of critical flaws in the statistical techniques used, as some of these studies did not use weighting of exacerbation according to difference in total person-time of follow-up duration, which produced biased estimates of the mean rate and exaggerated the influence of those subjects dropping out early [27].

In the TORCH study, patients in the FP group (1000 μg/day) demonstrated reduced annual rate of moderate or severe exacerbations compared to placebo (0.93/year vs. 1.13/year), resulting in a rate ratio for exacerbations of 0.82, which is a reduction of 18% in a year.

The pooled results from 11 randomized trials (8164 patients) showed that the use of ICS was associated with an 18% relative risk (RR) reduction in the occurrence of exacerbations (RR, 0.82; 95% CI: 0.73–0.92), which was not related to the level of baseline lung function on meta-regression analysis [28]. In a recent Cochrane meta-analysis, using both generic inverse variance and pooled means analysis, Yang and colleagues confirmed that long-term use of ICS significantly reduces the mean rate of exacerbations (generic inverse variance analysis: MD −0.26 exacerbation per patient per year, pooled means analysis: MD −0.19 exacerbations per patient per year) [16].

Effects of ICS on Mortality

For decades the topic of ICS effect on COPD mortality has been a subject for debate, with a lot of arguments from the case in favor and the case against.

No significant effects were found in early ICS trials including LHS, EUROSCOP, and ISOLDE trials [11–13]. But a meta-analysis published in 2005 by Sin et al. suggested overall survival benefit of ICS treatment, a 27% reduction in all-cause mortality (hazard ratio (HR), 0.73; 95% CI: 0.55–0.96) [29]. The mortality benefit was pronounced in females, former smokers, and patients with baseline post-bronchodilator $FEV_1 < 60\%$ predicted. Another large epidemiological study and *post hoc* analyses of RCTs have suggested that benefit of ICS may be associated with a reduction in cardiovascular mortality [30–32].

However, a subsequent systematic review and meta-analysis of 11 eligible RCTs (14,426 participants) by Drummond et al. in 2008, comparing ICS treatment for 6 or more months with nonsteroid inhaled treatment, revealed that ICS treatment did not affect 1-year all-cause mortality (RR, 0.86; 95% CI: 0.68–1.09; $P = 0.20$) [33]. Positive observational studies suggesting a reduction in mortality with ICS were criticized for immortal time bias [34], and a pooled analysis of 23 high-quality RCTs failed to show an apparent effect of ICS on reduction of cardiovascular mortality (RR, 0.96; 95% CI: 0.86–1.07; $P = 0.43$) [35].

In the TORCH study, fluticasone had no effect on mortality. It did not significantly differ between FP monotherapy and placebo arm (16 vs. 15.2%; $P = 0.53$) [24]. Recent Cochrane review analyzing mortality with nine long-term studies including TORCH also supported the evidence against the effect of ICS on mortality. ICS was not associated with significant effect on mortality (odds ratio (OR), 0.98; 95% CI: 0.83–1.16; 8390 participants) [16]. Therefore, the effect of ICS on COPD mortality is still far from conclusion.

Inhaled Corticosteroid and Long-Acting β2-Adrenergic Agonist Combination

Although COPD is a very heterogeneous disease, airway inflammation and bronchoconstriction are central features shared by many COPD patients [36]. Therefore, such two components have been important targets of COPD treatment. In this respect, combination of ICS as anti-inflammatory drug and LABA as bronchodilator is recommended for the crucial therapeutic strategy in current COPD guidelines [36, 37].

Scientific Rationale of ICS/LABA Combination

Molecular cross talk between corticosteroids and β2-adrenoreceptor (β2-AR) by reciprocal potentiation are responsible for pharmacologic benefits of combination treatment with ICS and LABAs [38, 39]. There is evidence that LABAs may affect GR and thus improve anti-inflammatory effect of ICS. LABAs increase the translocation of GR to the nucleus and subsequent GR-GRE binding, which induce the expression of a number of key anti-inflammatory gene transcriptions (Fig. 16.5) [2, 40].

Specifically, LABAs activate β2-AR coupled to stimulate G protein (Gs), which stimulates adenylate cyclase to catalyze the synthesis of cyclic adenosine monophosphate (cAMP) [41]. cAMP in turn activates cAMP-dependent protein kinase A (PKA), which contributes to enhance nuclear translocation of GR from cytoplasm. Subsequently, GRs interact with specific DNA sequences of GRE, thus inducing gene transcription and increasing β2-AR mRNA levels [41]. As a result, LABAs augment not only GR function but also GR-dependent gene expression, which eventually amplify the anti-inflammatory effects of ICS [42, 43].

In addition, LABAs appear to be able to potentiate corticosteroid-dependent histone deacetylation. Formoterol is capable of partially inhibiting the activity of phosphoinositide 3-kinase delta (PI3Kδ), thus reversing GC insensitivity caused by PI3Kδ-induced inactivation of HDAC2 under conditions of high oxidative stress such as COPD [38, 41].

Corticosteroids positively increase the gene transcription of β2-AR, resulting in increased expression of cell surface receptors [44]. In this way corticosteroids can play an important role in maintaining β2-AR density not to be downregulated by chronic exposure to LABAs [45].

Above findings suggest that the combination treatment of ICS and LABA appears to provide synergistic action; LABAs improve the anti-inflammatory effect of ICS, which in turn augments LABA responses in COPD. However, effect of ICS alone or in conjunction with LABAs on airway inflammation in COPD is still less than convincing, and there is currently no evidence that combination therapy with ICS/LABAs is more effective in improving systemic inflammation [46].

Clinical Evidence on the Role of ICS/LABA Combination in COPD

After the year 2000, majority of clinical studies have focused on the COPD outcomes of fixed-dose combination of ICS/LABA.

Effect of ICS/LABA Combination on Lung Function

Mahler et al. examined the benefits of fluticasone propionate (FP) and salmeterol (SAL) combination (SFC) in 691 patients for 24 weeks [47]. A significantly greater increase in pre-dose FEV_1 at the endpoint was observed after SFC (156 mL) compared with SAL (107 mL, $P = 0.012$) and placebo (−4 mL, $P < 0.001$). In the TRISTAN study, Calverley et al. also found that SFC increased pretreatment FEV_1 significantly more than did the placebo (treatment difference 133 mL; 95% CI: 105–161; $P < 0.0001$),

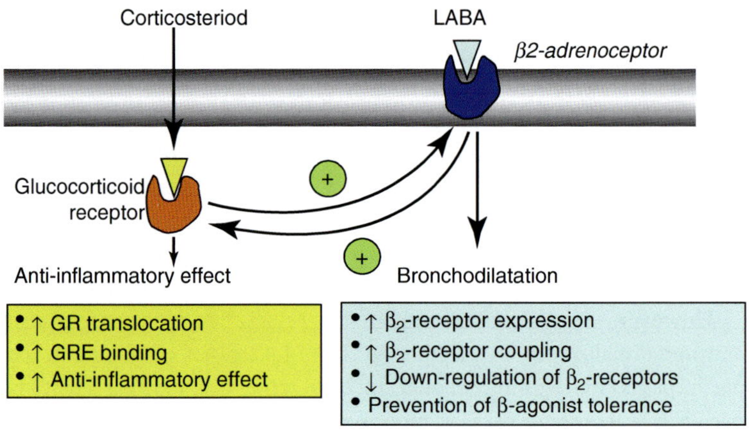

Fig. 16.5 Molecular cross talk between long-acting β2-agonists (LABA) and corticosteroids (reproduced from Barnes [40]). *GR* glucocorticoid receptor, *GRE* glucocorticoid response elements

SAL (treatment difference 73 mL; 95% CI: 46–101; $P < 0.001$), or FP alone (treatment difference 95 mL; 95% CI: 67–122, $P < 0.001$) [48]. The budesonide (BUD) and formoterol (FOR) combination (BUD/FOR) study also reported that BUD/FOR combination treatment maintained higher FEV_1 and pre-bronchodilator peak expiratory flow compared to placebo or either monocomponent [49].

Undoubtedly, the most important long-term trial that evaluated the effectiveness of ICS/LABA combination in COPD was the TORCH study [24]. In a post hoc analysis, after a 3-year treatment, the SFC combination increased the mean post-bronchodilator FEV_1 by 29 mL, and significantly reduced the rate of lung function decline compared to placebo (placebo decline of 55 mL/year, salmeterol decline of 42 mL/year, fluticasone decline of 42 mL/year, and salmeterol/fluticasone decline of 39 mL/year) (Table 16.1, Fig. 16.4) [17].

Although the rates of decline were significantly reduced for all active treatment arms vs. placebo, there were no significant differences between ICS-containing treatments and SAL monotherapy, which raises the question regarding the benefit of ICS in lung function decline [25]. One of the major methodologic limitations criticized in the TORCH trial is that the absence of a pure intent-to-treat analysis was not possible for FEV_1 decline because this could not be obtained after the subjects discontinued the study medication. 35% of subjects in ICS/LABA and 45% of placebo group did not complete the 3-year follow-up including the 21% dropped out in the first year [50]. Moreover, loss to follow-up was not random: dropout patients were older, and had a lower FEV_1, and greater exacerbation history [50, 51]. Therefore, FEV_1 decline using incomplete follow-up could be biased since the slope of FEV_1 decline in the remaining patients who had better lung function would have been affected by regression to mean, which could lead to an overestimation of FEV_1 decline in the placebo, eventually leading to false conclusion that ICS-containing treatment affects lung function decline [25, 50]. A recent Cochrane review examining between ICS and placebo revealed no significant effect of ICS to reduce lung function decline [16]. Another meta-analysis comparing ICS/LABA combination vs. LABA monotherapy, a borderline improvement in FEV_1 of 4–6 mL was observed in favor of ICS/LABA [52]. However, this small benefit did not satisfy the FEV_1 threshold of MCID (0.100 L or more); thus the implication of this minor improvement seems uncertain [25].

In a recent Cochrane network meta-analysis, combination ICS/LABA was the highest ranked class for trough FEV_1, with mean improvement over placebo of 133.3 mL at 6 months (95% CI: 100.6–164.0) and slightly less at 12 months (mean difference (MD), 100 mL; 95% CI: 55.5–140.1). LAMAs (MD, 103.5 mL; 95% CI: 81.8–124.9) and LABAs (MD, 99.4 mL; 95% CI: 72.0–127.8) showed roughly equivalent results at 6 months, and ICSs were the fourth ranked class (MD, 65.4 mL; 95% CI:33.1–96.9) [53]. The network has demonstrated the benefit of ICS when added to LABAs in participants who largely had an FEV_1 that was less than 50% predicted.

Recently, new ICS/LABA combinations have developed, including fluticasone furoate/vilanterol (FF/VI), mometasone furoate/formoterol fumarate (MF/FOR), and beclomethasone dipropionate/formoterol fumarate (BDP/FOR) [54].

A 24-week investigation compared the efficacy of different dosages of the once-daily FF (50, 100 μg)/VI (25 μg) combination with monocomponents (FF 100 μg, VI 25 μg) and placebo in patients with moderate-to-severe COPD. The combination of FF/VI significantly improved weighted mean (wm) FEV_1 (173 mL) and trough FEV_1 (115 mL) vs. placebo. Although all treatment arms significantly improved FEV_1 compared to placebo, there was no significant difference between FF/VI dosages and VI monotherapy [55]. Another 24-week trial of same design, but with double the strengths of FF/VI doses (200/25, 100/25 μg), found the same results [56]. The first trial comparing FF/VI (100/25 μg) once daily vs. FP/SAL 500/50 μg twice daily over 12 weeks reported that improvements in lung function were not different [57].

There is relatively few data investigating BDP/FF combination inhaler. In a 48-week RCT, BDP/FOR, BUD/FOR, and formoterol alone improved pre-dose morning FEV_1 by 0.077 (L), 0.080 (L), and 0.026 (L), respectively, in 718 patients with severe COPD (FEV_1 between 30 and 50% of predicted). BDP/FOR was shown to be non-inferior to BUD/FOR (the lower limit of the 97.5% CI was −0.052 (L), which is within the prespecified non-inferiority margin of −0.100 (L)) and statistically significantly better than formoterol alone ($P = 0.046$) [58].

MF/FOR combination also showed significantly greater increases in trough FEV_1. The increase was fourfold greater with MF/FOR (400/10 μg) than with FOR (10 μg) at 13-week endpoint ($P < 0.05$) [59]. In the 26-week treatment period, significantly greater increases in mean changes in FEV_1 area under the curve from 0 to 12 h post-dose (FEV_1 $AUC_{0-12\,h}$) occurred with MF/FOR (400/10 μg) vs. MF 400 μg and placebo at the weeks 13 and 26 endpoints ($P = 0.032$).

Comparison of lung function between ICS/LABA combinations with fixed-dose LAMA/LABA combinations was reported. In the ILLUMINATE study in symptomatic GOLD grade II and III patients without moderate-to-severe exacerbation in the previous year, glycopyrronium/indacaterol 50/110 μg (QVA149; Ultibro Breezhaler) provided significant improvements in lung function vs. b.i.d. SFC 500/50 μg [60]. At week 26, FEV_1 AUC_{0-12h} was significantly higher with QVA149 than with SFC (treatment difference, 0.138 L; 95% CI: 0.100–0.176; $P < 0.001$) (Fig. 16.6).

In the 6-month LANTERN study, comparing QVA149 with SFC 500/50 μg b.i.d. in patients with moderate-to-severe COPD with a history of ≤1 exacerbation in the previous year, QVA149

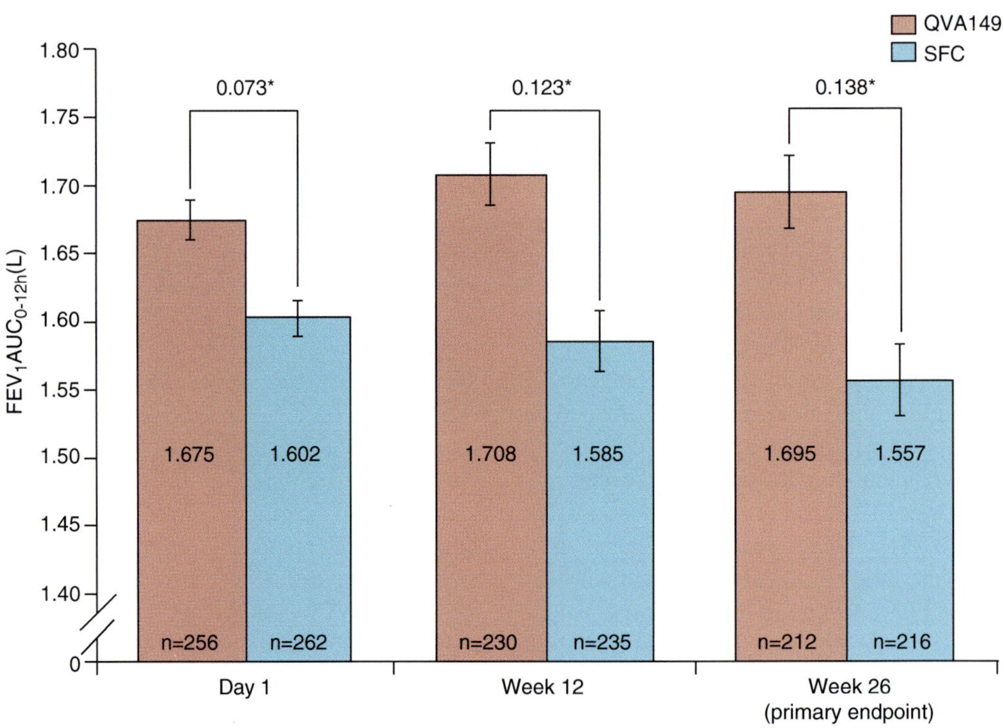

Fig. 16.6 FEV_1 AUC_{0-12h} in the ILLUMINATE study. Data are least squares mean (SE) (from Vogelmeier et al. [60], reproduced with kind permission) *FEV_1* forced expiratory volume in 1 s, *AUC_{0-12h}* area under the plasma concentration-time curve from 0 to 12 h, *SFC* salmeterol/fluticasone. *$p < 0.0001$ for comparisons between QVA149 and SFC

demonstrated statistically significant superiority to SFC for trough FEV_1 (treatment difference [Δ] = 75 mL; $P < 0.001$) [61]. Similar finding was reported in a 12-week study comparing umeclidinium/vilanterol with SFC [62].

Effect of ICS/LABA Combination on Exacerbation

Although no statistically significant differences between treatment groups (SFC 1000/100 μg, SAL 50 μg, FP 1000 μg, placebo) in time to exacerbation were found in the study by Mahler et al. [47] and Hannania et al. [63], combination treatment of ICS/LABA (SFC) reduced the frequency of exacerbation and exacerbation requiring steroid treatment compared to placebo in the TRISTAN study. However, there was no statistical difference in exacerbation rate between SFC and salmeterol [48].

In the TORCH study, a 25% reduction in the annual rate of exacerbations was noted in the SFC (0.85/year; 95% CI: 0.80–0.90) compared to placebo group (1.13/year; 95% CI: 1.07–1.20), with a number needed to treat (NNT) of four to prevent one exacerbation. Compared with salmeterol alone, the addition of fluticasone significantly reduced the rate of moderate exacerbations, but it did not have any significant beneficial effect on severe exacerbation requiring hospitalization (RR, 1.02; 95% CI: 0.87–1.20, $P = 0.79$) [24, 64] (Fig. 16.7).

Furthermore, in post hoc analysis of the TORCH study, early therapy with SFC in moderate grade of COPD demonstrated a better result with respect to the decrease in exacerbation rate: 31% (95% CI: 19–40) in GOLD II, 26% (95% CI: 17–34) in GOLD III, and 14% (95% CI: -4-29) in GOLD IV [18]. SFC reduced the annual rate of exacerbation as much as 31% (SFC 0.57/year vs. placebo 0.82/year) in GOLD II, 26% in GOLD III, and 14% in GOLD IV [18].

Besides fluticasone-containing combination trials, BUD/FOR has been shown to be effective in reduction of exacerbation. Two early studies evaluating the efficacy of combination treatment with BUD/FOR in patients with moderate and severe COPD were published in 2003. Szafranski and colleagues found that BUD/FOR exhibited significantly lower severe exacerbation by as much as 24% vs. placebo and 23% vs. formoterol [65]. Calverley et al. also showed that BUD/FOR was associated with reduced rate of exacerbations and prolonged the time to first exacerbation requiring medical intervention compared to placebo [49].

Despite the limitation of observational real-life COPD cohort studies, two large database studies suggested that differences in efficacy might exist between the ICS/LABA in favor of BUD/FOR. In a Canadian database study, the odds ratios (OR) for course of oral steroid (OR, 0.85; 95% CI: 0.72–1.0), emergency department

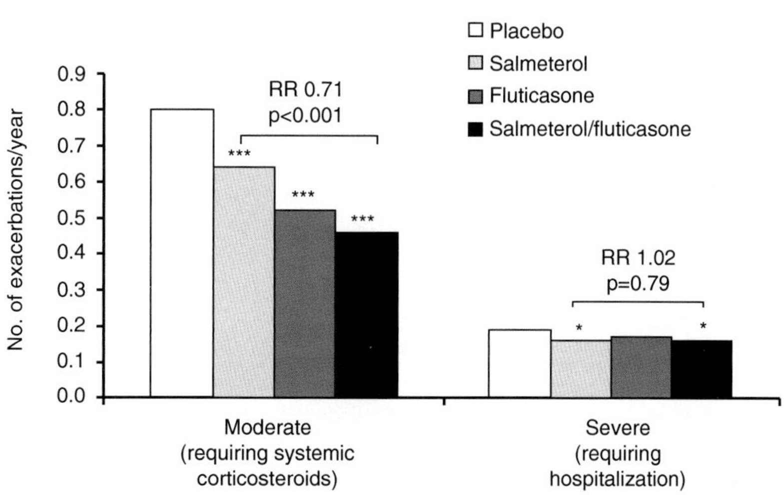

Fig. 16.7 Effect of treatment on the annual rate of exacerbation in the TORCH study (from Price et al. [64], reproduced with kind permission)

visit (OR, 0.75; 95% CI: 0.58–0.97, $P < 0.05$), hospital admission (OR, 0.61, 95% CI: 0.47–0.81, $P < 0.05$), and addition of tiotropium (OR, 0.71; 95% CI: 0.57–0.89) were all in favor of the BUD/FOR combination [66].

The result of the Canadian study has been confirmed by a large Swedish database observational PATHOS study [67]. Pairwise propensity score matching of 9893 COPD patients (7155 BUD/FOR and 2738 SFC) yielded two cohorts of 2734 patients. Compared with SFC, BUD/FOR was associated with a reduced risk of annual exacerbation by 26.6% (0.80 vs. 1.09, $P < 0.0001$), with a reduced hospitalization due to COPD by 29% (0.1 vs. 0.21, $P < 0.0001$) (Table 16.2).

Adding BUD/FOR to LAMA decreased morning symptom and exacerbation over the 3 months of the CLIMB trial [68], but further studies evaluating the benefits of ICS in addition to dual bronchodilator are warranted.

Comparative efficacy between ICS/LABA and LAMA in terms of reducing COPD exacerbations was investigated. In the INSPIRE study, 1323 patients were randomized to receive either SFC or tiotropium (TIO) for 2 years, but SFC arm failed to show superiority over TIO treatment, as the annual exacerbation rate was 1.28 in the SFC group and 1.32 in the TIO group (RR, 0.97; 95% CI: 0.84–1.12; $P = 0.66$) [69]. On the other hand, the nature of the exacerbations differed between the two groups in that a significantly higher rate of exacerbations treated with antibiotics was observed in the SFC than the TIO group (0.97 vs. 0.82; RR, 1.19; 95% CI: 1.02–1.38; $P = 0.028$), whereas SFC was better for exacerbation requiring systemic steroids (0.69 vs. 0.85; RR, 0.81; 95% CI: 0.67–0.99; $P = 0.039$). The plausible explanation for the higher exacerbations requiring antibiotics in the SFC group might be related to fluticasone-induced impairment of local immune resistance to lower respiratory infection. In addition, an increased exacerbation requiring steroids in the TIO group could have reflected the diminished beneficial effect of ICS among the ~50% of the TIO subjects who had previously received ICS prior to the trial [70].

In the POET-COPD study, once-daily TIO treatment was significantly associated with fewer exacerbations compared with twice-daily LABA, irrespective of the use of ICS [71]. It is not clear whether this reflects specific benefit of anti-inflammatory effect from blocking anti-muscarinic receptors.

Exacerbation results using newly developed ICS/LABA combinations have also been reported. Pooled data from two replicate 1-year trials of the once-daily new ICS/LABA formulation demonstrated that FF/VI (100/25 μg) significantly decreased the annual rate of moderate-to-severe exacerbations by 27% compared to vilanterol alone (Fig. 16.8) [72].

However, there were no differences in severe exacerbation rates between vilanterol alone and the various doses of the combination therapy. With regard to exacerbation, these studies suggest that addition of ICS to a 24-h LABA could further reduce exacerbation. Moreover, reduction of exacerbation was seen

Table 16.2 Yearly occurrence of exacerbation in propensity score-matched populations of COPD patients treated with budesonide/formoterol vs. fluticasone/salmeterol

Variable events, per patient-year	Fluticasone/salmeterol ($n = 2734$) Mean (95% CI)	Budesonide/formoterol ($n = 2734$) Mean (95% CI)	Treatment contrast Rate ratio (95% CI)	*P*-value
All exacerbations	1.09 (1.05–1.14)	0.80 (0.77–0.84)	0.74 (0.69–0.79)	<0.0001
COPD hospitalizations	0.21 (0.20–0.23)	0.15 (0.142–0.163)	0.71 (0.65–0.78)	<0.0001
COPD-related hospital stay, days	0.95 (0.88–1.02)	0.63 (0.58–0.67)	0.66 (0.62–0.71)	<0.0001
Emergency visits	0.034 (0.031–0.037)	0.027 (0.025–0.030)	0.79 (0.71–0.89)	0.0003
Oral steroid use	0.85 (0.81–0.90)	0.63 (0.60–0.67)	0.74 (0.68–0.81)	<0.0001
Antibiotic use	0.54 (0.52–0.57)	0.38 (0.37–0.40)	0.70 (0.66–0.75)	<0.0001

From Larsson et al. [66], reproduced with kind permission

even when ICS did not improve FEV_1, suggesting that the ICS effect may be mediated independent of lung function change [73]. In a post hoc analysis, patients with higher blood eosinophil count (≥ 2%) gained greater benefit from treatment with ICS (fluticasone furoate) to reduce exacerbation frequency than did those with a low eosinophil count [74], which provide evidence supporting the role of blood eosinophil counts as a biomarker with the potential to guide treatment decision in predicting potential benefit of ICS over bronchodilator in reducing exacerbations.

The other new ICS/LABA combination, BDP/FOR in the extra-fine formulation, has been demonstrated to be more effective, when compared with formoterol alone, in decreasing the yearly exacerbation rate (RR, 0.72; 95% CI: 0.62–0.84; $P < 0.001$), and prolonged the time to first exacerbation in patients with severe COPD with a history of exacerbation in the 48-week FORWARD (Foster 48-week trial to reduce exacerbation in COPD) study [75]. In a *post hoc* analysis on the FORWARD study, there was a pattern of increasing exacerbation frequency with increasing blood eosinophil count in patients treated with formoterol. There was a 46% reduction in adjusted exacerbation rate caused by BDP/FOR that was found in the highest eosinophil quartile (≥ 279.8 μl) [76].

In the LANTERN study, QVA149 showed a significantly reduced rate of moderate or severe exacerbation by 31% compared to SFC in patients with moderate-to-severe COPD and a history of up to one exacerbation in the previous year [61]. In the subgroup analysis, the annualized rate of all exacerbation was significantly lower with QVA149 vs. SFC (RR, 0.43; 95% CI: 0.25–0.76, $P = 0.003$). However, the annualized rate of moderate or severe exacerbations was not statistically different between QVA149 and SFC among patients with an exacerbation history (RR, 0.60; 95% CI: 0.33–1.08, $P = 0.086$).

Phase III FLAME head-to-head trial examining the rate of exacerbation between QVA149 and SFC during 52 weeks of treatment in 3362 patients with moderate-to-severe COPD and a history of exacerbations is also reported [77]. QVA149 was superior to SFC in reducing the annual rate of all COPD exacerbations by 11% (3.59 vs. 4.03; RR, 0.89; 95% CI: 0.83–0.96; $P = 0.003$) and moderate or severe exacerbations by 17% ($P < 0.001$). In this study, the effect of QVA149 in reducing the rate of COPD exacerbation was independent of the baseline blood eosinophil count. These findings provide evidence to support the use of LAMA/LABA regimen over the use of LABA plus ICS in preventing exacerbations in patients at high risk for COPD exacerbation (Table 16.3).

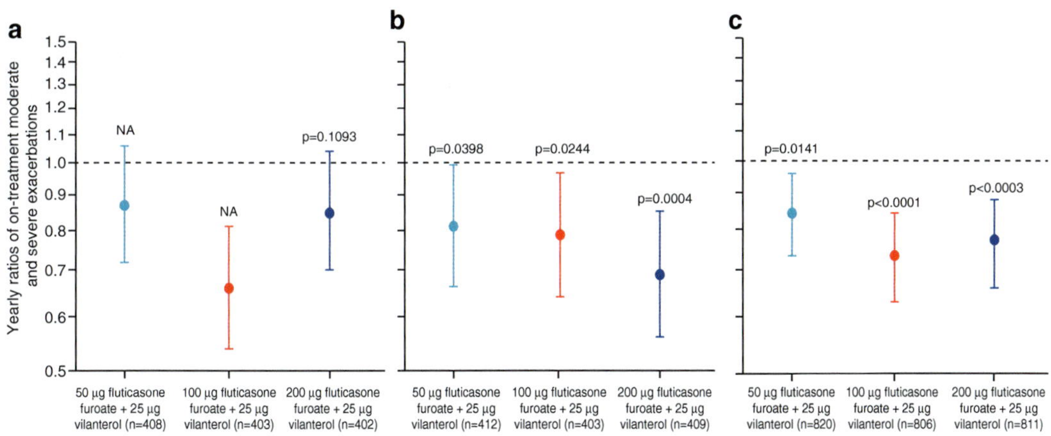

Fig. 16.8 Yearly ratio of moderate and severe exacerbations in the combined fluticasone furoate and vilanterol groups to moderate and severe exacerbations in the vilanterol-only group in study 1 (A), study 2 (B), and overall (C) (from Dransfield et al. [71], reproduced with kind permission)

Table 16.3 Effect of fixed-dose combination of ICS/LABA on the risk of COPD exacerbation (reproduced from Miravitlles et al. 2016 [78])

Treatment	Annual exacerbation rate	Comparator	Annual exacerbation rate	Reduction in exacerbation	Exacerbation endpoint	Patient population: Exacerbation entry (No./year)	Patient population: FEV_1% predicted
SFC [24]	0.85	Placebo salmeterol FP	1.13 0.97 0.93	25% 12% 9%	Secondary (moderate or severe)	NA	<60% (pre-BD)
SFC [48]	0.97	Placebo	1.30	25%	Secondary (moderate)	≥1	25–70% (pre-BD)
SFC [69]	1.28	Tiotropium	1.32	NS	Primary (moderate or severe)	NA	<50% (post-BD)
BUD/FOR [49]	1.38	Placebo Formoterol Budesonide	1.80 1.85 1.60	23.6% NS NS	Primary (all)	≥1	<50% (pre-BD)
BUD/FOR [65]	1.42	Placebo Formoterol Budesonide	1.87 1.84 1.59	24% 23% NS	Primary (severe)	≥1	<50%
FF/VI [72]	0.81	Vilanterol	1.11	30% (pooled data)	Primary (moderate or severe)	≥1	<70% (post-BD)
BDP/FOR [75]	0.80	Formoterol	1.12	28%	Primary (moderate or severe)	≥1	<50%
BDP/FOR [58]	0.41	Bud/Form Formoterol	0.42 0.43	NS	Primary	≥1	30–50% (post-BD)

Effect of ICS/LABA Combination on Quality of Life

TORCH trial reported an improvement of 3.0 units of the SGRQ in the SFC group, 1.8 units in the FP group, and 0.8 units in the SAL group. On the contrary, placebo group showed a deterioration of 0.2 units in the SGRQ [24]. Therefore, SFC improved SGRQ score by 2.2 units compared to SAL alone and by 3.2 units over the placebo group, which was below the MCID of 4 units. The greatest improvement compared to placebo was observed in those patients with more severe COPD—an improvement by 5.9 units in GOLD 4, and 3.3 units in GOLD 3. However, in less severe GOLD 2, the SGRQ improvement was less, but still significant (2.3 units) [18]. Compared with placebo, BUD/FOR also significantly improved SGRQ total score (mean difference, 3.9; $P = 0.009$) in a 12-month study. The review of the Cochrane Airways Group documented that ICS/LABA combination improved the health-related quality of life measured on the SGRQ compared with placebo or ICS, but the mean differences observed are relatively small in relation to the MCID [79, 80]. In addition, same group reported that ICS/LABA was more effective than LABA alone in improving SGRQ score (1.58 units lower with SFC; 2.69 units lower with BUD/FOR) [81].

Several studies reported the comparison results of health status between ICS/LABA combinations and fixed LAMA/LABA combinations. In the ILLUMINATE study, SGRQ-C total scores were not different between QVA149 and SFC groups, with both groups showing an improvement. Mean difference in SGRQ-C total score for QVA149 vs. SFC at week 26 was −1.24 ($p = 0.25$) [60]. Since the study population recruited was low-risk, non-exacerbating subjects, SGRQ-C scores might not have been significantly different. In the LANTERN study, recruiting patients

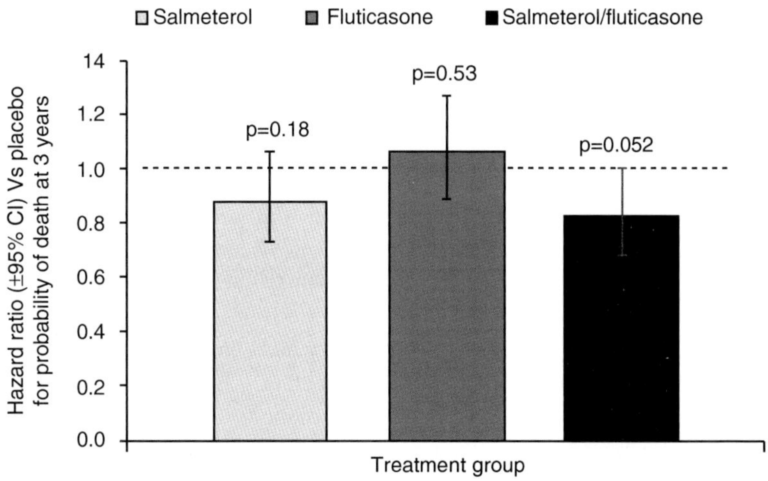

Fig. 16.9 Effects of therapy on mortality in the TORCH study (from Price et al. [64], reproduced with kind permission)

with a history of ≤1 exacerbation, there was also a similar improvement in the SGRQ total score between patients receiving QVA149 and SFC. However, the percentage of patients who achieved MCID was numerically higher with QVA149 vs. SFC [61].

The improvement in the SGRQ-C was greater in the QVA149 group than in the SFC group in the FLAME study [77]. The differences between the QVA149 group and the SFC group ranged from −1.2 points at week 12 to −1.8 points at week 52 ($P < 0.01$ for both comparisons). The percentage of patients who achieved MCID was significantly higher in the QVA149 group than in the SFC group (49.2% vs. 43.7%; odds ratio, 1.30; $P < 0.001$). Above results suggest that fixed LAMA/LABA combination therapy is similar or better than ICS/LABA treatment with regard to health-related quality of life in patients with COPD.

Effect of ICS/LABA Combination on Mortality

Although, the effect of ICS/LABA combination therapy on mortality has been studied for long times, but it is still a controversial issue.

The largest study specifically designed to investigate the effect of ICS with or without LABA on mortality over 3 years was TORCH trial. Although minimally decreased mortality was found with SFC compared to placebo (10.3 vs. 12.6%; HR 0.81; 95% CI: 0.67–0.98), SFC failed to reach statistical significance ($P = 0.052$) (Fig. 16.9) [24].

The addition of FP to SAL did not offer additional benefit over the LABA alone, but the HR for the SFC compared with FP was significant ($p = 0.007$), suggesting that the LABA might be conferring a protective effect [24, 64]. Two studies supported this finding that most of the beneficial effect of SFC on mortality is due to salmeterol [82, 83]. In their analyses, the salmeterol component was associated with a significant reduction in mortality, with a rate ratio of 0.83 (95% CI: 0.74–0.95) and hazard ratio of 0.81 (95% CI: 0.70–0.94). The fluticasone component had no effect on mortality (rate ratio and hazard ratio both 1.00). Rodrigo et al. also showed that ICS/LABA combination therapy did not decrease mortality (all-cause, respiratory, and cardiovascular) [52]. Another subsequent Cochrane meta-analysis suggested that all-cause mortality can be reduced with ICS/LABA combination therapy compared to placebo (OR 0.79; 95% CI: 0.65–0.98); however, it was not statistically different between ICS/LABA and LABA alone (OR 0.89; 95% CI: 0.73–1.08), suggesting a beneficial effect of LABA more than of ICS [84].

In a *post hoc* analysis of TORCH trial, treatment with SFC may be associated with reduced mortality compared with placebo in GOLD 2 patients (HR 0.67; 95% CI: 0.45–0.98; 11.4% of the patients died on placebo compared with 7.8% on SFC) [18]. A review by Zervas et al. has suggested that ICS/LABA combination might also reduce cardiovascular disease and all-cause mortality [25]. In addition, in a mixed treatment comparison meta-analysis that aimed to compare the risk of overall and cardiovascular death for inhaled medications in COPD patients, ICS/LABA was associated with the lowest risk of death among all treatments [85].

SUMMIT (study to understand mortality and morbidity in COPD) trial investigated whether new ICS/LABA formulation FF/VI can prolong survival in patients with COPD and history of, or increased risk for, cardiovascular disease [86]. The study aimed to show a mortality reduction of 30% with the FF/VI; however, mortality was 12.2% lower in the FF/VI group than in the placebo group (HR, 0.88; 95% CI: 0.74–1.04), and it did not reach statistical significance ($P = 0.137$) [87]. Based on these results of the SUMMIT study, although investigators claimed that a clinically meaningful difference in mortality has not been entirely excluded because the 95% CI for the HR encompasses a 26% reduction in the risk of dying, the uncertainty over the role of ICS in treating COPD continues. So far, there is no clear evidence that ICS delivered to the lungs has proven benefit in reducing cardiovascular or all-cause mortality.

In the INSPIRE study, SFC improved mortality compared to TIO (3% vs. 6% of patients during the 2-year study), although this was not a primary endpoint [69]. 2013 Cochrane Airway Group review reported that it was unable to conclude whether ICS/LABA or LAMA treatment had the lower mortality rate [88].

There is little available comparative information on mortality between ICS/LABA combination therapy and fixed LABA/LAMA combinations.

Triple-Inhaler Therapy (ICS + LABA + LAMA)

NICE guidelines in the UK recommend triple therapy in patients who remain breathless or have exacerbations despite maintenance therapy with LAMA or LABA + ICS irrespective of their FEV_1 [37]. GOLD recommends the triple therapy as first choice in group D patients [89]. Triple therapy might be useful in patients with severe to very severe COPD, particularly in those with high peripheral blood or sputum eosinophil count and asthma–COPD overlap syndrome (ACOS), or those who are frequent exacerbators [90]. However, it is often prescribed in real-life treatment of COPD, even in mild-to-moderate patients who are not suffering from severe COPD [91].

In patients with severe COPD in the Canadian OPTIMAL study, in which the primary endpoint was exacerbation requiring oral corticosteroids or antibiotics, it was found that the addition of SFC to tiotropium therapy compared to tiotropium alone was associated with significant improvements in lung function and disease-specific quality of life and a reduction in all-cause hospitalizations, but did not significantly influence the rates of COPD exacerbations [92].

In a 24-week randomized trial, 237 patients taking tiotropium plus SFC (250/50 ug twice daily) were compared to 242 taking tiotropium alone. The group taking triple-inhaler therapy had a significant improvement in pre-bronchodilator FEV_1 (L) and the total SGRQ-C score compared to the tiotropium-only group [93].

Although a recent meta-analysis has confirmed that the addition of SFC to subjects treated with tiotropium significantly improves lung function HRQoL, and exacerbation without increasing the risk of adverse events [94], the WISDOM trial has documented similar moderate or severe exacerbations between those who continued and discontinued ICS therapy in patients with severe COPD receiving tiotropium and salmeterol [95]. These findings show non-inferiority of dual-bronchodilator therapy as compared with triple therapy in reducing exacerbations in severe COPD patients.

Few data are available for the efficacy of single-inhaler triple therapy. New inhaled fixed drug combinations of ICS/LABA/LAMA, including fluticasone furoate/vilanterol/umeclidinium (FF/VI/UMEC), budesonide/formoterol/glycopyrronium (BUD/FOR/GB), and beclometasone/formoterol/glycopyrronium (BDP/FOR/GB), are in Phase III of clinical development for COPD [90].

The Trilogy study was the first large, long-term study aimed to compare the efficacy and safety of single-inhaler triple therapy comprising BDP/FOR/GB to that of BDP/FOR in patients with COPD who have severe or very severe air-flow limitation, symptoms, and an exacerbation history [96]. BDP/FOR/GB improved pre-dose FEV_1 by 0.081 (L) (95% CI: 0.052–0.109; $P < 0.001$) and 2-h post-dose FEV_1 by 0.117 (L) (0.086–0.147; $P < 0.001$) compared with BDP/FOR. This study also shows that a reduction of moderate-to-severe exacerbation can be achieved through triple therapy with the use of a single inhaler (RR, 0.77; 95% CI: 0.65–0.92; $P = 0.005$), corresponding to a 23% reduction in exacerbations compared with BDP/FOR.

It is still unclear when we should step up to or step down from triple therapy and whether there are potential phenotypes that would be more responsive to triple therapy. Future long-term studies should assess the efficacy and safety of triple ICS/LABA/LAMA therapy in selected COPD phenotypes.

Adverse Effects of ICS in COPD

Local and Systemic Side Effects

The frequent use of ICS as monotherapy, especially at higher doses, or in combination with long-acting bronchodilator has been accompanied by local and systemic adverse effects. Local side effects are most commonly seen in ICS treatment, including dysphonia and hoarseness, oropharyngeal candidiasis, perioral dermatitis, and cough during inhalation [97]. The incidence of these side effects ranges from 1 to 10%, and they occur in a minority of patients without major sequelae [21]. Although they are not usually serious, they may be more prone to affect the adherence of ICS therapy [98]. Compared with local side effects, systemic effects of ICS appear to be related with systemic absorption of ICS into the circulation through the pulmonary vasculature or GI tract [99]. Since a large proportion of COPD patients are elderly, high dose of ICS is commonly prescribed for prolonged period; thus they are more vulnerable to the increased risk of systemic side effects such as pneumonia [100].

Pneumonia

Increased risk of pneumonia associated with FDC containing ICS, particularly fluticasone, raised the major safety concerns in COPD [24, 101, 102]. TORCH was the first largest study that identified an increased risk of pneumonia in patients who were regularly treated with an ICS [24]. A greater rate of pneumonia was identified in the ICS and ICS/LABA treatment arms (84 and 88 per 1000 treatment-year, respectively) compared with LABA and placebo (52 and 52 per 1000 treatment-year, respectively). The Quebec health insurance database study including 163,514 patients, of which 20,344 had a serious pneumonia event during the 5.4 years of follow-up, showed that the risk of serious pneumonia was elevated with current use of ICS and sustained with long-term use but declined and disappeared after 6 months after discontinuation of ICS [102]. The risk for severe pneumonia with fluticasone was daily dose dependent and much higher (RR, 2.01; 95% CI: 1.93–2.10) than that with budesonide (RR, 1.17; 95% CI: 1.09–1.26). The INSPIRE study also reported double the rate of pneumonia with SFC (8%) than with tiotropium (4%) [69].

This finding of intra-class difference with regard to the risk of pneumonia between fluticasone- and budesonide-containing FDC of ICS/LABA was also documented in the PATHOS study [103]. Compared with BUD/FOR, rate of pneumonia was higher in patients treated with FP/SAL (RR 1.73; 95% CI 1.57–1.90; $P < 0.001$). The rate of admission to hospital was also significantly higher in the FP/SAL group (RR, 1.74; 95% CI: 1.56–1.94; $P < 0.001$, respectively). Moreover, mortality related to pneumonia was higher in the FP/SAL group (97 deaths) than in the BUD/FOR group (52 deaths) (HR, 1.76; 95% CI: 1.22–2.53; $P = 0.003$). A new once-daily ICS/LABA combination inhaler containing fluticasone furoate also found an excess of eight pneumonia deaths [72], seven received higher dose of ICS, suggesting that fluticasone itself may be associated with higher risk of any pneumonia.

Several mechanisms that link between ICS use and risk of developing pneumonia have been proposed. Impaired macrophage function, reduced bacterial adherence in the large airways, alteration of the pulmonary microbiome, and steroid-induced immune suppression may lead to increase in the probability of lower respiratory infection [64, 104].

These evidences suggest that it appears to be appropriate to limit the use of ICS to the specific subgroups of COPD patients who might benefit from ICS treatment.

Effect of ICS Withdrawal on Exacerbation and Pulmonary Function

In the GLUCOLD 5-year follow-up study (GL2) after 30-month treatment with fluticasone or fluticasone and salmeterol (GL1), patients using ICS during GL1, but only using ICS 0–50% of the time during GL2, had significantly accelerated annual FEV_1 decline compared with GL1 [105].

The WISDOM study was designed to investigate the effect of ICS withdrawal on exacerbation and pulmonary function [95]. 2485 patients were randomized to continued triple therapy or withdrawal of ICS in three steps over a 12-week period. Although exacerbation was similar among those who continued and discontinued ICS therapy, withdrawal of ICS was associated with mean reduction in trough FEV_1 over baseline at 18 weeks (−38 mL, $P < 0.001$) and at 52 weeks (−43 mL, $P = 0.001$) compared with ICS-continuation group.

In a post hoc analysis, moderate or severe exacerbation rate was higher in the ICS-withdrawal group vs. the ICS-continuation group in patients with high blood eosinophil counts [106]. 4% or greater or 300 cells per μL or more was significantly associated with a deleterious effect of ICS withdrawal.

Although these findings need to be confirmed in a prospective study, withdrawal of ICS can worsen lung function and should be conducted with caution in patients with higher blood eosinophil counts.

Phosphodiesterase-4 Inhibitor

Pharmacology

Roflumilast is a potent selective phosphodiesterase-4 (PDE4) inhibitor aimed to reduce the risk of COPD exacerbation in patients with severe COPD associated with chronic bronchitis and history of exacerbations [107]. Roflumilast inhibits the hydrolysis of cyclic adenosine monophosphate (cAMP) in inflammatory cells, which results in increased anti-inflammatory effects such as suppression of inflammatory mediators and cytokines (Fig. 16.10) [107–109].

Roflumilast is available in a once-daily oral dosage form (500 μg tablets). The absolute bioavailability of roflumilast following a 500 μg oral dose is 79%. The median time to reach maximum plasma concentrations of roflumilast (t_{max}) is 1 h, and the plasma half-life ranges from 8 to 31 h. Roflumilast is converted to roflumilast N-oxide (the major active metabolite of roflumilast), which is estimated to have about 90% of the total PDE4 inhibitory activity of roflumilast [110].

Clinical Efficacy of PDE4 Inhibitor in COPD

Pooled analysis of M2–111 and M2–112 studies of roflumilast showed significant reduction (14.3%) in moderate-to-severe exacerbation compared with placebo [111]. It showed that features associated with greater response to roflumilast were presence of chronic bronchitis with or without emphysema, elevated cough or sputum scores at baseline (≥1 average score per day), and concurrent use of ICS [111]. Subsequent M2–124 and M2–125 studies included patients with severe airflow limitation, chronic bronchitis symptoms, and a history of exacerbations. In these studies, roflumilast significantly reduced moderate or severe exacerbation (15% in M2–124 and 18% in M2–125) [112]. Concomitant administration of roflumilast and LABA reduced 20.7% of moderate-to-severe exacerbation compared with 14.6% reduction in patients taking roflumilast alone [113]. Treatment with roflumilast shifts patients from the frequent to the more stable infrequent exacerbator state. Pooled data from

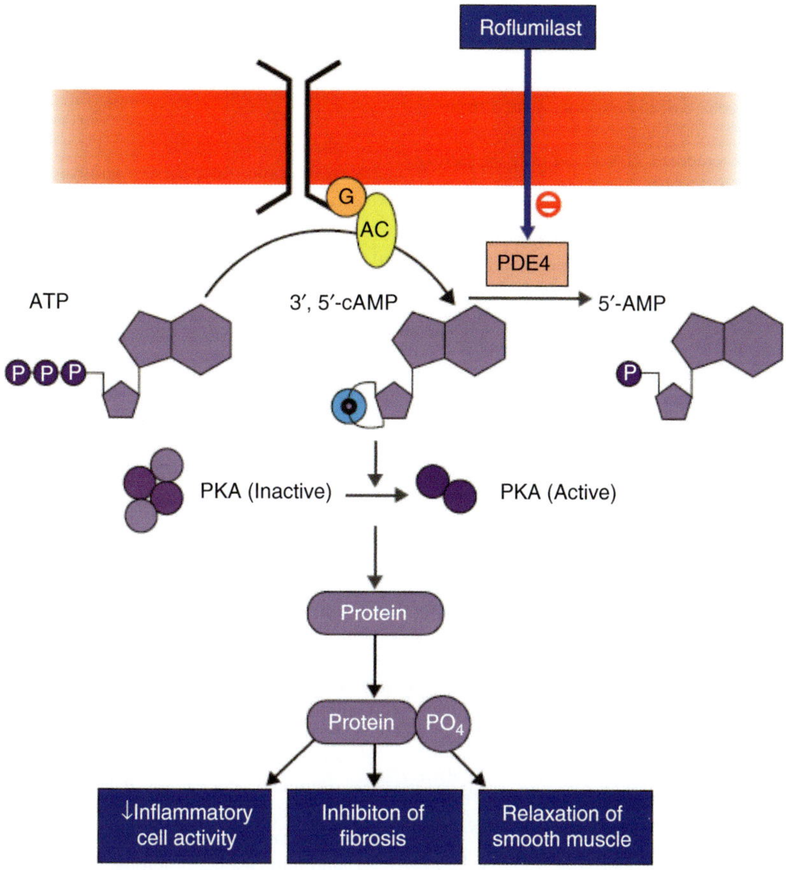

Fig. 16.10 Phosphodiesterase-4 inhibitors increase levels of cAMP through inhibition of its metabolism (from Klaus F. Rabe [109], reproduced with kind permission)

two M2–124 and M2–125 studies, among frequent exacerbators treated with roflumilast, show that 32.0% still had frequent exacerbations at year 1 compared with 40.8% of placebo-treated patients (risk ratio, 0.799; $P = 0.0148$) [114].

The REACT study, a Phase III/IV randomized, double-blind, multicenter study, aimed to investigate whether roflumilast further reduces exacerbations when added to ICS/LABA combination in patients with frequent exacerbations [115]. The rate of moderate-to-severe COPD exacerbations was 13.2% lower in the roflumilast group than in the placebo group in the Poisson regression analysis (RR, 0.868; 95% CI: 0.753–1.002; $P = 0.0529$) and was 14.2% lower in the negative binomial regression analysis (RR, 0.858; 95% CI: 0.740–0.995; $P = 0.0424$). Given this evidence, roflumilast, as part of a combination regimen with long-acting bronchodilators, appears to be a reasonable treatment option for patients with severe to very severe COPD associated with chronic bronchitis and a history of exacerbations [116].

Adverse Effects

In all clinical trials to date, roflumilast was generally considered safe and well tolerated. However, combining the data of roflumilast revealed that gastrointestinal adverse events, such as nausea, diarrhea, and weight loss, were the most common side effects [117]. The frequency and severity of gastrointestinal adverse events appeared to be dose dependent and up to 15% of the subjects are known to be intolerable to roflumilast treatment. Tentative ways to prevent initial adverse events include progressive increase of initial dosing, administration on alternate days, and symptomatic treatment particularly of diarrhea or headache [110].

References

1. Ito K, Chung KF, Adcock IM. Update on glucocorticoid action and resistance. J Allergy Clin Immunol. 2006;117:522–43.
2. Barnes PJ. Corticosteroid effects on cell signalling. Eur Respir J. 2006;27:413–26.
3. Adcock IM, Barnes PJ. Molecular mechanisms of corticosteroid resistance. Chest. 2008;134:394–401.
4. Ito K, Barnes PJ, Adcock IM. Glucocorticoid receptor recruitment of histone deacetylase 2 inhibits interleukin-1beta-induced histone H4 acetylation on lysines 8 and 12. Mol Cell Biol. 2000;20:6891–903.
5. Barnes PJ. New molecular targets for the treatment of neutrophilic diseases. J Allergy Clin Immunol. 2007;119:1055–62. quiz 63-4.
6. Jiang Z, Zhu L. Update on molecular mechanisms of corticosteroid resistance in chronic obstructive pulmonary disease. Pulm Pharmacol Ther. 2016;37:1–8.
7. Ito K, Ito M, Elliott WM, et al. Decreased histone deacetylase activity in chronic obstructive pulmonary disease. N Engl J Med. 2005;352:1967–76.
8. Barnes PJ. New anti-inflammatory targets for chronic obstructive pulmonary disease. Nat Rev Drug Discov. 2013;12:543–59.
9. Ito K, Yamamura S, Essilfie-Quaye S, et al. Histone deacetylase 2-mediated deacetylation of the glucocorticoid receptor enables NF-kappaB suppression. J Exp Med. 2006;203:7–13.
10. Vestbo J, Søorensen T, Lange P, Brix A, Torre P, Viskum K. Long-term effect of inhaled budesonide in mild and moderate chronic obstructive pulmonary disease: a randomised controlled trial. Lancet. 1999;353:1819–23.
11. Pauwels RA, Lofdahl CG, Laitinen LA, et al. Long-term treatment with inhaled budesonide in persons with mild chronic obstructive pulmonary disease who continue smoking. European Respiratory Society study on chronic obstructive pulmonary disease. N Engl J Med. 1999;340:1948–53.
12. Burge PS, Calverley PM, Jones PW, Spencer S, Anderson JA, Maslen TK. Randomised, double blind, placebo controlled study of fluticasone propionate in patients with moderate to severe chronic obstructive pulmonary disease: the ISOLDE trial. BMJ. 2000;320:1297–303.
13. Lung Health Study Research Group. Effect of inhaled triamcinolone on the decline in pulmonary function in chronic obstructive pulmonary disease. N Engl J Med. 2000;343:1902–9.
14. Sutherland ER, Allmers H, Ayas NT, Venn AJ, Martin RJ. Inhaled corticosteroids reduce the progression of airflow limitation in chronic obstructive pulmonary disease: a meta-analysis. Thorax. 2003;58:937–41.
15. Highland KB, Strange C, Heffner JE. Long-term effects of inhaled corticosteroids on FEV1 in patients with chronic obstructive pulmonary disease. A meta-analysis. Ann Intern Med. 2003;138:969–73.
16. Yang IA, Clarke MS, Sim EH, Fong KM. Inhaled corticosteroids for stable chronic obstructive pulmonary disease. Cochrane Database Syst Rev. 2012;7:CD002991.
17. Celli BR, Thomas NE, Anderson JA, et al. Effect of pharmacotherapy on rate of decline of lung function in chronic obstructive pulmonary disease: results from the TORCH study. Am J Respir Crit Care Med. 2008;178:332–8.
18. Jenkins CR, Jones PW, Calverley PM, et al. Efficacy of salmeterol/fluticasone propionate by GOLD stage of chronic obstructive pulmonary disease: analysis from the randomised, placebo-controlled TORCH study. Respir Res. 2009;10:59.
19. Lapperre TS, Snoeck-Stroband JB, Gosman MM, et al. Effect of fluticasone with and without salmeterol on pulmonary outcomes in chronic obstructive pulmonary disease: a randomized trial. Ann Intern Med. 2009;151:517–27.
20. Suissa S, Barnes PJ. Inhaled corticosteroids in COPD: the case against. Eur Respir J. 2009;34:13–6.
21. Telenga ED, Kerstjens HA, Postma DS, Ten Hacken NH, van den Berge M. Inhaled corticosteroids in chronic obstructive pulmonary disease: a review. Expert Opin Pharmacother. 2010;11:405–21.
22. Jones PW, Quirk FH, Baveystock CM. The St George's respiratory questionnaire. Respir Med. 1991;85(Suppl B):25–31. discussion 3-7.
23. Jones PW. Interpreting thresholds for a clinically significant change in health status in asthma and COPD. Eur Respir J. 2002;19:398–404.
24. Calverley PM, Anderson JA, Celli B, et al. Salmeterol and fluticasone propionate and survival in chronic obstructive pulmonary disease. N Engl J Med. 2007;356:775–89.
25. Zervas E, Samitas K, Gaga M, Beghe B, Fabbri LM. Inhaled corticosteroids in COPD: pros and cons. Curr Drug Targets. 2013;14:192–224.
26. Alsaeedi A, Sin DD, McAlister FA. The effects of inhaled corticosteroids in chronic obstructive pulmonary disease: a systematic review of randomized placebo-controlled trials. Am J Med. 2002;113:59–65.
27. Suissa S. Statistical treatment of exacerbations in therapeutic trials of chronic obstructive pulmonary disease. Am J Respir Crit Care Med. 2006;173:842–6.
28. Agarwal R, Aggarwal AN, Gupta D, Jindal SK. Inhaled corticosteroids vs placebo for preventing COPD exacerbations: a systematic review and metaregression of randomized controlled trials. Chest. 2010;137:318–25.
29. Sin DD, Wu L, Anderson JA, et al. Inhaled corticosteroids and mortality in chronic obstructive pulmonary disease. Thorax. 2005;60:992–7.
30. Macie C, Wooldrage K, Manfreda J, Anthonisen NR. Inhaled corticosteroids and mortality in COPD. Chest. 2006;130:640–6.

31. Lee TA, Pickard AS, Au DH, Bartle B, Weiss KB. Risk for death associated with medications for recently diagnosed chronic obstructive pulmonary disease. Ann Intern Med. 2008;149:380–90.
32. Lofdahl CG, Postma DS, Pride NB, Boe J, Thoren A. Possible protection by inhaled budesonide against ischaemic cardiac events in mild COPD. Eur Respir J. 2007;29:1115–9.
33. Drummond MB, Dasenbrook EC, Pitz MW, Murphy DJ, Fan E. Inhaled corticosteroids in patients with stable chronic obstructive pulmonary disease: a systematic review and meta-analysis. JAMA. 2008;300:2407–16.
34. Suissa S. Observational studies of inhaled corticosteroids in chronic obstructive pulmonary disease: misconstrued immortal time bias. Am J Respir Crit Care Med. 2006;173:464. author reply -5.
35. Loke YK, Kwok CS, Singh S. Risk of myocardial infarction and cardiovascular death associated with inhaled corticosteroids in COPD. Eur Respir J. 2010;35:1003–21.
36. Vestbo J, Hurd SS, Agusti AG, et al. Global strategy for the diagnosis, management, and prevention of chronic obstructive pulmonary disease: GOLD executive summary. Am J Respir Crit Care Med. 2013;187:347–65.
37. Gruffydd-Jones K, Loveridge C. The 2010 NICE COPD guidelines: how do they compare with the GOLD guidelines? Prim Care Respir J. 2011;20:199–204.
38. Barnes PJ. Scientific rationale for inhaled combination therapy with long-acting beta2-agonists and corticosteroids. Eur Respir J. 2002;19:182–91.
39. Newton R, Leigh R, Giembycz MA. Pharmacological strategies for improving the efficacy and therapeutic ratio of glucocorticoids in inflammatory lung diseases. Pharmacol Ther. 2010;125:286–327.
40. Barnes PJ. Inhaled corticosteroids. Pharmaceuticals (Basel). 2010;3:514–40.
41. Pelaia G, Muzzio CC, Vatrella A, Maselli R, Magnoni MS, Rizzi A. Pharmacological basis and scientific rationale underlying the targeted use of inhaled corticosteroid/long-acting beta2-adrenergic agonist combinations in chronic obstructive pulmonary disease treatment. Expert Opin Pharmacother. 2015;16:2009–21.
42. Sin DD, Man SF. Corticosteroids and adrenoceptor agonists: the compliments for combination therapy in chronic airways diseases. Eur J Pharmacol. 2006;533:28–35.
43. Usmani OS, Ito K, Maneechotesuwan K, et al. Glucocorticoid receptor nuclear translocation in airway cells after inhaled combination therapy. Am J Respir Crit Care Med. 2005;172:704–12.
44. Mak JC, Nishikawa M, Barnes PJ. Glucocorticosteroids increase beta 2-adrenergic receptor transcription in human lung. Am J Phys. 1995;268:L41–6.
45. Mak JC, Nishikawa M, Shirasaki H, Miyayasu K, Barnes PJ. Protective effects of a glucocorticoid on downregulation of pulmonary beta 2-adrenergic receptors in vivo. J Clin Invest. 1995;96:99–106.
46. Sin DD, Man SF, Marciniuk DD, et al. The effects of fluticasone with or without salmeterol on systemic biomarkers of inflammation in chronic obstructive pulmonary disease. Am J Respir Crit Care Med. 2008;177:1207–14.
47. Mahler DA, Wire P, Horstman D, et al. Effectiveness of fluticasone propionate and salmeterol combination delivered via the Diskus device in the treatment of chronic obstructive pulmonary disease. Am J Respir Crit Care Med. 2002;166:1084–91.
48. Calverley P, Pauwels R, Vestbo J, et al. Combined salmeterol and fluticasone in the treatment of chronic obstructive pulmonary disease: a randomised controlled trial. Lancet. 2003;361:449–56.
49. Calverley PM, Boonsawat W, Cseke Z, Zhong N, Peterson S, Olsson H. Maintenance therapy with budesonide and formoterol in chronic obstructive pulmonary disease. Eur Respir J. 2003;22:912–9.
50. Ernst P, Saad N, Suissa S. Inhaled corticosteroids in COPD: the clinical evidence. Eur Respir J. 2015;45:525–37.
51. Vestbo J, Anderson JA, Calverley PM, et al. Bias due to withdrawal in long-term randomised trials in COPD: evidence from the TORCH study. Clin Respir J. 2011;5:44–9.
52. Rodrigo GJ, Castro-Rodriguez JA, Plaza V. Safety and efficacy of combined long-acting beta-agonists and inhaled corticosteroids vs long-acting beta-agonists monotherapy for stable COPD: a systematic review. Chest. 2009;136:1029–38.
53. Kew KM, Dias S, Cates CJ. Long-acting inhaled therapy (beta-agonists, anticholinergics and steroids) for COPD: a network meta-analysis. Cochrane Database Syst Rev. 2014;3:CD010844.
54. Bateman ED, Mahler DA, Vogelmeier CF, Wedzicha JA, Patalano F, Banerji D. Recent advances in COPD disease management with fixed-dose long-acting combination therapies. Expert Rev Respir Med. 2014;8:357–79.
55. Kerwin EM, Scott-Wilson C, Sanford L, et al. A randomised trial of fluticasone furoate/vilanterol (50/25 mug; 100/25 mug) on lung function in COPD. Respir Med. 2013;107:560–9.
56. Martinez FJ, Boscia J, Feldman G, et al. Fluticasone furoate/vilanterol (100/25; 200/25 mug) improves lung function in COPD: a randomised trial. Respir Med. 2013;107:550–9.
57. Agusti A, de Teresa L, De Backer W, et al. A comparison of the efficacy and safety of once-daily fluticasone furoate/vilanterol with twice-daily fluticasone propionate/salmeterol in moderate to very severe COPD. Eur Respir J. 2014;43:763–72.
58. Calverley PM, Kuna P, Monso E, et al. Beclomethasone/formoterol in the management of COPD: a randomised controlled trial. Respir Med. 2010;104:1858–68.
59. Tashkin DP, Doherty DE, Kerwin E, et al. Efficacy and safety characteristics of mometasone furoate/formoterol fumarate fixed-dose combination in subjects

with moderate to very severe COPD: findings from pooled analysis of two randomized, 52-week placebo-controlled trials. Int J Chron Obstruct Pulmon Dis. 2012;7:73–86.
60. Vogelmeier CF, Bateman ED, Pallante J, et al. Efficacy and safety of once-daily QVA149 compared with twice-daily salmeterol-fluticasone in patients with chronic obstructive pulmonary disease (ILLUMINATE): a randomised, double-blind, parallel group study. Lancet Respir Med. 2013;1:51–60.
61. Zhong N, Wang C, Zhou X, et al. LANTERN: a randomized study of QVA149 versus salmeterol/fluticasone combination in patients with COPD. Int J Chron Obstruct Pulmon Dis. 2015;10:1015–26.
62. Donohue JF, Worsley S, Zhu CQ, Hardaker L, Church A. Improvements in lung function with umeclidinium/vilanterol versus fluticasone propionate/salmeterol in patients with moderate-to-severe COPD and infrequent exacerbations. Respir Med. 2015;109:870–81.
63. Hanania NA, Darken P, Horstman D, et al. The efficacy and safety of fluticasone propionate (250 microg)/salmeterol (50 microg) combined in the Diskus inhaler for the treatment of COPD. Chest. 2003;124:834–43.
64. Price D, Yawn B, Brusselle G, Rossi A. Risk-to-benefit ratio of inhaled corticosteroids in patients with COPD. Prim Care Respir J. 2013;22:92–100.
65. Szafranski W, Cukier A, Ramirez A, et al. Efficacy and safety of budesonide/formoterol in the management of chronic obstructive pulmonary disease. Eur Respir J. 2003;21:74–81.
66. Blais L, Forget A, Ramachandran S. Relative effectiveness of budesonide/formoterol and fluticasone propionate/salmeterol in a 1-year, population-based, matched cohort study of patients with chronic obstructive pulmonary disease (COPD): effect on COPD-related exacerbations, emergency department visits and hospitalizations, medication utilization, and treatment adherence. Clin Ther. 2010;32:1320–8.
67. Larsson K, Janson C, Lisspers K, et al. Combination of budesonide/formoterol more effective than fluticasone/salmeterol in preventing exacerbations in chronic obstructive pulmonary disease: the PATHOS study. J Intern Med. 2013;273:584–94.
68. Welte T, Miravitlles M, Hernandez P, et al. Efficacy and tolerability of budesonide/formoterol added to tiotropium in patients with chronic obstructive pulmonary disease. Am J Respir Crit Care Med. 2009;180:741–50.
69. Wedzicha JA, Calverley PM, Seemungal TA, et al. The prevention of chronic obstructive pulmonary disease exacerbations by salmeterol/fluticasone propionate or tiotropium bromide. Am J Respir Crit Care Med. 2008;177:19–26.
70. Tashkin DP. Preventing and managing exacerbations in COPD—critical appraisal of the role of tiotropium. Int J Chron Obstruct Pulmon Dis. 2010;5:41–53.
71. Vogelmeier C, Hederer B, Glaab T, et al. Tiotropium versus salmeterol for the prevention of exacerbations of COPD. N Engl J Med. 2011;364:1093–103.
72. Dransfield MT, Bourbeau J, Jones PW, et al. Once-daily inhaled fluticasone furoate and vilanterol versus vilanterol only for prevention of exacerbations of COPD: two replicate double-blind, parallel-group, randomised controlled trials. Lancet Respir Med. 2013;1:210–23.
73. De Soyza A, Calverley PM. Large trials, new knowledge: the changing face of COPD management. Eur Respir J. 2015;45:1692–703.
74. Pascoe S, Locantore N, Dransfield MT, Barnes NC, Pavord ID. Blood eosinophil counts, exacerbations, and response to the addition of inhaled fluticasone furoate to vilanterol in patients with chronic obstructive pulmonary disease: a secondary analysis of data from two parallel randomised controlled trials. Lancet Respir Med. 2015;3:435–42.
75. Wedzicha JA, Singh D, Vestbo J, et al. Extrafine beclomethasone/formoterol in severe COPD patients with history of exacerbations. Respir Med. 2014;108:1153–62.
76. Siddiqui SH, Guasconi A, Vestbo J, et al. Blood eosinophils: a biomarker of response to extrafine beclomethasone/formoterol in chronic obstructive pulmonary disease. Am J Respir Crit Care Med. 2015;192:523–5.
77. Wedzicha JA, Banerji D, Chapman KR, et al. Indacaterol-Glycopyrronium versus salmeterol-fluticasone for COPD. N Engl J Med. 2016;374:2222–34.
78. Miravitlles M, D'Urzo A, Singh D, Koblizek V. Pharmacological strategies to reduce exacerbation risk in COPD: a narrative review. Respir Res. 2016;17:112.
79. Nannini LJ, Poole P, Milan SJ, Holmes R, Normansell R. Combined corticosteroid and long-acting beta(2)-agonist in one inhaler versus placebo for chronic obstructive pulmonary disease. Cochrane Database Syst Rev. 2013;11:CD003794.
80. Nannini LJ, Poole P, Milan SJ, Kesterton A. Combined corticosteroid and long-acting beta(2)-agonist in one inhaler versus inhaled corticosteroids alone for chronic obstructive pulmonary disease. Cochrane Database Syst Rev. 2013;8:CD006826.
81. Nannini LJ, Lasserson TJ, Poole P. Combined corticosteroid and long-acting beta(2)-agonist in one inhaler versus long-acting beta(2)-agonists for chronic obstructive pulmonary disease. Cochrane Database Syst Rev. 2012;9:CD006829.
82. La Vecchia C, Fabbri LM. Prevention of death in COPD. N Engl J Med. 2007;356:2211–2. author reply 3-4.
83. Suissa S, Ernst P, Vandemheen KL, Aaron SD. Methodological issues in therapeutic trials of COPD. Eur Respir J. 2008;31:927–33.
84. Nannini LJ, Cates CJ, Lasserson TJ, Poole P. Combined corticosteroid and long-acting beta-agonist in one inhaler versus long-acting beta-agonists for chronic obstructive pulmonary disease. Cochrane Database Syst Rev. 2007:CD006829.

85. Dong YH, Lin HH, Shau WY, Wu YC, Chang CH, Lai MS. Comparative safety of inhaled medications in patients with chronic obstructive pulmonary disease: systematic review and mixed treatment comparison meta-analysis of randomised controlled trials. Thorax. 2013;68:48–56.
86. Vestbo J, Anderson J, Brook RD, et al. The study to understand mortality and morbidity in COPD (SUMMIT) study protocol. Eur Respir J. 2013;41:1017–22.
87. Vestbo J, Anderson JA, Brook RD, et al. Fluticasone furoate and vilanterol and survival in chronic obstructive pulmonary disease with heightened cardiovascular risk (SUMMIT): a double-blind randomised controlled trial. Lancet. 2016;387:1817–26.
88. Welsh EJ, Cates CJ, Poole P. Combination inhaled steroid and long-acting beta2-agonist versus tiotropium for chronic obstructive pulmonary disease. Cochrane Database Syst Rev. 2013;5:CD007891.
89. Global Initiative for Chronic Obstructive Lung Disease (GOLD). Global strategy for the diagnosis, management, and prevention of COPD. 2016. www.goldcopd.org. Accessed 21 Jan 2016.
90. Montuschi P, Malerba M, Macis G, Mores N, Santini G. Triple inhaled therapy for chronic obstructive pulmonary disease. Drug Discov Today. 2016;21:1820–7.
91. James GD, Donaldson GC, Wedzicha JA, Nazareth I. Trends in management and outcomes of COPD patients in primary care, 2000-2009: a retrospective cohort study. NPJ Prim Care Respir Med. 2014;24:14015.
92. Aaron SD, Vandemheen KL, Fergusson D, et al. Tiotropium in combination with placebo, salmeterol, or fluticasone-salmeterol for treatment of chronic obstructive pulmonary disease: a randomized trial. Ann Intern Med. 2007;146:545–55.
93. Jung KS, Park HY, Park SY, et al. Comparison of tiotropium plus fluticasone propionate/salmeterol with tiotropium in COPD: a randomized controlled study. Respir Med. 2012;106:382–9.
94. Liu Y, Shi H, Sun X, et al. Benefits of adding fluticasone propionate/salmeterol to tiotropium in COPD: a meta-analysis. Eur J Intern Med. 2014;25:491–5.
95. Magnussen H, Disse B, Rodriguez-Roisin R, et al. Withdrawal of inhaled glucocorticoids and exacerbations of COPD. N Engl J Med. 2014;371:1285–94.
96. Singh D, Papi A, Corradi M, et al. Single inhaler triple therapy versus inhaled corticosteroid plus long-acting beta2-agonist therapy for chronic obstructive pulmonary disease (TRILOGY): a double-blind, parallel group, randomised controlled trial. Lancet. 2016;388:963–73.
97. Roland NJ, Bhalla RK, Earis J. The local side effects of inhaled corticosteroids: current understanding and review of the literature. Chest. 2004;126:213–9.
98. Irwin RS, Richardson ND. Side effects with inhaled corticosteroids: the physician's perception. Chest. 2006;130:41S–53S.
99. Tattersfield AE, Harrison TW, Hubbard RB, Mortimer K. Safety of inhaled corticosteroids. Proc Am Thorac Soc. 2004;1:171–5.
100. Babu KS, Kastelik JA, Morjaria JB. Inhaled corticosteroids in chronic obstructive pulmonary disease: a pro-con perspective. Br J Clin Pharmacol. 2014;78:282–300.
101. Crim C, Dransfield MT, Bourbeau J, et al. Pneumonia risk with inhaled fluticasone furoate and vilanterol compared with vilanterol alone in patients with COPD. Ann Am Thorac Soc. 2015;12:27–34.
102. Suissa S, Patenaude V, Lapi F, Ernst P. Inhaled corticosteroids in COPD and the risk of serious pneumonia. Thorax. 2013;68:1029–36.
103. Janson C, Larsson K, Lisspers KH, et al. Pneumonia and pneumonia related mortality in patients with COPD treated with fixed combinations of inhaled corticosteroid and long acting beta2 agonist: observational matched cohort study (PATHOS). BMJ. 2013;346:f3306.
104. Finney L, Berry M, Singanayagam A, Elkin SL, Johnston SL, Mallia P. Inhaled corticosteroids and pneumonia in chronic obstructive pulmonary disease. Lancet Respir Med. 2014;2:919–32.
105. Kunz LI, Postma DS, Klooster K, et al. Relapse in FEV1 decline after steroid withdrawal in COPD. Chest. 2015;148:389–96.
106. Watz H, Tetzlaff K, Wouters EF, et al. Blood eosinophil count and exacerbations in severe chronic obstructive pulmonary disease after withdrawal of inhaled corticosteroids: a post-hoc analysis of the WISDOM trial. Lancet Respir Med. 2016;4:390–8.
107. Hatzelmann A, Morcillo EJ, Lungarella G, et al. The preclinical pharmacology of roflumilast—a selective, oral phosphodiesterase 4 inhibitor in development for chronic obstructive pulmonary disease. Pulm Pharmacol Ther. 2010;23:235–56.
108. Sanz MJ, Cortijo J, Morcillo EJ. PDE4 inhibitors as new anti-inflammatory drugs: effects on cell trafficking and cell adhesion molecules expression. Pharmacol Ther. 2005;106:269–97.
109. Rabe KF. Update on roflumilast, a phosphodiesterase 4 inhibitor for the treatment of chronic obstructive pulmonary disease. Br J Pharmacol. 2011;163:53–67.
110. Beghe B, Rabe KF, Fabbri LM. Phosphodiesterase-4 inhibitor therapy for lung diseases. Am J Respir Crit Care Med. 2013;188:271–8.
111. Rennard SI, Calverley PM, Goehring UM, Bredenbroker D, Martinez FJ. Reduction of exacerbations by the PDE4 inhibitor roflumilast—the importance of defining different subsets of patients with COPD. Respir Res. 2011;12:18.
112. Calverley PM, Rabe KF, Goehring UM, et al. Roflumilast in symptomatic chronic obstructive pulmonary disease: two randomised clinical trials. Lancet. 2009;374:685–94.

113. Bateman ED, Rabe KF, Calverley PM, et al. Roflumilast with long-acting beta2-agonists for COPD: influence of exacerbation history. Eur Respir J. 2011;38:553–60.
114. Wedzicha JA, Rabe KF, Martinez FJ, et al. Efficacy of roflumilast in the COPD frequent exacerbator phenotype. Chest. 2013;143:1302–11.
115. Martinez FJ, Calverley PM, Goehring UM, Brose M, Fabbri LM, Rabe KF. Effect of roflumilast on exacerbations in patients with severe chronic obstructive pulmonary disease uncontrolled by combination therapy (REACT): a multicentre randomised controlled trial. Lancet. 2015;385:857–66.
116. Wedzicha JA, Calverley PM, Rabe KF. Roflumilast: a review of its use in the treatment of COPD. Int J Chron Obstruct Pulmon Dis. 2016;11:81–90.
117. Michalski JM, Golden G, Ikari J, Rennard SI. PDE4: a novel target in the treatment of chronic obstructive pulmonary disease. Clin Pharmacol Ther. 2012;91:134–42.

Non-pharmacologic Management: LVR, Rehabilitation, and Nutrition

17

Sei Won Lee and Eun Mi Kim

Non-pharmacologic Management

Lung Volume Reduction in Severe Emphysema

Chronic obstructive pulmonary disease (COPD) is characterized by chronic airflow limitation that is caused by a mixture of small-airway disease and parenchymal destruction [1]. Lung parenchyma destruction, also known as emphysema, results in decreased elastic recoil, progressive hyperinflation, and air trapping, which in turn lead to dyspnea and decreased lung function. Currently, bronchodilators are the mainstay of COPD pharmacologic treatment. Although they can improve dyspnea and lung function, the degree of improvement has some limitation. Furthermore, bronchodilators are also less effective in emphysema-dominant phenotype [2].

Due to this limitation, a large number of patients with advanced emphysema have respiratory symptom and deteriorate despite appropriate medication. For the management of these patients, more invasive approaches including lung transplantation or lung volume reduction surgery (LVRS) can be suggested. Bronchoscopic lung volume reduction (BLVR) has been introduced lately and offered a new dimension to treatment modalities in COPD.

Lung volume reduction (LVR) has definite evidence in COPD. However, it can be applied in limited number of emphysema-dominant phenotype; it has no role in treatment of non-emphysematous COPD and no studies or trials have been done in this group. Therefore, it is important in personalized medicine in COPD to understand who the best candidate of this treatment is. BLVR has also various modalities to be applied and physician should decide the best option according to the clinical and radiographic characteristics. In this chapter, we will discuss current evidences and limitation of these treatments and its application in real practice.

Lung Volume Reduction Surgery

Historical Background

Excision and decompression of space occupying avascular bullae had been reported to relieve dyspnea and exercise tolerance significantly in patients with COPD. This surgery has been accepted and indicated when relatively normal underlying lung compressed by the bullae is

S.W. Lee, M.D. (✉)
Department of Pulmonary and Critical Care Medicine, Asan Medical Center, University of Ulsan College of Medicine, Ulsan, South Korea
e-mail: iseiwon@gmail.com

E.M. Kim, Ph.D.
Department of Dietetics, Kangbuk Samsung Hospital, Seoul, South Korea
e-mail: emkim82@gmail.com

S.-D. Lee (ed.), *COPD*, DOI 10.1007/978-3-662-47178-4_17

identified. This treatment became the basis for the current LVR.In 1950s, Dr. Otto C. Brantigan introduced different concept of pulmonary resection in patients with diffuse emphysema. He hypothesized that excision of the most destroyed portions of the lung could reduce airflow limitation by improvement of elastic recoil and mechanic of respiration [3, 4]. Significant clinical improvement was notified in 75% of patients, and this improvement continued for more than 5 years in some patients. However, high mortality rate (16% early mortality) and morbidity limit the wide acceptance of this procedure.Dr. Joel D. Cooper reintroduced this procedure with improved results in 1990s [5]. The lung function and hyperinflation showed marked improvement; FEV_1 increased by 51% and RV decreased by 28%. The improvements in measured pulmonary function were paralleled by a significant reduction in dyspnea and an improvement in the quality of life. Reevaluation at 1 and 2 years after operation showed the benefit to be well maintained. Furthermore, the mortality was reduced markedly to 4%. This report became an important suggestion for LVRS as the palliative treatment for severe emphysema and followed by several small group studies for LVRS. However, the effectiveness and safety were not certain and had not been determined by randomized trials. Therefore, the pivotal study, National Emphysema Treatment Trial (NETT) was designed and performed [6].

Clinical Evidences

NETT was the first multicenter trial including 1218 patients. The study design was open-label randomized comparing LVRS and medical therapy and aimed two main objectives: (1) to determine effectiveness and safety of LVRS in the treatment of emphysema, (2) to identify the characteristics which make difference in harm and risk by LVRS. The main contribution of this study in this field is to clarify the main population who get benefit from this procedure.

1. Effectiveness
   Changes in exercise capacity, distance walked in 6 min, percentage of the predicted value for FEV_1, quality of life, and degree of dyspnea at 6, 12, and 24 months all favored the surgery group.
2. Mortality
   In whole study period (29 months), total mortality was the same between LVRS and medical group. In the first 3 months, mortality was higher in surgery group (7.9% vs. 1.3%, $P < 0.001$). However, among patients with predominantly upper-lobe emphysema and lower exercise capacity, mortality was lower in patients with LVRS than those with medical therapy (18.7% vs. 33.8%, $P = 0.005$). Meanwhile, LVRS showed significant higher mortality in patients with predominantly non-upper lobe emphysema and high exercise capacity. In other group, LVRS did not make significant in overall mortality compared with medical therapy.
3. Complication
   After LVRS, 90% of patients developed an air leak with a median duration of 7 days, and 3.3% of total patients undertook reoperation for this problem. Sixty percent developed one or more postoperative problems including pneumonia (18.2%), reintubation (21.8%), arrhythmia (18.6%), tracheostomy (8.2%), and failure to wean (8.0%). Hospitalization of more than 30 days after LVRS reached to 28%.

This study showed that survival and clinical benefit of LVRS over medical therapy in selected population. However, relatively high mortality (7.9%) within 3 months and high complication rates became the main handicap for wide performance of LVRS in real practice. Unfortunately, there is no additional pivotal study which could develop LVRS after NETT, and the LVR technique had shifted to noninvasive bronchoscopy-assisted method. Currently, LVRS was performed in only limited cases.

Summary and Application in Personalized Medicine

The only individual baseline factors associated with differences in mortality favoring LVRS were upper lobe predominant emphysema and low baseline exercise capacity. The only individual baseline factor associated with differential improvement in the maximal workload at 24 months was the upper lobe predominant emphysema.Considering these factors and high complication rates, LVRS can be justified in limited cases when:

- Emphysema is upper-lobe predominant
- BLVR was not indicated due to incomplete fissure or unavailability
- Severe respiratory symptom despite all medical therapy available

Bronchoscopic Lung Volume Reduction (BLVR)

1. Why BLVR?
   LVRS can reduce hyperinflation and expand healthier lung by surgical removal of emphysematous portion. It can improve lung function and exercise capacity and even can improve long-term survival in selected emphysema. For these benefits, it is established as the palliative therapy for selective patients with emphysema. However, it is also associated with relevant postoperational morbidity and mortality, which cannot be negligible in real practice. It is not easy for patients to accept surgery with >50% of postoperative complication and 8% mortality within 3 months after surgery [6] although the complications seem to reduce nowadays.
2. Evidences and Techniques
   BLVR techniques include endobronchial valves (EBV), bronchoscopic thermal vapor ablation (BTVA), lung volume reduction coils (LVRC), and polymeric lung volume reduction. At this moment, EBV has the most efficacious and the largest amount of evidence. Basic principle is to reduce lung volume of the most diseased lobe and increase airway caliber in relatively healthier lung. Unfortunately, this treatment cannot be applied to emphysema with interlobar flow or without heterogeneity. To overcome this limitation, other treatment options are being developed, but they are still only available under clinical trials.

Endobronchial Valve (EBV)

Endobronchial valves are the check valve devices to allow airflow in only one way. After deployed, they allow air and secretion to come out, but block air reentry. Accordingly, the emphysematous lobe reduces in its volume and become excluded for ventilation. The Zephyr® EBVs is a polymer duck-bill valve mounted inside a stainless steel cylinder attached to a nitinol self-expanding retainer. It can be inserted with guidance of bronchoscopy and two sizes (4.0 for bronchus with 4–7 mm lumen diameter and 5.5 for 5.5–8.5) are available (Fig. 17.1).

After several studies with small population, a large randomized multicenter, Endobronchial Valve for Emphysema Palliation (VENT) trial made the important progress. This study showed BLVR with EBV had significant clinical efficacy in lung function and exercise capacity without a significant increase of complication. Functional improvements were relatively small in this study; 4.3% in FEV1 and 2.5% in 6-min walking distance (6MWD). Meanwhile, this study found parameters for response including complete fissure (lobar exclusion of target lobe) and heterogeneity of emphysema [7]. Following studies confirmed the importance of complete fissure and collateral ventilation. Patients with complete fissure on CT can have greater improvement (26% in FEV1 and 22% in 6MWD) and those with incomplete fissure can have only small or insignificant improvements [8]. Chartis™ is developed to measure collateral ventilation through incomplete fissure, and it showed role in the prediction of target lobe volume reduction (TLVR) [9]. Successful BLVR may have survival benefit, supported by indirect evidences [10–12] (Fig. 17.2).

Biological Bronchoscopic Lung Volume Reduction (Bio-BLVR)

Sealant is the most promising among bio-LVR material until now. The principle involves instillation of biologically active agents (chondroitin sulfate, polylysine-fibrin glue, and

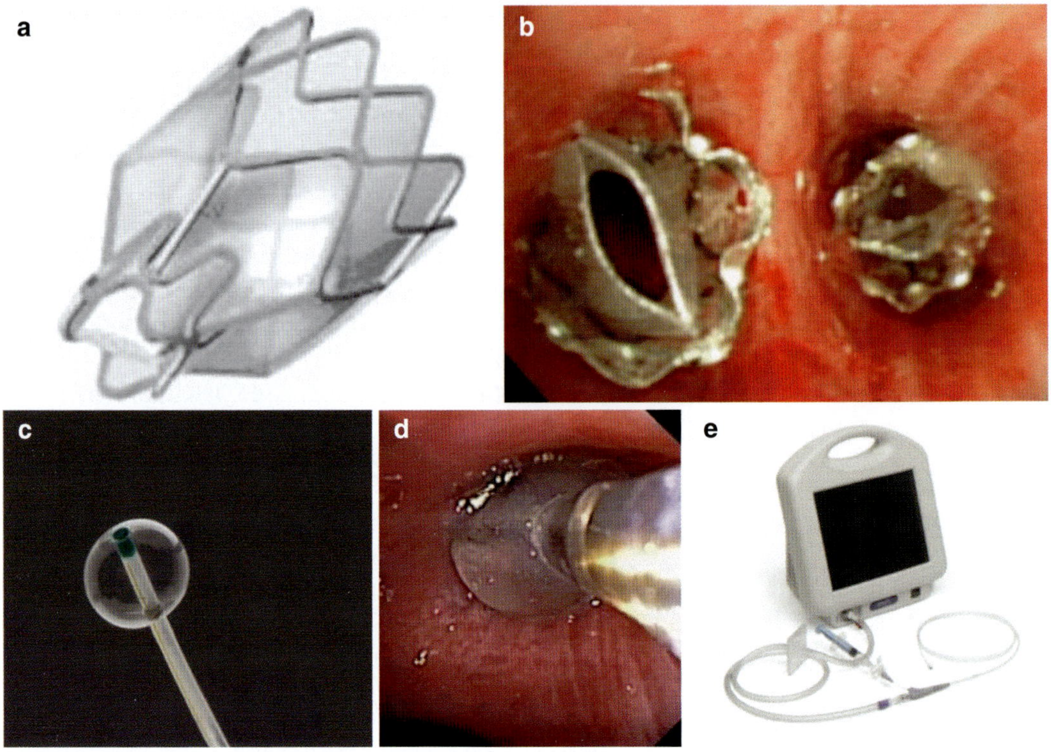

Fig. 17.1 Devices for EBV. (**a**) Zephyr® EBV (**b**) EBV inserted in bronchus. The mouth of EBV opens in expiration, whereas it closes in inspiration. (**c**) The tip of Chartis™ catheter. (**d**) Chartis™ is blocking the target lobe bronchus about collateral ventilation. (**e**) The Chartis™ system

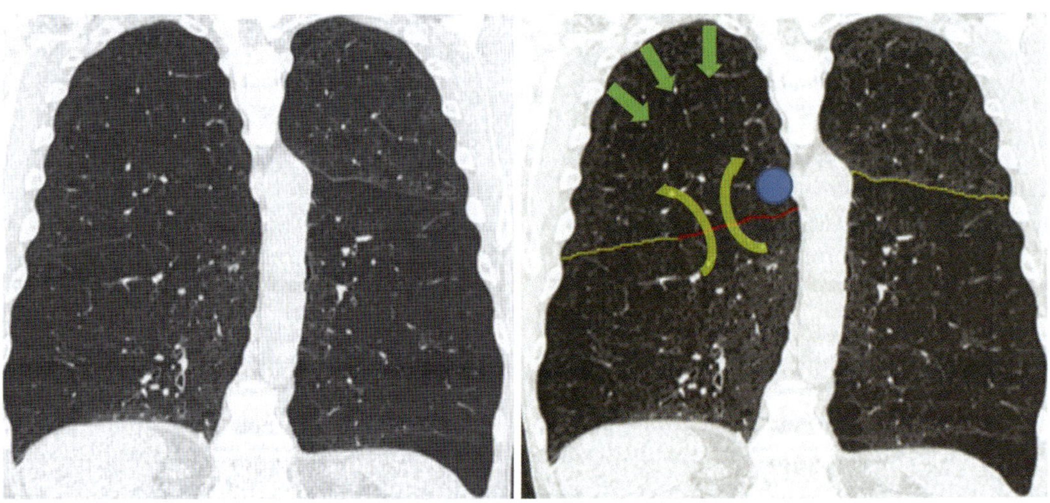

Fig. 17.2 Complete and incomplete fissure. Right major fissure has some incomplete portion (*red line*); if target lobe is right upper lobe, target lobe volume reduction may not be achieved after EBV insertion (*blue circle*) because airflow can enter into target lobe via incomplete portion. Meanwhile, left major is almost complete (*yellow line*)

thrombin solution), which contracts diseased emphysematous lung by formation of organized scar. Recent randomized trials showed significant improvement in FEV_1 (52.4 mL from baseline at 6 months) and exercise capacity (52.4 m from baseline at 6 months). Despite this effect, relatively large number of complication (15/61 cases of pneumonia, 12/61 cases of COPD exacerbation) associated with inflammation were reported, and these risks limit its current utility [13].

Bronchoscopic injection of autologous blood and fibrinogen into an emphysematous bulla has also effected volume reduction, but has not been evaluated except small pilot studies. However, they are promising because of no significant effect reported until now.

Lung Volume Reduction Coil (LVRC)

This is a self-activating metal nickel titanium (nitinol) coil delivered by bronchoscopy and underfluoroscopic guidance. It is designed to spring back to recover its predetermined coiled shape when released into the airway, compressing diseased tissue and increasing regional elastic tension. The device system consists of two components: the coil and the delivery system. Shape-memory nitinol wires are inserted to most diseased lung and 10–12 coils per upper lobe and 11–14 coils per lower lobe are usually inserted to optimize effect. Bilateral treatment, approximately 4–6 weeks apart, is recommended. The proposed mechanism is increase of airway caliber of healthier lung by compressing more diseased lung. However, the exact mechanisms are still need to be investigated.

To date, only several cohort or retrospective analyses are available, and there are no published trials compared with control or other LVR techniques. In the review of six trials, it showed FEV_1 improvement of 13.8–19.9% or 0.09–0.10 L at 3 months with acceptable safety. This improvement decreased over time, but maintained over 1 year in three trials [14]. This procedure showed some potential, especially for patients with incomplete fissure (Fig. 17.3).

Bronchoscopic Thermal Vapor Ablation (BTVA)

A specified quantity of steam is generated via a steam generator and delivered into diseased lung via bronchoscopy to reduce lung volume by contraction. Recent multicenter single arm study showed significant improvements in FEV_1 (141 mL, 17%), St. George's Respiratory Questionnaire (SGRQ, −11.0), 6MWD (18.5 m), residual volume (−302.8 mL), and modified Medical Research Council dyspnea scale score (mMRC, −0.83) at 6 months. These improvements diminished at 12 months and were greater in GOLD stage IV and higher heterogeneity. Further research compared to medical treatment is necessary for clinical validity.

Others

Other techniques including intrabronchial valve (IBV) and airway fenestration had been tried. However, these techniques are not practical until now, due to lack of efficacy.

Suggested Indication and Pre-procedural Evaluation

Considering recent clinical trials, the indication and contraindication of BLVR can be considered like below:

Indication

1. Hyperinflation: RV > 180%, TLC > 100%
2. Low lung function: FEV1 15–45%
3. Complete fissure of target lobe can be applied to endobronchial valve and intrabronchial valve
4. Exercise capacity (optional): 6-min walking 150–400 m

Contraindication

1. DLCO <20%
2. Giant bulla at lobe other than target lobe
3. Previous thoracotomy
4. Excessive sputum
5. Severe pulmonary hypertension
6. Unstable cardiac condition
7. Current smoker

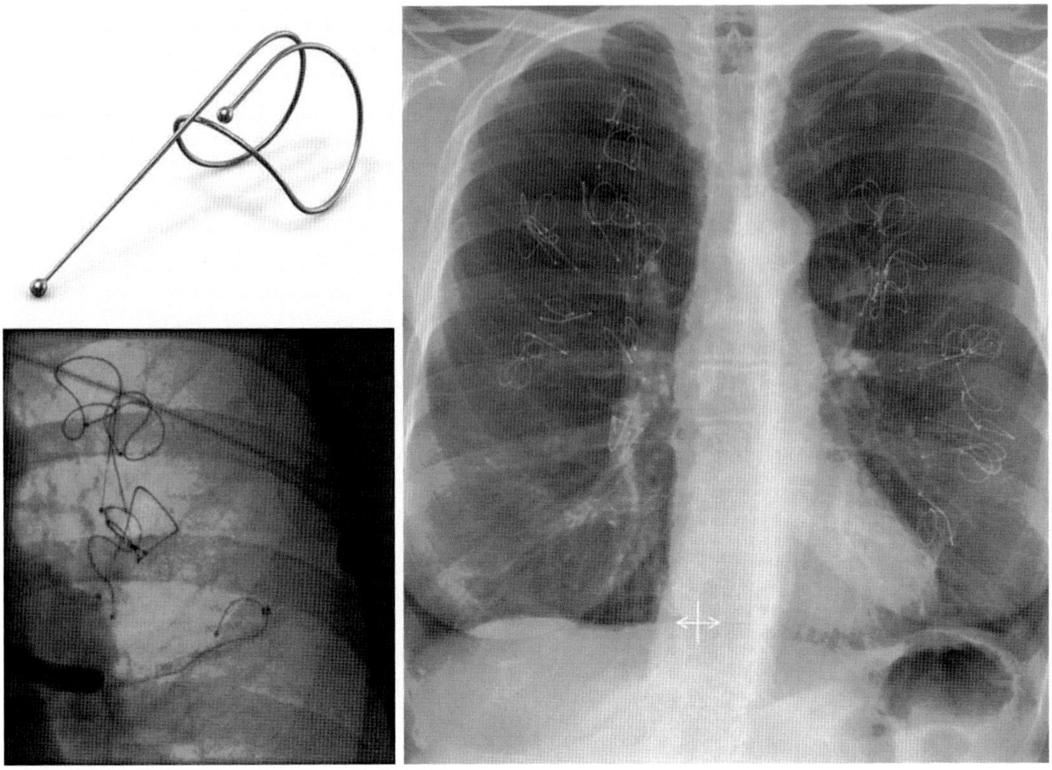

Fig. 17.3 Lung volume reduction coil (LVRC). Lung volume reduction coil (coil) (*upper left*). The image of a lung volume reduction coil. Image used with permission, PneumRx, Inc. a BTG International group company. (*Lower left*) The LVRCs are inserted via fluoroscopic guidance. (*Right*) Chest X-ray of post-procedure. Image courtesy of Dr. Dirk-Jan Slebos with permission

Every indication and contraindication has its meanings. The main benefit of this procedure comes from reducing hyperinflation, measured by RV or RV/TLC. The greater hyperinflation is, the greater possibility of clinical benefit can be anticipated. It should be noted that this procedure cannot be applied if hyperinflation is not evident on pulmonary function, even when emphysema is definitely present radiographically. This procedure can also be applied to patients with large bullae and persistent air leak.

Physician also should bear in mind contraindication to select appropriate candidates and avoid complication. The BLVR improve lung function by the change lung structure not by its regeneration. Therefore, we could not anticipate clinical benefit in patients whose lung reserve is too low (DLCO $< 20\%$). Giant bulla of ipsilateral side to target lobe is prone to pneumothorax, sometimes lethal because of tension. It should be avoided as the target lobe if giant bulla (usually >3 cm or a third of lung volume) is noted at adjacent ipsilateral lobes. However, giant bulla is not a problem if it is located in target lobe. Excessive sputum also can decrease the function of valves by blocking and be the source of infection.

Pulmonary Function Test

Not only FEV_1 or FVC, but also RV, RV/TLC, and DLCO are also important predictors for clinical response. Therefore, full examination about pulmonary function is crucial to decide appropriate candidates.

Radiographic Intervention

Radiographic imaging plays an important role in BLVR. Before procedure, several factors can predict successful results. Heterogeneity of emphysema and fissure completeness is the key factor for clinical response, and quantitative image can help analysis. Large bullae in ipsilateral side of target lobe is the predictor of major complication, intractable pneumothorax; therefore, the patients with this feature should be avoided for procedure. After procedure, radiographic evaluation is still important. The achievement of target lung volume reduction is the most important predictor for clinical improvement including survival. Chest X-ray should be followed for at least 2–5 days for detection pneumothorax. However, the criteria have not been determined clearly. The most commonly used criteria are:

- Complete fissure: 90% in two planes
- Target lobe reduction: 350 mL or 50% of the initial target lobe

Exercise Tests

Exercise capacity is the major outcome which BLVR can improve. The patients with good exercise capacity is not a contraindication, but clinical improvement can be limited if the exercise capacity is almost similar to normal level. In contrast, very low level of exercise capacity can be the indicator of poor general condition. These patients can be critical when complication develops. The criteria to indicate BLVR is hard to be determined by currently available evidences, but 150–450 m in 6-min walking distance may be acceptable criteria for this.

An Example of Good Candidate

A 66-year-old male with smoking history of 80-pack-year history had dyspnea of modified medical research council (mMRC) grade 4. He undertook BLVR with endobronchial valve and experienced marked improvement in lung function, quality of life, and exercise capacity 6 months after procedure as given below:

- FEV_1: 0.67 L → 1.22 L (182%)
- FVC: 2.37 L → 2.96 L (125%)
- Six minutes walking distance: 100 m → 230 m (230%)
- mMRC: grade 4 → grade 2
- Residual volume: 194% of predicted value → 111% of predicted value

The success for this patient can be explained by several factors (Fig. 17.4).

(a) Severe hyperinflation
(b) Heterogeneity of emphysema: definite target lobe with low function compared with volume
(c) Complete fissure on CT and no collateral ventilation on Chartis Console™
(d) Target lobe reduction achieved after procedure

Management of Major Complication

Major Complication

- Pneumothorax: most common
- Pneumonia
- Acute exacerbation
- Hemoptysis
- Empyema
- Death

Pneumothorax is the most common complication, and the management is important for procedural success. Pneumothorax happens during the inflation of ipsilateral lobes other than target one during reduction of the target lobe. Therefore, pneumothorax is suggested as an indicator for good clinical response. To reduce pneumothorax, the patients with large bullae at adjacent lobe of target should be avoided. When pneumothorax happens, the general guideline of pneumothorax management can be applied including O_2 inhalation or thoracostomy according to its size. However, the removal of BLVR device is considered if it is not resolved after treatment of several days and the device is removable (EBV or IBV). Several weeks after pneumothorax resolves, reinsertion can be considered carefully (Fig. 17.5).

Pneumonia and acute exacerbation can be managed like usual patients with COPD. If pneumonia of target lobe is not resolved with appropriate therapy of antibiotics, the removal of device should be considered in the case of BLVR with EBV or IBV.

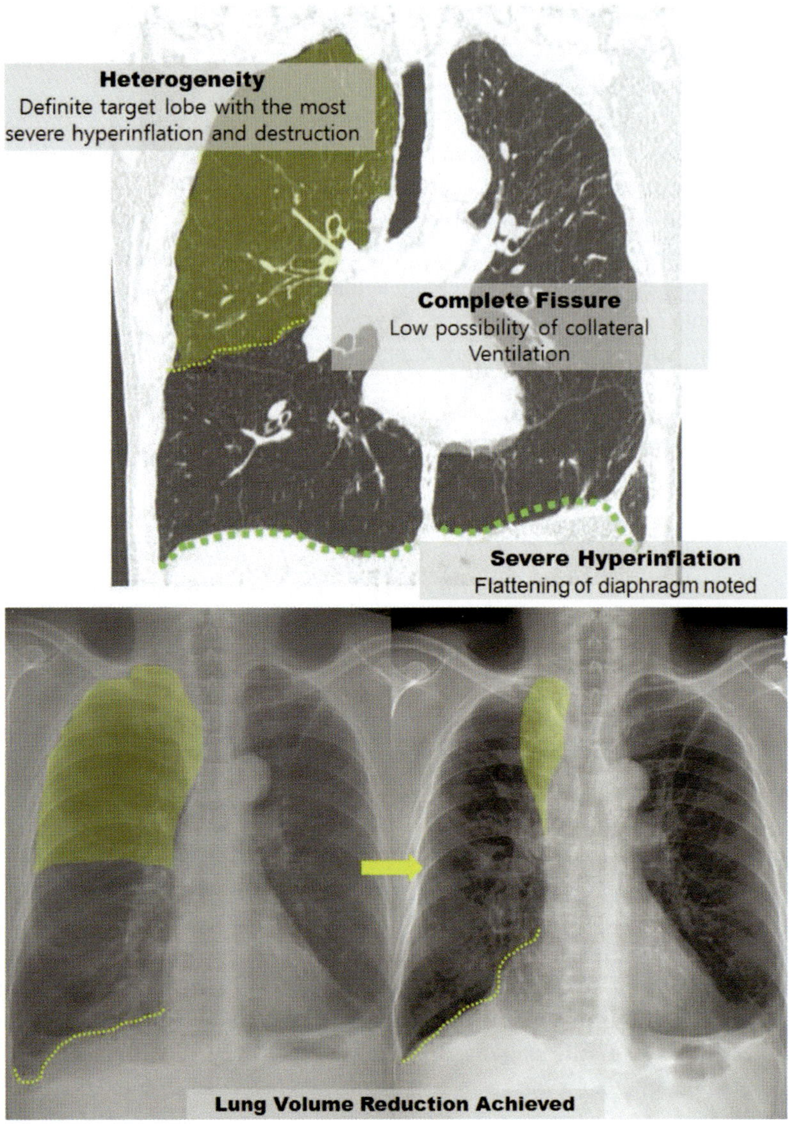

Fig. 17.4 An example of patients with a good clinical response. Right upper lobe (RUL) is the main target lobe and severe hyperinflation, heterogeneity of emphysema, complete fissure around RUL, and target lobe reduction were notified

Mortality was reported in 0–2.3%. Tension pneumothorax and migration of device can be its causes.

Summary and Application in Personalized Medicine

Severe emphysema with hyperinflation (large RV or RV/TLC) and preserved lung diffusion capacity (DLCO or DLCO/VA > 20%) can be the main candidates. EBVs are the most widely used and have shown promising results. However, these techniques can be applied only patients with definite target lobe with complete fissure. Several techniques including LVRC, BTVA, and bio-BLVR showed some possibility to overcome this limitation, but further research

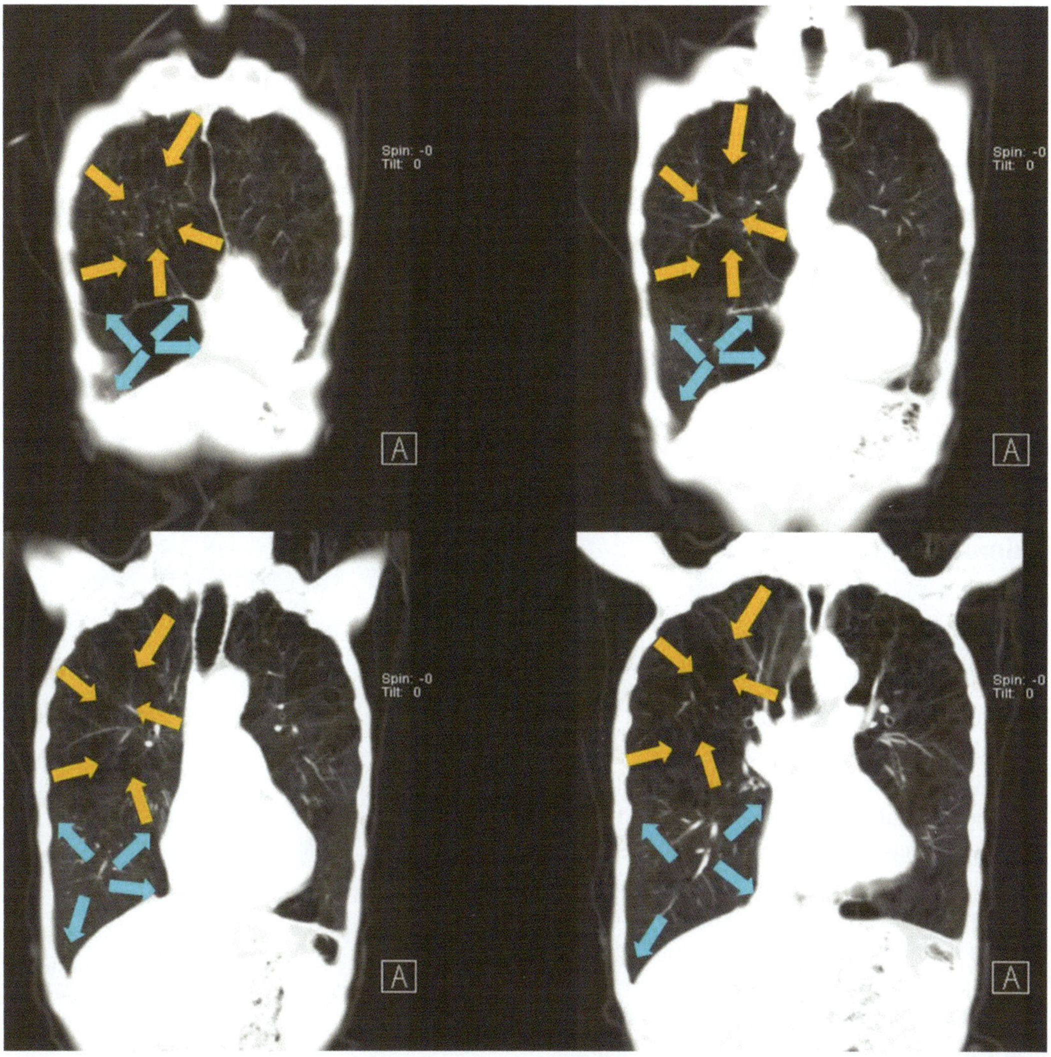

Fig. 17.5 The mechanism of pneumothorax after procedure. Pneumothorax is usually developed during inflation of adjacent ipsilateral lobe. In this patient, right upper lobe is the target lobe (RUL). If EBV was inserted at RUL, the volume of RUL start to decrease and those of right middle lobe and right lower lobe (RLL) start to increase. If there are bullae on RLL, it is prone to pneumothorax. Meanwhile, the bullae of RUL do not give a problem

is still necessary for practice. The application of BLVR should be personalized, and multiple techniques can be necessary sometimes in one patient. Considering the potential risks, BLVR should be considered when the clinical benefit is evident.

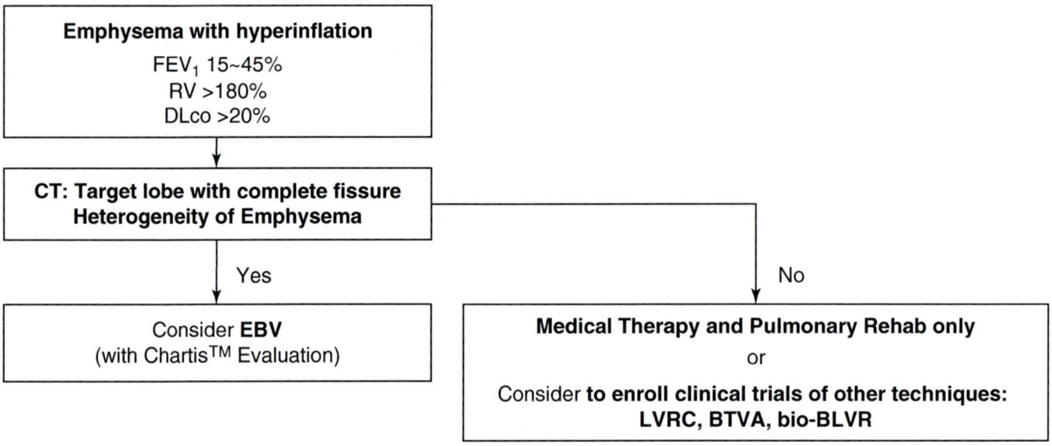

Pulmonary Rehabilitation

COPD is a treatable, but also incurable disease. Pharmacotherapy based on bronchodilators has marked progression recently, and it can improve lung function significantly. However, it is also limited by extent of improvement; even the most effective bronchodilator can increase FEV_1 by less than 200 mL. Patients with advanced COPD can have forced expiratory volume in one second (FEV_1) decline by more than 2 L sometimes, and they have severe respiratory symptom and difficulty in their daily life despite maximal pharmacotherapy. Considering this limitation of current treatment, we should recommend safe non-pharmacologic treatment, pulmonary rehabilitation in patients with COPD (Fig. 17.6).

Introduction: Multidisciplinary Approach

Pulmonary rehabilitation is multidisciplinary treatment program for chronic respiratory disease; it includes various aspects such as exercise, education, behavioral, and nutrition. All these factors are closely related, and if one problem starts to improve, other factors can follow to improve. This can finish vicious cycle of debilitation. The main purpose of pulmonary rehab is to relieve symptom, improve quality of life and exercise capacity, and expand physical and emotional activity in daily life. In the long term, it aims to maintain good health status (Fig. 17.7).

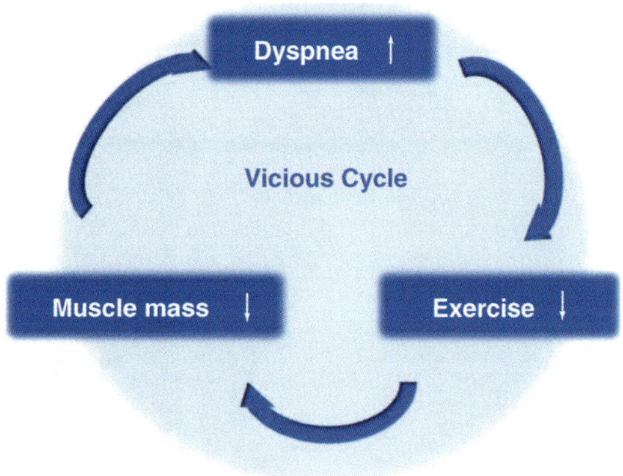

Fig. 17.6 Vicious cycle of COPD. Lung function is important in COPD, but it cannot explain all aspects of COPD. Decrease of muscle mass and inactivity are also the cause of debilitation and aggravation of COPD

Indication: Who Will Be the Candidates?

Every patient with COPD who have respiratory symptom and difficulty in daily life should be considered as candidates. COPD patients with mMRC grade I or GOLD stage I (FEV1 > 80%) had some evidence, [15, 16] but the most evidence is not enough. Therefore, most guidelines recommend pulmonary rehab for COPD of moderate patients with mMRC grade 2 or more [17,

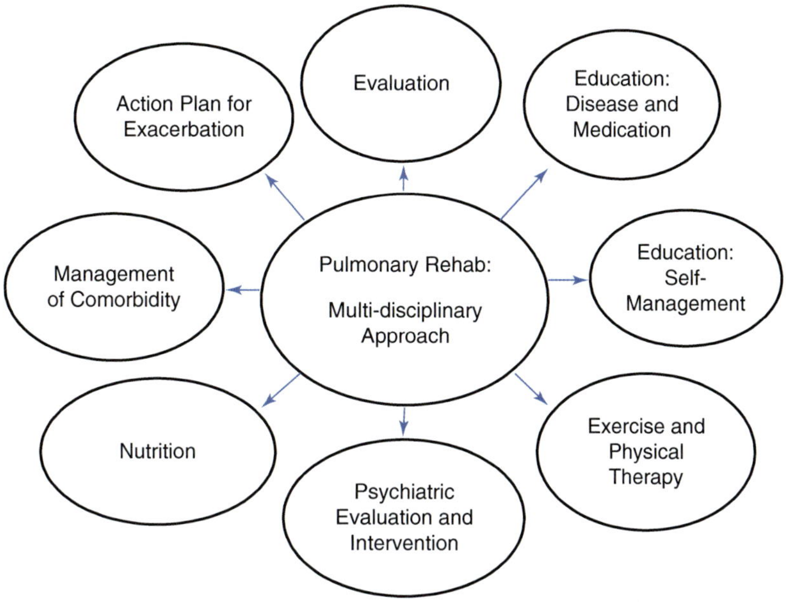

Fig. 17.7 Pulmonary rehab is mutidisciplinary and team-based approach

18]. Although the evidence for respiratory diseases other than COPD is not enough, personalized pulmonary rehab should be considered if patients have symptom and functional disability. The selection of patients should be decided by pulmonary rehab team in each hospital.

Evidences

Definite effect of pulmonary rehab (evidence A) on improvement of:

- Dyspea
- Exercise capacity
- Quality of life
- Anxiety and depression

1. Dyspnea
   Pulmonary rehab can improve respiratory symptom including dyspnea significantly. In meta-analysis, chronic respiratory questionnaire (CRQ) improved by 1.06 (95% confidence interval [CI] 0.85–1.26). This improvement exceeds the minimal clinical important difference (MCID) of CRQ which is 0.5. Six studies evaluating SGRQ score also showed improvement more than its MCID level of −4 [19]. COPD working group also reported definite dyspnea improvement after 4 weeks or more pulmonary rehabilitation [20].
2. Exercise Capacity
   Meta-analysis including 13 studies indicated that maximal exercise capacity of bicycle ergometer improved by 8.43 W (95% CI 3.4–13.4). Six minutes walking distance also increased significantly by 48 m [21]. In this analysis, the longer (≥6 months) and the more frequent (28 times or more) pulmonary rehab had increased the effect. Griffith et al. reported that pulmonary rehab incremental shuttle walk test (ISWT) by 75.9 m, which is more than its MCID of 47.5 m [22].
3. Quality of Life
   Quality of life can be evaluated for several components including symptom, body activity, social interaction, and emotional status. Pulmonary rehab improved all components of CRQ significantly including dysnea, fatigue, emotional function, and mastery. SGRQ includes total, symptom, impact, and activity, and pulmonary rehab improved these SGRQ areas except symptom [19]. In the largest number of study

included in this meta-analysis, both SGRQ and CRQ improved significantly after 6 weeks pulmonary rehab and the effect persists for 1 year compared with control [22]. Trooster et al. also reported that improvement after 6 months pulmonary rehab persisted for 18 months without decrease. Cochrane review about patients with COPD exacerbation showed improvement in all areas of CRQ and all areas of SGRQ except symptom [23].

4. Emotional and Social Effects
   Comprehensive pulmonary rehab improved significant improvement in anxiety and depression compared with control, but this effect was not significant if the program includes only exercise and education [24]. In the largest study included in this meta-analysis, pulmonary rehab improved hospital anxiety and depression scale (HADS) and this effect persisted after 1 year [22]. In another study, pulmonary rehab for 10 weeks decreased anxiety and improved cognitive function [25].
5. Survival
   The evidence for pulmonary rehab to improve survival is not enough until now, and most studies are small non-randomized observational studies. One randomized study including 119 patients with stable COPD reported that group with comprehensive pulmonary rehab improved survival by 11% (67% vs. 56%) compared with group with education only, but it did not reach statistical significance. Stav et al. reported that pulmonary rehab for 3 years improved survival predictor factors in COPD such as FEV_1 decline, exercise capacity, and body mass index (BMI) in a study including 80 patients with COPD [26]. Pulmonary rehab after COPD exacerbation was reported to improve survival in a meta-analysis [23]. However, a recent report suggested that unorganized pulmonary rehab without enough time periods after exacerbation can increase mortality [27].

Suggested Program

Supervised Exercise and Physical Therapy

Exercise is the most important factor and should be personalized for each patient. Aerobic exercise includes walking, bicycle ergometer, treadmill, and swimming. Aerobic exercise is usually recommended as 60% of maximal exercise capacity for 20–60 min, each session, 3–5 times per week. High and low intensity can be applied according to patients' performance. Muscle exercise can improve respiratory symptom and exercise capacity. It can be performed with 60–70% of maximal capacity, 10 times per session, 2–3 times per week.

Aerobic exercise program for patients with COPD

FITT	High intensity	Low intensity
Frequency	3–5/week or more	3–5/week or more
Intensity	Borg Scale 5–6	Borg Scale 3–5
Time	20–60 min/day, 6–8 weeks or more	20–60 min/day, 6–8 weeks or more
Type	Walking, bicycle, swimming	Walking, bicycle
Indication	Mild to moderate COPD	Severe COPD
Strength	Great improvement in exercise Great physiologic effect	Easy to perform at home Improvement in depression High compliance
Weakness	Difficult to apply to every patient High risk Need to observe Low compliance	Small improvement in exercise Longer duration is necessary

Strength of aerobic exercise should be decided ideally by VO_2max from cardiopulmonary exercise test (CPET). However, it is not easy to perform CPET for all patients with COPD. In these cases, 6MWD, Borg scale and maximal heart rate are helpful. Besides these methods, exercise intensity recommended to increase the degree of sweating and maintain the degree of being able to converse.

Education

Education is the essential part of pulmonary rehab. Appropriate education enables patients participate in their own treatment, and evaluate, cope with their health problems. Education should be personalized considering patients' interest, needs, severity, and comorbidity.

Education program includes the contents below:

- Techniques for inhaler
- Smoking cessation
- COPD action plan: exacerbation
- Vaccination: influenza and pneumococcus
- The impact of air pollution
- Nutrition

Evaluation: Patients-Centered Outcomes

Patients should be evaluated before and after pulmonary rehab. The evaluation includes:

- Symptom: history, physical exam, Borg scale, visual analogue scale, dyspnea, fatigue
- Quality of life: COPD assessment test (CAT), SGRQ
- Muscle: respiratory, upper and lower extremity
- Daily activity: monitoring tool or self-report can be utilized [28]
  Monitoring tool: Pedometer, activity monitor
  Functional status questionnaires: Pulmonary functional status and dyspnea questionnaire (PFSDQ), [29] PFSDQ-modified, [30] pulmonary functional status scale (PFSS) [31]
- Exercise capacity: 6-min walking distance (6MWD), incremental maximal exercise test
- Nutrition
- Depression and psychiatric problem can be monitored:
  Centers for epidemiologic studies depression scale (CES-D)
  Beck Anxiety Inventory (BAI)
  Mini-mental state examination (MMSE)

Summary and Suggestion in Personalized Medicine

Pulmonary rehab should be considered in all patients who have respiratory symptom due to COPD. Considering evidences available, patients with moderate COPD of dyspnea (mMRC grade 2 or more) may have more benefit. Physician should recommend and organize personalized pulmonary rehab program if the patients with COPD have difficulty in their daily life.

Nutrition

COPD is a disease that makes the significant impact on nutrition status of patients. Nutritional problems including weight loss, muscle depletion, and cachexia are observed often in COPD patients. Those problems are associated with poor nutrient intake, increased energy expenditure due to increased work of breathing, chronic systemic inflammation, chronic corticosteroid use, and so on. It was reported that 30–60% of inpatients and 10–45% of outpatients with COPD are malnourished state [32]. The prevalence of malnutrition depends on the severity of disease. Malnutrition can exert deleterious effects on respiratory function and immune function. Therefore, careful nutrition care for COPD patients to prevent malnutrition is needed. However, excessive intake should be avoided because over-nutrition is also harmful to COPD patients. Therefore, it is important to assess nutritional status and to carry out nutrition education for COPD patients. To refer patients to nutritional professionals can be helpful to implement comprehensive nutrition assessment and adequate nutrition interventions including nutrition education.

In addition, it is suggested that nutrition may be important modifiable factor for the progression and management of COPD [33].

Nutrition Assessment

Body Mass

Weight loss is common in COPD patients and is reported in 25–40% of all COPD [34]. Weight loss is accompanied with fat-free mass and loss of fat-free mass causes decreased muscle function. The prevalence of muscle atrophy in COPD patients is reported 20–40% although reported prevalence varies depending on definition and disease stage [35]. Weight loss, low BMI (body mass index), and muscle wasting are associated with increased mortality, regardless of disease severity. In a prospective multicenter study, it was reported that hospitalized COPD patients with BMI <20 kg/m^2 had higher mortality compared to patients with BMI >20 kg/m^2 [36]. BMI <20–22 kg/m^2 is suggested as cut-off point to define underweight status [37, 38] although BMI <18.5 kg/m^2 corresponds to underweight in WHO classification.

Although weight and BMI are useful tools to assess nutritional status, fat-free mass may be a better indicator [39]. In a large-scale study, it was suggested that the type of low body weight, not low body weight per se predicts outcome [40]. Depletion of fat-free mass can occur not only in underweight patients but also in patients with normal BMI or even obesity. Fat-free mass can measure using BIA (bioelectrical impedance analysis), or DEX (dual energy X-ray absorptiometry). However, measurement of body composition is not implemented routinely, and it makes to underestimate the muscle depletion in normal or obese patients. Fat-free mass is associated with pulmonary function [41, 42].

Involuntary weight loss is strongly associated with nutritional risk. In general, adult person is considered at nutritional risk when weight loss is more than 5% during a month or more than 10% during 6 months.

Excessive weight, particularly excessive body fat, may negatively affect COPD patients. Obesity can increase the workload of an already compromised respiratory system. Severe obese patients have difficulty in breathing caused by restrictions on the chest wall due to accumulated fat in and around the thoracic cage, diaphragm, and abdomen. As a result, lung volume is decreased and poor gas change is accompanied [39]. In addition, obesity may affect oxidative stress, inflammation response, and metabolic alteration.

Nutrition History, Laboratory Data, and Medical Test

Nutrition history is essential to assess the appropriateness of nutrient intake and to plan adequate nutrition interventions. Nutrition history includes various factors as follows.

- Meal frequency and pattern, snack pattern, current and previous diets, food preference, water and beverage drinking, use of medical nutrition supplements, any factors affecting access to food
- Problems related to eating: anorexia, changes in taste, difficulties in chewing or swallowing, nausea, vomiting, early satiety, shortness of breath, diarrhea, constipation, indigestion

Reviews on laboratory data (such as serum albumin, transferrin, prealbumin, CBC, vitamin D, calcium, magnesium, etc.) and results of tests related to nutrition such as bone mineral density are helpful to assess nutritional status of patient. In addition, it is needed to check on medication–nutrients interactions.

Nutritional Consideration

Energy and Protein

Energy intake should be individualized based on anthropometric data, physical activity, and medical status. Energy need is determined at the level that can maintain reasonable body weight. If the patient has low BMI, high calorie diet is recommended. In contrast, energy intake should be controlled to obese patients.

Indirect calorimetry is the most accurate method to measure resting energy expenditure (REE). In case that indirect calorimetry is not available, some predictive equations such as Harris-Benedict equation or Mifflin-St. Jeor equation can be used. In general, 25–30 kcal/kg body weight can meet energy need. In addition, some methods are available as given below [43, 44]:.

- Metabolic requirements for COPD: 1.25×REE
- COPD predictive equations [45]:
  11.5 × weight (kg) + 952 [male], 14.1 × weight (kg) + 515 [female]
- Ireton Jones equation

Adequate protein intake is important to maintain body mass and to produce various functional components. Protein intake of 1.2–1.7 g/kg body weight are recommended to avoid protein loss.

Carbohydrate and fat

There is limited evidence to support COPD-specific macronutrient composition. In case of hypercapnia, a diet moderate in carbohydrate and higher in fat may be considered [46]. However, excessive fat intake can make harmful effects including immune suppression.

Omega-3 polyunsaturated fatty acids (PUFA) have been shown to exert anti-inflammatory effect. Although there is no strong evidence, consumption of omega-3 PUFA (oily fish or fish oil) may have positive effects in COPD patients. Several studies using omega-3 PUFA supplementation to COPD patients are underway and are expected to provide evidences [33].

Vitamin, Mineral, and Fluid

Micronutrients intake should meet Dietary Reference Intakes (DRIs). It may be necessary to pay closer attention to the consumptions of several vitamins and minerals in COPD patients.

Adequate intake of antioxidant vitamins (vitamin C, vitamin E, and some carotenoids) may give beneficial effects on respiratory health via reducing oxidative stress. Also it has been suggested that there are some association between COPD and vitamin D in several studies. Vitamin D deficiency reported commonly in COPD patients. Poor diet, reduced vitamin D synthesis, and glucocorticoid use may contribute vitamin D deficiency in COPD patients [47].

Osteoporosis is often reported among COPD patient. Some factors including excess smoking, physical inactivity, and glucocorticoids medication have been suggested as the causes [48]. Inadequate calcium intake can exacerbate bone health in COPD patients. Excessive sodium intake can result in fluid retention or peripheral edema. These make difficulty in breathing [39].

Fluid intake should be adequate. If the patient is febrile, fluid intake has to be increased. As a rule, 1 mL/kg is recommended [39]. Enough water drinking may be helpful to keep mucus thin.

Nutritional Supplement

When the patient can't meet his or her nutritional need (mainly calorie and protein) with regular foods, use of nutritional supplements has been recommended. It was reported that use of nutritional supplements could make positive effects on nutritional status of undernourished COPD patients from several meta-analysis studies [34]. However, routine use of nutritional supplements to COPD patients is not recommended [37]. When patients can't eat regular foods, nutritional supplements can be used as a complete diet. If patients can't eat enough amounts, nutritional supplements can be added to regular meal.

Nutritional Tips

How to Resolve Some Problems Related to Eating

Problems	Recommendation
Chewing difficulties	– Use foods soft in texture such as cooked vegetable, moist ground meat, cooked cereal
Dyspnea and fatigue while eating	– Get enough rest before meal Eat slowly – Eat small and frequent meals
Abdominal distention	– Eat small amd frequent meals – Avoid gas-forming foods – Do not drink too much fluid during meal
Early satiety	– Eat small and frequent meals – Drink beverages at the end of the meal

Eating Tips for COPD Patients

- **Eat small, frequent meals instead of three large meals.** It helps that the stomach is not extremely full. Full stomach can interfere with breathing.
- **Plan meal that includes a variety of foods from different food groups** (grains, vegetables, fruits, protein foods, dairy, oils). It makes possible to eat nutritionally balanced meal.
- **Limit intake of gas-forming foods** such as carbonated beverages, heavily spiced foods, greasy foods, onions, cauliflower, broccoli, melon, pea, corn, cucumber, cabbage, brussels sprouts, turnip, beans, raw apple, and so on. They may bloat the abdomen and make breathing difficult.
- **Avoid excess salt intake.** High salt diet may cause edema and edema can make breathing difficult.
- **Eat slowly.** It may be helpful to avoid becoming short of breath.
- **Drink 6–8 cups of water daily.** Sufficient water drinking may help mucus thin. But don't try it at once.
- **Drink beverages after a meal.** It can help to reduce the feeling full or bloated.
- **Rest before eating.**
- **If you need to increase calorie and/or protein, add foods as follows:**
- Calorie: butter, whipped cream, sour cream, oils, mayonnaise, salad dressing, honey, jam, sugar, granola, dried fruits, cocoa powder, nut, seed, peanut butter, ice cream, margarine, or nutritional supplements
- Protein: cheeses including cottage or ricotta, powdered milk, eggs, yogurt, or nutritional supplements

References

1. Vestbo J, et al. Global strategy for the diagnosis, management, and prevention of chronic obstructive pulmonary disease: GOLD executive summary. Am J Respir Crit Care Med. 2013;187(4):347–65.
2. Lee JH, et al. Responses to inhaled long-acting beta-agonist and corticosteroid according to COPD subtype. Respir Med. 2009;104(4):542–9.
3. Brantigan OC, Mueller E. Surgical treatment of pulmonary emphysema. Am Surg. 1957;23(9): 789–804.
4. Brantigan OC, Mueller E, Kress MB. A surgical approach to pulmonary emphysema. Am Rev Respir Dis. 1959;80(1, Part 2):194–206.
5. Cooper JD, et al. Results of 150 consecutive bilateral lung volume reduction procedures in patients with severe emphysema. J Thorac Cardiovasc Surg. 1996;112(5):1319–29. discussion 1329–30
6. Fishman A, et al. A randomized trial comparing lung-volume-reduction surgery with medical therapy for severe emphysema. N Engl J Med. 2003;348(21):2059–73.
7. Sciurba FC, et al. A randomized study of endobronchial valves for advanced emphysema. N Engl J Med. 2010;363(13):1233–44.
8. Herth FJ, et al. Efficacy predictors of lung volume reduction with Zephyr valves in a European cohort. Eur Respir J. 2012;39(6):1334–42.
9. Herth FJ, et al. Radiological and clinical outcomes of using Chartis to plan endobronchial valve treatment. Eur Respir J. 2013;41(2):302–8.
10. Hopkinson NS, et al. Atelectasis and survival after bronchoscopic lung volume reduction for COPD. Eur Respir J. 2011;37(6):1346–51.

11. Kotecha S, et al. Long-term outcomes from bronchoscopic lung volume reduction using a bronchial prosthesis. Respirology. 2011;16(1):167–73.
12. Valipour A, et al. Target lobe volume reduction and COPD outcome measures after endobronchial valve therapy. Eur Respir J. 2014;43(2):387–96.
13. Come CE, et al. A randomised trial of lung sealant versus medical therapy for advanced emphysema. Eur Respir J. 2015;46(3):651–62.
14. Hartman JE, et al. Treatment of emphysema using bronchoscopic lung volume reduction coil technology: an update on efficacy and safety. Ther Adv Respir Dis. 2015;9(5):251–9.
15. Evans RA, Singh SJ, Collier R, Williams JE, Morgan MD. Pulmonary rehabilitation is successful for COPD irrespective of MRC dyspnoea grade. Respir Med. 2009;103(7):1070–5.
16. Man WD, Grant A, Hogg L, Moore J, Barker RD, Moxham J. Pulmonary rehabilitation in patients with MRC Dyspnoea scale 2. Thorax. 2011;66(3):263.
17. Decramer M, Vestbo J, Bourbeau J, Celi B, Hui D, Varela MV, et al. Global strategy for the diagnosis, management and the prevention of chronic obstructive pulmonary disease (updated 2014) .http://www.goldcopd.org/uploads/users/files/GOLD_Report_2014_Jun11.pdf. 2014.
18. Bolton CE, Bevan-Smith EF, Blakey JD, Crowe P, Elkin SL, Garrod R, et al. 2013 British Thoracic Society guideline on pulmonary rehabilitation in adults. Thorax. 68 Suppl 2:ii1–i30.
19. Lacasse Y, Martin S, Lasserson TJ, Goldstein RS. Meta-analysis of respiratory rehabilitation in chronic obstructive pulmonary disease. A Cochrane systematic review. Eura Medicophys. 2007;43(4):475–85.
20. Group CW. Pulmonary rehabilitation for patients with chronic pulmonary disease (COPD): an evidence-based analysis. Ont Health Technol Assess Ser. 2012;12(6):1–75.
21. Lacasse Y, Goldstein R, Lasserson TJ, Martin S. Pulmonary rehabilitation for chronic obstructive pulmonary disease. Cochrane Database Syst Rev. 2006;4:CD003793.
22. Griffiths TL, Burr ML, Campbell IA, Lewis-Jenkins V, Mullins J, Shiels K, et al. Results at 1 year of outpatient multidisciplinary pulmonary rehabilitation: a randomised controlled trial. Lancet. 2000;355(9201):362–8.
23. Puhan M, Scharplatz M, Troosters T, Walters EH, Steurer J. Pulmonary rehabilitation following exacerbations of chronic obstructive pulmonary disease. Cochrane Database Syst Rev. 2009;1:CD005305.
24. Coventry PA, Hind D. Comprehensive pulmonary rehabilitation for anxiety and depression in adults with chronic obstructive pulmonary disease: systematic review and meta-analysis. J Psychosom Res. 2007;63(5):551–65.
25. Emery CF, Schein RL, Hauck ER, MacIntyre NR. Psychological and cognitive outcomes of a randomized trial of exercise among patients with chronic obstructive pulmonary disease. Health Psychol. 1998;17(3):232–40.
26. Stav D, Raz M, Shpirer I. Three years of pulmonary rehabilitation: inhibit the decline in airflow obstruction, improves exercise endurance time, and body-mass index, in chronic obstructive pulmonary disease. BMC Pulm Med. 2009;9:26.
27. Greening NJ, Williams JE, Hussain SF, Harvey-Dunstan TC, Bankart MJ, Chaplin EJ, et al. An early rehabilitation intervention to enhance recovery during hospital admission for an exacerbation of chronic respiratory disease: randomised controlled trial. BMJ. 2014;349:g4315.
28. Steele BG, Belza B, Cain K, Warms C, Coppersmith J, Howard J. Bodies in motion: monitoring daily activity and exercise with motion sensors in people with chronic pulmonary disease. J Rehabil Res Dev. 2003;40(5 Suppl 2):45–58.
29. Lareau SC, Carrieri-Kohlman V, Janson-Bjerklie S, Roos PJ. Development and testing of the Pulmonary Functional Status and Dyspnea Questionnaire (PFSDQ). Heart Lung. 1994;23(3):242–50.
30. Lareau SC, Meek PM, Roos PJ. Development and testing of the modified version of the pulmonary functional status and dyspnea questionnaire (PFSDQ-M). Heart Lung. 1998;27(3):159–68.
31. Weaver TE, Narsavage GL, Guilfoyle MJ. The development and psychometric evaluation of the Pulmonary Functional Status Scale: an instrument to assess functional status in pulmonary disease. J Cardpulm Rehabil. 1998;18(2):105–11.
32. Stratton RJ, Green CJ, Elia M. Disease-related malnutrition: an evidence-based approach to treatment. Wallingford: CABI; 2003.
33. Berthon BS, Wood LG. Nutrition and respiratory health-feature review. Forum Nutr. 2015;7:1618–43.
34. Itoh M, Tsuji T, Nemoto K, Nakamura H, Aoshoba K. Undernutrition in patients with COPD and its treatment. Forum Nutr. 2013;5:1316–35.
35. Langen RCJ, Gosker HR, Remels AHV, Schols AMWJ. Triggers and mechanisms of skeletal muscle wasting in chronic obstructive pulmonary disease. Int J Biochem Cell Biol. 2013;45:2245–56.
36. Hallin R, Gudmundsson G, Ulrik CS, Nieminen MM, Gislason T, Linberg E, Brondum E, Aine T, Basle P, Janson C. Nutritional status and long-term mortality in hospitalised patients with chronic obstructive pulmonary disease (COPD). Respir Med. 2007;101:1954–60.
37. American Association of Cardiovascular and Pulmonary Rehabilitation. Guidelines for pulmonary

rehabilitation programs, 4th ed. American Association of Cardiovascular and Pulmonary Rehabilitation. 2011.
38. Van der Valk P, Monninkhof E, Van der Palen J, Zielhuis G, Van Herwaarden C. Management of stable COPD. Patient Educ Couns. 2004;52:225–9.
39. Escott-Stump S. Nutrition and diagnosis-related care. 7th ed. Philadelphia: Lippincott Williams & Wilkins; 2012.
40. Schols AM, Broekhuizen R, Weling-Scheepers CA, Wouters EF. Body composition and mortality in chronic obstructive pulmonary disease. Am J Clin Nutr. 2005;82:53–9.
41. Burchfiel CM, Enright PL, Sharp DS, Chyou PH, Rodriguez BL, Curb JD. Factors associated with variations in pulmonary function among elderly Japanese-American men. Chest. 1997;112:87–97.
42. Amara CE, Koval JJ, Paterson DH, Cunningham DA. Lung function in older human: the contribution of body composition, physical activity and smoking. Ann Hum Biol. 2001;25:522–36.
43. Academy of Nutrition and Dietetics. Chronic obstructive pulmonary disease toolkit. Academy of Nutrition and Dietetics. 2012.
44. American Society for Parenteral and Enteral Nutrition. The science and practice of nutrition support American Society for Parenteral and Enteral Nutrition: a case based core curriculum. Dubuque: Kendall/Hunt; 2001.
45. Moore JA, Angelillo VA. Equations for the prediction of resting energy expenditure in chronic obstructive lung disease. Chest. 1988;94:1260–3.
46. Width M, Reinhard T. The clinical dietitian's essential pocket guide. Philadelphia: Lippincott Williams & Wilkins; 2009.
47. Herr C, Greulich T, Koczulla RA, Meyer S, Zakharkina T, Bransch M, Eschmann R, Bals R. The role of vitamin D in pulmonary disease: COPD, asthma, infection, and cancer. Respir Res. 2011;12:31.
48. Jørgensen NR, Schwarz P. Osteoporosis in chronic obstructive pulmonary disease patients. Curr Opin Pulm Med. 2008;14:122–7.

Exacerbation of COPD

18

Jin Hwa Lee

Introduction [1–4]

COPD exacerbation is defined as an aggravation of the patient's respiratory symptoms such as dyspnea, cough, and sputum beyond normal day-to-day variations, which needs a change in medication. To diagnose COPD exacerbation, physicians should exclude other possible causes such as heart failure, pneumonia, pneumothorax, or pulmonary thromboembolism [5], which could be one of common comorbidities in COPD patients. Since COPD exacerbation has significant negative impacts on the patient's quality of life and lung function decline, it is one of the most important prognostic factors in COPD patients. Practically it is significantly associated with high in-hospital and subsequent mortality and large socioeconomic burden [6]. Nevertheless, useful biomarkers to predict and/or diagnose COPD exacerbation have not yet been developed. The diagnosis still depends on only symptomatic change. Moreover, precipitating factors for COPD exacerbation are not always identifiable, though bacterial or viral respiratory infection has been known as one of the most common causes. A previous study suggested four biologic COPD exacerbation clusters (bacterial, eosinophilic, viral, and paus-inflammatory) and their corresponding biomarkers [7]. However, they need to be validated.

Predictors of COPD Exacerbation

Severe airflow limitation defined as low forced expiratory volume in one second (FEV_1) is a well-known risk factor for COPD exacerbation [8]. A large prospective cohort study showed that history of prior exacerbations is the best predictor of COPD exacerbations [9]. This study served as an evidence that a "frequent exacerbator" is one of COPD phenotypes. In two large COPD cohorts, pulmonary artery enlargement gauged by computed tomography scan of the chest [a ratio of the diameter of pulmonary artery to the diameter of aorta (PA/A) > 1] was the most significant predictor of COPD exacerbation [10]. Gastroesophageal reflux was also associated with COPD exacerbation in several prospective and retrospective cohort studies [9, 11, 12]. Chronic bronchitis [13] and emphysema phenotypes [14] were associated with frequent exacerbation.

Systemic Corticosteroids

Systemic corticosteroids are well-established treatment of COPD exacerbations. Systemic corticosteroid by the oral or parenteral route

J.H. Lee
Division of Pulmonary and Critical Care Medicine, Department of Internal Medicine, College of Medicine, Ewha Womans University, Seoul, South Korea
e-mail: jinhwalee@ewha.ac.kr

S.-D. Lee (ed.), *COPD*, DOI 10.1007/978-3-662-47178-4_18

decreases risk of recurrence and treatment failure, shortens length of hospital stay, and improves lung function and symptoms. Compared with oral corticosteroid, parenteral treatment has no benefit on treatment failure, relapse, or mortality. Parenteral administration rather than oral treatment increases adverse effects of corticosteroid [15].

Even though 10–14 days of oral corticosteroids have been recommended for treatment of COPD exacerbations, recent studies suggest that 5 days of oral corticosteroids (40 mg of prednisolone or equivalent) would be sufficient for treatment of COPD exacerbations [16, 17]. Also nebulized budesonide showed similar efficacy to prednisone in terms of both lung function and hypoxemia [18]. However, it is controversial whether patients with acute exacerbation hospitalized in an intensive care unit (ICU) have benefit from systemic corticosteroids. Previous studies showed rather adverse effect of corticosteroids such as hyperglycemia than a reduction of mortality in patients with COPD exacerbation admitted in the ICU [19]. In critically ill patient with COPD exacerbation, lower-dose (methylprednisolone, ≤240 mg/day) corticosteroid did not show mortality reduction compared to higher-dose (methylprednisolone, >240 mg/day) [20]. However, lower-dose corticosteroid was associated with shorter hospital and ICU stay, shorter length of invasive ventilation, lower medical cost, and lower insulin requirement [20].

Antibiotics

Half of COPD exacerbations are likely to be involved by bacterial infection of respiratory tract. However, sputum culture and/or documentation of pathogen before initiation of antibiotic treatment are not required particularly in outpatient setting [21]. Since bacterial colonization of tracheobronchial tree is common even in patients with stable COPD, prescription of empirical antibiotics has high priority [21]. Whether to decide to give antibiotics to COPD patients with exacerbation still depends on clinical symptoms such as dyspnea and purulent sputum, though several biomarkers including procalcitonin have been tested to detect bacterial exacerbation.

Recent meta-analysis demonstrated beneficial effects of antibiotics for COPD exacerbations on outcomes of hospitalized patients, particularly reduction of treatment failure [22]. However, outpatient antibiotic treatment did not reduce treatment failure risk [22]. Unfortunately, antibiotics did not show any mortality reduction and shortening of length of hospital stay in hospitalized patients with COPD exacerbation [22]. Therefore further studies are needed to identify patients with benefit from antibiotics.

The choice of the antibiotic depends on the local bacterial resistance pattern. Since the most common pathogens are *Haemophilus influenzae, Moraxella catarrhalis,* and *Streptococcus pneumonia* [23], amoxicillin with or without clavulanate, macrolide, or doxycycline are usually initial choice. Other less frequently isolated potential pathogens are *Haemophilus parainfluenzae, Staphylococcus aureus, Pseudomonas aeruginosa,* and *gram-negative Enterobacteriaceae.* Patients at high risk i.e., frequent exacerbators, severe airway obstruction, or admission to an intensive care unit need broad-spectrum antibiotics with activity to *Pseudomonas aeruginosa* [24], such as piperacillin with or without tazobactam or cyprofloxacin.

The duration of the antibiotic treatment for COPD exacerbation has not been well defined. However, a meta-analysis for exacerbation of chronic bronchitis revealed that short course of antibiotic treatment is likely to be as effective as and safer than long-duration treatment [25].

If a COPD patient with exacerbation requiring hospitalization has high probability of influenza infection, antiviral agent such as oseltamivir should be given [26]. Zanamivir inhalation is not recommended because of bronchoconstriction risk.

Inhaled Short-Acting Bronchodilators

Inhaled short-acting beta 2-agonists with or without inhaled short-acting anticholinergics are almost always used to treat acute exacerbation of

COPD though their effects have not yet been validated. A systematic review of delivery methods of short-acting bronchodilators did not find any significant differences in FEV_1 between nebulizers and metered-dose inhalers (with or without a spacer device) [27]. However, nebulizers are more convenient for patients with tachypnea and dyspnea.

Oxygen [28]

Oxygen supplementation is one of key elements of hospital treatment of COPD exacerbations since hypoxemia is common and one of reasons for hospitalization. Thirty to sixty minutes after O_2 supplementation, arterial blood gas analysis should be performed to confirm appropriate oxygenation without respiratory acidosis. High oxygen supplementation can exaggerate ventilation/perfusion mismatch because oxygen dilates pulmonary vessels, resulting in respiratory acidosis and diminished mental status. Therefore O_2 supplementation should be titrated to target 88% and over on peripheral O_2 saturation. High-flow devices such as Optiflow™ can provide more accurate and higher fraction of inspired O_2 than do nasal prongs or masks [29], and COPD patients with high O_2 requirement and no hypercarbia may have benefit without mechanical ventilation. If a patient shows no clinical improvement and/or decreased consciousness despite oxygen supplementation, mechanical ventilation should be applied to reduce breathing work and improve hypoxemia.

Mechanical Ventilation

COPD patients with impending respiratory failure, altered mental status, or hemodynamic instability need intensive care. Sometimes intermediate unit is more appropriate for COPD patients with exacerbation, who do not need immediate mechanical ventilation but need more careful monitoring. This unit should have specialized personnel and respiratory equipment.

Non-invasive Ventilation (NIV)

NIV is an attractive alternative option for COPD patients with severe exacerbation, who do not need immediate invasive mechanical ventilation (e.g., severe dyspnea with alert mental status and hemodynamic stability) [30]. COPD exacerbation, particularly associated with hypercapneic respiratory failure, shows the best outcome among diseases requiring NIV. Also, NIV is frequently used for patients who still need ventilator support after weaning of invasive mechanical ventilation, which prompts early weaning, reduces the risk of ventilator-associated pneumonia, and shortens length of ICU stay [31]. Recent meta-analysis emphasizes early adoption of NIV for survival benefit since late apply of NIV failed to show survival benefit [32]. One prospective cohort study demonstrated that primary NIV use and its success, but not empirical antibiotic therapy, are associated with a favorable outcome [33].

Invasive Mechanical Ventilation

Invasive mechanical ventilation is necessary for COPD patients with severe exacerbation who do not tolerate NIV. Indications for invasive mechanical ventilation during acute exacerbation of COPD are the same as general indications, i.e., at least one of severe hypoxemic respiratory failure, altered mental status, aspiration, excessive secretions with inability of self-expectoration, severe hemodynamic instability, and severe arrhythmias.

Although patients with severe COPD have high mortality of respiratory failure, acute mortality of COPD patients with respiratory failure is relatively low compared to mortality of patients with respiratory failure and without COPD [34]. Nevertheless, COPD patients and their families sometimes deny endotracheal intubation and admission to an ICU since they have suffered dyspnea for a long time and most of them are very old. Decision of withholding and/or withdrawal of treatment should be based on the patient's performance status including other comorbidities and reversibility of respiratory failure cause.

Other Treatments Without Definite Evidence

Mucolytics such as N-acetylcysteine showed no benefit in patients with COPD exacerbation [35]. Randomized controlled studies of methylxanthines exhibited significant adverse effects rather than therapeutic effects [36, 37]. Although intravenous magnesium plays a role in bronchodilation during asthma attack, magnesium inhalation failed to show any benefit for COPD exacerbations [38]. Chest physiotherapy with percussion, vibration and postural drainage have not yet demonstrated any benefit for COPD exacerbation [39], though some patients with bronchiectasis may have benefit.

Management of Exacerbations in Emergency Room

If a COPD patient visits emergency room with aggravation of respiratory symptoms, short-acting bronchodilator inhalation should be applied with or without oxygen supplementation. Other possible causes of symptom aggravation such as heart failure, pneumonia, or pulmonary thromboembolism should be excluded [5]. When COPD exacerbation is diagnosed, systemic corticosteroids could be prescribed. If the patient complains recent increase of sputum amount and/or purulence, antibiotic treatment should be given [40]. If the above management relieves symptoms and there is no hypoxemia at room air, the patient will be discharged with an appointment of outpatient clinic. Otherwise, hospitalization is mandatory. Particularly high requirement of supplemental oxygen and the presence of respiratory acidosis indicate the need of ventilator support.

Home Care of Exacerbations

While self-care strategies could relieve asthma symptoms during an asthma attack, COPD exacerbations usually need hospital care because hypoxemia is commonly accompanied and some patients need the other's help even during their stable period. Nevertheless, recent meta-analysis demonstrated that nurse-guided home care is one of effective and practical alternatives to admission in selected COPD patients with exacerbation without hypercarbic respiratory failure [41]. However, telemonitoring has not showed any benefits for COPD exacerbation [42–44].

References

1. Aaron SD. Management and prevention of exacerbations of COPD. BMJ. 2014;349:g5237.
2. Mackay AJ, Hurst JR. COPD exacerbations: causes, prevention, and treatment. Med Clin North Am. 2012;96(4):789–809.
3. Qureshi H, Sharafkhaneh A, Hanania NA. Chronic obstructive pulmonary disease exacerbations: latest evidence and clinical implications. Ther Adv Chronic Dis. 2014;5(5):212–27.
4. Dixit D, Bridgeman MB, Andrews LB, Narayanan N, Radbel J, Parikh A, et al. Acute exacerbations of chronic obstructive pulmonary disease: diagnosis, management, and prevention in critically ill patients. Pharmacotherapy. 2015;35(6):631–48.
5. Zvezdin B, Milutinov S, Kojicic M, Hadnadjev M, Hromis S, Markovic M, et al. A postmortem analysis of major causes of early death in patients hospitalized with COPD exacerbation. Chest. 2009;136(2):376–80.
6. Soler-Cataluna JJ, Martinez-Garcia MA, Roman Sanchez P, Salcedo E, Navarro M, Ochando R. Severe acute exacerbations and mortality in patients with chronic obstructive pulmonary disease. Thorax. 2005;60(11):925–31.
7. Bafadhel M, McKenna S, Terry S, Mistry V, Reid C, Haldar P, et al. Acute exacerbations of chronic obstructive pulmonary disease: identification of biologic clusters and their biomarkers. Am J Respir Crit Care Med. 2011;184(6):662–71.
8. Niewoehner DE, Lokhnygina Y, Rice K, Kuschner WG, Sharafkhaneh A, Sarosi GA, et al. Risk indexes for exacerbations and hospitalizations due to COPD. Chest. 2007;131(1):20–8.
9. Hurst JR, Vestbo J, Anzueto A, Locantore N, Mullerova H, Tal-Singer R, et al. Susceptibility to exacerbation in chronic obstructive pulmonary disease. N Engl J Med. 2010;363(12):1128–38.
10. Wells JM, Washko GR, Han MK, Abbas N, Nath H, Mamary AJ, et al. Pulmonary arterial enlargement and acute exacerbations of COPD. N Engl J Med. 2012;367(10):913–21.
11. Kim J, Lee JH, Kim Y, Kim K, Oh YM, Yoo KH, et al. Association between chronic obstructive pulmonary disease and gastroesophageal reflux disease: a national cross-sectional cohort study. BMC Pulm Med. 2013;13:51.
12. Martinez CH, Okajima Y, Murray S, Washko GR, Martinez FJ, Silverman EK, et al. Impact of self-

reported gastroesophageal reflux disease in subjects from COPDGene cohort. Respir Res. 2014;15:62.
13. Burgel PR, Nesme-Meyer P, Chanez P, Caillaud D, Carre P, Perez T, et al. Cough and sputum production are associated with frequent exacerbations and hospitalizations in COPD subjects. Chest. 2009;135(4):975–82.
14. Oh YM, Sheen SS, Park JH, Jin UR, Yoo JW, Seo JB, et al. Emphysematous phenotype is an independent predictor for frequent exacerbation of COPD. Int J Tuberc Lung Dis. 2014;18(12):1407–14.
15. Walters JA, Tan DJ, White CJ, Gibson PG, Wood-Baker R, Walters EH. Systemic corticosteroids for acute exacerbations of chronic obstructive pulmonary disease. Cochrane Database Syst Rev. 2014;9:CD001288.
16. Walters JA, Tan DJ, White CJ, Wood-Baker R. Different durations of corticosteroid therapy for exacerbations of chronic obstructive pulmonary disease. Cochrane Database Syst Rev. 2014;12:CD006897.
17. Woods JA, Wheeler JS, Finch CK, Pinner NA. Corticosteroids in the treatment of acute exacerbations of chronic obstructive pulmonary disease. Int J Chron Obstruct Pulmon Dis. 2014;9:421–30.
18. Gunen H, Hacievliyagil SS, Yetkin O, Gulbas G, Mutlu LC, In E. The role of nebulised budesonide in the treatment of exacerbations of COPD. Eur Respir J. 2007;29(4):660–7.
19. Abroug F, Ouanes I, Abroug S, Dachraoui F, Abdallah SB, Hammouda Z, et al. Systemic corticosteroids in acute exacerbation of COPD: a meta-analysis of controlled studies with emphasis on ICU patients. Ann Intensive Care. 2014;4:32.
20. Kiser TH, Allen RR, Valuck RJ, Moss M, Vandivier RW. Outcomes associated with corticosteroid dosage in critically ill patients with acute exacerbations of chronic obstructive pulmonary disease. Am J Respir Crit Care Med. 2014;189(9):1052–64.
21. Wilson R, Sethi S, Anzueto A, Miravitlles M. Antibiotics for treatment and prevention of exacerbations of chronic obstructive pulmonary disease. J Infect. 2013;67(6):497–515.
22. Vollenweider DJ, Jarrett H, Steurer-Stey CA, Garcia-Aymerich J, Puhan MA. Antibiotics for exacerbations of chronic obstructive pulmonary disease. Cochrane Database Syst Rev. 2012;12:CD010257.
23. Sethi S. Bacteria in exacerbations of chronic obstructive pulmonary disease: phenomenon or epiphenomenon? Proc Am Thorac Soc. 2004;1(2):109–14.
24. Gallego M, Pomares X, Espasa M, Castaner E, Sole M, Suarez D, et al. Pseudomonas Aeruginosa isolates in severe chronic obstructive pulmonary disease: characterization and risk factors. BMC Pulm Med. 2014;14:103.
25. Falagas ME, Avgeri SG, Matthaiou DK, Dimopoulos G, Siempos II. Short- versus long-duration antimicrobial treatment for exacerbations of chronic bronchitis: a meta-analysis. J Antimicrob Chemother. 2008;62(3):442–50.
26. Wesseling G. Occasional review: influenza in COPD: pathogenesis, prevention, and treatment. Int J Chron Obstruct Pulmon Dis. 2007;2(1):5–10.
27. Turner MO, Patel A, Ginsburg S, FitzGerald JM. Bronchodilator delivery in acute airflow obstruction. A meta-analysis. Arch Intern Med. 1997;157(15):1736–44.
28. Brill SE, Wedzicha JA. Oxygen therapy in acute exacerbations of chronic obstructive pulmonary disease. Int J Chron Obstruct Pulmon Dis. 2014;9:1241–52.
29. Spoletini G, Alotaibi M, Blasi F, Hill NS. Heated humidified high-flow nasal oxygen in adults: mechanisms of action and clinical implications. Chest. 2015;148(1):253–61.
30. Ramsay M, Hart N. Current opinions on non-invasive ventilation as a treatment for chronic obstructive pulmonary disease. Curr Opin Pulm Med. 2013;19(6):626–30.
31. White DP, Criner GJ, Dreher M, Hart N, Peyerl FW, Wolfe LF, et al. The role of noninvasive ventilation in the management and mitigation of exacerbations and hospital admissions/readmissions for the patient with moderate to severe COPD (multimedia activity). Chest. 2015;147(6):1704–5.
32. Cabrini L, Landoni G, Oriani A, Plumari VP, Nobile L, Greco M, et al. Noninvasive ventilation and survival in acute care settings: a comprehensive systematic review and metaanalysis of randomized controlled trials. Crit Care Med. 2015;43(4):880–8.
33. Ouanes I, Ouanes-Besbes L, Ben Abdallah S, Dachraoui F, Abroug F. Trends in use and impact on outcome of empiric antibiotic therapy and non-invasive ventilation in COPD patients with acute exacerbation. Ann Intensive Care. 2015;5(1):30.
34. Esteban A, Anzueto A, Frutos F, Alia I, Brochard L, Stewart TE, et al. Characteristics and outcomes in adult patients receiving mechanical ventilation: a 28-day international study. JAMA. 2002;287(3):345–55.
35. Black PN, Morgan-Day A, McMillan TE, Poole PJ, Young RP. Randomised, controlled trial of N-acetylcysteine for treatment of acute exacerbations of chronic obstructive pulmonary disease [ISRCTN21676344]. BMC Pulm Med. 2004;4:13.
36. Barr RG, Rowe BH, Camargo CA Jr. Methylxanthines for exacerbations of chronic obstructive pulmonary disease: meta-analysis of randomised trials. BMJ. 2003;327(7416):643.
37. Duffy N, Walker P, Diamantea F, Calverley PM, Davies L. Intravenous aminophylline in patients admitted to hospital with non-acidotic exacerbations of chronic obstructive pulmonary disease: a prospective randomised controlled trial. Thorax. 2005;60(9):713–7.
38. Edwards L, Shirtcliffe P, Wadsworth K, Healy B, Jefferies S, Weatherall M, et al. Use of nebulised magnesium sulphate as an adjuvant in the treatment of acute exacerbations of COPD in adults: a randomised double-blind placebo-controlled trial. Thorax. 2013;68(4):338–43.
39. Bach PB, Brown C, Gelfand SE, McCrory DC, American College of Physicians-American Society of Internal M, American College of Chest P. Management of acute exacerbations of chronic obstructive pulmo-

nary disease: a summary and appraisal of published evidence. Ann Intern Med. 2001;134(7):600–20.
40. Anthonisen NR, Manfreda J, Warren CP, Hershfield ES, Harding GK, Nelson NA. Antibiotic therapy in exacerbations of chronic obstructive pulmonary disease. Ann Intern Med. 1987;106(2):196–204.
41. Jeppesen E, Brurberg KG, Vist GE, Wedzicha JA, Wright JJ, Greenstone M, et al. Hospital at home for acute exacerbations of chronic obstructive pulmonary disease. Cochrane Database Syst Rev. 2012;5:CD003573.
42. Cartwright M, Hirani SP, Rixon L, Beynon M, Doll H, Bower P, et al. Effect of telehealth on quality of life and psychological outcomes over 12 months (whole systems demonstrator telehealth questionnaire study): nested study of patient reported outcomes in a pragmatic, cluster randomised controlled trial. BMJ. 2013;346:f653.
43. Henderson C, Knapp M, Fernandez JL, Beecham J, Hirani SP, Cartwright M, et al. Cost effectiveness of telehealth for patients with long term conditions (whole systems demonstrator telehealth questionnaire study): nested economic evaluation in a pragmatic, cluster randomised controlled trial. BMJ. 2013;346:f1035.
44. Pinnock H, Hanley J, McCloughan L, Todd A, Krishan A, Lewis S, et al. Effectiveness of telemonitoring integrated into existing clinical services on hospital admission for exacerbation of chronic obstructive pulmonary disease: researcher blind, multicentre, randomised controlled trial. BMJ. 2013;347:f6070.

Comorbidities: Assessment and Treatment

19

Nurdan Kokturk, Ayse Baha, and Nese Dursunoglu

Introduction

COPD is an umbrella term that is associated with several systemic manifestation, lung involvement, and comorbidities [1, 2]. Currently, the description of comorbidity is complicated and has three different domains: "(1) the coexistence of one or more diseases with no other causation, (2) coexistence of diseases that share common risk factors and pathogenic pathways, (3) coexistence of diseases that are complicated by the interaction with the lung and systemic manifestation of COPD" [3]. In a very recent study, BODE Investigator Group suggested that COPD is interlinked with several comorbidities larger than non-COPD controls indicating common pathobiological process [4]. The importance of comorbidities is their impact on clinical outcomes of a patient life. COPD is a life-threatening and disabling disease and comorbidities cause additional impact revealing impairment in quality of life and increasing mortality [3].

N. Kokturk, M.D. (✉)
Department of Pulmonary Medicine, School of Medicine, Gazi University, Ankara, Turkey
e-mail: kokturk.nurdan@gmail.com

A. Baha, M.D.
Department of Pulmonary Medicine, Ufuk University Faculty of Medicine, Ankara, Turkey
e-mail: dr_aysedemir@hotmail.com

N. Dursunoglu, M.D.
Department of Pulmonary Medicine, School of Medicine, Pamukkale University, Denizli, Turkey
e-mail: ndursunoglu@yahoo.com

COPD patients have higher number of comorbidities (3.7) than controls (1.8). Studies showed that 94% of COPD patients had at least one comorbidity and up to 46% had three or more comorbidities [3]. Comorbidities have significant impact on health status, health care utilization, readmission, and mortality [1, 5, 6]. The National Health and Nutrition Examination Survey (NHANES I) study showed that each increase in comorbidities is associated with 43% higher chance of worse self-rated quality of life [7]. They increase the use of health care resources, the risk of readmission and mortality. Gastroesophageal reflux disease (GERD), depression, anxiety, cardiovascular disease, and pulmonary embolism are associated with exacerbations [6, 8]. Comorbidities have significant impact of clinical outcomes of exacerbations, hospitalization numbers, and the length of stay [6, 9, 10]. Studies showed that the presence of three or more comorbidities was a better predictor of impaired health status than any other demographic or clinical variable [3]. The impact of comorbidities in exacerbations whether they mimic exacerbations or they precipitate the intensity of exacerbation is still a matter of debate [6]. Comorbidities increase economic burden in COPD. The direct costs have escalated from 18 billion dollars in 2002 to 29.5 billons in 2010, the largest part consisting of hospital expenses [3]. Most of the annual direct costs of COPD are associated with comorbidities [3]. According to a recent trial, the chronic kidney disease and the anemia had greater impact on

S.-D. Lee (ed.), *COPD*, DOI 10.1007/978-3-662-47178-4_19

health care cost [11]. Comorbidities are not only related with hospitalization. COPD patients use approximately 50% more cardiovascular agents than age-matched and sex-matched controls, and almost twice as many antibiotics, analgesics, and psychotherapeutic medications [3, 12].

Finally, comorbidities are related with higher mortality. In our cohort of severe COPD, Charlson comorbidity index and lung cancer are related with mortality [9]. Toward a Revolution in COPD Health (TORCH) and Understanding Potential Long-term Impacts on Function with Tiotropium (UPLIFT) studies showed that the almost 70% of causes of deaths in COPD were non-respiratory. The major non-respiratory reasons of death were cancer and cardiovascular diseases particularly in mild-to-moderate disease [13–16]. The numbers of comorbidities are related with mortality [9, 16]. The mortality was 2.2-fold increased for patients with 4 and higher points of COPD Specific Comorbidity Test (COTE) index [17].

The most common comorbidities associated with COPD are hyperlipidemia, hypertension, ischemic heart disease, diabetes, skeletal muscle wasting, cachexia, osteoporosis, depression, and lung cancer [1, 2]. Recently, COTE index and COMCOLD (Comorbidities in Chronic Obstructive Lung Disease) are designed to address comorbidities that impacted in morbidity and mortality in COPD [17, 18].

The frequent coexistence of those diseases suggests that they might have common mechanistic pathways or shared risk factors such as smoking, reduced physical activities, and ageing [2]. One of the suggested underlying mechanisms is shared systemic inflammation. The systemic inflammation could arise from smoking, other risk factors, or ageing itself. Ageing is related with comorbidities better than forced expiratory flow rate in one second (FEV_1) itself [19].

Some of the causal mechanisms are attributed to systemic effects of COPD [16]. Accordingly, COPD can cause a systemic inflammation so called "spill-over inflammation" and other diseases may develop triggered by that inflammation [1]. Comorbidities are important because they might be the reason of actual mortality, may result in difficulties in controlling COPD and sometimes they might be the actual problem underlying exacerbation. Some comorbidities, i.e., lung cancer, depression, anxiety, and pulmonary embolism, could be easily overlooked under the condition of uncontrolled COPD. The quality of life and the risk of mortality could be increased due to somehow manageable conditions [1] and should be actively searched and aggressively treated according to their own treatment strategies [1].

COPD medication may also contribute to the development and worsening of comorbidities [3]. Bronchodilators could contribute cardiovascular morbidity such as arrhythmias and tremor. Anticholinergics can affect intraocular pressure and bladder functions. Inhaled steroids may increase the risk of cataracts, skin bruising, osteoporosis, and pneumonia. Systemic steroids can contribute to diabetes, hypertension, osteoporosis, muscle dysfunction, and adrenal insufficiency [3].

However, important data are lacking regarding comorbidities. There is no convincing evidence to suggest that treatment of COPD would reduce comorbidities, the treatment of comorbidities improves COPD and that the presence of COPD alters the treatment modalities of comorbidities. Large-scale prospective studies are needed to address those clinical questions. The best suggested approach in reduction of comorbidities in COPD is reduction of common risk factors. Whether reduction of so-called spill-over inflammation with anti-inflammatory treatment of COPD would also reduce COPD-related comorbidities is still doubtful [5].

Herein we categorized the frequent comorbidities that were described as if the prevalence was greater than 5% in COPD population (Table 19.1) [6].

Table 19.1 Summary of frequent and important comorbidities in COPD [6]

Comorbidity	Prevalence %	Shared risk factors
Respiratory system		
Asthma	20	Small airway obstruction, inflammation
Lung cancer	15–20	Systemic inflammation (NF-KB)
Pulmonary fibrosis	6	Systemic inflammation
PHT	10–91	Hypoxia, endothelial dysfunction, pulmonary arterial dysfunction
Endocrine system		
DM	10–19	Corticosteroid use, systemic inflammation, insülin resistance
Obesity	16–24	Hormones, systemic inflammation
Metabolic syndrome	25–57	Systemic inflammation, insülin resistance
Vitamin D deficiency	60	Aging, low food intake, corticosteroid use, immobilization
Musculoskeletal system		
Muscle dysfunction	36	Low physical activity, corticosteroid use, hypoxia, hypercapnia, inflammation, smoking
Osteoporosis	4–59	Corticosteroid use, systemic inflammation, vitamin D deficiency
Cardiovascular system		
IHD	16–53	Systemic inflammation, vascular endothelial dysfunction
HF	20–32	Systemic inflammation, dynamic hyperinflation
Systemic hypertension	40–60	Loss connective tissue, high arterial stiffness, aging
VTE	3–29	Endothelial dysfunction, immobilization, coagulopathy
Gastrointestinal system		
GERD	7.7–30	Decrease low esophageal sphincter relaxations
Malnutrition	10–15	Nutritional imbalance, systemic inflammation
Sleep disorders		
Overlap syndrome	0.5–3	Obesity, systemic inflammation
Hematologic system		
Anemia	7.5–33	Renal impairment, malnutrition, low testosterone levels, growth hormone level abnormalities
Urinary system		
CKD	16–39	
Anxiety-depression	8–80	Immobilization, hypoxia, increased number of comorbidities, poor quality of life, living alone

NK-KB nuclear factor KB, *PHT* pulmonary hypertension, *DM* diabetes mellitus, *IHD* ischemic heart disease, *HF* heart failure, *VTE* venous thromboembolism, *CKD* chronic kidney disease.

COPD and Respiratory System

Asthma

Asthma COPD Overlap (ACOS) has a prevalence of 20% of patients with obstructive lung diseases (asthma or COPD) and 2% in general population. The coexistence of both diseases causes significant impairment in health status, increased exacerbation, and increased hospitalization. Treatment should cover both inhaled steroids and bronchodilators in ACOS patients. There is limited evidence for treatment recommendation because ACOS patients are excluded from randomized controlled trials [20]. The detailed information of ACOS has been covered elsewhere in this textbook.

Lung Cancer

Both COPD and lung cancer have developed in 15–20% of chronic smokers and expected to increase in prevalence and mortality to 2030 [21, 22]. Although ageing, smoking, and family history have been identified as key risk factors, host susceptibility has been indicated in both diseases. The question of whether COPD and lung cancer are linked independent of shared risk factors has been investigated for more than a decade. The first National Health and Nutrition Examination Survey (NHANES I) showed that moderate to severe airway obstruction increased the risk of lung cancer (Hazard Ratio: 2.8) [23]. Later studies showed that both emphysema and airflow obstruction are related with increased lung cancer incidence after adjusting for potential confounders [23–25]. Data have shown that COPD prevalence in a population of lung cancer is 9% up to 50% [17, 26]. COPD prevalence in newly diagnosed lung cancer patients was found to be sixfold greater than in matched smokers [26]. The major impact of lung cancer in COPD is management difficulties and increased mortality [3, 9]. Vice versa COPD has impact on lung cancer in a similar manner with limiting the chance of surgery, increasing postoperative complications and finally increasing the chance of mortality [3, 6, 27].

The underlying mechanisms under COPD and lung cancer are very complex. Genetic factors, ageing, epigenetic mutations, and common inflammatory mechanisms have been identified [5, 22, 28]. Recent advances in genetic epidemiology demonstrate several number of loci are overlapping both in COPD and lung cancer. CHRNA 3/5 (Chr15q25) and FAM13A are among them [22]. Those data have raised two important questions: (1) Do COPD patients or emphysema patients need early screening for lung cancer detection and (2) Is there any place for a genetic-based risk stratification of smokers that might help better targeted therapy, prevention, and early diagnosis? The answer is probably YES for both questions [22, 29]. Supporting that concept, in a posthoc analysis of National Lung Screening Trial, in a subgroup of screened patients who demonstrate airflow limitation, the risk of lung cancer increased twofold, the overdiagnosis was minimal, and they had stage shift favorable for screening [30]. New screening risk models including the information about COPD is under validation [31].

Pulmonary Fibrosis

The association of combined pulmonary fibrosis and emphysema (CPFE) was first described as a syndrome by Cottin in 2005 as upper lobe emphysema, lower lobe fibrosis, subnormal lung volume and diminished carbon monoxide diffusion capacity (DLCO) and high prevalence of pulmonary hypertension [32]. The combined appearance was first interpreted as a coincidence of two smoking-related diseases; however, in reality, most idiopathic pulmonary fibrosis (IPF) patients do not have emphysema and most COPD patients do not show overt fibrosis either. Therefore the actual pathobiology would be different from what it was historically though and might indicate an individual susceptibility [33].

The prevalence of pulmonary fibrosis has found to be 6.1% in 1664 COPD patients in a recent landmark study performed by BODE group [17]. Pulmonary fibrosis was found to be related with higher mortality (HR: 1.51, CI 95% (1.13–2.03)) [17]. The prevalence of detectable CPFE patients in IPF patients are varied depending on methodology (8–51%) [34].

The patients have heavy smoking history. Telomerase abnormalities can be considered to explain genetic susceptibility [34]. The symptoms of CPFE are more likely to resemble IPF showing progressive dyspnea and dry cough [34]. Paraseptal emphysema is typical for CPFE [32, 34]. Thick walled cystic lesions, lower lobe fibrosis, honeycombing, and traction bronchiectasis are common imaging findings [34]. In respect to associated findings, emphysema is more extended in CPFE patients than IPF patients. The difference of fibrosis scores between CPFE and IPF is controversial [34].

Those patients have higher risk of pulmonary hypertension. The pulmonary hypertension prevalence was reported as 47–90%. Likewise, lung cancer has been detected with a prevalence of 35.8–46.8% indicating higher prevalence than either COPD or IPF [34]. Both pulmonary hypertension and lung cancer have contributed to worse prognosis of CPFE [34].

Treatment of CPFE

There is no specific therapy for CPFE. Patients should be treated as either disease alone. Hypoxemia should be corrected by long-term oxygen therapy. Bronchodilation could be an option for CPFE patients with airflow obstruction. It is currently unknown whether pirfenidone or nintedanib is efficacious in CPFE [34]. Lung transplantation is the only therapeutic option [6].

Chronic Kidney Disease (CKD)

The prevalence of CKD has been shown as 16.7, 22.2, and 39% in different COPD cohorts [17, 35, 36]. The risk of renal diseases is greater in COPD group than non-COPD control groups [37]. Chronic renal failure may exist with the normal serum creatinine level in COPD [3, 35]. The arterial stiffness and endothelial dysfunction could lead to a renal dysfunction [3]. In NHANES III study, all cause of mortality was associated with albumin/creatinine ratio and estimated GFR [38]. CKD has also impact on treatment of COPD and its complications [3, 6].

Treatment: CKD in COPD is treated as the same for patients without COPD [1].

COPD and Endocrinology and Metabolism

Weight loss and muscle wasting are present in 20% of stable COPD patients. This reaches to 40% for patients with respiratory failure and 70% of patients requiring mechanical ventilation [39]. There is a decrease in fat-free mass with decrease in muscle mass (sarcopenia). The muscle mass is influenced by inflammatory cytokines, mechanical load on the muscles, and anabolic axes. There are four anabolic axes: somatotropic, gonadal, adrenal, and insulin [39].

COPD and Somatotropic Axis

The major component of somatotropic axis is growth hormone (GH) and insulin-like growth factor (IGF-I). IGF-I stimulates muscle protein synthesis and hypertrophy and inhibits protein catabolism [39]. Aging, malnutrition, inactivity, and administration of glucocorticoids are associated with downregulation of the GH/IGF-I system; however, hypoxemia and hypercapnia may result in an increased level of GH/IGF-I levels. Depressed level of IGF-I in COPD may contribute to the decreased muscle mass in COPD; however, resistance to GH or ghrelin action may also be the case in cachexia in COPD.

Treatment: The administration of recombinant human GH has produced conflicting results. There are important questions on selection criteria, monitoring and safety of the studies of recombinant GH/IGF-I supplementation in COPD [39].

COPD and Gonadal Axis

Gonadal axis is a complex network of hormones that includes testosterone and other anabolic hormones. In both men and women, testosterone is responsible for libido, sexual hair, and muscle and bone health. The level of testosterone and its precursor adrenal steroid dehydroepiandrosterone (DHEA) is declined with advanced age. That is called "late-onset hypogonadism" and it accompanies with decreased energy level, libido, bone density, and muscle mass. The research in that field is more focused on men; however, women have similar declined level of androgens [39].

Ageing, chronic comorbidities, hypoxemia, hypercapnia, smoking, administration of glucocorticoids, systemic inflammation, and obesity are the risk factors of late-onset hypogonadism in COPD. The prevalence of late-onset hypogonadism in normal population is about 3% and in COPD is reported between 22 and 69%. Different results may be due to different sample size and population [39]. Studies did not find a relation between testosterone level and sexual difficulties, health quality surveys, and respiratory muscle performance. In some studies, low level of testosterone has found to be related with a decrease in quadriceps strength and testosterone administration has caused an increase in strength. However, there are also negative studies and the doses and the duration of testosterone administration is not known. Current studies have not shown a difference in exercise performance in hypogonadal and eugonadal COPD patients. Testosterone administration has not made any improvement in exercise performance [39].

Diagnosis: The late-onset hypogonadism should be searched when patients concern about erectile dysfunction and other related symptoms. When it happens the repetitive testosterone levels are measured and should be lower than 8 nmol/L or in borderline level (8–11 nmol/L) in order to initiate advance evaluation [41]. ANDROTEST is designed for the purpose of diagnosis showing a sensitivity and specificity close to 70% in detecting low total or free testosterone [40].

Treatment: Testosterone therapy should be considered for sexual dysfunction regardless with COPD. However, it is not known that the symptoms are related with normal aging or related with low testesteron [40]. Although hypogonadism is related with obesity, metabolic syndrome and diabetes Type 2, hypertension and cardiovascular disease, testesteron should not be offered for potential additional benefits regarding muscle functions and insulin resistance, if there is no symptoms of sexual dysfunction [41]. We do not know now if there is a causal relationship with low testosterone with those conditions or low testosterone is basically a result of those conditions. For instance, studies showed that losing weight resulted in an increase in serum testosterone levels [42]. There is no clear indication for administration of testosterone in COPD. Testesteron replacement can be related with potential obstacles. The absolute contraindication for testosterone replacement includes prostate and breast carcinoma. The relative contraindications are serum prostate specific antigen >4 ng/mL, a hematocrit >50%, severe lower urinary tract symptoms caused by benign prostatic hypertrophy, untreated or poorly controlled congestive heart failure, and untreated sleep apnea [41]. Late-onset hypogonadism is underdiagnosed, under researched area. Further large randomized studies are needed.

COPD and Adrenal Axis

The adrenal gland produces a vast array of hormones: cortisol, DHEA and its metabolite, DHEAS. The high levels of cortisol/DHEA or cortisol/DHEAS ratios are thought to create an imbalance between protein synthesis and degradation favoring catabolism. Cortisol mobilizes glucose, free fatty acids, and amino acid; increases appetite; and induces insulin resistance. Studies found that DHEAS levels are lower in COPD patients than in controls. There is no data regarding cortisol levels are altered in COPD [40, 41]. However, it is known that systemic steroids and high dose inhaled steroids increase the risk of adrenal insufficiency. Neither glucocorticoid dose nor duration of treatment can be used to predict adrenal insufficiency [43].

In COPD, the cortisol/DHEAS ratio was greater among patients with reduced muscle mass. On the other hand, administration of DHEA had no effect on body composition, muscle strength or quality of life, and bone mineral density in people without COPD [43].

Treatment: There is no evidence that DHEA administration has a significant benefit in COPD [40–42].

Diabetes Mellitus

Insulin is an anabolic hormone that exerts its action binding to its receptors throughout the body including lung, liver, and skeletal muscle. Insulin improves hypoxia-induced vasoconstriction and causes pulmonary artery vasodilation [39].

Diabetes Mellitus (DM) can result from destruction of pancreatic beta cells. There is insulin deficiency (type 1) and insulin resistance (type 2) in patients with diabetes.

The prevalence of diabetes in patients with COPD is 10–18.7% [39]. The relation between impaired pulmonary function and the risk of diabetes is controversial. In the Framingham Heart Study and NHANES study, there was no association between COPD and the development of diabetes [39]. However, other studies showed contrasting results. In a large nationwide twin cohort in Denmark, patients with chronic bronchitis and COPD had an increased risk of type 2 diabetes after adjusting for age, sex, smoking, and body mass index (BMI) (OR: 1.57 for chronic bronchitis or OR: 2.62 for COPD). The prevalence of type 2 diabetes in COPD group was 6.6% while it was 2.3% in non-COPD control group [44]. In a Women's Health Study, 38,570 women were followed for 12.2 years; during follow-up, 2472 incident type 2 diabetes events were accounted and asthma or COPD was found to be associated with diabetes (RR: 1.37 for asthma and 1.38 for COPD) [45]. In a primary care setting, analyzing the primary care records of 1,204,100 individuals, the physician diagnosed COPD has increased the risk of new onset type 2 DM [46].

Glucose metabolism is more disturbed in COPD patients than non-COPD patients. The etiology behind this phenomenon is not known well. However, shared risk factors and common inflammatory pathophysiology could be reason behind it. Advanced age, hereditary factors, smoking, and low birth weight are the shared risk factors of both diabetes and COPD [47].

Obesity and Adipose Tissue

Obesity is one of the major risk factors of new onset type 2 diabetes and metabolic syndrome. Obesity could be associated with decreased respiratory volumes. In addition to this, central obesity can enhance systemic inflammatory cytokines such as interleukin-6 (IL-6) and tumor necrosis factor α (TNF-α). Obesity is also associated with reduced adiponectin which has anti-inflammatory properties [47].

Abdominal obesity is more prevalent in mild-to-moderate COPD (16–24%) than severe disease (6%) and that is associated with airflow obstruction independently from smoking [48, 49]. In a study performed in California, 54% of the COPD patients were obese (BMI > 30 kg/m^2) and this rate was higher than the general population. Obesity was more associated with chronic bronchitis than emphysema [50, 51]. On the other hand, low BMI is considered a worse prognostic marker and related with all cause of mortality [52]. However, low BMI seen in advanced COPD is a result of loss of fat-free mass and pathophysiologically similar to cancer cachexia [47]. Supporting these results, another study showed that low BMI was associated with greater mortality compared with normal or high BMI. The loss of three BMI units was associated with increase in all cause of mortality in controls and COPD groups, whereas weight gain was associated with increased mortality only in controls [53]. In a Korean cohort, increased BMI is related with mortality from cardiovascular disease [54]. However in a European cohort, low BMI is related with increased mortality [55]. It seems that in early stages of COPD, obesity is accompanied with cardiovascular disease and insulin resistance leading mortality and in the severe stages the obesity is a protective effect for mortality [56]. It is called obesity paradox and the pathogenesis behind it is not known. Future studies are needed to explain "obesity paradox." Fat-free mass loss could be an explanation behind low BMI seen more in emphysema related with higher mortality [47].

Adipose tissue is an active endocrine organ producing several substances. Leptin and adiponectin are more studied [47, 57, 58]. Resistin may contribute to the dysglycemia and insulin resistance in COPD [59]. More studies are needed if there is a true mechanistic interaction between those markers and COPD [47].

Systemic Inflammation and Oxidative Stress

Both COPD and type 2 diabetes are related with both enhanced oxidative stress and systemic inflammation. TNF-alpha, IL-6, IL-1B, CRP, and fibrinogen are most studied [47].

Hypoxia could have contribution on COPD. Pancreatic B cells may be damaged by hypoxia. The pathophysiology could be mediated by hypoxia inducible factor 1 family (HIF). Hypoxia-mediated increase in HIF-1alpha can induce adipose tissue fibrosis and resistance to insulin at the level of skeletal muscle [47].

Moreover, COPD is associated with hypogonadism, increased catecholamines, and RAAS (renin–angiotensin–aldosterone systems) and they all related with glucose metabolism [47].

The Impact of DM Type 2 in COPD

DM has impact on pulmonary vasculature leading to pulmonary microangiopathy showing detrimental effect on alveolar capillary bed. That results in reduced diffusion capacity of carbon monoxide [60]. Studies showed that DM-related nephropathy is significantly associated with the presence of pulmonary capillary dysfunction [47].

DM is associated with the development of muscle dysfunction. Diaphragm could be targeted by DM which could be probably mediated by phrenic neuropathy [47]. In Copenhagen City Study, Framingham Heart Study, and Fremantle studies, subjects with DM had lower values of FEV_1 and forced vital capacity (FVC) [61–63]. In Fremantle study, DM is associated with greater lung decline and DM-related airflow limitation was associated with increased mortality [63]. In Normative Aging Study, DM is not associated with accelerated decline of lung function [64].

DM also associated with increased risk of exacerbations. DM-associated inflammation can cause increase risk of pro-inflammatory state that can increase the risk of exacerbation. The systemic glucocorticosteroids are used in exacerbation and that can induce diabetes. Glucocorticosteroids can cause hyperglycemia by increasing gluconeogenesis in the liver and decreasing glucose uptake in the liver and adipose tissue [65]. The estimated DM prevalence among chronic systemic CS user is about 11% within 3 years following treatment [66]. There is evidence that particularly high dose inhaled steroids can increase the risk of type 2 diabetes and can worsen the glycemic control [65, 67].

DM associated the increased risk of infections. Hyperglycemia may particularly increase the risk of methicillin resistant *Staphylococcus aureus* (MRSA). Hyperglycemia is related with increased morbidity and mortality in COPD exacerbation [68]. Comorbid DM prolongs length of stay and increases risk of death in patients with COPD exacerbations (AECOPD) [69, 70].

The Impact on DM Therapies in COPD

The goal of diabetic care is to achieve glucose levels close to normal levels [39]. Patients should be cared as standard DM patients in achieving this goal [1, 71]. Inhaled steroids in diabetic patients with COPD are conflicting. The studies showed that systemic insulin therapy may be beneficial for DLCO. Oral antidiabetics such as metformin or thiazolidinedione improve FVC that was thought to be due to improved respiratory muscle function [47]. Moreover, metformin has some antitumor effects [47]. Metformin is thought to increase the risk of lactic acidosis, and is considered contraindication for chronic hypoxemic conditions. However, recent studies showed no significant acidosis in metformin users [72].

COPD and Metabolic Syndrome

Metabolic syndrome is defined as several criteria (Table.19.2) [73]. These criteria are given as an indirect measurement of insulin resistance. The direct measurement of insulin is less established in the routine clinic [73]. Homeostasis Model Assessment of Insulin Resistance (HOMA-IR) is the most widely used. It requires measurement of fasting plasma glucose and insulin levels [73].

The prevalence of metabolic syndrome is reported to be 25, 42.9–57% [74–76]. It seems that metabolic syndrome accompanied milder COPD than severe disease [76]. The impact of metabolic syndrome in COPD is not well studied. However, studies showed that COPD patients with metabolic syndrome have more complaints

Table 19.2 Metabolic syndrome definition criteria [73]

	NCEP ATP III	IDF
	3 out of 5	Waist +2 out of 4
Waist circumference		
Males	≥102 cm	≥94
Females	≥88 cm	≥80
Fasting glucose[a,b]	≥5.6 mmol/L	≥5.6 mmol/L
High-density lipoproteins[b]		
Males	<1 mmol/L	<1 mmol/L
Females	<1.3 mmol/L	<1.3 mmol/L
Triglycerides	≥1.7 mmol/L	≥1.7 mmol/L
Blood pressure	≥130/85 mmHg	≥130/85 mmHg

NCEP ATP III national cholesterol education program adult treatment panel III, *IDF* international diabetes federation
[a]Either above cutoff or established diabetes mellitus or specific treatment
[b]Either above cutoff or specific treatment

and more comorbidities [75, 76]. The cardiovascular mortality seen in mild COPD could be related with metabolic syndrome [73].

Treatment: Reducing weight, exercise, testesteron, and insulin sensitizers are beneficial in metabolic syndrome. However, there is no specific guideline for the treatment of comorbidities including metabolic syndrome with COPD [73]. It should be treated according to the endocrinological principals [77].

COPD and Thyroid Disease

The thyroid hormones regulate the metabolism of proteins, lipids, and carbohydrates, and increase the metabolic rate as a result of respiratory drive. Limited data are available on thyroid disease and COPD. The prevalence of thyroidal disease in COPD is not known [39].

COPD and Hypothyroidism

Impaired thyroid function can present as subclinical hypothyroidism, manifest hypothyroidism, and nonthyroidal illness syndrome. Nonthyroidal illness syndrome is described as low T3, decreased or normal T4, and normal TSH. This was called as euthyroid sick syndrome in the past but that nomenclature is abandoned now. Severe obstruction, hypoxemia, systemic glucocorticosteroid usage, and systemic inflammation can be the etiology behind hypothyroidism. When present hypothyroidism can decrease respiratory drive, respiratory muscle function, exercise capacity and increase the risk for sleep disorder.

Treatment: Hypothyroidism in patients with COPD should be treated in the same manner as in patients without COPD [39, 78].

COPD and Hyperthyroidism

Hyperthyroidism may impair respiratory muscle function, respiratory mechanics, and exercise capacity. As a result, inspiratory and expiratory muscle weakness, decreased lung compliance, and respiratory failure can occur [39].

Treatment: Hyperthyroidism in patients with COPD should be treated in the same manner as in patients without COPD [78].

COPD and Renin–Angiotensin–Aldosterone System

Patients with COPD can develop fluid retention when stable or during exacerbation. Right heart pressure can be normal or increased. Traditionally, volume overload is thought to be caused by right ventricular failure caused by hypoxia-induced pulmonary vasoconstriction. Growing evidence suggests that renal vasoconstriction is central in the fluid retention and that can be triggered by hypercapnia. Development of sodium and water retention in COPD implies poor prognosis [39].

Treatment: Although the renin–angiotensin–aldosterone system has been studied for more than 30 years in COPD, few investigations have assessed aiming to reduce fluid retention. Postponing diuretics as long as possible can be one approach because diuretics can aggravate sodium and water retention by several mechanisms. Some authors suggest the use of angiotensin-converting enzyme inhibitors for increasing sodium excretion. However, the results are inconsistent in different studies [39].

COPD and Vitamin D

Vitamin D has long been known as essential for musculoskeletal health. However, more recently there has been increased interest in vitamin D regarding its potential noncalcemic effects and its relationship with chronic disease, particularly COPD, since vitamin D hypovitaminosis is a common status throughout the world including socioeconomically underdeveloped and developed countries [79]. There has been interest in a possible link between vitamin D hypovitaminosis and COPD pathogenesis, progression, exacerbations and associated comorbidities.

Vitamin D synthesized in skin under the effect of UV light. It is converted to active form in kidney. Vitamin D regulates calcium and phosphorus metabolism. The desired vitamin D level is above 30 ng/mL. Vitamin D deficiency is described as if the 25(OH) vitamin D level is under 20 ng/mL. Insufficiency is between 20 and 29 ng/mL [80]. The noncalcemic effects are expected with higher levels.

An age-matched controlled study showed that COPD patients had significantly lower vitamin D levels when compared to controls, which might suggest that COPD patients have a higher risk of vitamin D deficiency [81].

COPD itself may comprise additional risks for vitamin D deficiency due to the fact that low food intake, aging, staying indoors, increased vitamin D catabolism due to glucocorticosteroids, impaired activation by renal dysfunction, lower storage capacity in muscles or fat tissues due to wasting [81, 82].

Vitamin D deficiency is related with osteoporosis, muscle weakness, infection, and cardiovascular events in COPD. Several studies showed that vitamin D deficiency is related with COPD onset, COPD progression and exacerbation.

Treatment: Direct sun exposure without sunscreen is needed for skin to produce vitamin D3. The recent Endocrinology Guideline in vitamin D deficiency recommends that adults above age 50 require daily 600–800 IU vitamin D for bone and muscle health. However, in order to raise blood vitamin D level over 30 mg/dL 1500–2000 IU/d vitamin D will be needed [80].

The guideline suggests that all vitamin D deficient adults should be treated with 50,000 IU of vitamin D2 or vitamin D3 once a week for 8 weeks or its equivalent of 6000 IU of vitamin D2 or vitamin D3 daily to achieve a blood level of 25(OH)D above 30 ng/mL, followed by maintenance therapy of 1500–2000 IU/day. Higher doses are needed in obese patients and patients with malabsorption syndromes. The serum vitamin D level should not exceed 100 ng/mL. There is no clear evidence to recommend higher dose Vitamin D supplementation for noncalcemic benefits in COPD [80].

COPD and Musculoskeletal Functions

COPD and Muscle Dysfunction

Skeletal muscle dysfunction is an important systemic consequence of COPD because of its impact on physical activity, exercise tolerance, quality of life, and survival on the disease [83]. Skeletal muscle function is described by muscle strength (the ability to generate force production), muscle endurance (the ability to sustain a given contraction over time), and muscle fatigue (a physiological sense defined as the failure of force generation resulting from activity under load). Skeletal muscle weakness is characterized by reduced muscle strength, reduced muscle endurance, and the presence of muscle fatigue [84]. Muscle weakness is mainly observed in the lower limb muscle of patients with COPD.

Lower limb muscle weakness is found to be more severe in patients with cachexia and worsens during exacerbations [85–87]. In lower limb muscles, several adaptations develop with COPD; these include muscle fiber type shift from type I towards type IIx muscle fibers resulting in reduced oxidative and increased glycolytic capacity, fiber atrophy, loss of muscle mass, and decreased capillary density [88]. Importantly, reduced quadriceps strength is found to be a useful predictor for mortality in patients with COPD [89] and the quadriceps muscle weakness is a common feature in patients within all stages of COPD [84, 90].

Reduced quadriceps strength in COPD is associated with reduced exercise capacity [91, 92], compromised health status [93], increased need for health care resources [94], and mortality independent of airflow obstruction [88].

Eighteen to 36% of COPD patients present with net detriment of muscle mass, which is responsible for weight loss in 17–35% of these patients [95]. The estimated overall prevalence of skeletal muscle weakness in patients was shown to be 20–30% [84, 96]. Although skeletal muscle weakness is a feature of cachexia, quadriceps weakness in COPD is not simply an epiphenomenon; indeed, weakness is frequent with a ratio of approximately 2:1 compared with loss of fat-free mass [90].

Seymour et al. have demonstrated that a significant proportion of patients in GOLD stages 1 and 2, or with an MRC dyspnea score of 1 and 2, had quadriceps weakness (28% and 26%, respectively); these values rose to 38% in GOLD stage 4, and 43% in patients with an MRC score of 4 and 5 [97].

The physiopathological interaction between COPD and alterations in limb muscle tissue is still poorly understood. Several factors, such as smoking, corticosteroids, hypoxia, hypercapnia, inflammation, oxidative stress, reduced daily physical activity, vitamin D deficiency, and nutritional deficits, have been proposed to explain the initiation and the progression of muscle dysfunction in COPD [84].

Etiology

Smoking: Smoking was shown to be related to decreased skeletal muscle strength and physical performance in healthy adults [98, 99]. In healthy smokers and patients with COPD, cigarette smoke was shown to induce muscle atrophy, reduce muscle protein synthesis, induce oxidative modifications on muscle proteins [100], and increase the expression of genes involved in muscle catabolism and associated with inhibition of muscle growth [101].

Corticosteroid use: Corticosteroids are frequently used in patients with COPD to reduce pulmonary symptoms and to treat exacerbations [102]. Although a short course of systemic corticosteroids may not alter limb muscle function in COPD [103], these anti-inflammatory agents have a trophism for the muscles, and their chronic or repeated use can potentiate muscle atrophy and weakness in patients with COPD [104]. Morphological changes have been reported in the quadriceps in patients with COPD presenting with a corticosteroids-related myopathy [105].

Hypoxia: Hypoxia may contribute to muscle wasting in COPD by a variety of mechanisms, including reduced anabolic hormone levels [106], increased levels of pro-inflammatory cytokines [107] and by the generation of ROS (reactive oxygen species) that contribute to oxidative stress [108].

Hypercapnia: The phosphocreatine (PCr)/phosphate (Pi) ratio is significantly lower [109] during exercise in COPD patients, with faster PCr depletion [110], and postexercise recovery is slower in patients compared with healthy controls. The ratio of PCr to Pi is closely related to that of adenosine-tri-phosphate (ATP) to adenosine-di-phosphate (ADP) and, hence, is a useful marker of muscle energy status. Acute hypercapnia leads to intracellular acidosis that has marked effects upon muscle cell metabolism, including decreases in ATP, PCr, and adenosine nucleotides [111, 112]. Furthermore, acute hypercapnia in healthy humans reduces limb muscle and diaphragm contractility [113, 114].

Inflammation: Systemic inflammation has been postulated as a major etiological factor in the skeletal muscle dysfunction commonly seen in COPD. TNF-α levels are elevated in patients who fail to gain weight during a rehabilitation and re-feeding program, whereas increased blood levels of IL-6 (interleukin-6), interleukin-8 (IL-8), TNF-α, and CRP (C-reactive protein) in COPD patients have been associated with increased resting energy expenditure, giving support to the concept that pro-inflammatory cytokines play a role in COPD-associated cachexia [90].

Oxidative Stress: The most important triggers for the development of oxidative stress in patients with COPD are cigarette smoke and systemic inflammation [84]. Oxidative stress was found to be associated with decreased quadriceps muscle strength and was shown to cause increased bone resorption during severe COPD exacerbations [115].

Vitamin D deficiency: Vitamin D was shown to play an important role in the growth of skeletal muscles, muscle contractility, and myogenesis [116] as well as in the development of the growth plate, mineralized bone, and osteoclastogenesis [117]. Therefore vitamin D deficiency may contribute to limb muscle dysfunction [84].

Inactivity: Physical inactivity was found to be crucial in the development of skeletal muscle weakness in patients with COPD. It is believed to result in quadriceps weakness due to mechanical unloading of the muscle and due to muscle wasting [118, 119].

Also, nutritional depletion is associated with reduced upper and lower limb muscle force, a loss of force at higher stimulation frequencies, slowing of muscle relaxation rate, and a reduction in muscle endurance [90].

Treatment

Several interventions have been used in an attempt to improve muscle function in patients with COPD. These and their respective effects on limb muscles are summarized in Table 19.3 [83].

Pharmacological (testosterone replacement therapy, vitamin D and calcium supplementation) and non-pharmacological treatments (exercise training, prevention of falls and balance training and nutritional counseling) are applied in the management of musculoskeletal problems in patients with COPD [83, 84].

Aerobic exercise training, resistance/strength training, and inspiratory muscle training are done in exercise training taking into account overload, specialization, individual differences, and reversibility principles [83, 120]. Supplemental oxygen given during exercise reduces ventilatory requirements for a given workload and increases oxygen supply to muscles exercising at high exercise levels and maximal exercise tolerance [83]. Transcutaneous neuromuscular electrical stimulation (NMES) is suitable for severe deconditioned patients with COPD, during exacerbation periods, transferred to intensive care or bedridden patients with COPD [83, 84]. Water exercises are useful for severe dyspneic patients with COPD with advanced age and physical comorbidities. Muscle strength, functional capacity,

Table 19.3 Effects of treatments for limb muscle dysfunction in chronic obstructive pulmonary disease [83]

Treatment	Mass	Strength	Exercise tolerance	Survival
Exercise	+	+	+	?
Oxygen	?	?	+	+
Nutrition alone	–	–	–	?
Nutrition + exercise	+	+	+	?
Nutrition + exercise + anabolic hormones	+	+	+	?
Testosterone	+	+	–	?
Growth hormones	+	–	–	?
Ghrelin	?	?	?	?
Megestrol	–	?	–	?
Creatinine	?	?	–	?
Antioxidants	?	?	?	?
Vitamin D alone	?	?	?	?
Vitamin D + exercise	?	?	?	?

(+): Studies support that the treatment has a favorable effect on the outcome; (–): studies support that the treatment has no favorable effect on the outcome; (?): there are no supporting data for a treatment effect on the outcome and quality of life have been improved with whole body vibration therapy in patients with COPD and it increased benefits obtained by pulmonary rehabilitation program [84].

Effects of nutritional supplementation are controversial in stable COPD patients. Improvements were observed in body composition, muscle function, exercise capacity, and health status with pulmonary rehabilitation programs with additional nutritional supplementation in COPD patients with nutritional deficiency. Response to nutritional supplementation is very variable and is associated with patient characteristics, type of treatment, and treatment compliance [83, 120]. Testosterone and its analogs are anabolic agents that increase muscle protein synthesis and muscle mass and reduce muscle protein degradation and fat mass. Their benefits increase when combined with resistance training. They are not routinely recommended because of possible side effects. Growth hormone and secretagogues provide significant weight and lean body mass gain in patients with COPD and malnutrition but their results on respiratory and limb muscle strength and exercise capacity are still controversial. They are not recommended due to possibility of carcinogenic effects, side effects, and high costs in COPD patients with muscle dysfunction [83]. Positive effects in terms of disease prognosis are achieved in patients with COPD with early intervention for comorbidities. Future studies should focus on mechanisms of muscle dysfunction and mechanisms-based treatment.

COPD and Osteoporosis

Osteoporosis is a systemic skeletal disorder characterized by low bone mineral density (BMD) and microarchitectural changes, leading to impaired bone strength and increased risk of fracture [121]. Osteoporosis is a well-recognized comorbidity of COPD patients and is an important area of consideration for therapeutic interventions. The most commonly used tool to measure BMD is dual-energy x-ray absorptiometry (DEXA), which is used to define osteoporosis and provides a useful estimate of fracture risk [122]. According to the World Health Organization (WHO), a T-score greater than −1 is accepted as normal, T-scores between −1 and −2.5 are classified as osteopenia, and T-scores of less than −2.5 are defined as osteoporosis [122].

The prevalence of osteoporosis in COPD varies between 4 and 59%, depending on the diagnostic methods used and the severity of the COPD population [123]. More than half of the patients with COPD recruited for the large TORCH trial (6000 patients) had osteoporosis or osteopenia as determined by DEXA scan [124]. COPD could be a risk factor for osteoporosis. In NHANES study including 14,828 subjects over 45 years, osteoporosis prevalence was found 16.9% in subjects with COPD and 8.5% in subjects without COPD [125, 126]. In another cross-sectional study, the prevalence of osteoporosis was 75% in patients with Global Initiative for Chronic Obstructive Lung Disease (GOLD) stage IV disease, and strongly correlated with reduced fat-free mass (FFM). Another important finding in this study was that the prevalence rate was high even for males, with an even higher incidence in postmenopausal women [127, 128].

Recently, in COPD Gene cohort with 3321 current or ex-smoker COPD patients, male smokers had significantly greater risk for osteoporosis and fracture. The osteoporosis prevalence was greater in severe COPD reaching 84%. Emphysema was found to be associated with osteoporosis [129].

Etiology

Corticosteroids use: Oral glucocorticosteroids (OGCs) have both direct adverse effects on bone and indirect effects attributable to muscle weakening and atrophy [130]. These effects are both dose-dependent and duration-dependent. At supraphysiologic concentration GCs profoundly inhibit osteoblast function and bone formation. Prolonged GC use leads to reduction in bone turnover impaired bone renewal and bone loss [66]. Bone mineral loss can be as high as 15.8% among inhaled corticosteroids (ICS) users. The fracture risk is 75% higher among OGCs users [131]. However, the ICS studies have not shown consistent findings regarding bone mineral loss. Some studies showed no aggragation in bone loss; however, others showed excess bone loss with high doses [65, 132–134].

Chronic inflammation: Studies suggest that COPD and associated systemic inflammation is a risk factor for osteoporosis independent of other potentiators [135, 136]. In Liang et al. study, the presence of systemic inflammation was associated with a greater likelihood of low BMD, and multivariate logistic regression analysis showed that TNF-a and IL-6 were independent predictors of low BMD [136].

Vitamin D deficiency: Vitamin D along with PTHs plays a key role in regulating calcium and bone homeostasis [125]. Vitamin D deficiency increases the susceptibility to osteoporotic fractures because of low BMD. It also increases the fracture risk by causing swaying of the body and falls because of muscle weakness [125]. Various factors that have been implicated for the deficiency of vitamin D in COPD patients include poor diet, less exposure to sunlight because of decreased physical activity, accelerated skin ageing, renal dysfunction, depression, and treatment with corticosteroids [137].

Anemia: Anemia is a common entity in COPD patients, and its prevalence varies from 7.5 to 34%, depending upon the selected populations and the diagnostic tools to determine the hemoglobin level [138]. Korkmaz et al. demonstrated significantly higher prevalence of anemia in patients with low BMD of the femur and spine [139]. Rutten et al. reported 20% prevalence of anemia among 321 COPD patients admitted for pulmonary rehabilitation, and anemia was also found to be an independent predictor of low BMD [140]. The pathophysiological nexus between anemia and osteoporosis is not clear; however, human and animal experiments suggest the role of anemia-associated hypoxia as the potential mechanisms for the development of osteoporosis [141].

Smoking: Smoking induces osteoporosis by several potential mechanisms: altered metabolism of calciotropic hormone; dysregulation in the production, metabolism, and binding of estradiol; altered metabolism of adrenal cortical hormone; and effects on collagen metabolism and bone angiogenesis [142].

Hypogonadism: Sex steroids play a crucial role in maintaining skeletal integrity via stimulating bone formation and inhibiting bone resorption [143]. The reported prevalence of hypogonadism in men with COPD varies from 22% to 69% and has been associated with osteoporosis, depression, and muscle weakness [144].

The Impact of Osteoporosis

Osteoporosis is related with vertebral compression fractures. Lumbal and thoracal regions are most affected. Every single compression causes 9% reduction in vital capacity. Osteoporosis could be progressive over the years in COPD. In a study with 3-years follow-up, the prevalence of osteoporosis increased from 47 to 61% [145]. Vertebral compression fractures increase the risk of hip fractures [125]. The prevalence of hip fractures is not exactly known in COPD. However in a Danish cohort hip fracture in COPD patients showed poor prognosis with 60–70% higher risk of death [125, 146].

The Diagnosis of Osteoporosis

The diagnosis of osteoporosis relies on the quantitative assessment of bone mineral density (BMD), usually by central dual-energy X-ray absorptiometry (DXA). BMD at the femoral neck provides the reference site [147]. An individual's BMD is presented as the standard deviation above or below the mean BMD of the reference population, as outlined in Table 19.4 [148].

Table. 19.4 WHO Definition of Osteoporosis Based on BMD [148]

Classification	BMD	T-score
Normal	Within 1 SD of the mean level for a young-adult reference population	T-score at –1.0 and above
Low bone mass (osteopenia)	Between 1.0 and 2.5 SD below that of the mean level for a young-adult reference population	T-score between –1.0 and –2.5
Osteoporosis	2.5 SD or more below that of the mean level for a young-adult reference population	T-score at or below –2.5
Severe or established osteoporosis	2.5 SD or more below that of the mean level for a young-adult reference population	T-score at or below –2.5 with one or more fractures

Prevention and Treatment of Osteoporosis

Non-pharmacological Management

Active smoking cessation should be instituted at the earliest. Weight-bearing and strengthening exercise should be encouraged. Overuse of ICS in COPD must be avoided. ICS use should be restricted to COPD patients with forced expiratory volume (FEV1), 50% of predicted. Unnecessary prolonged use of oral steroids during COPD exacerbations should be avoided [125].

Pharmacological Management

Pharmacological interventions consist of calcium and vitamin D supplementation and antiresorptive therapy. Vitamin D and calcium supplementation is an integral part in the prevention and treatment of osteoporosis [125], but there is no worldwide consensus on optimal dietary intakes and optimal levels of serum vitamin D level.

All symptomatic COPD patients should be evaluated for the presence of following minor criteria:

- BMI <21 kg/m^2
- Current smoking
- Use of ethanol >3 units/day
- Age > 65 years
- Parent hip fracture
- Rib fracture
- Menopause
- Inactivity
- FEV1, 50% predicted

and major criteria:

- Systemic corticosteroids (3 months/year)
- Major fragility fracture (spine/hip) [125]

BMD of the hip and lumbar spine should be measured by DEXA scan along with serum 25-OH D if at least three minor or one major criterion is present. Pharmacologic therapy is indicated in the following conditions [149]:

1. COPD with documented fragility hip or vertebral fractures,
2. T-score below −2.5SD, and
3. $-2, 5 < T\text{-score} < -1$ and one major criterion.

Also the FRAX tool uses updated, evidence-based estimates of absolute fracture risk and was created for the purpose of quantitatively integrating numerous clinical factors into a clinically useful risk prediction model [150].

Readers are referred to American College of Rheumatology 2010 Recommendations for the Prevention and Treatment of Glucocorticoid-Induced Osteoporosis Guidelines for the treatment of glucocorticoid-induced osteoporosis [150].

COPD and Cardiovascular Diseases

COPD and cardiovascular diseases (CVD) are leading causes of mortality globally. In 2005, COPD and CVD caused an estimated 120,000 and 830,000 deaths, respectively, in the United States. Clinicians have long recognized that there is a very high prevalence of CVD among patients with COPD, and, indeed, CVD is the major contributor to morbidity and mortality in patients with COPD [151]. COPD and coronary artery disease (CAD) are both highly prevalent and share common risk factors, such as exposure to cigarette smoke, older age, sex, and inactivity [152]. However, it is also thought that systemic inflammatory changes related to COPD may increase the risk of CVD independently [153]. Additionally, pathophysiologic changes associated with COPD can directly impact heart function; for instance, emphysema and lung hyperinflation may impair left ventricular filling and lower cardiac output or cause pulmonary hypertension and right-sided heart failure [151].

Ischemic Heart Disease

Cardiovascular diseases are the leading causes of death in patients with mild-to-moderate COPD, chief among which is ischemic heart disease (IHD). The prevalence of IHD in COPD patients ranges between 16.1 and 53% and includes various descriptions (coronary artery disease, angina, and myocardial infarction (MI)) [6].

There are multiple sources of evidence demonstrating a high prevalence of IHD in COPD patients. In the Evaluation of COPD Longitudinally to Identify Predictive Surrogate Endpoints (ECLIPSE) study, "heart trouble" as opposed to IHD was reported in 26% of 2164 COPD patients compared with 11% of 337 smoking controls ($p < 0.001$), with a MI reported in 9% versus 3% ($p < 0.001$) [154].

A combination of increased risk factors in patients with COPD, chronic systemic inflammation accelerating atherosclerosis, vascular endothelial dysfunction, physiological stress from comorbidities, and acute inflammation following exacerbation are likely to be involved [155].

Though the exact mechanisms are yet to be elucidated, the temporal relationship of ischemic events with acute exacerbations and correlation of systematic inflammatory markers such as C-reactive protein and fibrinogen with increased IHD implicate inflammation as a significant contributor [155].

Arterial stiffness (measured by aortic pulse wave velocity), an independent predictor of cardiovascular events and mortality, is increased in patients with COPD and was correlated with computed tomography-quantified emphysema and airflow obstruction [6].

Sex-related differences have been investigated in most chronic diseases, including COPD and IHD. Disparity between men and women is mostly a result of behavioral and environmental factors, coupled with biological and gender-based genetic factors [156].

Imbalance of thrombotic/antithrombotic mechanisms, with increased procoagulant activity, has been postulated in COPD [157]. Accordingly, comorbidities related to altered thrombotic status, such as cardiovascular disorders, myocardial infarction and pulmonary embolism, are fairly common in patients with COPD [158].

Heart Failure

Chronic obstructive pulmonary disease (COPD) and heart failure (HF) frequently coexist in clinical practice [159]. The diagnosis of heart failure in COPD patients requires careful clinical history taking including symptoms of orthopnea and paroxysmal nocturnal dyspnea, in addition to cardiovascular examination. Biomarkers such as N-terminal precursor of Brain Natriuretic Peptide (NT-proBNP) have proved useful in differentiating COPD from heart failure both in the stable state and in the acute setting [160]. Both conditions share some risk factors including cigarette smoking, advanced age, and systemic inflammation [161].

The prevalence of COPD among individuals with HF ranges from 20 to 32% of cases, and 10% of hospitalized HF patients also suffer COPD. The hospital HF adjusted prevalence is three times greater among patients discharged with COPD when compared with patients without this disease [160]. COPD is a predictor of mortality in heart failure; indeed, 5-year survival in heart failure patients with COPD is 31% compared with 71% in its absence [162].

Shared etiological factors such as increased age and smoking, together with the high prevalence of hypertension and IHD in patients with COPD, confer much of the increased risk of heart failure in COPD patients. Systemic inflammation is thought to accelerate atherosclerosis and thereby increase the risk of heart failure [6].

Hypertension

Hypertension is generally asymptomatic and thus would not be expected to particularly impact on COPD patients [160]. Overall the prevalence of hypertension appears to be around 30–45% of the general population, with a steep increase with ageing [163]. However, hypertension is consistently one of the most prevalent comorbid diagnoses in COPD patients reported in 40–60% [160]. The pathophysiological links of COPD and hypertension are not yet well described. However, it seems feasible that accelerated aging, loss of connective tissue, and increased arterial stiffness may predispose patients to systemic hypertension and an increased risk of cardiovascular disease in COPD patients.

Venous Thromboembolism (VTE)

Acute pulmonary embolism (PE) and deep venous thrombosis (DVT) are manifestations of the overall disease known as venous thromboembolism (VTE) [158]. Chronic obstructive pulmonary disease (COPD) is a moderate predisposing factor for VTE, principally when associated with hospitalization [164]. The presentation of pulmonary embolism is similarly subtle with nonspecific clinical features such as acute dyspnea, tachycardia, and pleuritic chest pain. While COPD remains a clinical diagnosis, PE requires objective confirmation of clot by an imaging study to warrant appropriate anticoagulation therapy [165].

In the absence of typical symptoms such as productive cough, fever, or decreased breath sounds diffusely, obtaining laboratory and diagnostic studies such as D-dimer, B-type natriuretic peptide, troponin, and arterial blood gas may be helpful in defining other underlying pathologies. Similarly, a nonresponse to aggressive COPD treatment with beta-agonists, antibiotics, and steroids in patients with typical presentations supports evaluation for other causes of dyspnea [165].

During COPD exacerbations, VTE is found in 3–29% of cases [166, 167]. The former consideration may particularly apply during COPD exacerbation, a situation in which undiagnosed PE was found in an autopsy study in up to 30% of COPD patients who died [168]. The prevalence of PE in patients with COPD is important because of combined morbidity and mortality. In a follow-up of 1487 patients from the Prospective Investigation of Pulmonary Embolism Diagnosis (PIOPED) study, Carson et al. found an adjusted estimated relative risk of death at 1 year with COPD and PE of 1.94, compared with 1.1 for patients with PE alone. The 1-year mortality of those with COPD and PE was 53.3%, in contrast to 15% of those with PE alone [169].

The three factors of Virchow's triad are observed in COPD (systemic venous endothelial dysfunction, coagulopathy, and venous stasis due to a physical inactivity), which explains their predisposition to venous thromboembolism (VTE) [170]. Also platelet activation has been shown to be increased in stable COPD as detected by platelet-monocyte aggregates and further increased during exacerbations. Fibrinogen levels are directly as well as related to the incidence of cardiovascular events, and are higher in stable COPD patients than in healthy controls [160].

Treatment of Heart Disease

Despite having similar disease mechanisms, there are substantial differences between IHD and COPD in their current treatment strategies.

The most striking difference in these treatment strategies is the use of beta-agonists in COPD and beta-blockers in heart disease. This has led to contrasting indications and subsequent underuse, particularly of beta-blockers, of some classes of drug [156]. Recent data, such as the TORCH trial, suggest that drugs used to treat COPD, such as long-acting beta2-agonists, are tolerated and have an acceptable safety cardiovascular profile [171, 172]. Beta-blockers, on the other hand, are most important of coronary artery disease (CAD) treatment, but their use in patients with COPD remains uncertain. The main concern is that these drugs might induce bronchospasm and worsen lung function. However, data have shown that beta-blockers, especially if cardioselective, may also be beneficial and related with lower mortality in patients with COPD, with the only exception in the most severe requiring long-term oxygen treatment [171–174].

Recent studies have suggested that the use of beta-blockers in inpatients with exacerbations of COPD is well tolerated and may be associated with reduced mortality [175, 176]. Also, the findings of a meta-analysis confirmed that beta-blocker use in patients with COPD may not only decrease the risk of overall mortality but also reduced the risk of exacerbation of COPD [177].

Angiotensin-converting enzyme (ACE) inhibitors have been associated with reduced exacerbations and mortality in COPD. Furthermore, lowering of ACE levels has been postulated to decrease lung inflammation and improve respiratory muscle function. At present, this data is mainly limited to observational studies. Therefore, guidelines suggest their use in COPD and cardiovascular disease but not yet for COPD alone [93].

COPD and Gastroesophageal Reflux Disease

Gastroesophageal reflux disease (GERD) is one of the most common causes of chronic cough and a potential risk factor for exacerbation of COPD [178–180]. Use of PPI/H2RA and self-reported history of GERD were associated with an increased risk of moderate-to-severe exacerbations and hospitalized exacerbations [181]. The ECLIPSE study identified a history of heartburn or reflux as an independent predictor of frequent exacerbator status. Old age, female gender, medical aid insurance type, and many COPD medications except inhaled muscarinic antagonists were associated with GERD [160]. The prevalence of GERD in COPD patients ranged between 7.7 and 30%. However, Casanova et al. used 24-h pH monitoring to assess acid GERD prevalence and demonstrated that 62% of patients with severe COPD (FEV_1 range 20–49%) versus 19% of controls had acid GERD [182]. Importantly, 58% of the COPD patients with GERD were asymptomatic [6].

The key underlying mechanism of GERD is transient relaxations of the lower esophageal sphincter allowing stomach contents to move into the esophagus and often as high as the larynx and mouth, particularly when intra-abdominal pressure is raised [160]. Also laryngopharyngeal sensitivity is important in preventing pulmonary aspiration. Patients with cough and GERD have significantly reduced laryngopharyngeal sensitivity to air stimuli compared with healthy subjects [183]. In addition, medications such as theophylline and inhaled beta2-agonists may decrease the lower esophageal sphincter pressure, could facilitate GER [184, 185].

Treatment of Gastroesophageal Reflux Disease

Treatment of the GERD is not altered by the presence of COPD, that it should be treated more aggressively [6]. Regarding treatment of the peptic ulcer disease in the context of COPD, no alteration to standard acid suppression therapy is required. The severity of COPD may, however, complicate the ability to perform endoscopic or surgical procedures in terms of anesthetic safety. With regard to the treatment of COPD, steroids can delay the healing of ulcers, and thus minimization of oral steroids in the context of recent ulcer is prudent [6].

COPD and Malnutrition

Changes in body composition are frequently seen in COPD. Decreased weight and muscle mass effect COPD patients undesirably and malnutrition is related with increased mortality and morbidity [186, 187]. BMI below 20 kg/m^2 is defined as malnutrition for COPD patients. Weight loss has been reported in about 50% of patients with severe COPD and, although less common, it is observed in about 10–15% of mild-to-moderate COPD [188].

Malnutrition in COPD is the consequence of an imbalance between energy intake and consumption. Inadequate intake is caused by dyspnea resulting from the effort of eating and by impaired leptin regulation, a hormone that reduces food intake [189]. Energy consumption for respiration is 36–76 kkal in healthy individuals and 430–720 kkal in COPD patients, respectively. Moreover, low intake and steroid therapy increase muscle wasting. Impaired muscle strength worsens respiratory failure, treatment response during exacerbations and prolongs weaning time from mechanical ventilation [186, 190].

Treatment of Malnutrition

Nutritional supplementation especially for undernourished COPD patients provides weight gain, improves respiratory muscle strength, exercise capacity, quality of life, and anthropometric measurements [191]. Energy consumptions of COPD patients are 20–25 kkal/kg/day for females and 25–30 kkal/kg/day for males. 7–8% of daily energy from saturated fatty acids, 12–15% of daily energy from monounsaturated fatty acids, and 7–8% of daily energy from polyunsaturated fatty acids should be met. There has been no strict criteria about protein content of diet in COPD patients. Amount of protein should be 1.2–1.5 g/kg/day (15–20% of total energy) to have positive nitrogen balance and support immune system.

Oral nutritional supplements (as powders, puddings or liquids) can be used to supplement the diet when nutrient requirements cannot be satisfied through normal food and drink [186]. Enteral (nasogastric, naso-jejunal, gastrostomy) or parenteral nutrition can be used for COPD patients without oral intake. Early enteral nutrition protects tissue damage and gastrointestinal system, improves immune system and decreases bacterial translocation. Therefore early enteral nutrition accelerates recovery and improves survival in critically ill patients [192].

COPD and Sleep Disorders

Recent International Classification of Sleep Disorders, 3rd edition (ICSD-3) was published by The American Academy of Sleep Medicine Board in 2014. This guide identifies seven major categories of sleep disorders that include insomnia disorders, sleep-related breathing disorders, central disorders of hypersomnolence, circadian rhythm sleep-wake disorders, sleep-related movement disorders, parasomnias, and other sleep disorders. COPD is associated with the heading of sleep-related breathing disorders and more closely the subheading of sleep hypoventilation syndromes [193].

Patients with COPD have a higher prevalence of insomnia, nightmares, and daytime sleepiness than the general population, with close to 50% of patients are reporting significant disturbance in sleep quality [194].

Sleep has negative effects on breathing such as changes in central respiratory control (chemosensitivity decreases even in 20–25%), airway resistance (Raw increases and respiratory secretions accumulate), and muscle contractility (decreases especially in REM sleep). During sleep, partial carbon dioxide ($PaCO_2$) increases 2–8 mmHg while partial oxygen pressure (PaO_2) decreases 3–10 mmHg and oxyhemoglobin saturation (SpO2) decreases ~2%. All those changes do not have an adverse effect in healthy individuals but may cause trouble in patients with COPD.

Sleep is typically fragmented with diminished slow wave and rapid-eye-movement (REM), which likely represents an important contributing factor to daytime symptoms such as fatigue and lethargy. Furthermore, normal physiological adaptations during sleep, which result in mild hypoventilation in normal subjects, are more profound in COPD, which can result in clinically important nocturnal oxygen desaturation (NOD). The coexistence of OSA and COPD is common; however, there is little convincing evidence that one disorder predisposes to the other [195].

In the literature, nocturnal COPD symptoms such as nocturnal cough and wheezing were reported up to 53%, and also difficulty initiating or maintaining sleep and excessive daytime sleepiness as 23% [196]. In addition, those have been reported in a significant number of patients and may affect sleep quality in those patients. Several studies have shown that sleep quality is worse in people with COPD compared to healthy individuals. Beyond symptoms, there are nocturnal alterations in ventilation and gas control in patients with COPD [197].

Sleep-induced hypoxemia-nocturnal oxygen desaturation (NOD) is defined as "an SpO_2 (oxyhemoglobin saturation) during sleep of <90% for more than 5 min with a nadir of at least 85%" or "> 30% of total sleep time with an SpO_2 of <90%" in subject with a baseline awake SpO_2 of ≥90%. [198, 199]. Proposed mechanisms for NOD are ventilation/perfusion mismatch, hypoventilation, increased upper airway resistance, reduced chemoresponsiveness, REM-related muscle atonia, and greater reduction in functional residual capacity during sleep [195]. Hypoxic pulmonary vasoconstriction is considered a major driver of the development of pulmonary hypertension and cor pulmonale in COPD, NOD also could cause nocturnal cardiac arrhythmias and nocturnal sudden cardiac death [200, 201]. In another study, daytime hypoxemia, hypercapnia, and reduced FEV_1 were found to be predictors of right-heart failure

[202]. McNicholas et al. described nocturnal death was highest among "blue-bloater" type of COPD patients with type 2 respiratory failure, which is more associated with sleep-disordered breathing [203].

Hypoventilation causes the most important gas-exchange alteration during sleep in COPD patients, leading to hypercapnia and hypoxemia, especially during REM sleep. Blood gases alterations lead to increased arousals, sleep disruption, pulmonary hypertension, and higher mortality [198]. Sleep-induced hypoventilation is characterized by elevated levels of $PaCO_2$ while asleep, defined in the ICSD-3 as a level≥45 mmHg or "disproportionately increased relative to levels during wakefulness" [199].

Overlap syndrome first described by Flenley almost 30 years ago, as a coexistence of two diseases: obstructive sleep apnea (OSA) and chronic obstructive pulmonary disease (COPD) [204]. While OSA and COPD carry its own comorbidities and complications, it has been surmised that patients with overlap syndrome may have a worse prognosis than patients with only one of either disease [204]. Taking into account the individual prevalences of COPD and OSA, it has also been suggested that the prevalence of overlap syndrome in adults aged 40 years and over is 0.5%–1% [205]. The combination of obstructive sleep apnea and COPD does have implications with respect to outcome. The "overlap syndrome" is associated with lower and longer nocturnal oxyhemoglobin desaturations, and produces more severe pulmonary hemodynamic complications. Patients with the overlap syndrome have been reported to exhibit diurnal hypercapnia more frequently, and concomitant COPD patients at risk for overlap syndrome (those with polycythemia, cor pulmonale, or neuropsychological impairment) should be appropriately screened. Oximetry will show sawtoothing oxygen desaturation during NREM periods, with persistently low SpO2 during REM.

There are some indirect data about the prevalence of overlap syndrome. In the Sleep Heart Health Study, a large community-based cohort study which included polysomnography and spirometry, 0.5% of the participants had airflow obstruction [206]. In a European study with predominantly mild COPD patients, OSA occurred in 3% [207].

Diagnosis

General consensus statements suggest screening for sleep-disordered breathing in COPD patients who complain of symptoms typically associated with sleep-disordered breathing such as excessive daytime somnolence and frequent nocturnal arousals from sleep [208]. Additionally, it has been suggested that patients with COPD who develop morning headaches following nocturnal oxygen supplementation should undergo a diagnostic polysomnogram. Nocturnal oxymetry is recommended to evaluate gas exchange during sleep in COPD patients. However, the utility of overnight oxygen saturation measurements in suggesting OSA in COPD is quite limited. Nocturnal oximetry may be more useful for evaluating the effectiveness of nocturnal oxygen therapy. Sleep studies are usually indicated when there is a possibility of sleep apnea or obesity-hypoventilation syndrome. Unattended overnight polysomnograms performed in an ambulatory setting (also known as "portable" or "home" sleep studies) have been a common modality for screening for OSA in high-risk patient populations. These studies utilize a limited number of channels, and exact sleep time and arousals from sleep as determined by electroencephalography are often not available [209]. The American Academy of Sleep Medicine (AASM) defines OSA by at least five events per hour of sleep with associated symptoms such as daytime sleepiness, respiratory pauses during sleep, or gasping arousals [199].

Treatment

The first management principle of sleep-related breathing disturbances in COPD should be to optimize oxygenation. But the concentration of added oxygen should be carefully titrated to bring the arterial oxygen tension (PaO_2) up into the mildly hypoxemic range in order to minimize the tendency towards carbon dioxide retention, particularly during sleep [209].

The Global Initiative for Chronic Obstructive Lung Disease (GOLD) guidelines recommend that supplemental oxygen therapy be provided to patients whose oxygen saturations fall below 88% or who have a PO_2 less than 55 mmHg during wakefulness or PO_2 between 55 and 60 mmHg with evidence of pulmonary hypertension, congestive heart failure, or polycythemia [208].

In particular, there appears to be a low risk of serious carbon dioxide retention with carefully controlled oxygen therapy during exacerbations of COPD even when relatively high flow oxygen supplementation is required to bring the SaO_2 into the region of 90–92% [210]. Thus, the priority in oxygen supplementation should be to provide sufficient oxygen to bring the SaO_2 level above 90%, but doing so in a controlled fashion to avoid excessive supplementation. Oxygen supplementation during sleep is best delivered via nasal cannulae, since face masks are more likely to become dislodged during sleep [211]. In the chronic setting, indications for supplemental oxygen are best determined by measures that indicate the overall magnitude of hypoxemia during sleep, such as the cumulative time spent with $SaO_2 < 90\%$.

In addition to correction of hypoxemia is particularly important and in recent years considerable interest has focused on the potential benefits of noninvasive ventilation (NIV). Nocturnal positive pressure ventilation (NPPV) is the delivery of mechanically assisted breaths without placement of an artificial airway, usually with the use of a fitted nasal mask. According to consensus report, indications for usage of NPPV include: (a) symptoms (e.g., fatigue, dyspnea, or morning headache); (b) physiologic criteria ($PaCO_2 > 55$ or 50–54 mmHg with NOD), or (c) $PaCO_2$ 50–54 mmHg with recurrent hospitalization related to episodes of hypercapnic respiratory failure [212]. NPPV appears to decrease the inspiratory work of breathing, reduce diaphragmatic electromyogram activity, improve PaO_2, decrease $PaCO_2$, and increase minute ventilation [213]. Either volume or pressure modes are equally effective, but pressure support appears to be better tolerated and more comfortable. Sleep quality and diurnal PaO_2 and $PaCO_2$ levels are better with NIV plus supplemental oxygen than with oxygen alone [214]. Patients with the overlap syndrome should also be treated by nocturnal pressure support and the choice between continuous positive airway pressure (CPAP) or bilevel positive airway pressure (BIPAP) can be determined based on the pattern of sleep-disordered breathing. In cases where OSA predominates, CPAP may be most appropriate, whereas in cases where there is evidence of significant nocturnal hypoventilation with associated periods of sustained hypoxemia, BIPAP may be more appropriate. Newer modalities of pressure support, such as adaptive servo ventilation, may be particularly suited to patients with the overlap syndrome [215].

Anxiety and Depression in COPD

Patients with COPD who have perceptions of poor health are likely to experience anxiety, depression, sleep disturbance, and problems with daily functioning like patients with any chronic disease. Depending on the methodology and the definition, the prevalence of anxiety and depression are varied between 8 and 80% of COPD patients who report depression and/or anxiety [216–218]. Depression and anxiety are more prevalent in COPD than other diseases and than general population. There is a bidirectional relation between anxiety (RR:1.83), depression (RR:1.27), and COPD. While anxiety and depression increase the worse prognosis in COPD, COPD increases the risk of depression (RR: 1.69) [219]. Hence, $FEV_1\%$ predicted has been correlated with increased risk of depression [218]. The known risk factors of anxiety and depression include physical disability, oxygen dependence, respiratory symptoms, increased number of comorbidities, female sex, current smoking, low socioeconomic class, marital status, living alone, and poor quality of life [216, 218].

Comorbid depressive symptoms in patients with COPD are associated with poorer survival, longer hospitalization stay, persistent smoking, increased symptom burden, and poorer physical and social functioning. Interventions that reduce depressive symptoms may potentially affect COPD outcomes [220]. In its final stages, COPD is a severely disabling condition that is characterized by dyspnea, which causes substantial anxiety. Anxiety is associated with an impaired quality of life and increased hospital admissions. Untreated comorbid anxiety can have devastating consequences for both patients and their relatives [221].

It is not easy to diagnose depression in COPD patients because of the overlapping symptoms between COPD and depression. However, the six-item Hamilton Depression Subscale (HAM-D-6) appears to be a useful screening tool. Quality of life is strongly impaired in COPD patients and patients' quality of life emerges to be more correlated with the presence of depressive symptoms than with the severity of COPD [222]. Whether patients with a history or family history of psychiatric disorders might be predisposed to developing anxious or depressed responses, and whether these responses are especially difficult to treat among those with premorbid conditions, remains to be evaluated. However, it is likely that an improved understanding of the psychiatric history in patients and their families, as well as the role of anxiety or depressive reactions to illness, will influence the management of psychological impairments and ultimately improve health-related quality of life (QoL).

Treatment

Management of comorbid depression and/or insomnia complaints in COPD patients requires careful consideration of the effects of medications. In addition to medications, alternative non-pharmacologic treatments should also be considered, such as cognitive behavioral therapy [223, 224].

Pulmonary rehabilitation programs have gained increased acceptance in the treatment of COPD, mainly due to their capacity to stabilize and, in some instances, to reverse many physio-pathogenic factors involved in airway obstruction [225, 226]. However, studies exploring the role of psychotherapy in the pulmonary rehabilitation program as a way to alter subject anxiety and depression levels have yielded ambiguous results [227–229].

Pulmonary rehabilitation programs have also been described for COPD patients for comorbid anxiety and depression. By means of progressive exercise, training of respiratory function, and psycho-education, patients obtained better exercise tolerance, less dyspnea, and better quality of life [230].

In a study it was shown that in patients with severe COPD, pulmonary rehabilitation induces important changes on depression and anxiety independent of changes in dyspnea and health-related quality of life [231].

In another study comparing cognitive behavioral group treatment and COPD education for anxiety and depression symptoms in COPD patients, it was found that both therapies achieved sustainable improvements in QoL for COPD patients experiencing moderate-to-severe symptoms of depression or anxiety [232].

COPD and Anemia

World Health Organization (WHO) defines anemia as an hematocrit level, 39% in males and 36% in females [233]. Iron deficiency is common in patients with congestive heart failure, where it has been identified as an independent predictor of mortality [234]. In COPD, iron deficiency could be particularly deleterious since hypoxemia is common, is a marker of disease severity and is important in the pathophysiology and extrapulmonary manifestations of the condition [235]. Hypoxemia and pulmonary hypertension in COPD are both predictors of mortality [235, 236].

The prevalence of anemia in patients with COPD varies from 7.5 to 33%. Anemia of chronic disease (ACD) is probably the most common type of anemia associated with COPD. ACD is driven by COPD-mediated systemic inflammation [237]. Systemic inflammation seems to be an important factor for its establishment and repeated bursts of inflammatory mediators during COPD exacerbations could further inhibit erythropoiesis. However, renal impairment, malnutrition, low testosterone levels, growth hormone level abnormalities, oxygen supplementation, theophylline treatment, inhibition of angiotensin-converting enzyme, and aging itself are additional factors that could be associated with the development of anemia [238].

Fatigue and dyspnea are the major symptoms of anemia, and these can be related to reduced oxygen carrying capacity of blood. Furthermore, this symptom complex in patients with COPD will inevitably contribute the morbidity and mortality associated with impaired quality of life and reduced exercise capacity. Anemia in COPD is associated with greater health care resource utilization, impaired quality of life, decreased survival, and a greater likelihood of hospitalization [239].

In a study, a linear relationship was found between hemoglobin levels, exercise capacity, and quality of life [240]. In a database cohort of 2524 COPD patients being prescribed long-term oxygen therapy for the first time, authors reported a prevalence of anemia of 12.6% in males and 8.2% in females, higher than that of polycythemia (8.4% of the patients) defined by an hematocrit level 54% [241]. The ANTADIR hematocrit study suggests that low hematocrit values are associated with an increased morbidity [241].

Schönhofer et al. demonstrated that correction of anemia with blood transfusions among 20 patients with severe COPD significantly reduced disease-related elevations in minute ventilation and work of breathing, suggesting that anemia correction may be beneficial in alleviating dyspnea and improving exercise capacity [242]. They also demonstrated that among five patients with severe anemia, successful treatment of anemia resulted in an increased ability to wean patients from mechanical ventilation [243].

In a recent study, it has been demonstrated that a high prevalence of non-anemic iron deficiency in COPD may be driven by inflammation. Inflammation elevates hepcidin, which reduces serum iron and dietary iron absorption. Hepcidin is therefore important in the pathogenesis of the anemia of chronic disease [244].

Treatment

As in other chronic conditions, anemia predicts a worse outcome in COPD, both in the setting of admission with an acute exacerbation and in the long term so it is very important to manage anemia in management of COPD. Therapeutic possibilities include both the manipulation of iron status through intravenous iron therapy and hepcidin antagonists becoming available in recent years [244].

References

1. Global Initiative for Chronic Obstructive Lung Disease (GOLD). Pocket Quide to COPD Diagnosis, Management and Prevention, Updated 2015. http://www.goldcopd.org/.
2. Decramer M, Janssens W, Miravitlles M. Chronic obstructive pulmonary disease. Lancet. 2012;379:1341–51.
3. Hillas G, Perlikos F, Tsiligianni I, Tzanaki N. Managing comorbidities in COPD. Int J COPD. 2015;10:95–109.
4. Divo MJ, Casanova C, Marin JM, Pinto-Plata VM, de Torres JP, Zulueta JJ. Chronic obstructive pulmonary disease comorbidities network. Eur Respir J. 2015;46(3):640–50.
5. Decramer M, Janssens W. Chronic obstructive pulmonary disease and comorbidities. Lancet Respir Med. 2013;1:73–83.
6. Smith MC, Wrobel JP. Epidemiology and clinical impact of major comorbidities in patients with COPD. Int J COPD. 2014;9:871–88.
7. Putcha N, Puhan MA, Hansel NN, Drummond MB, Boyd CM. Impact of co-morbidities on self-rated health in self-reported COPD: an analysis of NHANES 2001–2008. COPD. 2013;10(3):324–32.
8. Ozyilmaz E, Kokturk N, Teksut G, Tatlicioglu T. Unsuspected risk factors of frequent exacerbations requiring hospital admission in chronic obstructive pulmonary disease. Int J Clin Pract. 2013;67(7):691–7.
9. Kokturk N, Teksut G, Bakir H, Ozkan S. What affects mortality in patients with chronic obstructive pulmonary disease: ado indices and charlson comorbidity score. In: C47. Asthma and COPD. San Diego: ATS Annual Congress; 2014. p. A4617.
10. Soler-Cataluña JJ, Martínez-García MA, Román Sánchez P, Salcedo E, Navarro M, Ochando R. Severe acute exacerbations and mortality in patients with chronic obstructive pulmonary disease. Thorax. 2005;60:925–31.
11. Mannino DM, Higuchi K, Yu TC, Zhou H, Li Y, Tian H, et al. Economic burden of COPD in the presence of comorbidities. Chest. 2015;148(1):138–50.

12. Mapel DW, Hurley JS, Frost FJ, Petersen HV, Picchi MA, Coultas DB. Health care utilization in chronic obstructive pulmonary disease. A case-control study in health maintenance organization. Arch Intern Med. 2000;160:2653–8.
13. Sin DD, Anthonisen NR, Soriano JB, Agusti AG. Mortality in COPD: role of comorbidities. Eur Respir J. 2006;28:1245–57.
14. McGarvey LP, Magder S, Burkhart D, Kesten S, Liu D, Manuel RC, Niewoehner DE. Cause-specific mortality adjudication in the UPLIFT® COPD trial: findings and recommendations. Respir Med. 2012;106:515–21.
15. McGarvey LP, John M, Anderson JA, Zvarich M, Wise RA. Ascertainment of cause-specific mortality in COPD: operations of the TORCH clinical endpoint committee. Thorax. 2007;62:411–5.
16. Miller J, Edwards LD, Agusti A, Bakke P, Calverley PM, Celli B, et al. Comorbidity, systemic inflammation and outcomes in the ECLIPSE cohort. Respir Med. 2013;107:1376–84.
17. Divo M, Cote C, de Torres JP, Casanova C, Marin JM, Pinto-Plata V. Comorbidities and risk of mortality in patients with COPD. Am J Respir Crit Care Med. 2012;186(2):155–61.
18. Frei A, Muggensturmc P, Putchad N, Siebelinge L, Zollerb M, Boydf CM, et al. Five comorbidities reflected the health status in patients with chronic obstructive pulmonary disease: the newly developed COMCOLD index. J Clin Epidemiol. 2014;67:904–11.
19. Burgel PR, Paillasseur JL, Caillaud D, et al. Clinical COPD phenotypes: a novel approach using principal component and cluster analyses. Eur Respir J. 2010;36:531–9.
20. Gibson PG, McDonald VM. Asthma–COPD overlap 2015: now we are six. Thorax. 2015;70:683–91.
21. www.who.org
22. Young RP, Hopkins RJ, Gamble GD, Etzel C, El-Zein R, Crapo JD. Genetic evidence linking lung cancer and COPD: a new perspective. Appl Clin Genet. 2011;4:99–111.
23. Mannino DM, Aguayo SM, Petty TL, Redd SC. Low lung function and incident lung cancer in the United States data from the first national health and nutrition examination survey follow-up. Arch Intern Med. 2003;163:1475–80.
24. de Torres JP, Bastarrika G, Wisnivesky JP, Alcaide AB, Campo A, Seijo LM, et al. Assessing the relationship between lung cancer risk and emphysema detected on low-dose CT of the chest. Chest. 2007;132:1932–8.
25. Wilson DO, Weissfeld JL, Balkan A, Schragin JG, Fuhrman CR, Fisher SN, et al. Association of radiographic emphysema and airflow obstruction with lung cancer. Am J Respir Crit Care Med. 2008;178:738–44.
26. Young RP, Hopkins RJ, Christmas T, Black PN, Metcalf P, Gamble GD. COPD prevalence is increased in lung cancer, independent of age, sex and smoking history. Eur Respir J. 2009;34:380–6.
27. Kiria VA, Sorianob JB, Visickc G, Fabbri LM. Recent trends in lung cancer and its association with COPD: an analysis using the UK GP research database. Prim Care Respir J. 2010;19(1):57–61.
28. Young RP, Hopkins RJ, Gamble GD. Clinical applications of gene-based risk prediction for lung cancer and the central role of chronic obstructive pulmonary disease. Front Genet. 2012;16(3):210.
29. Lowry KP, Gazelle GS, Gilmore ME, Johanson C, Munshi V, Choi SE, et al. Personalizing annual lung cancer screening for patients with chronic obstructive pulmonary disease: a decision analysis. Cancer. 2015;121(10):1556–62.
30. Young RP, Duan F, Chiles C, Hopkins RJ, Gamble GD, Greco EM, et al. Airflow limitation and histology shift in the National Lung Screening Trial. The NLST-ACRIN cohort substudy. Am J Respir Crit Care Med. 2015;192(9):1060–7.
31. Young RP, Hopkins RJ. Lung cancer risk prediction to select smokers for screening CT—letter. Cancer Prev Res. 2012;5:697.
32. Cottin V, Nunes H, Brillet PY, Delaval P, Devouassou G, Tillie-Leblond I, et al. Combined pulmonary fibrosis and emphysema: a distinct underrecognised entity. Eur Respir J. 2005;26:586–93.
33. Katzenstein AA, Mukhopadhyay S, Zanardi C, Dexter E. Clinically occult interstitial fibrosis in smokers: classification and significance of a surprisingly common finding in lobectomy specimens. Hum Pathol. 2010;41:316–25.
34. Lin H, Jiang S. Combined pulmonary fibrosis and emphysema (CPFE): an entity different from emphysema or pulmonary fibrosis alone. J Thorac Dis. 2015;7(4):767–79.
35. Incalzi RA, Corsonello A, Pedone C, Battaglia S, Paglino G, Bellia V, et al. Chronic renal failure: a neglected comorbidity of COPD. Chest. 2010;137(4):831–7.
36. Yoshizawa T, Okada K, Furuichi S, Ishiguro T, Yoshizawa A, Akahoshi T, et al. Prevalence of chronic kidney diseases in patients with chronic obstructive pulmonary disease: assessment based on glomerular filtration rate estimated from creatinine and cystatin C levels. Int J COPD. 2015;10:1283–9.
37. Mapel DW, Marton JP. Prevalence of renal and hepatobiliary disease, laboratory abnormalities, and potentially toxic medication exposures among persons with COPD. Int J COPD. 2013;8:127–34.
38. Ford ES. Urinary albumin-creatinine ratio, estimated glomerular filtration rate, and all-cause mortality among US adults with obstructive lung function. Chest. 2015;147(1):56–67.
39. Laghi F, Adiguzel N, Tobin MJ. Endocrinological derangements in COPD. Eur Respir J. 2009;34:975–96.
40. Corona G, Rastrelli G, Maggi M. Diagnosis and treatment of late-onset hypogonadism: systematic review and meta-analysis of TRT outcomes. Best Pract Res Clin Endocrinol Metab. 2013;27(4):557–9.
41. Huhtaniemi I. Late-onset hypogonadism: current concepts and controversies of pathogen-

esis, diagnosis and treatment. Asian J Androl. 2014;16(2):192–202.
42. Corona G, Vignozzi L, Sforza A, Maggi M. Risks and benefits of late onset hypogonadism treatment: an expert opinion. World J Mens Health. 2013;31(2):103–25.
43. Dinsen S, Baslund B, Klose M, Rasmussen AK, Friis-Hansen L, Hilsted L, et al. Why glucocorticoid withdrawal may sometimes be as dangerous as the treatment itself. Eur J Intern Med. 2013;24(8):714–20.
44. Meteran H, Backer V, Kyvik KO, Skytthe A, Thomsen SF. Comorbidity between chronic obstructive pulmonary disease and type 2 diabetes: a nation-wide cohort twin study. Respir Med. 2015;109(8):1026–30.
45. Song Y, Klevak A, Manson JE, Buring JE, Liu S. Asthma, chronic obstructive pulmonary disease, and type 2 diabetes in the Women's health study. Diabetes Res Clin Pract. 2010;90(3):365–71.
46. Feary JR, Rodrigues LC, Smith CJ, Hubbard RB, Gibson JE. Prevalence of major comorbidities in subjects with COPD and incidence of myocardial infarction and stroke: a comprehensive analysis using data from primary care. Thorax. 2010;65:956–62.
47. Mirrakhimov AE. Chronic obstructive pulmonary disease and glucose metabolism: a bitter sweet symphony. Cardiovasc Diabetol. 2012;11:132.
48. Suratt PM, Wilhoit SC, Hsiao HS, et al. Compliance of chest wall in obese subjects. J Appl Physiol. 1984;57:403–7.
49. Ofir D, Laveneziana P, Webb KA, et al. Ventilatory and perceptual responses to cycle exercise in obese women. J Appl Physiol. 2007;102:2217–26.
50. Ferretti A, Giampiccolo P, Cavalli A, et al. Expiratory flow limitation and orthopnea in massively obese subjects. Chest. 2001;119:1401–8.
51. Rubinstein I, Zamel N, DuBarry L, et al. Airflow limitation in morbidly obese, nonsmoking men. Ann Intern Med. 1990;112:828–32.
52. Holley HS, Milic-Emili J, Becklake MR, et al. Regional distribution of pulmonary ventilation and perfusion in obesity. J Clin Invest. 1967;46:475–81.
53. Landbo C, Prescott E, Lange P, Vestbo J, Almdal TP. Prognostic value of nutritional status in chronic obstructive pulmonary disease. Am J Respir Crit Care Med. 1999;160:1856–61.
54. Jee SH, Sull JW, Park J, Lee SY, Ohrr H, Guallar E, Samet JM. Body-mass index and mortality in Korean men and women. N Engl J Med. 2006;355:779–8.
55. Doehner W, Erdmann E, Cairns R, Clark EL, Dormandy JA, Ferrannini E, et al. Inverse relation of body weight and weight change with mortality and morbidity in patients with type 2 diabetes and cardiovascular co-morbidity: an analysis of the PROactive study population. Int J Cardiol. 2012;162(1):20–6.
56. Franssen FME, O'Donnell DE, Goossens GH, Blaak EE, Schols AMWJ. Obesity and the lung: 5 obesity and COPD. Thorax. 2008;63(12):1110–7.
57. Calikoglu M, Sahin G, Unlu A, Ozturk C, Tamer L, Ercan B, Kanik A, Atik U. Leptin and TNF-alpha levels in patients with chronic obstructive pulmonary disease and their relationship to nutritional parameters. Respiration. 2004;71(1):45–50.
58. Kirdar S, Serter M, Ceylan E, Sener AG, Kavak T, Karadağ F. Adiponectin as a biomarker of systemic inflammatory response in smoker patients with stable and exacerbation phases of chronic obstructive pulmonary disease. Scand J Clin Lab Invest. 2009;69(2):219–24.
59. Schols AM, Creutzberg EC, Buurman WA, Campfield LA, Saris WH, Wouters EF. Plasma leptin is related to proinflammatory status and dietary intake in patients with chronic obstructive pulmonary disease. Am J Respir Crit Care Med. 1999;160(4):1220–6.
60. Guvener N, Tutuncu NB, Akcay S, Eyuboglu F, Gokcel A. Alveolar gas exchange in patients with type 2 diabetes mellitus. Endocr J. 2003;50(6):663–7.
61. Walter RE, Beiser A, Givelber RJ, O'Connor GT, Gottlieb DJ. Association between glycemic state and lung function: the Framingham heart study. Am J Respir Crit Care Med. 2003;167(6):911–6.
62. Lawlor DA, Ebrahim S, Smith GD. Associations of measures of lung function with insulin resistance and type 2 diabetes: findings from the British Women's heart and health study. Diabetologia. 2004;47(2):195–203.
63. Davis WA, Knuiman M, Kendall P, Grange V, Davis TM. Glycemic exposure is associated with reduced pulmonary function in type 2 diabetes: the Fremantle diabetes study. Diabetes Care. 2004;27(3):752–7.
64. Litonjua AA, Lazarus R, Sparrow D, Demolles D, Weiss ST. Lung function in type 2 diabetes: the normative aging study. Respir Med. 2005;99(12):1583–90.
65. Pandya D, Puttanna A, Balagopal V. Systemic effects of inhaled corticosteroids: an overview. Open Respir Med J. 2014;8:59–65.
66. Henneicke H, Gasparini SJ, Brennan-Speranza TC, Zhou H, Seibel MJ. Glucocorticoids and bone: local effects and systemic implications. Trends Endocrinol Metab. 2014;25(4):197–211.
67. Suissa S, Kezouh A, Ernst P. Inhaled corticosteroids and the risks of diabetes onset and progression. Am J Med. 2010;123(11):1001–6.
68. Baker EH, Janaway CH, Philips BJ, Brennan AL, Baines DL, Wood DM, Jones PW. Hyperglycaemia is associated with poor outcomes in patients admitted to hospital with acute exacerbations of chronic obstructive pulmonary disease. Thorax. 2006;61(14):284–9.
69. Parappil A, Depczynski B, Collett P, Marks GB. Effect of comorbid diabetes on length of stay and risk of death in patients admitted with acute exacerbations of COPD. Respirology. 2010;15(6):918–22.
70. Burt MG, Roberts GW, Aguilar-Loza NR, Quinn SJ, Frith PA, Stranks SN. Relationship between glycaemia and length of hospital stay during an acute exacerbation of chronic obstructive pulmonary disease. Intern Med J. 2013;43(6):721–4.

71. Handelsman Y, Bloomgarden ZT, Grunberger G, Umpierrez G, Zimmerman RS, Bailey TS, et al. American association of clinical endocrinologists and American College of endocrinology—clinical practice guidelines for developing a diabetes mellitus comprehensive care plan—2015. Endocr Pract. 2015;21(1):1–87.
72. Hitchings AW, Archer JRH, Srivastava SA, Baker EH. Safety of metformin in patients with chronic obstructive pulmonary disease and type 2 diabetes mellitus. COPD. 2015;12(2):126–31.
73. Doehnera W, Haeuslera KG, Endresa M, Ankerb SD, MacNeee W, Lainscak M. Neurological and endocrinological disorders: orphans in chronic obstructive pulmonary disease. Respir Med. 2011;105(1):12–9.
74. Breyer MK, Spruit MA, Hanson CK, Franssen FME, Vanfleteren LEGW, Groenen MTJ, et al. Prevalence of metabolic syndrome in copd patients and its consequences. PLoS One. 9(6):e98013.
75. Díez-Manglano J, Barquero-Romero J, Almagro P, Cabrera FJ, López García F, Montero L, et al. COPD patients with and without metabolic syndrome: clinical and functional differences. Intern Emerg Med. 2014;9(4):419–25.
76. Mekov E, Slavova Y, Tsakova A, Genova M, Kostadinov D, Minchev D, et al. Metabolic syndrome in hospitalized patients with chronic obstructive pulmonary disease. PeerJ. 2015;3:e1068.
77. Alberti KG, Zimmet P, Shaw J, IDF Epidemiology Task Force Consensus Group. The metabolic syndrome—a new worldwide definition. Lancet. 2005;366(9491):1059–62.
78. Garber JR, Cobin RH, Gharib H, Hennessey JV, Klein I, Mechanick JI. Clinical practice guidelines for hypothyroidism in adults: cosponsored by the Amercan Association of Clinical Endocrinologists and the American Thyroid Association. Endocr Pract. 2012;18(6):988–1028.
79. Van Schoor NM, Lips P. Worldwide vitamin D status. Best Pract Res Clin Endocrinol Metab. 2011;25(4):671–80.
80. Holick MF, Binkley NC, Bischoff-Ferrari HA, Gordon CM, Hanley DA, Heaney RP, et al. Evaluation, treatment, and prevention of vitamin D deficiency: an Endocrin Society clinical practice guideline. J Clin Endocrinol Metab. 2011;96(7):1911–30.
81. Janssens W, Lehouck A, Carremans C, Bouillon R, Mathieu C, Decramer M. Vitamin D beyond bones in chronic obstructive pulmonary disease: time to act. Am J Respir Crit Care Med. 2009;179(8):630–6.
82. Holick MF. Vitamin D deficiency. N Engl J Med. 2007;357(3):266–81.
83. Maltais F, Decramer M, Casaburi R, Barreiro E, Burelle Y, Debigare R, et al. An official ATS/ERS satatement: update on limb muscle dysfunction in COPD. Am J Respir Crit Care Med. 2014;189(9):15–62.
84. Cielen N, Maes K, Gayan-Ramirez G. Musculoskeletal disorders in chronic obstructive pulmonary disease. BioMed Res Int. 2014;2014:965764.
85. Crul T, Spruit MA, Gayan-Ramirez G, Quarck R, Gosselink R, Troosters T, et al. Markers of inflammation and disuse vastus lateralis of chronic obstructive pulmonary disease patients. Eur J Clin Investig. 2007;37(11):897–904.
86. Spruit MA, Gosselink R, Troosters T, Kasran A, Gayan-Ramirez G, Bogaerts P, et al. Muscle force during an acute exacerbation in hospitalised patients with COPD and its relationship with CXCL8 and IGF-I. Thorax. 2003;58(9):752–6.
87. American Thoracic Society/European Respiratory Society. Skeletalmuscle dysfunction in chronic obstructive pulmonary disease: a statement of the American Thoracic Society and European Respiratory Society. Am J Respir Crit Care Med. 1999;159(4):1–40.
88. Swallow EB, Reyes D, Hopkinson NS, et al. Quadriceps strength predicts mortality in patients with moderate to severe chronic obstructive pulmonary disease. Thorax. 2007;62(2):115–20.
89. Choudhury G, Rabinovich R, MacNee W. Comorbidities and systemic effects of chronic obstructive pulmonary disease. Clin Chest Med. 2014;35:101–30.
90. Man WD, Kemp P, Moxham J, Polkey MI. Skeletal muscle dysfunction in COPD: clinical and laboratory observations. Clin Sci. 2009;117:251–64.
91. Agusti AG, Noguera A, Sauleda J, et al. Systemic effects of chronic obstructive pulmonary disease. Eur Respir J. 2003;21:347–60.
92. Gosselink R, Troosters T, Decramer M. Peripheral muscle weakness contributes to exercise limitation in COPD. Am J Respir Crit Care Med. 1996;153:976–80.
93. Shrikrishna D, Hopkinson NS. Chronic obstructive pulmonary disease: consequences eyond the lung. Clin Med. 2012;12:71–4.
94. Decramer M, Gosselink R, Troosters T, et al. Muscle weakness is related to utilization of health care resources in COPD patients. Eur Respir J. 1997;10:417–23.
95. Schols AM, Soeters PB, Dingemans AM, et al. Prevalence and characteristics of nutritional depletion in patients with stable COPD eligible for pulmonary rehabilitation. Am Rev Respir Dis. 1993;147:1151–6.
96. Donaldson AV, Maddocks M, Martollini D, et al. Muscle function in COPD: a complex interplay. Int J Chron Obstruct Pulmon Dis. 2012;7:523–35.
97. Seymour JM, Spruit MA, Hopkinson NS, et al. The prevelance of quadriceps weakness in COPD and the relationship with disease severity. Eur Respir J. 2010;36:81–8.
98. Kok MO, Hoekstra T, Twisk JWR. The longitudinal relation between smoking and muscle strength in healthy adults. Eur Addict Res. 2012;18(2):70–5.
99. Rapuri PB, Gallagher JC, Smith LM. Smoking is a risk factor for decreased physical performance

in elderly women. J Gerontol A Biol Sci Med Sci. 2007;62(1):93–100.
100. Barreiro E, Peinado VI, Galdiz JB, et al. Cigarette smoke induced oxidative stress: a role in chronic obstructive pulmonary disease skeletal muscle dysfunction. Am J Respir Crit Care Med. 2010;182(4):477–88.
101. Rom O, Kaisari S, Aizenbud D, Reznick AZ. Identification of possible cigarette smoke constituents responsible for muscle catabolism. J Muscle Res Cell Motil. 2012;33(3–4):199–208.
102. Renkema TEJ, Schouten JP, Koëter GH, Postma DS. Effects of long-term treatment with corticosteroids in COPD. Chest. 1996;109(5):115–62.
103. Decramer M, Lacquet LM, Fagard R, Rogiers P. Corticosteroids contribute to muscle weakness in chronic airflow obstruction. Am J Respir Crit Care Med. 1994;150(1):11–6.
104. Hopkinson NS, Man WD, Dayer MJ, Ross ET, Nickol AH, Hart N, et al. Acute effect of oral steroids on muscle function in chronic obstructive pulmonary disease. Eur Respir J. 2004;24(1):137–42.
105. Decramer M, de Bock V, Dom R. Functional and histologic picture of steroid-induced myopathy in chronic obstructive pulmonary disease. Am J Respir Crit Care Med. 1996;153(6–1):1958–64.
106. Semple PD, Beastall GH, Watson WS, Hume R. Serum testosterone depression associated with hypoxia in respiratory failure. Clin Sci. 1980;58(1):105–6.
107. Takabatake N, Nakamura H, Abe S, Inoue S, Hino T, Saito H, et al. The relationship between chronic hypoxemia and activation of the tumor necrosis factor-α system in patients with chronic obstructive pulmonary disease. Am J Respir Crit Care Med. 2000;161(4–1):1179–84.
108. Heunks LM, Vina J, van Herwaarden CL, Folgering HT, Gimeno A, Dekhuijzen PN. Xanthine oxidase is involved in exercise-induced oxidative stress in chronic obstructive pulmonary disease. Am J Phys. 1999;277(6–2):1697–704.
109. Kutsuzawa T, Shioya S, Kurita D, Haida M, Ohta Y, Yamabayashi H. Muscle energy metabolism and nutritional status in patients with chronic obstructive pulmonary disease. A 31P magnetic resonance study. Am J Respir Crit Care Med. 1995;152(2):647–52.
110. Thompson CH, Davies RJ, Kemp GJ, Taylor DJ, Radda GK, Rajagopalan B. Skeletal muscle metabolism during exercise and recovery in patients with respiratory failure. Thorax. 1993;48(5):486–90.
111. Gertz I, Hedenstierna G, Hellers G, Wahren J. Muscle metabolism in patients with chronic obstructive lung disease and acute respiratory failure. Clin Sci Mol Med. 1977;52(4):396–403.
112. Pouw EM, Schols AM, van der Vusse GJ, Wouters EF. Elevated inosine monophosphate levels in resting muscle of patients with stable chronic obstructive pulmonary disease. Am J Respir Crit Care Med. 1998;157(2):453–7.
113. Vianna LG, Koulouris N, Lanigan C, Moxham J. Effect of acute hypercapnia on limb muscle contractility in humans. J Appl Physiol. 1990;69(4):1486–93.
114. Juan G, Calverley P, Talamo C, Schnader J, Roussos C. Effect of carbon dioxide on diaphragmatic function in human beings. N Engl J Med. 1984;310(14):874–9.
115. Stanojkovic I, Kotur-Stevuljevic J, Milenkovic B, Spasic S, Vujic T, Stefnovic A, et al. Pulmonary function, oxidative stress and inflammatory markers in severe COPD exacerbation. Respir Med. 2011;105(1):31–7.
116. Girgis CM, Clifton-Bligh RJ, Hamrick MW, Holick MF, Gunton JE. The roles of vitamin D in skeletal muscle: form, function, andmetabolism. Endocr Rev. 2013;34(1):33–83.
117. St-Arnaud R. The direct role of vitamin D on bone homeostasis. Arch Biochem Biophys. 2008;473(2):225–30.
118. Bernard S, Leblanc P, Whittom F, Carrier G, Jobin J, Belleau R, et al. Peripheral muscle weakness in patients with chronic obstructive pulmonary disease. Am J Respir Crit Care Med. 1998;158(2):629–34.
119. Shrikrishna D, Patel M, Tanner RJ, Symour JM, Connolly BA, Puthucheary ZA, et al. Quadriceps wasting and physical inactivity in patients with COPD. Eur Respir J. 2012;40(5):1115–22.
120. Spruit MA, Singh SJ, Garvey C, ZuWallack R, Nici L, Rochester C, et al. An official American Thoracic Society/European Respiratory Society statement: key concepts and advances in pulmonary rehabilitation. Am J Respir Crit Care Med. 2013;188(8):13–64.
121. MacNee W. Systemic inflammatory biomarkers and co-morbidities of chronic obstructive pulmonary disease. Ann Med. 2012;45(3):291–300.
122. Kanis JA. Assessment of fracture risk and its application to screening for postmenopausal osteoporosis: synopsis of a WHO report. WHO study group. Osteoporos Int. 1994;4(6):368–81.
123. Graat-Verboom L, Wouters EF, Smeenk FW, van den Borne BE, Lunde R, Spruit MA. Current status of research on osteoporosis in COPD: a systematic review. Eur Respir J. 2009;34(1):209–18.
124. Calverley PM, Anderson JA, Celli B, Ferguson GT, Jenkins C, Jones PW, et al. Salmeterol and fluticasone propionate and survival in chronic obstructive pulmonary disease. N Engl J Med. 2007;356(8):775–89.
125. Sarkar M, Bhardwaj R, Madabhavi I, Khatana J. Osteoporosis in chronic obstructive pulmonary disease. Clin Med Insights Circ Respir Pulm Med. 2015;9:5–21.
126. Schnell K, Weiss CO, Lee T, Krishnan JA, Leff B, Wolff JL, et al. The prevalence of clinically-relevant comorbid conditions in patients with physician-diagnosed COPD: a cross-sectional study using data from NHANES 1999–2008. BMC Pulm Med. 2012;12:26.
127. Vrieze A, de Greef MH, Wijkstra PJ, Vempe JB. Low bone mineral density in COPD patients related to worse lung function, low weight and decreased fat-free mass. Osteoporos Int. 2007;18(9):1197–202.

128. Jorgensen NR, Schwarz P, Holme I, Henriksen BM, Petersen VJ, Backer V. The prevalence of osteoporosis in patients with chronic obstructive pulmonary disease: across sectional study. Respir Med. 2007;101(1):177–85.
129. Jaramillo JD, Wilson C, Stinson DJ, Lynch DA, Bowler RP, Lutz S, et al. Reduced bone density and vertebral fractures in smokers. Men and COPD patients at increased risk. Ann Am Thorac Soc. 2015;12(5):648–56.
130. Mazokopakis EE, Starakis IK. Recommendations for diagnosis and management of osteoporosis in COPD men. ISRN Rheumatol. 2011;2011:901416.
131. Chee C, Sellahewa L, Pappachan JM. Inhaled corticosteroids and bone health. Open Respir Med J. 2014;8:85–92.
132. Kelly HW, Sternberg AL, Lescher R, Fuhlbrigge AL, Williams P, Zeiger RS, et al. Effect of inhaled glucocorticoids in childhood on adult height. N Engl J Med. 2012;367:904–12.
133. Buehring B, Viswanathan R, Binkley N, Busse W. Glucocorticoid-induced osteoporosis: an update on effects and management. J Allergy Clin Immunol. 2013;132(5):1019–30.
134. Ferguson GT, Calverley PM, Anderson JA, Jenkins CR, Jones PW, Willits LR, et al. Prevalence and progression of osteoporosis in patients with COPD: results from the TOwards a revolution in COPD health study. Chest. 2009;136(6):1456–65.
135. Sabit R, Bolton CE, Edwards PH, Pettit RJ, Evns WD, McEniery CM, et al. Arterial stiffness and osteoporosis in chronic obstructive pulmonary disease. Am J Respir Crit Care Med. 2007;175(12):1259–65.
136. Liang B, Feng Y. The association of low bone mineral density with systemic inflammation in clinically stable COPD. Endocrine. 2012;42(1):190–5.
137. Persson LJ, Aanerud M, Hiemstra PS, Hardie JA, Bakke PS, Eagan TM. Chronic obstructive pulmonary disease is associated with low levels of vitamin D. PLoS One. 2012;7:e38934.
138. Yohannes AM, Ershler WB. Anemia in COPD: a systematic review of the prevalence, quality of life, and mortality. Respir Care. 2011;56(5):644–52.
139. Korkmaz U, Korkmaz N, Yazici S, et al. Anemia as a risk factor for low bone mineral density in postmenopausal Turkish women. Eur J Intern Med. 2012;23(2):154–8.
140. Rutten EP, Franssen FM, Spruit MA, Wouters EF. Anemia is associated with bone mineral density in chronic obstructive pulmonary disease. COPD. 2013;10(3):286–92.
141. Fujimoto H, Fujimoto K, Ueda A, Ohata M. Hypoxemia is a risk factor for bone mass loss. J Bone Miner Metab. 1999;17(3):211–6.
142. Yoon V, Maalouf NM, Sakhaee K. The effects of smoking on bone metabolism. Osteoporos Int. 2012;23:2081–92.
143. Compston JE. Sex steroids and bone. Physiol Rev. 2001;81:419–47.
144. Balasubramanian V, Naing S. Hypogonadism in chronic obstructive pulmonary disease: incidence and effects. Curr Opin Pulm Med. 2012;18(2):112–7.
145. Graat-Verboom L, Smeenk FW, van den Borne BE, et al. Progression of osteoporosis in patients with COPD: a 3 year follow-up study. Respir Med. 2012;106(6):861–70.
146. de Luise C, Brimacombe M, Pedersen L, Sørensen HT. Chronic obstructive pulmonary disease and mortality following hip fracture: a population-based cohort study. Eur J Epidemiol. 2008;23(2):115–22.
147. Compston J, Cooper A, Cooper C, Francis R, Kanis JA, Marsh D, et al. Guideline for the diagnosis and management of osteoporosis in postmenopausal women and men from the age of 50 years in the UK. Maturitas. 2009;62(2):105–8.
148. Cosman F, de Beur SJ, LeBoff MS, Lewiecki EM, Tanner B, Randall S. Clinician's guide to prevention and treatment of osteoporosis. Osteoporos Int. 2014;25(10):2359–81.
149. Lehouck A, van Remoortel H, Troosters T, Decramer M, Janssens W. COPD and bone metabolism: a clinical update. Rev Mal Respir. 2010;27(10):1231–42.
150. Grossman JM, Gordon R, Ranganath VK, Deal C, Caplan L, Chen W. American College of Rheumatology 2010 recommendations for the prevention and treatment of glucocorticoid-induced osteoporosis. Arthritis Care Res. 2010;62(11):1515–26.
151. Mullerova H, Agusti A, Erqou S, Mapel DW. Cardiovascular comorbidity in COPD: systematic literature review. Chest. 2013;144(4):1163–78.
152. Barnes PJ, Celli BR. Systemic manifestations and comorbidities of COPD. Eur Respir J. 2009;33(5):1165–85.
153. Agustí A, Edwards LD, Rennard SI, MacNee W, Tal-Singer R, Miller BE, et al. Persistent systemic inflammation is associated with poor clinical outcomes in COPD: a novel phenotype. PLoS One. 2012;7(5):e37483.
154. Agusti A, Calverley PMA, Celli B, Coxson HO, Edwards LD, Lomas DA, et al. Characterisation of COPD heterogeneity in the ECLIPSE cohort. Respir Res. 2010;11:122.
155. Barger G, Dale HH. Chemical structure and sympathomimetic action of amines. J Physiol. 1910;41(1–2):19–59.
156. Roversi S, Roversi P, Spadafora G, Rossi R, Fabbri LM. Coronary artery disease concomitant with chronic obstructive pulmonary disease. Eur J Clin Investig. 2014;44(1):93–102.
157. Maclay JD, Macnee W. Cardiovascular disease in COPD: mechanisms. Chest. 2013;143(3):798–807.
158. Bertoletti L, Quenet S, Mismetti P, Hernandez L, Martin-Villasclaras JJ, Tolosa C, et al. Clinical presentation and outcome of venous thromboembolism in COPD. Eur Respir J. 2012;39(4):862–8.
159. de Miguel DJ, Chancafe Morgan J, Jiménez GR. The association between COPD and heartfailure risk: a review. Int J Chron Obstruct Pulmon Dis. 2013;8:305–12.
160. Patel AR, Hurst JR. Extrapulmonary comorbidities in chronic obstructive pulmonary disease: state of the art. Expert Rev Respir Med. 2011;5(5):647–62.

161. Hawkins NM, Petrie MC, Jhund PS, Chalmers GW, Dunn FG, McMurray JV. Heart failure and chronic obstructive pulmonary disease: diagnosis pitfalls and epidemiology. Eur J Heart Fail. 2009;11(2):130–9.
162. Rusinaru D, Saaidi I, Godard S, Mahjoub H, Battle C, Tribouilloy C. Impact of chronic obstructive pulmonary disease on long-term outcome of patients hospitalized for heart failure. Am J Cardiol. 2008;101(3):353–8.
163. Mancia G, Fagard R, Narkiewicz K. 2013 ESH/ESC guidelines for the management of arterial hypertension. J Hypertens. 2013;31:1281–357.
164. Torbicki A, Perrier A, Konstantinides S, et al. Guidelines on the diagnosis and management of acute pulmonary embolism: the task force for the diagnosis and management of acute pulmonary embolism of the European Society of Cardiology (ESC). Eur Heart J. 2008;29:2276–315.
165. Sharma GVRK, Sasahara AA. Diagnosis of pulmonary embolism in patients with chronic obstructive pulmonary disease. J Chronic Dis. 1975;28:253–7.
166. Tillie-Leblond I, Marquette CH, Perez T, Scherpereel A, Zanetti C, Tonnel AB, et al. Pulmonary embolism in patients with unexplained exacerbation of chronic obstructive pulmonary disease: prevalence and risk factors. Ann Intern Med. 2006;144(6):390–6.
167. Gunen H, Gulbas G, In E, Yetkin O, Hacievliyagil SS. Venous thromboemboli and exacerbations of COPD. Eur Respir J. 2010;35(6):1243–8.
168. Neuhaus A, Bentz RR, Weg JG. Pulmonary embolism in respiratory failure. Chest. 1978;73(4):460–5.
169. Moua T, Wood K. COPD and PE: a clinical dilemma. Int J Chron Obstruct Pulmon Dis. 2008;3(2):277–84.
170. Cavaillès A, Brinchault-Rabin G, Dixmier A, Goupil F, Gut-Gobert C, Marchand-Adam S. Comorbidities of COPD. Eur Respir Rev. 2013;22(130):454–75.
171. Calverley PM, Anderson JA, Celli B, Ferguson GT, Jenkins C, Jones PW, et al. Cardiovascular events in patients with COPD: TORCH study results. Thorax. 2010;65(8):719–25.
172. Decramer ML, Hanania NA, Lotvall JO, Yawn BP. The safety of long-acting beta2-agonists in the treatment of stable chronic obstructive pulmonary disease. Int J Chron Obstruct Pulmon Dis. 2013;8:53–64.
173. Etminan M, Jafari S, Carleton B, FitzGerald JM. Beta-blocker use and COPD mortality: a systematic review and meta-analysis. BMC Pulm Med. 2012;12:48.
174. Ekstrom MP, Hermansson AB, Strom KE. Effects of cardiovascular drugs on mortality in severe chronic obstructive pulmonary disease. Am J Respir Crit Care Med. 2013;187(7):715–20.
175. Dransfield MT, Rowe SM, Johnson JE, Bailey WC, Gerald LB. Use of beta blockers and the risk of death in hospitalised patients with acute exacerbations of COPD. Thorax. 2008;63(4):301–5.
176. Bhatt SP, Wells JM, Kinney GL, Washko GR Jr, Budoff M, Kim YI, et al. β-blockers are associated with a reduction in COPD exacerbations. Thorax. 2016;71(1):8–14.
177. Du Q, Sun Y, Ding N, Lu L, Chen Y. Beta-blockers reduced the risk of mortality and exacerbation in patients with COPD: a meta-analysis of observational studies. PLoS One. 2014;9(11):e113048.
178. Hurst JR, Vestbo J, Anzueto A, Locantore N, Müllerova H, Tal-Singer R, et al. Susceptibility to exacerbation in chronic obstructive pulmonary disease. N Engl J Med. 2010;363(12):1128–38.
179. Rascon-Aguilar IE, Pamer M, Wludyka P, Cury J, Coultas D, Lambiase LR, et al. Role of gastroesophageal reflux symptoms in exacerbations of COPD. Chest. 2006;130(4):1096–101.
180. Lin YH, Tsai CL, Chien LN, Chiou HY, Jeng C. Newly diagnosed gastroesophageal reflux disease increased the risk of acute exacerbation of chronic obstructive pulmonary disease during the first year following diagnosis—a nationwide population-based cohort study. Int J Clin Pract. 2015;69(3):350–7.
181. Benson VS, Müllerova H, Vestbo J, Wedzicha JA, Patel A, Hurst JR. Associations between gastro-oesophageal reflux, its management and exacerbations of chronic obstructive pulmonary disease. Respir Med. 2015;109(9):1147–54.
182. Casanova C, Baudet JS, del Valle VM, Martin JM, Aquiree-Jaime A, de Torres JP, et al. Increased gastro-oesophageal reflux disease in patients with severe COPD. Eur Respir J. 2004;23(6):841–5.
183. Savarino E, Bazzica M, Zentilin P, Pohl D, Parodi A, Cittadini G, et al. Gastroesophageal reflux and pulmonary fibrosis in scleroderma: a study using pH-impedance monitoring. Am J Respir Crit Care Med. 2009;179(5):408–13.
184. Stein MR, Towner TG, Weber RW, Mansfield LE, Jacobson KW, McDonnell JT, et al. The effect of theophylline on the lower esophageal sphincter pressure. Ann Allergy. 1980;45(4):238–41.
185. Crowell MD, Zayat EN, Lacy BE, Schettler-Duncan A, Liu MC. The effects of an inhaled beta(2)-adrenergic agonist on lower esophageal function: a dose–response study. Chest. 2001;120(4):1184–9.
186. Schols AM, Ferreira IM, Franssen FM, Gosker HR, Janssens W, Muscaritoli M, et al. Nutritional assessment and therapy in COPD: a European Respiratory Society statement. Eur Respir J. 2014;44(6):1504–20.
187. Akbulut G, Gezmen-Karadag M, Ertas Y, Barut Uyar B, Yassibas E, Turkozu D, et al. Plasma orexin-a and ghrelin levels in patients with chronic obstructive pulmonary disease: interaction with nutritional status and body composition. Exp Ther Med. 2014;7(6):1617–24.
188. Agusti AG. Systemic effects of chronic obstructive pulmonary disease. Proc Am Thorac Soc. 2005;2(4):367–70.
189. Wagner PD. Possible mechanisms underlying the development of cachexia in COPD. Eur Respir J. 2008;31(3):492–501.
190. Cavailles A, Brinchault-Robin G, Dixmier A, et al. Comorbidites of COPD. Eur Respir Rev. 2013;22(130):454–75.

191. Ferreira IM, Brooks D, White J, Goldstein R. Nutritional supplementation for stable COPD. Cochrane Database Syst Rev. 2012;12:CD000998.
192. Schols AM. Nutrition as a metabolic modulator in COPD. Chest. 2013;144(4):1340–5.
193. Sateia MJ. International classification of sleep disorders-third edition: highlights and modifications. Chest. 2014;146(5):1387–94.
194. Collop N. Sleep and sleep disorders in chronic obstructive pulmonary disease. Respiration. 2010;80(1):78–86.
195. Budhiraja R, Siddiqi TA, Quan SF. Sleep disorders in chronic obstructive pulmonary disease: etiology, impact, and management. J Clin Sleep Med. 2015;11(3):259–70.
196. Klink ME, Dodge R, Quan SF. The relation of sleep complaints to respiratory symptoms in a general population. Chest. 1994;105(1):151–4.
197. Crinion SJ, McNicholas WT. Sleep-related disorders in chronic obstructive pulmonary disease. Expert Rev Respir Med. 2014;8(1):79–88.
198. Casey KR, Cantillo KO, Brown LK. Sleep-related hypoventilation/hypoxemic syndromes. Chest. 2007;131(6):1936–48.
199. American Academy of Sleep Medicine. International classification of sleep disorders. 3rd ed. Darien: American Academy of Sleep Medicine; 2014.
200. Sidney S, Sorel M, Quesenberry CP Jr, DeLuise C, Lanes S, Eisner MD. COPD and incident cardiovascular disease hospitalizations and mortality: Kaiser Permanente medical care program. Chest. 2005;128(4):2068–75.
201. Sin DD, Wu L, Man SF. The relationship between reduced lung function and cardiovascular mortality: a population-based study and a systematic review of the literature. Chest. 2005;127(6):1952–9.
202. Chaouat A, Weitzenblum E, Kessler R, Charpentier C, Ehrhart M, Levi-Valensi P, et al. Sleep-related O2 desaturation and daytime pulmonary haemodynamics in COPD patients with mild hypoxaemia. Eur Respir J. 1997;10(8):1730–5.
203. McNicholas WT, FitzGerald MX. Nocturnal death among patients with chronic bronchitis and emphysema. BMJ. 1984;289(6449):878.
204. Flenley DC. Sleep in chronic obstructive lung disease. Clin Chest Med. 1985;6(4):651–61.
205. Chaouat A, Weitzenblum E, Krieger J, Ifoundza T, Oswald M, Kessler R. Association of chronic obstructive pulmonary disease and sleep apnea syndrome. Am J Respir Crit Care Med. 1995;151(1):82–6.
206. Sanders MH, Newman AB, Haggerty CL, Redline S, Lebowitz M, Samet J, et al. Sleep and sleep-disordered breathing in adults with predominantly mild obstructive airway disease. Am J Respir Crit Care Med. 2003;167(1):7–14.
207. Bednarek M, Plywaczewski R, Jonczak L, Zielinski J. There is no relationship between chronic obstructive pulmonary disease and obstructive sleep apnea syndrome: a population study. Respiration. 2005;72(2):142–9.
208. Mieczkowski B, Ezzie ME. Update on obstructive sleep apnea and its relation to COPD. Int J Chron Obstruct Pulmon Dis. 2014;9:349–62.
209. GOLD Committee. Global strategy for the diagnosis management and prevention of COPD. NewYork: Global Initiative for Chronic Obstructive Lung Disease (GOLD); 2014.
210. Moloney ED, Kiely JL, McNicholas WT. Controlled oxygen therapy and carbon dioxide retention during exacerbations of chronic obstructive pulmonary disease. Lancet. 2001;357(9255):526–8.
211. Costello RW, Liston R, McNicholas WT. Compliance at night with low flow oxygen therapy: a comparison of nasal cannulae and Venturi face masks. Thorax. 1995;50(4):405–6.
212. Clinical indications for noninvasive positive pressure ventilation in chronic respiratory failure due to restrictive lung disease, COPD, and nocturnal hypoventilation—a consensus conference report. Chest. 1999;116(2):521–34.
213. Renston JP, DiMarco AF, Supinski GS. Respiratory muscle rest using nasal BiPAP ventilation in patients with stable severe COPD. Chest. 1994;105(4):1053–60.
214. Meecham Jones DJ, Paul EA, Jones PW, Wedzicha JA. Nasal pressure support ventilation plus oxygen compared with oxygen therapy alone in hypercapnic COPD. Am J Respir Crit Care Med. 1995;152(2):538–44.
215. McNicholas WT, Verbraecken J, Marin JM. Sleep disorders in COPD: the forgotten dimension. Eur Respir Rev. 2013;22(129):365–75.
216. Ng TP, Niti M, Tan WC, Cao Z, Ong KC, Eng P. Depressive symptoms and chronic obstructive pulmonary disease: effect on mortality, hospital readmission, symptom burden, functional status, and quality of life. Arch Intern Med. 2007;167(1):60–7.
217. Smith MC, Wrobel J. Epidemiology and clinical impact of major comorbidities in patients with COPD. Int J Chron Obstruct Pulmon Dis. 2014;9:871–88.
218. Maurer J, Rebbapragada V, Borson S, Goldstein R, Kunik ME, Yohannes AM, Hanania A, et al. Anxiety and depression in COPD: current understanding, unanswered questions, and research needs. Chest. 2008;134(4):43–56.
219. Atlantis E, Fahey P, Cochrane B, Smith S. Bidirectional associations between clinically relevant depression or anxiety and COPD: a systematic review and meta-analysis. Chest. 2013;144(3):766–77.
220. Cully JA, Graham DP, Stanley MA, Ferguson CJ, Sharafkhaneh A, Souchek J, et al. Quality of life in patients with chronic obstructive pulmonary disease and comorbid anxiety or depression. Psychosomatics. 2006;47(4):312–9.
221. Hill K, Geist R, Goldstein RS, Lacasse Y, Anxiety and depression in end-stage COPD. Eur Respir J 2008;31(3):667–677.
222. Stage KB, Middelboe T, Stage TB, Sørensen CH. Depression in COPD—management and quality

of life considerations. Int J Chron Obstruct Pulmon Dis. 2006;1(3):315–20.
223. Steens RD, Pouliot Z, Millar TW, Kryger MH, George CF. Effects of zolpidem and triazolam on sleep and respiration in mild to moderate chronic obstructive pulmonary disease. Sleep. 1993;16(4):318–26.
224. Yohannes AM, Baldwin RC, Connolly MJ. Depression and anxiety in elderly outpatients with chronic obstructive pulmonary disease: prevalence, and validation of the BASDEC screening questionnaire. Int J Geriatr Psychiatry. 2000;15(12):1090–6.
225. Leatherman N. Pulmonary rehabilitation. In: Dantzker D, MacIntyre NR, Bakow ED, editors. Comprehensive respiratory care. Philadelphia: WB Saunders; 1955. p. 925–48.
226. Fahy B. Pulmonary rehabilitation: nuts and bolts. Clin Pulm Med. 2000;7:319–25.
227. Emery C, Hauck ER, Schein RL, MacIntyre NR. Psychological and cognitive outcomes of a randomized trial of exercise among patients with chronic obstructive pulmonary disease. Health Psychol. 1998;17(3):232–40.
228. Gayle R, Spitler DL, Karper WB, Jaeger RM, Rice SN. Psychological changes in exercising COPD patients. Int J Rehabil Res. 1988;11(4):335–42.
229. Ries AL, Carlin BW, Carrieri-Kholman V. Pulmonary rehabilitation joint ACCP/AACVPR evidence-based guidelines. Chest. 1997;112(5):1363–96.
230. de Godoy DV, de Godoy RF. A randomized controlled trial of the effect of psychotherapy on anxiety and depression in chronic obstructive pulmonary disease. Arch Phys Med Rehabil. 2003;84(8):1154–7.
231. Paz-Diaz H, Montes de Oca M, Lopez JM, Celli BR. Pulmonary rehabilitation improves depression, anxiety, dyspnea and health status in patients with COPD. Am J Phys Med Rehabil. 2007;86(1):30–6.
232. Kunik ME, Veazey C, Cully JA, Souchek J, Graham DP, Hopko D, et al. COPD education and cognitive behavioral therapy group treatment for clinically significant symptoms of depression and anxiety in COPD patients: a randomized controlled trial. Psychol Med. 2008;38(3):385–96.
233. World Health Organization. Nutritional anemias: report of a WHO scientific group. In: WHO technical report series 405. Geneva: World Health Organization; 1968. p. 1–37.
234. Klip IT, Comin-Colet J, Voors AA, Ponikowski P, Enjuanes C, Banasiak W, et al. Iron deficiency in chronic heart failure: an international pooled analysis. Am Heart J. 2013;165(4):575–82.
235. Kent BD, Mitchell PD, McNicholas WT. Hypoxemia in patients with COPD: cause, effects, and disease progression. Int J Chron Obstruct Pulmon Dis. 2011;6:199–208.
236. Chaouat A, Naeije R, Weitzenblum E. Pulmonary hypertension in COPD. Eur Respir J. 2008;32(5):1371–85.
237. Sarkar M, Rajta PN, Khatana J. Anemia in chronic obstructive pulmonary disease: prevalence, pathogenesis, and potential impact. J Lung India. 2015;32(2):142–51.
238. Hopkinson NS, Polkey MI. Anaemia in chronic obstructive pulmonary disease: an insight into its prevalence and pathophysiology. Clin Sci (Lond). 2015;128(5):283–95.
239. Hoepers AT, Menezes MM, Fröde TS. Systematic review of anaemia and inflammatory markers in chronic obstructive pulmonary disease. Clin Exp Pharmacol Physiol. 2015;42(3):231–9.
240. Ferrari M, Manea L, Anton K, Bruzzone P, Meneghello M, Zamboni F, et al. Anemia and hemoglobin serum levels are associated with exercise capacity and quality of life in chronic obstructive pulmonary disease. BMC Pulm Med. 2015;15:58.
241. Chambellan A, Chailleux E, Similowski T, ANTADIR Observatory Group. Prognostic value of the hematocrit in patients with severe COPD receiving long-term oxygen therapy. Chest. 2005;128(3):1201.
242. Schönhofer B, Wenzel M, Geibel M, Köhler D. Blood transfusion and lung function in chronically anemic patients with severe chronic obstructive pulmonary disease. Crit Care Med. 1998;26(11):1824–8.
243. Schönhofer B, Böhrer H, Köhler D. Blood transfusion facilitating difficult weaning from the ventilator. Anaesthesia. 1998;53(2):181–4.
244. Nickol AH, Frise MC, Cheng HY, McGahey A, McFadyen BM, Harris-Wright T, et al. A cross-sectional study of the prevalence and associations of iron deficiency in a cohort of patients with chronic obstructive pulmonary disease. BMJ Open. 2015;5(7):e007911.

Personalized Treatment in COPD

20

Jae Seung Lee and Sang-Do Lee

Definition of Personalized Medicine

Patients typically have variability in response to many drugs that are currently available. It can be difficult to predict who will benefit from a medication, who will not respond. The concept of personalized medicine (PM) dates back many hundreds of years. However, it has received much attention in recent years after rapid developments in genomics which had enabled scientists and medical practitioners to develop personalized diagnosis and treatment. PM is based on the scientific understanding on how a person's unique genetic and molecular profile helps in determining his or her different treatment response [1]. The definition and scope of the term "PM" varies widely, ranging from the narrow "the right patient with the right drug at the right dose at the right time" to the extremely broad "tailoring of medical treatment to the individual characteristics, needs and preferences of a patient during all stages of care, including prevention, diagnosis, treatment and follow-up" [2]. Furthermore, several terms, including "pharmacogenomics," "precision medicine," and "stratified medicine" are sometimes used interchangeably with "personalized medicine." Pharmacogenomics—the study of variations of DNA and RNA characteristics as related to drug response [3]—is one of the most exciting areas of PM today. Pharmacogenomics uses genetic information for purposes of explaining interindividual differences in pharmacodynamics and pharmacokinetics, identifying responders to a drug, and predicting the efficacy and/or toxicity of a drug. In the respiratory disease area, genetic information about non-small cell lung cancer is increasingly being used. Gefitinib and erlotinib are both agents which are effective only in patients whose tumors have specific epidermal growth factor receptor (EGFR) mutation [4]. Precision medicine has been defined as "the use of genomic, epigenomic, exposure and other data to define individual patterns of disease, potentially leading to better individual treatment [5]." "Stratified medicine" is the grouping of patients based on the risk of disease or response to therapy by using diagnostic tests or techniques [6]. The factors which can be used to aid this process are varied; typically, this might include the use of specific clinical features, biomarkers, or genetic information.

COPD is in fact a very heterogeneous disease characterized by a wide range of symptoms, clinical findings, radiologic and pathologic abnormalities, and varied responses to treatment [7]. Recognition of COPD heterogeneity and identifying subgroups, the so-called clinical phenotypes of COPD patients, is especially important for the development of stratified medicine in COPD [8]. And there is a critical need to

J.S. Lee, M.D. (✉) • S.-D. Lee, M.D.
Department of Pulmonary and Critical Care Medicine, Asan Medical Center, University of Ulsan College of Medicine, Ulsan, South Korea
e-mail: jsdoc1186@daum.net; sdlee@amc.seoul.kr

S.-D. Lee (ed.), *COPD*, DOI 10.1007/978-3-662-47178-4_20

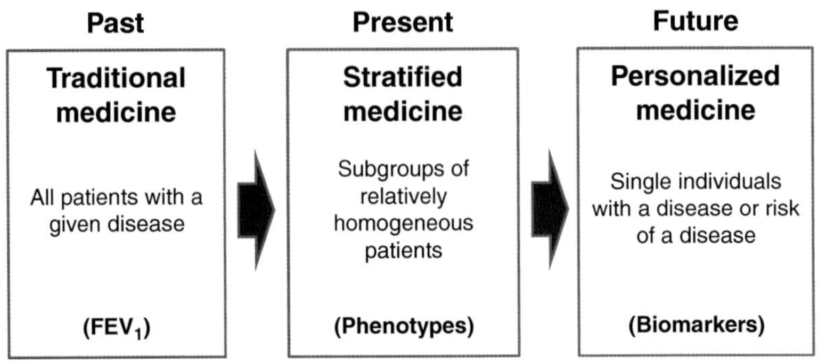

Fig. 20.1 Paradigm evolution of treatment of COPD. Modified from Agusti A. The path to personalized medicine in COPD. Thorax 2014;69:857–864

understand the molecular pathways that underlie the heterogeneity within COPD for better personalized management (Fig. 20.1, [9]).

Paradigm Shift of Treatment of COPD

COPD was recognized as a self-inflicted disease for which basically nothing could be done other than persuading the patient to quit smoking. To combat this nihilistic attitude toward COPD and improve management of COPD, the Global Initiative for Chronic Obstructive Lung Disease (GOLD) was initiated in 1998 and the first GOLD document was released in 2001. The first GOLD document used four-stage classification of COPD severity for providing an educational tool and a general indication of the approach to management [10]. The staging was based on airflow limitation as measured by the post-bronchodilator forced expiratory volume in 1 s (FEV_1). The principle for the pharmacological treatment of COPD in first GOLD guideline was characterized by a stepwise increase in treatment, depending on the severity of disease. The recommendations for initial choice of pharmacological treatment were based solely on the FEV_1. Bronchodilators were central to improve lung function and recommended for all symptomatic patients. Based on the FEV_1, as-needed treatment with short-acting bronchodilators or regular treatment with one or more long-acting bronchodilators was recommended. Inhaled corticosteroids (ICSs) were only considered for symptomatic COPD patients with a documented spirometric response to ICSs or in those with an $FEV_1 < 50\%$ predicted and repeated exacerbations [11]. Although improvement in both symptoms and health status was a GOLD treatment objective, symptom assessment did not have a direct relation to the initial choice of management.

A second major change in the field of COPD occurred in 2011 when the third revision of the GOLD document was released [12]. This change was caused by the acceptance of the concept that COPD was a complex and heterogeneous disease with a number of intrapulmonary and extrapulmonary components. FEV_1 was an insufficient marker of the severity of breathlessness, exercise limitation, and health status impairment [13, 14]. Furthermore, arbitrary stratifications of severity by FEV_1 are not necessarily indicative of treatment efficacy [15, 16]. GOLD 2011 document abandoned the concept of staging system and replace the term "stage" with "grade" and proposed a three-dimensional assessment of COPD which, while still considering the severity of airflow limitation (FEV_1), also includes the level of symptoms and the previous history of exacerbations to predict the risk of future exacerbations [12]. The four-quadrant system was introduced with the goal to match assessment with treatment choice, thus moving COPD treatment toward more personalized medicine. This proposed system is not strictly evidence based but rather close to "expert opinion." No therapeutic trial reported before the 2011 GOLD document date did use selection criteria that strictly matched the present GOLD classification.

Clinical Phenotype-Based Personalized Treatment in Stable COPD

Originally, the term "phenotype" refers to the composite of an organism's observable characteristics or traits such as its morphology, development, biochemical or physical properties, as opposed to genotype. In the field of COPD, an international group of experts has defined the term "COPD phenotype" as "a single or combination of disease attributes that describe differences between individuals with COPD as they relate to clinically meaningful outcomes (symptoms, exacerbations, response to therapy, rate of disease progression, or death) [17]." This definition provides a framework of categorizing unique characteristics of patients with COPD into distinct prognostic and therapeutic subgroups. The two extreme classic clinical phenotypes of "blue bloater" or "pink puffer" are not sufficient for categorizing various COPD phenotypes. A variety of clinical, physiologic, and radiologic parameters have been used to explore the different phenotypes of COPD [18]. Yet there is no consensus on the number and definition of the different COPD phenotypes. The phenotype should be able to classify patients into subgroups with prognostic value and to determine the most appropriate therapy to achieve better results from a clinical standpoint. This constitutes the basis of a personalized approach for the pharmacological treatment of COPD. Until now, frequent exacerbator, emphysema, chronic bronchitis, and asthma-COPD overlap syndrome (ACOS) have been regarded as clinically relevant phenotypes which could be used for personalized treatment [19, 20].

Frequent Exacerbator

COPD is often associated with exacerbations described as an acute worsening of respiratory symptoms associated with a variable degree of physiological deterioration [21]. Exacerbations of COPD are associated with poorer quality of life, accelerated decline of lung function, and increased mortality [22]. The COPD frequent exacerbator phenotype is defined by the occurrence of two or more exacerbations per year [23]. Exacerbations of COPD become more frequent as airflow limitation becomes more severe. However, there are large differences in exacerbation frequency among individuals [24]. The best predictor of exacerbations is the patient's own history of exacerbations [23]. Thus, "frequent exacerbators" appear to be a distinct phenotype. Strategies that are currently used to prevent COPD exacerbations include pharmacological interventions with long-acting bronchodilators alone or combination with ICSs, phosphodiesterase inhibitors and mucolytics, and non-pharmacological interventions such as smoking cessation, influenza vaccination, and pulmonary rehabilitation [25]. Fixed-dose ICS/long-acting β_2 agonist (LABA) combinations are recommended in patients with severe airflow limitation (FEV_1 < 50% predicted value) and two or more COPD exacerbations per year [12]. The ICS improves lung function, decreases the rate of exacerbations, and seems to improve the survival when combined with bronchodilators, but must be weighed against the potential for increased vulnerability to pneumonia [26]. Lower airway bacterial colonization and a new strain of a bacterial pathogen in COPD patients were known to be related to the frequency of exacerbations [27, 28]. These studies have led to renewed interest in long-term antibiotic treatment to prevent COPD exacerbations. Recent clinical trials have demonstrated that long-term prophylactic macrolide treatment was associated with a reduction in COPD exacerbations [29]. However, long-term prophylactic antibiotic treatment could increase the emergence of antibiotic-resistant bacteria [30]. Thus, prophylactic antibiotic treatment should be considered with caution for patients with COPD who have experienced frequent exacerbations despite other optimal treatments.

Emphysema

Emphysema is defined pathologically as the presence of permanent enlargement of the airspaces distal to the terminal bronchioles, accompanied by destruction of alveolar walls and without obvious fibrosis [31]. Computed tomography (CT) can detect earlier emphysema that can be detected by spirometry or diffusing capacity and many studies have addressed the ability of CT to accurately quantify the extent and severity of pulmonary emphysema [32]. CT emphysema severity is associated with lower body mass index, worse health status, BODE index, and a rapid decline in FEV_1 [33–36]. Expiratory flow limitation, air trapping, and hyperinflation are well-known problems in COPD patients. Hyperinflation correlates more directly with patient-centered outcomes such as dyspnea and exercise limitation than FEV_1 [37, 38]. The reduction in elastic recoil due to emphysema is responsible for static hyperinflation. Bronchodilators induce a relaxation of smooth muscle tone in airways and consequently reduce the flow limitation and promote lung emptying, as demonstrated by an increase in inspiratory capacity and reduction of residual volume on spirometry [39, 40]. This bronchodilator's effects lead to improvement in symptoms, exercise capacity, and the state of health as perceived by the patient. CT emphysema extent was shown to be predictive of a poorer pulmonary function in response to treatment with a short-acting bronchodilator and ICS/LABA [41, 42]. Besides the extent of emphysema, the distribution of emphysema is associated with therapeutic effect of lung volume reduction surgery [43, 44]. Lung volume reduction surgery (LVRS) is more effective than medical therapy for patients with predominantly upper-lobe emphysema and low exercise capacity prior to LVRS. By contrast, LVRS results in more mortality than medical management when it is used to treat severe emphysema patients with lower FEV_1 and either homogeneous emphysema on CT [45].

Chronic Bronchitis

Chronic bronchitis, defined by the presence of productive cough or expectoration for more than 3 months a year and more than two consecutive years [46], has been associated with elevated risk of airway colonization and respiratory infection. Chronic bronchitis is associated with multiple clinical consequences, including hastening lung function decline, increasing risk of exacerbations, reducing health-related quality of life, and possibly raising all-cause mortality [47–50]. In these patients, ICS and PDE-4 inhibitors can be indicated on top of regular long-lasting bronchodilator treatment [12]. PDE-4 inhibitor was shown to reduce moderate-to-severe exacerbations treated with corticosteroids by 15–20% and to improve pulmonary function in a subgroup of patients with chronic bronchitis, severe or very severe COPD, and a history of exacerbation [51, 52]. Acquired dysfunction of the cystic fibrosis transmembrane conductance regulator (CFTR) in airway epithelial cells can delay mucociliary transport and has been associated with chronic bronchitis [53]. Roflumilast activates CFTR-mediated anion transport [54] which may be at least one mechanism of its benefit in chronic bronchitis. Selected cases of frequent exacerbators might respond to long-term treatment with prophylactic antibiotics [30]. Independent of their antibiotic properties, macrolides have been shown to reduce neutrophil elastase-induced mucus stasis, suggesting benefit in chronic bronchitis [55]. When ICS cannot be used, mucolytics might be effective in reducing exacerbations [56, 57].

Asthma-COPD Overlap Syndrome (ACOS)

ICS is highly effective in asthma and have become the mainstay of therapy in all patients with persistent symptoms [58]. ICS is also widely used in COPD patients. However, there are still controversies about the ICS's clinical benefit and increasing evidence that ICS can increase the risk of pneumonia [26]. Therefore, it is necessary to distinguish between asthma and COPD to provide appropriate therapy for patients. However, within the spectrum of chronic airway obstruction, there are individuals with asthma-COPD overlap syndrome (ACOS) [59, 60] and around 15–20% of COPD patients may have an ACOS [61–63]. ACOS has been defined as the coexistence of increased variability of airflow in a patient with incompletely reversible airway obstruction [64]. Recent GOLD-Global Initiative for Asthma (GINA) document described the ACOS as persistent airflow limitation with several features usually associated with asthma and several features usually associated with COPD [65]. Unfortunately, there is no consensus on a unified definition or diagnostic criteria for ACOS. Recent Spanish guideline proposed experts consensus diagnostic criteria for ACOS but it requires prospective validation [66].

Patients with ACOS report worse health-related quality of life and experience more frequent and severe exacerbations than those without ACOS [62, 67]. Moreover, patients with coexisting COPD and asthma have a higher risk of death than those with COPD or asthma singly [68]. Patients with ACOS have been systematically excluded from both COPD and asthma pharmacological trials. As a consequence, there is no clear information about the response of these patients to most of the current pharmacological therapies. Individuals with ACOS are more likely to respond to ICS, and this justifies their use associated with a bronchodilator as a first treatment option in symptomatic individuals [69, 70]. Patients with the ACOS, in comparison with subjects with COPD alone, have higher peripheral and sputum eosinophil counts, preserved diffusing capacity, higher prevalence of bronchial thickening on chest HRCT, and better reversibility response to treatment with ICS [70]. In particular, the lung function improvement after treatment with ICS correlated significantly with sputum eosinophil counts and the grade of bronchial wall thickening [71–73]. These studies suggest that short-term treatment with ICS in patients with COPD and sputum eosinophilia, which is a component of ACOS, might improve lung function and symptoms by reducing airway inflammation. However, larger prospective controlled studies are required to establish the long-term effects of maintenance treatment with ICS in patients with ACOS in terms of reduction of exacerbations and lung function decline. Because airway inflammation in ACOS resembles that in asthma, it has been suggested that the use of long-acting bronchodilator alone in this population should be avoided [74]. In one clinical trial in patients with COPD and concomitant asthma, the use of tiotropium had a beneficial effect in improving lung function [75]. These trials provide a foundation to further explore the role of existing and future long-acting muscarinic antagonist (LAMA) agents in individuals with ACOS.

Biomarker Guided Personalized Treatment in COPD

Sputum and Serum Biomarker

Biomarker is defined as a "characteristic that is objectively measured and evaluated as an indicator of normal biologic processes, pathogenic processes, or pharmacologic responses to a therapeutic intervention" [76]. FEV_1 is thus a good marker for risk stratification and prognosis, but a suboptimal surrogate for assessing the therapeutic potential of novel drugs. Noninvasive biomarkers that aid phenotyping of COPD are crucial to the development of personalized treatment. A large amount of biomarkers has been evaluated in COPD patients [77]. However, there are still no well-validated biomarkers or surrogate endpoints that can be used to establish efficacy of novel drugs for COPD. Sputum and peripheral blood eosinophil counts and factional exhaled nitric oxide (FeNO) as the most investigated phenotypic biomarkers in airway disease. Induced sputum eosinophils have been considered the gold standard method to measure eosinophilic airway inflammation. Peripheral blood eosinophil counts may also be useful for monitoring eosinophilic airway inflammation. In COPD, sputum eosinophils may be a feature of ACOS and have been shown to be associated with a positive response to corticosteroid treatment [71–73].

FeNO has been extensively studied in the past 10 years for its biomarker potential in airway disease, and has been shown to be a useful and reproducible surrogate marker for airway inflammation, mediated by interleukin (IL)-4 and IL-13 [78]. In asthma, FeNO is reproducible, responsive to changes in ICS therapy, and can reflect uncontrolled asthma and predict future exacerbations [79]. The role of FeNO in COPD is less clear, as current smoking can influence FeNO readings unpredictably and independently of eosinophilic inflammation [80, 81]. However, elevated FeNO in COPD may indicate better response to ICS [82].

Recently, there have been attempts to phenotype the biological profiles of COPD exacerbations and biomarker-guided therapy for COPD exacerbations. Bacterial, viral, eosinophilic, and pauci-inflammatory phenotypes of COPD exacerbations have been identified, and these phenotypes are stable and related to the clinical phenotype in stable COPD [83, 84]. Peripheral blood eosinophils have emerged as a biomarker to guide oral corticosteroid treatment in COPD exacerbation. A recent randomized trial showed that a biomarker-directed treatment strategy using the peripheral blood eosinophil count to guide corticosteroid prescription can be safely used to treat outpatient exacerbations of COPD. Subjects without an eosinophilia treated with systemic corticosteroids had more adverse events and a poorer rate of recovery [85]. Antibiotics for COPD exacerbations showed large and consistent benefits in patients admitted to intensive care, but for outpatients and inpatients the results were inconsistent [86]. It is desirable to be able to reliably identify bacterial exacerbations and target antibiotics to this subgroup of patients. Current evidence suggests that procalcitonin and C-reactive protein have a role as a biomarker for bacterial exacerbations of COPD and that it can be safely used to reduce inappropriate antibiotics in acute exacerbations of COPD [87–89].

CT Biomarker

Recent advances in CT allow precise assessment of anatomic alterations in COPD, such as emphysema and airways disease. Furthermore, inspiratory and expiratory CT can provide functional parameters that can be used as imaging biomarkers for the diagnosis of phenotypes and disease progression [90]. Recently, there has been increasing interest in developing CT-based biomarkers which can be used to predict response to current and novel therapies. Kitaguchi et al. [34] reported that emphysema score and the grade of bronchial wall thickening were significant determinants for bronchodilator responsiveness and for the responsiveness to the treatment with an ICS. Another study group has shown that emphysema-dominant COPD patients responded poorly to the 3 months of combination ICS/LABA treatment [91]. However, other two studies found no significant differences in bronchodilator responsiveness among groups classified according to severity of emphysema [33, 92]. Patients with COPD show different response patterns to bronchodilator, such that some patients show improvement principally in expiratory flow, whereas others respond by improvement of lung volume [93]. The degrees of emphysema and air trapping may contribute to the different response patterns to bronchodilator in patients with COPD [41]. Expiratory flow limitation and lung hyperinflation are crucial pathophysiological mechanisms in the development of dyspnea, exercise intolerance, and respiratory failure in patients with COPD [94]. The degree of lung hyperinflation is a predictor of functional improvements after bronchodilator therapy and LVRS [95, 96]. Combined assessment of lung volume and disease components of COPD with CT can be valuable decision-making tools in the management of severe COPD patients. Lobar lung volume measurement is important in assessing the efficacy of lung volume reduction treatments [97]. Lobar lung volume measurements on both inspiratory and expiratory scans may reveal the heterogeneous severity of air trapping in each lobe, and it may be useful for the determination of target lobes for lung volume reduction treatments.

Genetic Biomarker

Severe α1- antitrypsin (AAT) deficiency is the only clearly defined genetic cause of COPD, accounting for 1–2% of COPD cases in the USA

[98]. α1-Antitrypsin deficiency also provides an example of the significance of COPD subtypes in COPD pharmacogenetics. Intravenous infusion of pooled human AAT is indicated for augmentation therapy in patients with severe AAT deficiency and COPD, but not in COPD patients without this genetic subtype [99]. There are likely to be other genes that define additional relevant COPD phenotype. Most COPD pharmacogenetics studies of acute bronchodilator responsiveness have focused on the β2-adrenergic receptor, the target for short- and long-acting β2-agonists.

At this point, the evidence for the role of *ADRB2* variants as pharmacogenetic determinants of response to bronchodilators is conflicting [100, 101]. Kim et al. followed 104 Korean COPD patients who were treated with a combination of inhaled ICS/LABA [102]. The codon 16 and 27 variants were not associated with bronchodilator response at baseline or change in FEV_1 over 12 weeks of treatment. The role of *ADRB2* variants as pharmacogenetic determinants of response to short-acting bronchodilators and LAMA remains unclear [103, 104]. In addition to *ADRB2*, other candidate genes have been analyzed in COPD pharmacogenetics studies. In patients with asthma, variants of the corticotropin-releasing hormone receptor-1 (*CRHR1*) are an important determinant of response to ICS treatment [105]. One intronic variant (rs242941) was associated with change in FEV_1 after 12 weeks of treatment with ICS/LABA in Korean COPD patients [106].

Kim et al. also examined SNPs in five candidate genes—*EPHX1*, *SFTPB*, *TGFB1*, serpin peptidase inhibitor E2 (*SERPINE2*) and glutathione *S*-transferase pi (*GSTP1*). Three SNPs in *EPHX1* and three SNPs in *SERPINE2* were associated with various bronchodilator response phenotypes, in addition to the associations found for the two synonymous variants in *ADRB2* [103]. Molecular phenotyping of COPD through "omics" data is likely to lead to an even more personalized pharmacological treatment of individual patients with COPD. Genomic approaches such as genome-wide association studies and gene expression studies have discovered several genes and molecular pathways involved in COPD pathogenesis; however, these "first generation" omics studies have explained a small portion of the COPD heritability [107]. High-throughput "next generation" sequencing method may become a powerful tool for characterizing the molecular changes underlying COPD as well as the heterogeneity among patients with COPD. Novel transcriptomic approaches to study the airway and lung tissue in COPD hold the potential to improve our understanding of the molecular mechanisms of heterogeneous clinical phenotypes [108, 109]. The GLUCOLD investigators have recently demonstrated that a more pronounced ICS treatment-induced alteration in airway gene expression was significantly associated with a lower rate of decline in FEV_1 [110]. This new understanding can be contributed to develop targeted COPD therapies and ultimately personalize treatment of COPD patients.

Future Perspective

Many COPD patients remain symptomatic despite maximal medical therapy. COPD is a complex disease with various clinical phenotypes; thus, there are likely to be drugs that are more or less effective for patients with a particular phenotype. Future clinical trials are likely to focus on patients with specific disease-related phenotypes. We now know that emerging phenotypes in COPD are dependent on the dynamics of interaction between genes and broader environmental, epigenetic influences. To develop novel biomarkers and targeted therapeutic interventions in COPD, it is necessary to improve our understanding of the interrelationships between phenotypes and their environmental, genetic, molecular, and cellular basis (Fig. 20.2 [111]). An integrated approach will be critical for the development of genetic profiles based on the complex molecular mechanisms underlying treatment responses to eventually deliver truly precise and personalized medicine.

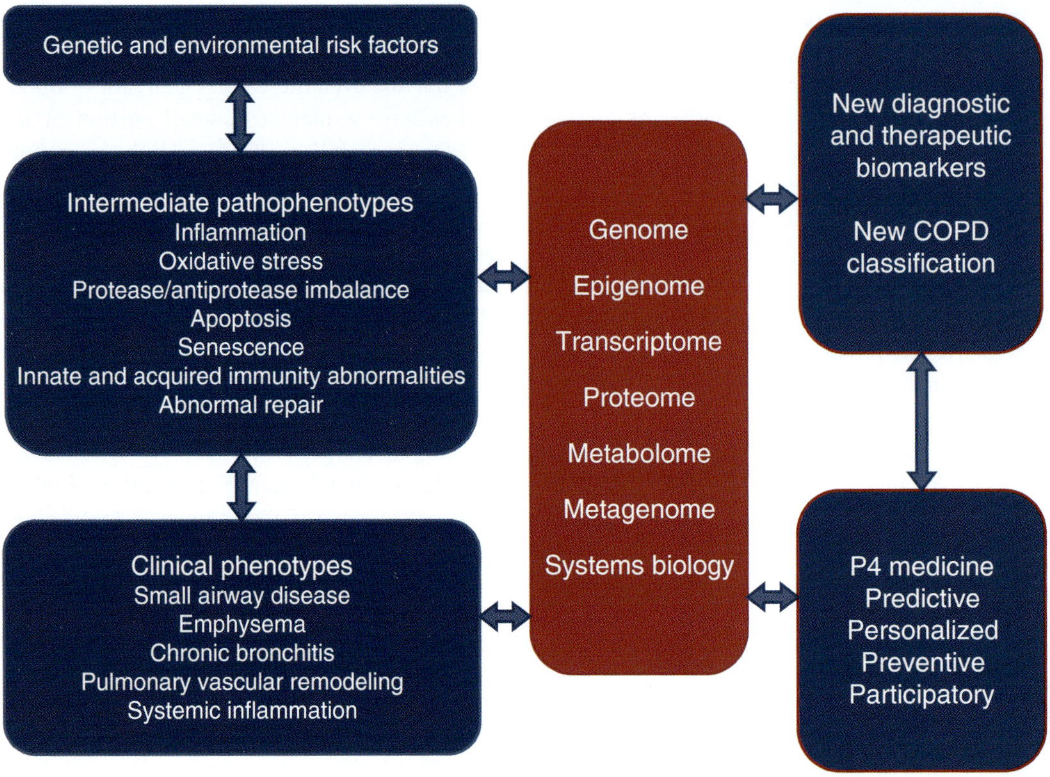

Fig. 20.2 The interaction between genetic and environmental factors leads to clinical phenotypes through intermediate pathophenotypes. Integrative analysis of multi-omics data may help us to discover new diagnostic and therapeutic biomarker and to develop personalized treatment. Reprinted with permission of the Springer (Park TS et al. Curr Respir Care Rep (2012) 1:189–198)

References

1. Sadee W, Dai Z. Pharmacogenetics/genomics and personalized medicine. Hum Mol Genet. 2005;14(2):R207–14.
2. FDA. Paving the way for personalized medicine. FDA's role in a new of medical product development; 2013.
3. FDA. Guidance for Industry: E15 definitions for genomic biomarkers, pharmacogenomics, pharmacogenetics, genomic data and sample coding categories; 2008.
4. Sequist LV, Bell DW, Lynch TJ, Haber DA. Molecular predictors of response to epidermal growth factor receptor antagonists in non-small-cell lung cancer. J Clin Oncol. 2007;25:587–95.
5. National Research Council (US) Committee on a Framework for Developing a New Taxonomy of Disease. Toward precision medicine: building a knowledge network for biomedical research and a new taxonomy of disease. Washington, DC: The National Academies Press; 2011.
6. The Academy of Medical Sciences. Realising the potential of stratified medicine. London: The Academy of Medical Sciences; 2013.
7. Park TS, Lee JS, Seo JB, Hong YK, Lee SW, Oh YM, Lee SD. Phenotyping of chronic obstructive pulmonary disease: heterogeneity and its clinical relevance. Curr Respir Care Rep. 2012;1:189–98.
8. Agusti A, Vestbo J. Current controversies and future perspectives in chronic obstructive pulmonary disease. Am J Respir Crit Care Med. 2011;184:507–13.
9. Agusti A, Sobradillo P, Celli B. Addressing the complexity of chronic obstructive pulmonary disease: from phenotypes and biomarkers to scale-free networks, systems biology, and P4 medicine. Am J Respir Crit Care Med. 2011;183:1129–37.
10. Pauwels RA, Buist AS, Calverley PM, Jenkins CR, Hurd SS. Global strategy for the diagnosis, management, and prevention of chronic obstructive pulmonary disease. NHLBI/WHO Global Initiative for chronic obstructive lung disease (GOLD) workshop summary. Am J Respir Crit Care Med. 2001 Apr;163(5):1256–76.
11. Rabe KF, Hurd S, Anzueto A, Barnes PJ, Buist SA, Calverley P, Fukuchi Y, Jenkins C, Rodriguez-Roisin R, van Weel C, Zielinski J, Global Initiative for Chronic Obstructive Lung Disease. Global strategy for the diagnosis, management, and prevention

of chronic obstructive pulmonary disease: GOLD executive summary. Am J Respir Crit Care Med. 2007;176:532–55.
12. Vestbo J, Hurd SS, Agusti AG, Jones PW, Vogelmeier C, Anzueto A, Barnes PJ, Fabbri LM, Martinez FJ, Nishimura M, Stockley RA, Sin DD, Rodriguez-Roisin R. Global strategy for the diagnosis, management, and prevention of chronic obstructive pulmonary disease: GOLD executive summary. Am J Respir Crit Care Med. 2013;187:347–65.
13. Agusti A. Chronic obstructive pulmonary disease: beyond the forced expiratory manoeuvre. Respiration. 2008;75:136–7.
14. Rennard SI, Vestbo J, Agusti A. What is chronic obstructive pulmonary disease anyway? Continua, categories, cut points, and moving beyond spirometry. Am J Respir Crit Care Med. 2013;187:1036–7.
15. Calverley PMA, Pauwels RA, Jones PW, Anderson JA, Vestbos J. The severity of airways obstruction as a determinant of treatment response in COPD. Int J Chron Obstruct Pulmon Dis. 2006;1:209–18.
16. Jenkins CR, Jones PW, Calverley PMA, et al. Efficacy of salmeterol/fluticasone propionate by GOLD stage of chronic obstructive pulmonary disease: analysis from the randomised, placebo-controlled TORCH study. Respir Res. 2009;10:59.
17. Han MK, Agusti A, Calverley PM, et al. Chronic obstructive pulmonary disease phenotypes: the future of COPD. Am J Respir Crit Care Med. 2010;182:598–604.
18. Friedlander AL, Lynch D, Dyar LA, et al. Phenotypes of chronic obstructive pulmonary disease. COPD. 2007;4:355–84.
19. Segreti A, Stirpe E, Rogliani P, Cazzola M. Defining phenotypes in COPD: an aid to personalized healthcare. Mol Diagn Ther. 2014;18(4):381–8.
20. Montuschi P, Malerba M, Santini G, Miravitlles M. Pharmacological treatment of chronic obstructive pulmonary disease: from evidence-based medicine to phenotyping. Drug Discov Today. 2014;19(12):1928–35.
21. Seemungal TAR, Donaldson GC, Bhowmik A, Jeffries DJ, Wedzicha JA. Time course and recovery of exacerbations in patients with chronic obstructive pulmonary disease. Am J Respir Crit Care Med. 2000;161:1608–13.
22. Wedzicha JA, Seemungal TAR. COPD exacerbations: defining their cause and prevention. Lancet. 2007;370:786–96.
23. Hurst JR, Vestbo J, Anzueto A, et al. Susceptibility to exacerbation in chronic obstructive pulmonary disease. N Engl J Med. 2010;363:1128–38.
24. Donaldson GC, Wedzicha JA. COPD exacerbations. I: epidemiology. Thorax. 2006;61:164–8.
25. Hurst JR, Wedzicha JA. Management and prevention of chronic obstructive pulmonary disease exacerbations: a state of the art review. BMC Med. 2009;7:40.
26. Falk JA, Minai OA, Mosenifar Z. Inhaled and systemic corticosteroids in chronic obstructive pulmonary disease. Proc Am Thorac Soc. 2008;5(4):506–12.
27. Patel IS, Seemungal TAR, Wilks M, Lloyd-Owen SJ, Donaldson GC, Wedzicha JA. Relationship between bacterial colonization and the frequency, character and severity of COPD exacerbations. Thorax. 2002;57:759–64.
28. Sethi S, Evans N, Grant BJ, Murphy TF. New strains of bacteria and exacerbations of chronic obstructive pulmonary disease. N Engl J Med. 2002;347:465–71.
29. Albert RK, Connett J, Bailey WC, Casaburi R, Cooper JA Jr, Criner GJ, et al. Azithromycin for prevention of exacerbations of COPD. N Engl J Med. 2011;365(8):689–98.
30. Lee JS, Park DA, Hong Y, Jo KW, Lee SW, Huh JW, Oh YM, Lee SD. Systematic review and meta-analysis of prophylactic antibiotics in COPD and/or chronic bronchitis. Int J Tuberc Lung Dis. 2013;72(2):153–62.
31. The definition of emphysema. Report of a National Heart, Lung, and Blood Institute, division of lung diseases workshop. Am Rev Respir Dis. 1985;132(1):182–5.
32. Friedman PJ. Imaging studyies in emphysema. Proc Am Thorac Soc. 2008;5:494–500.
33. Boschetto P, Miniati M, Miotto D, Braccioni F, De Rosa E, Bononi I, et al. Predominant emphysema phenotype in chronic obstructive pulmonary. Eur Respir J. 2003;21(3):450–4.
34. Kitaguchi Y, Fujimoto K, Kubo K, et al. Characteristics of COPD phenotypes classified according to the findings of HRCT. Respir Med. 2006;100:1742–52.
35. Lee JS, Ra SW, Chae EJ, Seo JB, Lim SY, Kim TH, Lee SD, Oh YM. Validation of the lower limit of normal diffusing capacity for detecting emphysema. Respiration. 2011;81:287–93.
36. Yuan R, Hogg JC, Pare PD, et al. Prediction of the rate of decline in FEV1 in smokers using quantitative computed tomography. Thorax. 2009;64:944–9.
37. Mahler DA, Harver A. A factor analysis of dyspnea ratings, respiratory muscle strength, and lung function in patients with chronic obstructive pulmonary disease. Am Rev Respir Dis. 1992;145:467–70.
38. Foglio K, Carone M, Pagani M, et al. Physiological and symptom determinants of exercise performance in patients with chronic airway obstruction. Respir Med. 2000;94:256–63.
39. Tashkin DP, Celli B, Decramer M, Liu D, Burkhart D, Cassino C, Kesten S. Bronchodilator responsiveness in patients with COPD. Eur Respir J. 2008;31:742–50.
40. Walker PP, Calverley PM. The volumetric response to bronchodilators in stable chronic obstructive pulmonary disease. COPD. 2008;5:147–52.
41. Lee JS, Huh JW, Chae EJ, Seo JB, Ra SW, Lee JH, Kim EK, Lee YK, et al. Response patterns to bronchodilator and quantitative computed tomography in chronic obstructive pulmonary disease. Clin Physiol Funct Imaging. 2012;32:12–8.
42. Lee JS, Huh JW, Chae EJ, et al. Predictors of pulmonary function response to treatment with salmeterol/

fluticasone in patients with chronic obstructive pulmonary disease. J Korean Med Sci. 2011;26:379–85.
43. Haruna A, Muro S, Nakano Y, et al. CT scan findings of emphysema predict mortality in COPD. Chest. 2010;138:635–40.
44. Martinez FJ, Foster G, Curtis JL, et al. Predictors of mortality in patients with emphysema and severe airflow obstruction. Am J Respir Crit Care Med. 2006;173:1326–34.
45. Fishman A, Martinez F, Naunheim K, et al. A randomized trial comparing lung-volume-reduction surgery with medical therapy for severe emphysema. N Engl J Med. 2003;348:2059–73.
46. Anonymous. Terminology, definitions, and classification of chronic pulmonary emphysema and related conditions. A report of the conclusions of a Ciba guest symposium. Thorax. 1959;14:286–99.
47. Vestbo J, Prescott E, Lange P. Association of chronic mucus hypersecretion with FEV1 decline and chronic obstructive pulmonary disease morbidity. Copenhagen City Heart Study Group. Am J Respir Crit Care Med. 1996;153:1530–5.
48. Pelkonen M, Notkola IL, Nissinen A, et al. Thirty-year cumulative incidence of chronic bronchitis and COPD in relation to 30-year pulmonary function and 40-year mortality: a follow-up in middle-aged rural men. Chest. 2006;130:1129–37.
49. Guerra S, Sherrill DL, Venker C, et al. Chronic bronchitis before age 50 years predicts incident airflow limitation and mortality risk. Thorax. 2009;64:894–900.
50. Kim V, Han MK, Vance GB, et al. The chronic bronchitic phenotype of COPD: an analysis of the COPDGene study. Chest. 2011;140:626–33.
51. Calverley PM, Rabe KF, Goehring UM, et al. Roflumilast in symptomatic chronic obstructive pulmonary disease: two randomized clinical trials. Lancet. 2009;374:685–94.
52. Lee SD, Hui DS, Mahayiddin AA, et al. Roflumilast in Asian patients with COPD: a randomized placebo-controlled trial. Respirology. 2011;16:1249–57.
53. Dransfield MT, Wilhelm AM, Flanagan B, et al. Acquired cystic fibrosis transmembrane conductance regulator dysfunction in the lower airways in COPD. Chest. 2013;144:498–506.
54. Lambert JA, Raju SV, Tang LP, et al. Cystic fibrosis transmembrane conductance regulator activation by roflumilast contributes to therapeutic benefit in chronic bronchitis. Am J Respir Cell Mol Biol. 2014;50:549–58.
55. Tarran R, Sabater JR, Clarke TC, et al. Nonantibiotic macrolides prevent human neutrophil elastase-induced mucus stasis and airway surface liquid volume depletion. Am J Physiol Lung Cell Mol Physiol. 2013;304:L746–56.
56. Decramer M, et al. Effects of N-acetylcysteine on outcomes in chronic obstructive pulmonary disease (bronchitis randomized on NAC cost-utility study, BRONCUS): a randomized placebo-controlled trial. Lancet. 2005;365:1552–60.
57. Zheng JP, et al. Effect of carbocisteine on acute exacerbation of chronic obstructive pulmonary disease (PEACE study): a randomised placebo-controlled study. Lancet. 2008;371:2013–8.
58. Global Initiative for Asthma. Global Strategy for Asthma Management and Prevention; 2014. www.ginasthma.com.
59. Jo KW, Ra SW, Chae EJ, et al. Three phenotypes of obstructive lung disease in the elderly. Int J Tuberc Lung Dis. 2010;14:1481–8.
60. Kim TB, YM O, Chang YS, et al. The reality of an intermediate type between asthma and COPD in practice. Respir Care. 2012;57(8):1248–53.
61. Soriano JB, Davis KJ, Coleman B, Visick G, Mannino D, Pride NB. The proportional Venn diagram of obstructive lung disease: two approximations from the United States and the United Kingdom. Chest. 2003;124(2):474–81.
62. Hardin M, Silverman EK, Barr RG, et al. The clinical features of the overlap between COPD and asthma. Respir Res. 2011;12:127.
63. Diaz-Guzman E, Khosravi M, Mannino DM. Asthma, chronic obstructive pulmonary disease, and mortality in the U.S. population. COPD. 2011;8:400–7.
64. Gibson PG, Simpson JL. The overlap syndrome of asthma and COPD: what are its features and how important is it? Thorax. 2009;64:728–35.
65. GINA-GOLD. Diagnosis of disease of chronic airflow limitation: asthma, COPD and asthma-COPD overlap syndrome (ACOS). www.goldcopd.org/asthma-copd-overlap.html.
66. Soler-Cataluna JJ, Cosio B, Izquierdo JL, Lopez-Campos JL, Marin JM, Aguero R. Consensus document on the overlap phenotype COPD-asthma in COPD. Arch Bronconeumol. 2012;48(9):331–7.
67. Kim MA, Noh CS, Chang YJ, Hong YK, Lee JS, Lee SW, Lee SD, Oh YM. Asthma and COPD overlap syndrome is associated with increased risk of hospitalisation. Int J Tuberc Lung Dis. 2015 Jul;19(7):864–9.
68. Menezes AM, de Oca MM, Pérez-Padilla R, et al. Increased risk of exacerbation and hospitalization in subjects with an overlap phenotype: COPD-asthma. Chest. 2014;145:297–304.
69. Chanez P, Vignola AM, O'Shaugnessy T, et al. Costicosteroid reversibility in COPD is related to features of asthma. Am J Respir Care Med. 1997;155:1529–34.
70. O'Donnell DE, Aaron S, Bourbeau J, Hernandez P, Marciniuk DD, Balter M. Canadian thoracic society recommendations for management of chronic obstructive pulmonary disease—2007 update. Can Respir J. 2007;14(Suppl B):5B–32B.
71. Kitaguchi Y, Komatsu Y, Fujimoto K, Hanaoka M, Kubo K. Sputum eosinophilia can predict responsiveness to inhaled corticosteroid treatment in patients with overlap syndrome of COPD and asthma. Int J Chron Obstr Pulm Dis. 2012;7:283–9.
72. Brightling CE, Monteiro W, Ward R, Parker D, Morgan MD, Wardlaw AJ, et al. Sputum eosinophilia

and short-term response to prednisolone in chronic obstructive pulmonary disease: a randomised controlled trial. Lancet. 2000;356(9240):1480–5.
73. Siva R, Green RH, Brightling CE, Shelley M, Hargadon B, McKenna S, et al. Eosinophilic airway inflammation and exacerbations of COPD: a randomised controlled trial. Eur Respir J. 2007;29(5):906–13.
74. Miravitlles M, Soler-Cataluna JJ, Calle M, Molina J, Almagro P, Quintano JA. Spanish COPD guidelines (GesEPOC): pharmacological treatment of stable COPD. Spanish Society of Pulmonology and Thoracic Surgery. Arch Bronconeumol. 2012;48(7):247–57.
75. Magnussen H, Bugnas B, van Noord J, Schmidt P, Gerken F, Kesten S. Improvements with tiotropium in COPD patients with concomitant asthma. Respir Med. 2008;102(1):50–6.
76. De Gruttola VG, Clax P, DeMets DL, Downing GJ, Ellenberg SS, Friedman L, Gail MH, Prentice R, Wittes J, Zeger SL. Considerations in the evaluation of surrogate endpoints in clinical trials. Summary of a national institutes of health workshop. Control Clin Trials. 2001;22:485–502.
77. Sin DD, Vestbo J. Biomarkers in chronic obstructive pulmonary disease. Proc Am Thorac Soc. 2009;6:543e5.
78. Pavord ID, Bafadel M. Exhaled nitric oxide and blood eosinophilia: independent markers of preventable risk. J Allergy Clin Immunol. 2013;132:828–9.
79. Price D, Ryan D, Burden A, et al. Using fractional exhaled nitric oxide (FeNO) to diagnose steroid-responsive disease and guide asthma management in routine care. Clin Transl Allergy. 2013;3:37.
80. Antus B, Barta I. Relationship between exhaled nitric oxide and the frequency of severe acute exacerbation of COPD: 3-year follow-up. Acta Physiol Hung. 2013;100:469–77.
81. Bazeghi N, Gerds TA, Budtz-Jørgensen E, Hove J, Vestbo J. Exhaled nitric oxide measure using multiple flows in clinically relevant subgroups of COPD. Respir Med. 2011;105:1338–44.
82. Kunisaki K, Rice K, Janoff E, Rector T, Niewoehner D. Exhaled nitric oxide, systemic inflammation, and the spirometric response to inhaled fluticasone propionate in severe chronic obstructive pulmonary disease: a prospective study. Ther Adv Respir Dis. 2008;2:55–64.
83. Bafadhel M, McKenna S, Terry S, Mistry V, Reid C, Haldar P, McCormick M, Haldar K, Kebadze T, Duvoix A. Acute exacerbations of chronic obstructive pulmonary disease: identification of biologic clusters and their biomarkers. Am J Respir Crit Care Med. 2011;184:662–71.
84. Hurst J. Exacerbation phenotyping in chronic obstructive pulmonary disease. Am J Respir Crit Care Med. 2011;184:625–6.
85. Bafadhel M, McKenna S, Terry S, et al. Blood eosinophils to direct corticosteroid treatment of exacerbations of chronic obstructive pulmonary disease: a randomized placebo-controlled trial. Am J Respir Crit Care Med. 2012;186:48–55.
86. Vollenweider DJ, Jarrett H, Steurer-Stey CA, Garcia-Aymerich J, Puhan MA. Antibiotics for exacerbations of chronic obstructive pulmonary disease. Cochrane Database Syst Rev. 2012;12:CD010257.
87. Christ-Crain M, Jaccard-Stolz D, Bingisser R, Gencay MM, Huber PR, Tamm M, Müller B. Effect of procalcitonin-guided treatment on antibiotic use and outcome in lower respiratory tract infections: cluster-randomised, single-blinded intervention trial. Lancet. 2004;363:600–7.
88. Bafadhel M, Clark TW, Reid C, Medina MJ, Batham S, Barer MR, Nicholson KG, Brightling CE. Procalcitonin and C-reactive protein in hospitalized adult patients with community-acquired pneumonia or exacerbation of asthma or COPD. Chest. 2011;139:1410–8.
89. Schuetz P, Christ-Crain M, Thomann R, Falconnier C, Wolbers M, Widmer I, Neidert S, Fricker T, Blum C, Schild U, et al. Effect of procalcitonin-based guidelines vs standard guidelines on antibiotic use in lower respiratory tract infections: the ProHOSP randomized controlled trial. JAMA. 2009;302:1059–66.
90. Galban CJ, Han MK, Boes JL, et al. Computed tomography-based biomarker provides unique signature for diagnosis of COPD phenotypes and disease progression. Nat Med. 2012;18:1711–5.
91. Lee JH, Lee YK, Kim EK, et al. Responses to inhaled long-acting beta-agnoist and corticosteroid according to COPD subtype. Respir Med. 2010;104:542–9.
92. Makita H, Nasuhara Y, Nagai K, Ito Y, Hasegawa M, Betsuyaku T, Onodera Y, Hizawa N, Nishimura M, Hokkaido COPD Cohort Study Group. Characterisation of phenotypes based on severity of emphysema in chronic obstructive pulmonary disease. Thorax. 2007;62:932–7.
93. Paré PD, Lawson LM, Brooks LA. Patterns of response to inhaled bronchodilators in asthmatics. Am Rev Respir Dis. 1983;127:680–5.
94. Cooper CB. The connection between chronic obstructive pulmonary disease symptoms and hyperinflation and its impact on exercise and function. Am J Med. 2006;119:S21–31.
95. Washko GR, Martinez FJ, Hoffman EA, Loring SH, Estepar RS, Diaz AA, Sciurba FC, Silverman EK, Han MK, Decamp M, Reilly JJ. National Emphysema Treatment Trial Research Group: physiological and computed tomographic predictors of outcome from lung volume reduction surgery. Am J Respir Crit Care Med. 2010;181:494–500.
96. Lee JS, Huh JW, Chae EJ, Seo JB, Ra SW, Lee JH, Kim EK, Lee YK, Kim TH, Kim WJ, Lee JH, Lee SM, Lee S, Lim SY, Shin TR, Yoon HI, Sheen SS, Oh YM, Lee SD. Different therapeutic responses in chronic obstructive pulmonary disease subgroups. Int J Tuberc Lung Dis. 2011;15:1104–10.
97. Coxson HO, Nasute Fauerbach PV, Storness-Bliss C, Muller NL, Cogswell S, Dillard DH, Finger CL, Springmeyer SC. Computed tomography assessment

of lung volume changes after bronchial valve treatment. Eur Respir J. 2008;32:1443–50.
98. Lieberman J, Winter B, Sastre A. α1-Antitrypsin Pi-types in 965 COPD patients. Chest. 1986;89(3):370–3.
99. Sandhaus RA, Turino G, Stocks J, et al. α1-Antitrypsin augmentation therapy for PI*MZ heterozygotes: a cautionary note. Chest. 2008;134(4):831–4.
100. Joos L, Weir TD, Connett JE, et al. Polymorphisms in the β2 adrenergic receptor and bronchodilator response, bronchial hyperresponsiveness, and rate of decline in lung function in smokers. Thorax. 2003;58(8):703–7.
101. Hizawa N, Makita H, Nasuhara Y, et al. β2-Adrenergic receptor genetic polymorphisms and short term bronchodilator responses in patients with COPD. Chest. 2007;132(5):1485–92.
102. Kim WJ, Oh YM, Sung J, et al. Lung function response to 12-week treatment with combined inhalationof long-acting β2 agonist and glucocorticoid according to *ADRB2* polymorphism in patients with chronic obstructive pulmonary disease. Lung. 2008;186(6):381–6.
103. Kim WJ, Hersh CP, DeMeo DL, Reilly JJ, Silverman EK. Genetic association analysis of COPD candidate genes with bronchodilator responsiveness. Respir Med. 2009;103(4):552–7.
104. Umeda N, Yoshikawa T, Kanazawa H, Hirata K, Fujimoto S. Association of β2-adrenoreceptor genotypes with bronchodilatory effect of tiotropium in COPD. Respirology. 2008;13(3):346–52.
105. Tantisira KG, Lake S, Silverman ES, et al. Corticosteroid pharmacogenetics: association of sequence variants in CRHR1 with improved lung function in asthmatics treated with inhaled corticosteroids. Hum Mol Genet. 2004;13(13):1353–9.
106. Kim WJ, Sheen SS, Kim TH, et al. Association between *CRHR1* polymorphism and improved lung function in response to inhaled corticosteroid in patients with COPD. Respirology. 2009;14(2):260–3.
107. Cho MH, McDonald ML, Zhou X, et al. Risk loci for chronic obstructive pulmonary disease: a genome-wide association study and meta-analysis. Lancet Respir Med. 2014;2(3):214–25.
108. Steiling K, van den Berge M, Hijazi K, Florido R, Campbell J, Liu G, Xiao J, Zhang X, Duclos G, Drizik E, et al. A dynamic bronchial airway gene expression signature of COPD and lung function impairment. Am J Respir Crit Care Med. 2013;187:933–42.
109. Kim WJ, Lim JH, Lee JS, Lee SD, Kim JH, Oh YM. Comprehensive analysis of transcriptome sequencing data in the lung tissues of COPD subjects. Int J Genomics. 2015;2015:206937.
110. van den Berge M, Steiling K, Timens W, Hiemstra PS, Sterk PJ, Heijink IH, Liu G, Alekseyev Y, Lenburg ME, Spira A, et al. Airway gene expression in COPD is dynamic with inhaled corticosteroid treatment and reflects biological pathways associated with disease activity. Thorax. 2013;187:933–42.
111. Silverman EK, Loscalzo J. Network medicine approaches to the genetics of complex diseases. Discov Med. 2012;14:143–52.

Part V

Prospectives

21 Cohort Study in COPD: Introduction to COPD Cohorts (The KOLD and COPDGene Study) and Collaborative Approaches

Deog Kyeom Kim

Introduction

COPD is a heterogeneous disease which is defined with the airflow limitation in spirometry irrespective of its causes. Despite the similar pathologic findings of chronic small airway inflammation and parenchymal destruction, COPD is regarded as an umbrella term containing heterogeneous clinical, radiographic, and physiological features, because patients with similar level of FEV_1 showed various clinical manifestations in the aspect of dyspnea, emphysema extent, exercise capacity, etc. [1] Heterogeneous phenotypes and even endotypes of COPD have been identified and characterized through various COPD cohort studies [2–4]. Therefore, our current knowledge on COPD can't be discussed without mentioning cohort studies.

In this part, the roles of COPD cohorts and what have been accomplished with them (e.g., COPDGene study (NCT00608764), KOLD study (Korean Obstructive Lung Disease), and ANOLD (Asian Network of Obstructive Lung Diseases) study) will be reviewed, and the needs for collaborative approaches in COPD study also should be discussed.

Cohort(s) in COPD Study

In a demographic study, "cohort" is a group of individuals having a statistical factor such as age or class membership in common. Traditionally, using the cohorts without epidemiological outcomes, we can compare the incidence and differences according to the presence of the "exposure" after passing the "time." It can indicate the temporal sequence between exposure and outcomes, and it allows to calculate the incidence of disease and enables examination of multiple outcomes. Nevertheless, cohort study is not easy to apply in clinical field in the limitations of large numbers of subjects for a long time, the high cost, time-consuming study, and bias such as differential loss to follow up.

In COPD studies, population-based observational cohorts such as birth cohorts are available but, as an expanded concept, the specific population including the disease, the common factor, COPD, is regarded as a cohort. Now, more commonly, study cohorts including patients COPD were established.

While observational cohorts including birth cohorts may have merits on identifying etiologic exposure and incidence of targeted disease, majority of currently active COPD cohorts including

D.K. Kim
Division of Pulmonary and Critical Care Medicine, Department of Internal Medicine, Seoul National University College of Medicine, SMG-SNU Boramae Medical Center, Seoul, South Korea
e-mail: kimdkmd@snu.ac.kr

S.-D. Lee (ed.), *COPD*, DOI 10.1007/978-3-662-47178-4_21

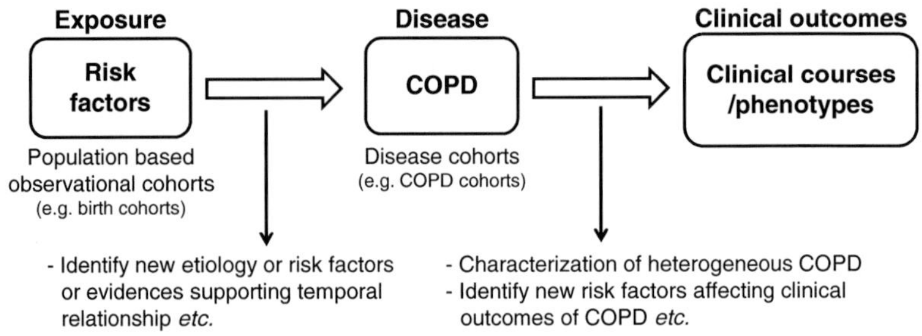

Fig. 21.1 Examples of the cohort in COPD study

COPDGene study (NCT00608764), ECLIPSE study (Evaluation of COPD Longitudinally to Identify Surrogate Endpoints), KOLD study, ANOLD study, etc. showed great outcomes in clarifying the clinical characteristics of COPD (i.e., phenotypes) as a COPD cohort itself (Fig. 21.1) and additionally combining case-control design and comparing with the healthy smokers, they revealed new findings contributing to the development and disease progression of COPD. Some cohorts such as lung health study (LHS, phase I, NCT00000568) and TESRA (Treatment of Emphysema With a Gamma-Selective Retinoid Agonist, NCT00413205) may be constructed being related to therapeutic interventions.

Examples of Representative COPD Cohorts: The Strength of Each Cohort

Until now, numerous COPD cohorts have been developed and each country tried to construct its original COPD cohort as the ethnical and environmental components may contribute to the development, progression, and heterogeneity of COPD [5]. Most of them are established in European and American countries. The COPDGene study and ECLIPSE study are representative cohorts in the number of recruited patients and their productivity in publication. Recently, some cohorts such as KOLD, ANOLD, and TCGS (Trans-Continental COPD Genetics) cohort recruiting Asian patients with COPD have been activated. Each cohort has some differential points from preexisting western cohorts according to the purpose of recruiting target population.

The KOLD Cohort

KOLD study is a well-organized Korean COPD cohort, and it is one of the leading long-term prospective cohort investigating heterogeneity of COPD in Asia. KOLD was activated to overcome the lack of prospective longitudinal cohort study of COPD in Asian countries, and it was aimed to clarify the heterogeneity of chronic obstructive airway disease [6]. It included the patients over 18 years of age with chronic respiratory symptoms as well as one or both of the criteria, airflow limitation (prebronchodilator $FEV_1/FVC < 0.7$) or bronchial hyper-responsiveness (measured with methacholine provocation test, $PC20 \leq 16$ mg/mL). Comparing with other western COPD cohorts, KOLD cohort did not use smoking history as inclusion criteria. Additionally, prebronchodilator FEV1/FVC ratio and bronchial hyper-responsiveness were adopted as inclusion criteria. As a result, it allows to recruit the patients with asthma and other unclassified obstructive lung disease including non-smoking COPD. They collected clinical samples (blood, DNA, and urine) and radiographic data (quantitative volumetric CT scan) as well as clinical data from 1117 patients with obstructive lung disease and 871 controls from 24 hospitals. Using this cohort, Korean researchers revealed the heterogeneity of COPD in terms of imaging parameters (e.g., airway dominant or emphysema dominant COPD) [7–9] and they showed that responses to inhaled corticosteroids and beta-agonist were different according to COPD subtype [10, 11]. This cohort study also suggested that "vascular type" of COPD associated with increased systolic pulmonary arterial pressure (sPAP) measured with echocardiography and the lower level of hemoglobin [10, 12].

KOLD cohort showed strengths in collecting and analyzing imaging data. Researchers in radiologic division of this cohort reported numerous articles relating to quantitative assessment of emphysema, air trapping, and airway thickening [9], slope of emphysema index [8], quantitative assessment of emphysema using dynamic contrast-enhanced magnetic resonance imaging, and texture-based quantification. The cohort enabled to perform genetic analysis and genomic study of COPD and the associated genes with COPD were validated in Korean patients with COPD [13–17].

In summary, KOLD cohort is the first large Korean COPD cohort and it identified the heterogeneity of COPD in phenotypes and therapeutic responses. New clinical, radiographic, and genomic studies can be performed in Korea through the KOLD cohort.

The COPDGene Cohort

The COPDGene study (http://www.copdgene.org/) is one of the largest studies to investigate the genetic factors of COPD. It is a multicenter observational study to identify genetic factors associated with COPD and characterize the phenotypes of COPD subjects by collecting CT images [18]. These phenotypes are used in a comprehensive genome-wide association studies GWAS to identify the susceptibility genes. This cross-sectional prospective cohort enrolled from 2008 to 2011 at 21 clinical centers in the USA. It plans for 4500 smoker controls (FEV1/FVC ratio $\geq$ 0.7, FEV1 $\geq$ 80% predicted) and 1500 GOLD 1 subjects and 4500 subjects in GOLD Stages 2–4 (1500 for each of the three GOLD stages) for a total of 10,500. Now, phase 2 study is ongoing. This large nationwide cohort reported more than 100 publications covering the characteristics of CT images in COPD in terms of emphysema, airway wall thickness, pulmonary vascular changes, and physiologic changes in COPD. This cohort extensively has been contributing to identify and validate the new genetic loci associated with COPD susceptibility [19–24] and other related characteristics such as low body mass index [21], radiographic findings [22, 25–28], clinical diagnosis of chronic bronchitis [29], and circulating biomarkers of COPD [19] as a developing cohort and validation cohort. Through COPDGene cohort, our knowledge on COPD phenotype and heterogeneity as well as susceptibility genetic loci has been expanded and various radiographic characterization of COPD could be achieved.

Next Steps in COPD Cohort Study: Collaborative Approaches

Needs for Collaborative Approaches in COPD Cohort Study

Even though many study cohorts have been established, there is some limitation in solving issues of clinical researches in COPD.

First of all, it is derived from the characteristics of COPD itself, i.e., heterogeneity of COPD. We now agree with that FEV_1 is not all of COPD. Patients with similar level of FEV_1 showed various clinical manifestations in terms of dyspnea, emphysema extent, exercise capacity, etc. Beyond smoking, there are also many other causes leading to COPD. Therefore, it is necessary to collect more people to cluster the subgroups and characterize specific features. As for example, in a single COPD cohort, various clinical subgroups (e.g., rapid lung function decliner, frequent exacerbator, bronchitis dominant COPD) and radiographic subgroups (e.g., emphysema dominant, small airway dominant) can be classified and larger study population will be necessary to clarify each characteristic.

Second, the limitations of traditional cohort study will require more cases. Larger number of subject is necessary to compensate the cases who are lost during follow-up and to achieve sufficient statistical power and even to validate or replicate the elucidated findings. This relationship between statistical power and required sample size is well described in GWAS study [30, 31]. In GWAS study, generally thousands of subjects will be necessary to differentiate the small effect of common genetic variants [32].

Third, many changes have been generalized in research fields. Technical advances in methodologies in research enable to perform collaborative studies more efficiently. Expansion of phenotypic information on COPD also contributes to the needs for collaborative researches.

In summary, based on the technical advances and expansion of our knowledge on COPD, a collaborative cohort study has become to be mandatory in COPD research area to overcome the heterogeneity of COPD and achieve the sufficient statistical power.

How Can We Collaborate in COPD Cohort Study?

Collaboration among cohort study can be activated entire the course of cohort study from designing the cohort to final analysis (Fig. 21.2).

In the step of designing and building a cohort, collaborative works can be initiated. The study design, target population, inclusion criteria, and methodology can be standardized and shared among collaborative researchers when the new collaborative cohort is activated. KOLD cohort and COPDGene cohort are the examples of nationwide collaborative cohort in Korea and the USA. Also international cooperation can build a new collaborative cohort such as ANOLD which is described in detail.

Another approach to build a collaborative cohort is to make a consortium of existing cohorts. This approach can make a large cohort more quickly because it will use the preexisting established cohorts. However, a variety of methodological issues including variable definition and measures can be an obstacle.

This approach has been already performed beyond COPD, and the international cancer genome consortium (https://icgc.org/) was established and enabled to find new genetic variants in the larger cohort. CHARGE (the Cohorts for Heart and Aging Research in Genomic Epidemiology) consortium is an example of a consortium to facilitate GWAS meta-analysis [33] and replication opportunities among multiple large population-based cohort studies. Recently, the NIH proposes to create a national cohort of at least one million Americans and with a central infrastructure, it may lead to harmonize data types and data collection and provide resources for explaining new scientific queries and develop new technologies.

There are some barriers and challenges in building a collaborative large cohort such as expense, time, feasibility, privacy, coordination, transparency, and governance. Therefore, a common infrastructure to bring together information from various studies is essential in the development and maintenance period of a collaborative cohort. Committees of COPDGene and KOLD cohort might play the role of minimizing the obstacles.

Additionally, the importance of effective communications should be emphasized to maintain the large cohort. Effective communications are essential within each cohort, between cohorts,

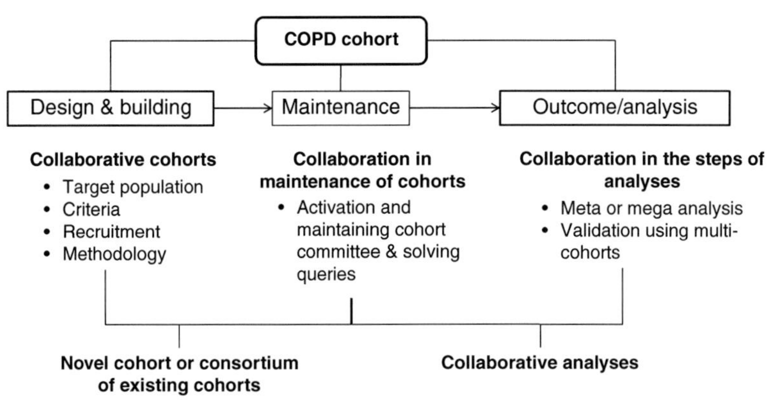

Fig. 21.2 Collaborative approaches in COPD cohort study

within the consortium working groups, and among the major consortium committees. Transparency, disclosure, and professional collaborative attitude of all investigators are critical for successful consortium.

Collaborative works can be performed in the step of analysis, and this collaboration is active in COPD genetic analysis. Meta-analysis or mega-analysis in COPD genomic study is an example of collaborative analysis. Major risk loci of COPD in GWAS was identified and validated in collaborative analysis in preexisting cohorts. Recently, Dr. Cho confirmed the three genetic loci including *CHRNA3, FAM13A,* and *HHIP* and identify the novel loci near *RIN3, MMP12*, and *TGFB2* by using the data from NETT, ICGN, ECLIPSE, and COPDGene cohorts. Dr. Cheng and Kim also reported AGER genetic variants associated with systemic biomarker of emphysema by collaborative analysis in different cohorts.

More ideally, collaborative analysis may be facilitated and can be more productive with sharing raw data of study cohorts.

Examples of Collaborative Cohort

ANOLD Cohort: A Novel International Collaborative Cohort

As better understanding COPD heterogeneity and overcoming COPD requires collaborative COPD research in various Asian countries, ANOLD, a collaborative Asian COPD cohort was constructed to characterize the COPD heterogeneity by genes, etiology, and clinical manifestations [34]. In Asia, risk factors for COPD such as high smoking prevalence, poverty, high prevalence of TB, and indoor air pollution including biomass are known to be more prevalent compared with western country; therefore, it would be necessary to paint an evolving COPD landscape for Asian countries. Beginning with 11 countries in 2008, now, 14 countries including South Korea, Japan, China, Taiwan, India, Malaysia, Thailand, Singapore, Philippines, Sri Lanka, Vietnam, and Hong Kong are participated. The collaborative findings from this cohort are published in 2013. It revealed that overall history of exposure to biomass fuel and dusty jobs were 32 and 44% and exposure to dusty job remained as an independent risk factor for chronic bronchitis after adjusting age, gender, GOLD grade, and city and diabetes mellitus was the most common comorbidity in this area. A recent analysis of 1022 patients from ten cities in ANOLD cohort showed three subtypes with distinct phenotypes by factor analysis—milder severity (59%), milder severity but more comorbidity (14%), and severe severity (27%). The phenotypes are distributed differentially by the region. This cohort is maintained in its phase 2 and more than 1500 patients from 14 sites were recruited and a centralized database in a research center in Asan Medical Center, Seoul, South Korea is responsible for quality control and governance of data. This cohort collected the longitudinal data on mortality, standardized lung imaging and blood DNA for genomic studies.

In summary, ANOLD cohort is a successful example of cooperative cohort which is constructed with a standardized protocol from many countries to identify the heterogeneity of COPD and region- or ethnic-specific contributing factors for COPD. It identified the characteristics of Asian COPD.

International COPD Genetics Consortium: A Consortium with Preexisting Cohorts

In the area of COPD genetic analysis, as GWAS can provide unbiased and comprehensive search for common susceptibility loci, GWAS-based genetic study changed the landscape of COPD genetics and it revealed new loci such as *HHIP, FAM13A*, and *IREB2* gene. Nevertheless, multiple additional COPD susceptibility genetic determinants may have not been identified in COPD, a complex disease as genetic polymorphism identified with GWAS showed small genetic effect and statistical power may not be achieved with a small population analysis. Therefore, as new single nucleotide polymorphisms (SNPs) were identified in Asian population by establishing the international lung cancer consortium and ENGAGE consortium, International COPD genetics consortium was proposed by Dr. Edwin Silverman in 2011 [32]. In this consortium, 38 study populations (20 case-control studies and 16 population-based cohort studies) have a much larger number of subjects more than 130,000 in total although each study recruited smaller number of subjects. Among them, about 14,700 cases and 37,600 controls have genome-wide SNP genotyping. Large fraction of studies included chest CT scan data and assessment of COPD exacerbation. This large COPD genetics consortium could improve the statistical power in genetic analysis and increased the chance to identify the new loci uncovered in smaller studies. Additionally, this cooperative approaches could provide a framework of future collaborative approaches and decrease the possibility of duplicated research efforts in COPD studies despite the limitation of variability of each study protocols and ethnic heterogeneity and difference in data platform.

Conclusion

COPD is a heterogeneous disease and we can't help admit that one single cohort can't solve the complex puzzle of COPD. Additionally, international human networking and methodological issues in cohort study are rapidly improving by technical development. Therefore, collaborative approaches in COPD cohort study are mandatory from the step of design/building to final analysis.

References

1. Agusti A. Systemic effects of chronic obstructive pulmonary disease: what we know and what we don't know (but should). Proc Am Thorac Soc. 2007;4:522–5.
2. Agusti A, Calverley PM, Celli B, Coxson HO, Edwards LD, Lomas DA, MacNee W, Miller BE, Rennard S, Silverman EK, Tal-Singer R, Wouters E, Yates JC, Vestbo J. Evaluation of CLtIPSEi. Characterisation of COPD heterogeneity in the ECLIPSE cohort. Respir Res. 2010;11:122.
3. Vestbo J, Agusti A, Wouters EF, Bakke P, Calverley PM, Celli B, Coxson H, Crim C, Edwards LD, Locantore N, Lomas DA, MacNee W, Miller B, Rennard SI, Silverman EK, Yates JC, Tal-Singer R. Evaluation of CLtIPSESI. Should we view chronic obstructive pulmonary disease differently after ECLIPSE? A clinical perspective from the study team. Am J Respir Crit Care Med. 2014;189:1022–30.
4. Rennard SI. The promise of observational studies (ECLIPSE, SPIROMICS, and COPDGene) in achieving the goal of personalized treatment of chronic obstructive pulmonary disease. Semin Respir Crit Care Med. 2015;36:478–90.
5. Han MK, Agusti A, Calverley PM, Celli BR, Criner G, Curtis JL, Fabbri LM, Goldin JG, Jones PW, Macnee W, Make BJ, Rabe KF, Rennard SI, Sciurba FC, Silverman EK, Vestbo J, Washko GR, Wouters EF, Martinez FJ. Chronic obstructive pulmonary disease phenotypes: the future of COPD. Am J Respir Crit Care Med. 2010;182:598–604.
6. Park TS, Lee JS, Seo JB, Hong Y, Yoo JW, Kang BJ, Lee SW, Oh YM, Lee SD, Group KS. Study design and outcomes of Korean Obstructive Lung Disease (KOLD) cohort study. Tuberc Respir Dis (Seoul). 2014;76:169–74.
7. Jo KW, Ra SW, Chae EJ, Seo JB, Kim NK, Lee JH, Kim EK, Lee YK, Kim TH, Huh JW, Kim WJ, Lee JH, Lee SM, Lim SY, Shin TR, Yoon HI, Sheen SS, Lee JS, Lee SD, Oh YM. Three phenotypes of obstructive lung disease in the elderly. Int J Tuberc Lung Dis. 2010;14:1481–8.
8. Chae EJ, Seo JB, Song JW, Kim N, Park BW, Lee YK, Oh YM, Lee SD, Lim SY. Slope of emphysema index: an objective descriptor of regional heterogeneity of emphysema and an independent determinant of pulmonary function. AJR Am J Roentgenol. 2010;194:W248–55.
9. Lee YK, Oh YM, Lee JH, Kim EK, Lee JH, Kim N, Seo JB, Lee SD, Group KS. Quantitative assessment of emphysema, air trapping, and airway thickening on computed tomography. Lung. 2008;186:157–65.
10. Lee JS, Huh JW, Chae EJ, Seo JB, Ra SW, Lee JH, Kim EK, Lee YK, Kim TH, Kim WJ, Lee JH, Lee SM, Lee S, Lim SY, Shin TR, Yoon HI, Sheen SS, Oh YM, Lee SD. Different therapeutic responses in chronic obstructive pulmonary disease subgroups. Int J Tuberc Lung Dis. 2011;15:1104–10.
11. Lee JH, Lee YK, Kim EK, Kim TH, Huh JW, Kim WJ, Lee JH, Lee SM, Lee S, Lim SY, Shin TR, Yoon HI, Sheen SS, Kim N, Seo JB, Oh YM, Lee SD. Responses to inhaled long-acting beta-agonist and corticosteroid according to COPD subtype. Respir Med. 2010;104:542–9.
12. Lee JH, Oh YM, Seo JB, Lee YK, Kim WJ, Sheen SS, Kim TH, Lee JH, Kim EK, Lee JS, Huh JW, Lim SY, Yoon HI, Shin TR, Lee SM, Lee SY, Lee SD. Pulmonary artery pressure in chronic obstructive pulmonary disease without resting hypoxaemia. Int J Tuberc Lung Dis. 2011;15:830–7.
13. Kim WJ, Lee MK, Shin C, Cho NH, Lee SD, Oh YM, Sung J. Genome-wide association studies identify locus on 6p21 influencing lung function in the Korean population. Respirology. 2014;19:360–8.
14. Kim WJ, Lim MN, Hong Y, Silverman EK, Lee JH, Jung BH, Ra SW, Choi HS, Jung YJ, Park YB, Park

MJ, Lee SW, Lee JS, Oh YM, Lee SD. Association of lung function genes with chronic obstructive pulmonary disease. Lung. 2014;192:473–80.
15. Kim WJ, Oh YM, Sung J, Kim TH, Huh JW, Jung H, Lee JH, Kim EK, Lee JH, Lee SM, Lee S, Lim SY, Shin TR, Yoon HI, Kwon SY, Lee SD. Lung function response to 12-week treatment with combined inhalation of long-acting beta2 agonist and glucocorticoid according to ADRB2 polymorphism in patients with chronic obstructive pulmonary disease. Lung. 2008;186:381–6.
16. Kim WJ, Oh YM, Sung J, Lee YK, Seo JB, Kim N, Kim TH, Huh JW, Lee JH, Kim EK, Lee JH, Lee SM, Lee S, Lim SY, Shin TR, Yoon HI, Kwon SY, Lee SD. CT scanning-based phenotypes vary with ADRB2 polymorphisms in chronic obstructive pulmonary disease. Respir Med. 2009;103:98–103.
17. Kim WJ, Sheen SS, Kim TH, Huh JW, Lee JH, Kim EK, Lee JH, Lee SM, Lee S, Lim SY, Shin TR, Yoon HI, Oh YM, Lee SD. Association between CRHR1 polymorphism and improved lung function in response to inhaled corticosteroid in patients with COPD. Respirology. 2009;14:260–3.
18. Regan EA, Hokanson JE, Murphy JR, Make B, Lynch DA, Beaty TH, Curran-Everett D, Silverman EK, Crapo JD. Genetic epidemiology of COPD (COPDGene) study design. COPD. 2010;7:32–43.
19. Kim DK, Cho MH, Hersh CP, Lomas DA, Miller BE, Kong X, Bakke P, Gulsvik A, Agusti A, Wouters E, Celli B, Coxson H, Vestbo J, MacNee W, Yates JC, Rennard S, Litonjua A, Qiu W, Beaty TH, Crapo JD, Riley JH, Tal-Singer R, Silverman EK, Eclipse I, Investigators CO. Genome-wide association analysis of blood biomarkers in chronic obstructive pulmonary disease. Am J Respir Crit Care Med. 2012;186:1238–47.
20. Kim DK, Hersh CP, Washko GR, Hokanson JE, Lynch DA, Newell JD, Murphy JR, Crapo JD, Silverman EK, Investigators CG. Epidemiology, radiology, and genetics of nicotine dependence in COPD. Respir Res. 2011;12:9.
21. Wan ES, Cho MH, Boutaoui N, Klanderman BJ, Sylvia JS, Ziniti JP, Won S, Lange C, Pillai SG, Anderson WH, Kong X, Lomas DA, Bakke PS, Gulsvik A, Regan EA, Murphy JR, Make BJ, Crapo JD, Wouters EF, Celli BR, Silverman EK, DeMeo DL, Evaluation of Chronic Obstructive Pulmonary Disease Longitudinally to Identify Predictive Surrogate E-P, Norway-Bergen C, National Emphysema Treatment T, investigators CG. Genome-wide association analysis of body mass in chronic obstructive pulmonary disease. Am J Respir Cell Mol Biol. 2011;45:304–10.
22. Kim WJ, Hoffman E, Reilly J, Hersh C, Demeo D, Washko G, Silverman EK. Association of COPD candidate genes with computed tomography emphysema and airway phenotypes in severe COPD. Eur Respir J. 2011;37:39–43.
23. Cho MH, Boutaoui N, Klanderman BJ, Sylvia JS, Ziniti JP, Hersh CP, DeMeo DL, Hunninghake GM, Litonjua AA, Sparrow D, Lange C, Won S, Murphy JR, Beaty TH, Regan EA, Make BJ, Hokanson JE, Crapo JD, Kong X, Anderson WH, Tal-Singer R, Lomas DA, Bakke P, Gulsvik A, Pillai SG, Silverman EK. Variants in FAM13A are associated with chronic obstructive pulmonary disease. Nat Genet. 2010;42:200–2.
24. Pillai SG, Ge D, Zhu G, Kong X, Shianna KV, Need AC, Feng S, Hersh CP, Bakke P, Gulsvik A, Ruppert A, Lodrup Carlsen KC, Roses A, Anderson W, Rennard SI, Lomas DA, Silverman EK, Goldstein DB, Investigators I. A genome-wide association study in chronic obstructive pulmonary disease (COPD): identification of two major susceptibility loci. PLoS Genet. 2009;5:e1000421.
25. Galban CJ, Han MK, Boes JL, Chughtai KA, Meyer CR, Johnson TD, Galban S, Rehemtulla A, Kazerooni EA, Martinez FJ, Ross BD. Computed tomography-based biomarker provides unique signature for diagnosis of COPD phenotypes and disease progression. Nat Med. 2012;18:1711–5.
26. Wells JM, Washko GR, Han MK, Abbas N, Nath H, Mamary AJ, Regan E, Bailey WC, Martinez FJ, Westfall E, Beaty TH, Curran-Everett D, Curtis JL, Hokanson JE, Lynch DA, Make BJ, Crapo JD, Silverman EK, Bowler RP, Dransfield MT, Investigators CO, Investigators ES. Pulmonary arterial enlargement and acute exacerbations of COPD. N Engl J Med. 2012;367:913–21.
27. Diaz AA, Come CE, Ross JC, San Jose Estepar R, Han MK, Loring SH, Silverman EK, Washko GR, Investigators CO. Association between airway caliber changes with lung inflation and emphysema assessed by volumetric CT scan in subjects with COPD. Chest. 2012;141:736–44.
28. Washko GR, Hunninghake GM, Fernandez IE, Nishino M, Okajima Y, Yamashiro T, Ross JC, Estepar RS, Lynch DA, Brehm JM, Andriole KP, Diaz AA, Khorasani R, D'Aco K, Sciurba FC, Silverman EK, Hatabu H, Rosas IO, Investigators CO. Lung volumes and emphysema in smokers with interstitial lung abnormalities. N Engl J Med. 2011;364:897–906.
29. Kim V, Han MK, Vance GB, Make BJ, Newell JD, Hokanson JE, Hersh CP, Stinson D, Silverman EK, Criner GJ, Investigators CO. The chronic bronchitic phenotype of COPD: an analysis of the COPDGene study. Chest. 2011;140:626–33.
30. Wain LV, Shrine N, Miller S, Jackson VE, Ntalla I, Artigas MS, Billington CK, Kheirallah AK, Allen R, Cook JP, Probert K, Obeidat M, Bosse Y, Hao K, Postma DS, Pare PD, Ramasamy A, Consortium UKBE, Magi R, Mihailov E, Reinmaa E, Melen E, O'Connell J, Frangou E, Delaneau O, OxGSKC, Freeman C, Petkova D, McCarthy M, Sayers I, Deloukas P, Hubbard R, Pavord I, Hansell AL, Thomson NC, Zeggini E, Morris AP, Marchini J, Strachan DP, Tobin MD, Hall IP. Novel insights into the genetics of smoking behaviour, lung function, and chronic obstructive pulmonary disease (UK

BiLEVE): a genetic association study in UK Biobank. Lancet Respir Med. 2015;3(10):769–81.
31. Moonesinghe R, Khoury MJ, Liu T, Ioannidis JP. Required sample size and nonreplicability thresholds for heterogeneous genetic associations. Proc Natl Acad Sci U S A. 2008;105:617–22.
32. Silverman EK, Vestbo J, Agusti A, Anderson W, Bakke PS, Barnes KC, Barr RG, Bleecker ER, Boezen HM, Burkart KM, Celli BR, Cho MH, Cookson WO, Croxton T, Daley D, DL DM, Gan W, Garcia-Aymerich J, Hall IP, Hansel NN, Hersh CP, Kalsheker N, Kiley JP, Kim WJ, Lambrechts D, Lee SD, Litonjua AA, Lomas DA, London SJ, Nishimura M, Nordestgaard BG, O'Donnell CJ, Postma DS, Puhan MA, Tesfaigzi Y, Tobin MD, Vogelmeier C, Wilk JB, Wouters E, Young RP, Ziegler-Heitbrock L, MacNee W, Crapo JD. Opportunities and challenges in the genetics of COPD 2010: an International COPD Genetics Conference report. COPD. 2011;8:121–35.
33. Psaty BM, Sitlani C. The ohorts for Heart and Aging Research in Genomic Epidemiology (CHARGE) Consortium as a model of collaborative science. Epidemiology. 2013;24:346–8.
34. Loh LC, Oh YM, Lee SD. The Asian Network for Obstructive Lung Disease (ANOLD)-COPD from an Asian perspective. QJM. 2015;108(12):921–2.

Big Data and Network Medicine in COPD

22

Edwin K. Silverman

Introduction

Personalized and precision medical care that is specific to an individual's disease subtype, stage, and comorbidities is an appropriate yet challenging goal for complex diseases like COPD [1]. Despite the well-documented need for improved treatment approaches in COPD, standard drug development strategies have been disappointingly slow and ineffective. This failure in therapeutic advances relates both to inadequate understanding of COPD pathogenesis and to traditional reductionist approaches to drug development which do not focus on the network of interacting genes and proteins that influence COPD susceptibility and severity. In this perspective, I will discuss the potential of Big Data and Network Medicine to provide progress in COPD diagnosis, prognosis, and treatment.

This work was supported by NIH Grants R01 HL089856, P01 HL105339, R01 HL113264, P01 HL114501, and R01 HL111759 to EKS.

E.K. Silverman, M.D., Ph.D.
Channing Division of Network Medicine, Brigham and Women's Hospital, Harvard Medical School, Boston, MA 02115, USA

Big Data: Can it Help Us to Understand COPD?

"Big Data" is a widely used buzz word in current medical research, but is there substance beyond the hype? Big Data provides substantial technical challenges related to organizing, moving, storing, and analyzing vast amounts of information [2]. Some scientific research areas, like astronomy and particle physics, have been dealing with the challenges of Big Data for many years [3]. In medical research, the exponentially increasing amounts of DNA sequencing data have driven much of the interest and concern about Big Data. Importantly, useful "Big Data" needs to be more than just a lot of data; it needs to have complex, accurate, and relevant information. We could weigh every grain of sand on a beach, but that would not provide a data set to help us to understand an ocean's ecological structure. Useful Big Data needs to include the right measurements of the right things at the right time.

Genetic research in COPD has already generated substantial amounts of Big Data. Over the past 30 years, COPD genetics research has undergone enormous changes, as the Human Genome Project and other large public resources have enabled genetic studies of unprecedented scope and power. In the 1980s, before single nucleotide polymorphism (SNP) genotyping was feasible, geneticists were limited to studies of familial aggregation and patterns of phenotype segregation in families. The era of short tandem repeat, or

S.-D. Lee (ed.), *COPD*, DOI 10.1007/978-3-662-47178-4_22

microsatellite, marker genotyping enabled linkage analysis studies in families; although several genomic regions with significant linkage to COPD and airflow obstruction were identified [4, 5], these studies did not lead to validated novel genetic determinants of COPD. The leading study design in COPD genetics today involves genome-wide association analysis (GWAS) [6] (Fig. 22.1), which typically requires genotyping hundreds of thousands of SNPs and statistical imputation of millions of other SNPs. These Big Data resources require careful quality control at both the level of the SNP marker and the subject. Since so many statistical tests are performed in GWAS, stringent levels of statistical significance (typically $p < 5 \times 10^{-8}$) are required to declare a genome-wide significant result. Large sample sizes, which may involve meta-analysis of multiple study populations, are often needed. Nonetheless, these Big Data approaches have led to the identification of eight genome-wide significant genomic regions for COPD and/or emphysema [7–11]. With the impending tsunami of data from whole exome and whole genome DNA sequencing, the challenges of Big Data management and analysis in COPD genetics will multiply.

Imaging, typically with chest CT scans, is another key source of Big Data in COPD research. Chest CT scanners provide a densitometric histogram of the lung, with very low density regions enriched for emphysema. Although chest CT scan information can be simplified using analytical approaches that assess the fraction of the lung below a designated density mask threshold (e.g., −950 HU), such approaches ignore much of the information about emphysema pattern and distribution within the CT scan. A Big Data approach to utilize chest CT scans more efficiently is based on the texture-based local histogram patterns related to different pathological types of

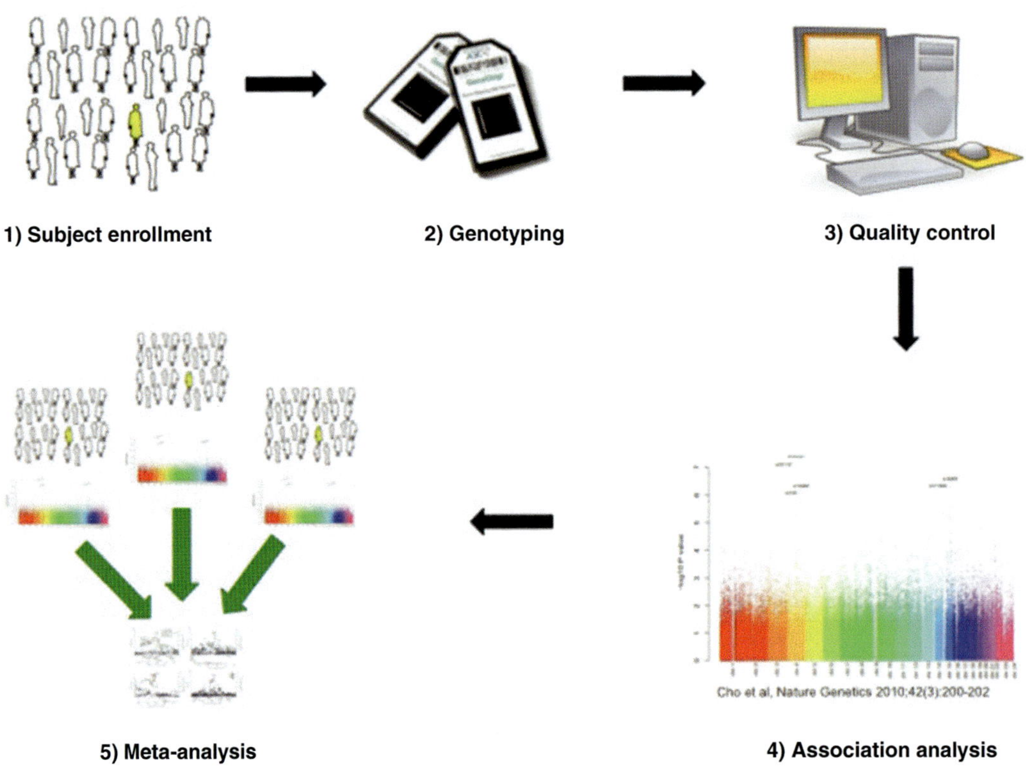

Fig. 22.1 *Approach for genome-wide association studies* [6]. After collecting DNA samples and phenotypic information from a study population, standard single nucleotide polymorphism (SNP) genotyping panels are tested. Quality control is performed at the level of both the subject and the SNP, and then statistical association between genotype and phenotype is assessed (typically with adjustment for genetic ancestry in case-control or population-based studies). In order to achieve genome-wide statistical significance, meta-analysis of multiple study populations is often required (From Hardin, J COPDF 2014, with permission)

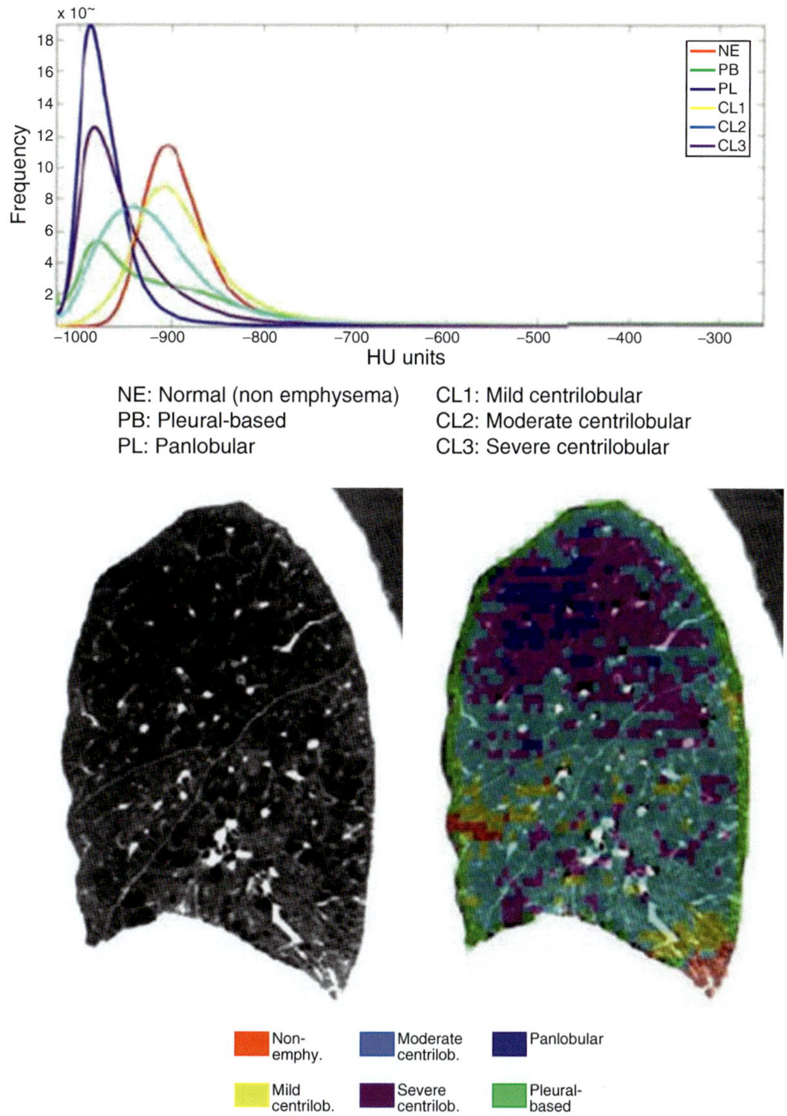

Fig. 22.2 *Texture-based assessment of emphysema* [12]. Emphysema patterns can be assessed by the local histogram pattern of densities within a region of interest on chest CT (From Castaldi, American Journal of Respiratory and Critical Care Medicine 2013; 188: 1083–90, with permission)

emphysema, such as centrilobular (graded as mild/moderate/severe) and panlobular emphysema [12] (Fig. 22.2). These local histogram patterns, which can be quantified using an automated pipeline, have stronger associations with clinically relevant COPD features than densitometrically defined emphysema. In addition, GWAS of these local histogram emphysema phenotypes led to the identification of novel genomic regions that met genome-wide significance [13].

In addition to genetics and imaging, transformative opportunities for COPD research are available based on technological advances in the generation of other types of Omics Big Data. Gene expression analysis has evolved from microarray assessment to RNA-Seq, which provides a more comprehensive view of transcriptional profiles, potentially including alternative splicing of the gene (leading to multiple isoforms of the same gene) and noncoding RNAs such as microRNA and other noncoding RNAs. For example, Ryan and colleagues have applied RNA-Seq to airway basal epithelial cells in seven healthy smokers and ten healthy nonsmokers [14]. They found large differences in gene expression between these groups, with significant enrichment for the differentially expressed genes located at the COPD and nicotine addiction GWAS region on chromosome 19q [15]. Kim and colleagues performed RNA-Seq in lung tissue samples from 98 COPD cases and 91 control subjects; they found 2312 differentially expressed genes, and they found evidence for significant dysregulation of the mitochondrial oxidative phosphorylation pathway in COPD subjects [16].

Metabolomics has evolved from assessment of small sets of known molecules to large panels of known metabolites and even to approaches that agnostically identify all small molecule metabolites in a biological sample. Telenga and colleagues studied a panel of more than 1500 lipids, a subset of the metabolome, in induced sputum samples from 19 COPD cases and 20 smoking controls [17]. They identified higher levels of multiple sphingolipids in the sputum samples from COPD cases, thus implicating sphingolipids as a potential biomarker of COPD. Subsequently, Bowler and colleagues performed a focused study of sphingolipids in plasma from 250 COPD cases and controls, and they found that multiple sphingomyelins were inversely associated with emphysema while trihexosylceramides were positively associated with COPD exacerbations [18].

Individual protein biomarkers have been studied in COPD for decades, with reasonable support for differences between COPD cases and controls for surfactant protein D [19], Club Cell Protein 16 [20], PARC [21], and fibrinogen [22]. sRAGE appears to be a useful biomarker for emphysema [23, 24]. Improvements in mass spectrometric approaches now can identify and quantify the proteome comprehensively; however, these Big Data approaches have had limited applications thus far in COPD research [25].

Finally, epigenetics, which involves genomic alterations that do not change the DNA nucleotide sequence, could be especially relevant for COPD since epigenetic marks may be induced by environmental exposures such as cigarette smoke. DNA methylation has been studied using microarray approaches, and methylation marks have been identified that differ between COPD cases and controls; in addition, methylation marks related to cigarette smoking have been found which gradually revert toward the nonsmoking pattern after smoking cessation [26, 27]. DNA sequencing approaches to methylation analysis (methylseq) have the potential to provide more comprehensive assessments of DNA methylation changes.

Network Medicine and COPD

Although genetics, imaging, and other Omics provide Big Data resources for COPD research, our analytical approaches to these data types need to evolve to meet the opportunities provided. Standard association analyses in epidemiology and genetics relate a single outcome to a predictor variable of interest, using approaches like multiple linear regression for quantitative outcomes and logistic regression for categorical outcomes. Multivariable models allow incorporation of multiple predictor variables, but assumptions about linear relationships persist. Interactions are typically either ignored or analyzed in a simplistic manner by including cross-product terms in the regression analysis. Methods to recognize and quantify nonlinear relationships and interactions will be essential to derive the maximal benefit from Big Data in COPD.

Network science provides approaches that can assist in the analysis of Big Data in complex diseases like COPD. Based on graph theory, networks provide a useful structure to visualize and analyze relationships—both linear and nonlinear—between variables of interest. The network is composed of entities, represented by nodes, and edges, which indicate a relationship between the nodes (Fig. 22.3). For example, in a social network, the nodes can represent individual people, and the edges can represent whether there is a specific type of relationship between those two people. In a protein–protein interaction network, the nodes represent individual proteins and an edge is placed if there is a physical interaction between those two proteins (e.g., yeast 2-hybrid assay). While in a gene coexpression network, the nodes represent the mRNA level of a specific gene, and edges are placed if a statistically significant correlation between those expression levels is identified. In addition to visualizing relationships between nodes, properties of the network such as the number of connections to different nodes can provide important information about network structure and response to perturbations. The multiple interactions encoded within networks can lead to network responses to perturbation that cannot be predicted from studying isolated nodes or pairs of nodes; these complex responses are referred to as emergent properties.

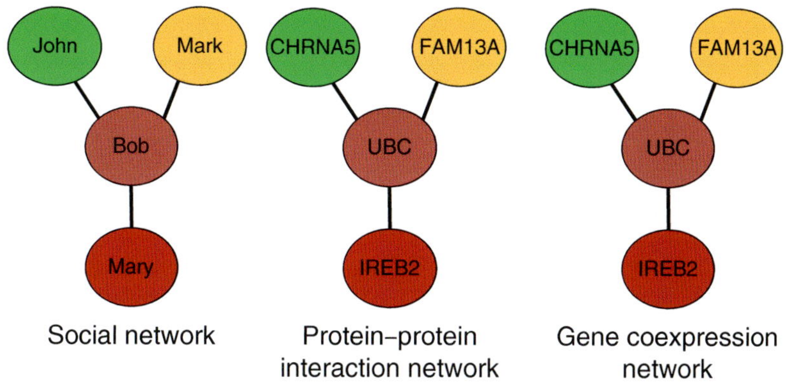

Fig. 22.3 *Examples of different types of networks.* In a social network, nodes represent people, and the edges connecting nodes represent a relationship (e.g., friendship). In a protein–protein interaction network, nodes represent proteins, and edges are placed if a physical interaction is demonstrated between proteins (e.g., yeast 2-hybrid assay, tandem affinity purification assay). The gene coexpression network, which in this case looks identical to the protein–protein interaction network, includes mRNA levels as nodes and edges if correlations between expression levels exceed a set threshold

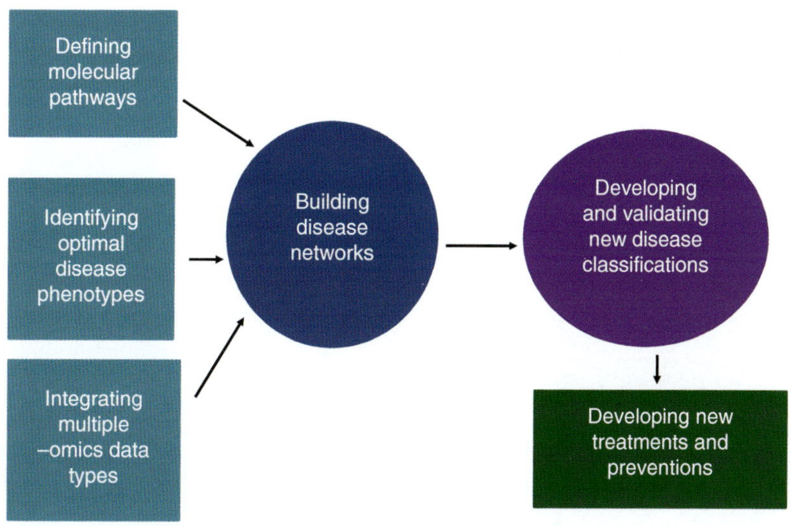

Fig. 22.4 *Network Medicine approaches to complex diseases.* The key activities required to apply Network Medicine to complex diseases like COPD

When network science approaches are applied to diseases, the term "Network Medicine" has been used [28, 29]. Network Medicine is not limited to a single type of network or a single source of data. The approaches envisioned for the developing field of Network Medicine are shown in Fig. 22.4. Since many molecular pathways remain poorly defined, creating a molecular wiring diagram of these pathways and interactions is an important part of Network Medicine. Defining optimal disease phenotypes, based on imaging, physiological, and clinical assessments, is required. Measuring and integrating multiple Omics data types is a key part of Network Medicine. These three approaches are utilized to define disease-related networks. These disease-related networks will be utilized to reclassify diseases like COPD based on their etiology instead of end-stage physiological and pathological manifestations—our current approach for classifying most diseases. Finally, new treatments and preventative strategies will be developed using systems pharmacology approaches. Although this road map for Network Medicine has great potential, substantial methodological and technical advances will be needed to turn it from aspiration to reality.

A variety of specific network types are utilized in Network Medicine. Protein–protein interactions within the cellular molecular interactome [30] have been utilized to identify interconnected subsets of the interactome related to specific diseases, known as disease modules. One approach to identify such disease modules is based on genetic association evidence. Using the dmGWAS method [31], McDonald and colleagues found a consensus module for COPD within the protein–protein interaction network that was enriched in IL7 pathway members [32]. Correlation networks based on gene expression levels can identify gene modules based on similar gene expression patterns, using approaches like weighted gene coexpression network analysis [33]. Gene regulatory networks have been developed based on relating transcription factor binding site information and gene expression levels using approaches such as PANDA [34]. PANDA analysis of mice heterozygous for deficiency of the *Hhip* COPD GWAS gene demonstrated network rewiring related to the Klf4 transcription factor [35].

Networks of clinical and imaging phenotypes can also be built; by using partial correlations, the edges in such phenotypic networks represent pairwise effects adjusted for all of the other network relationships [36]. Comparisons between the phenotypic networks created in different groups of subjects can potentially identify key differences between those subjects. In Fig. 22.5, the differences in phenotypic

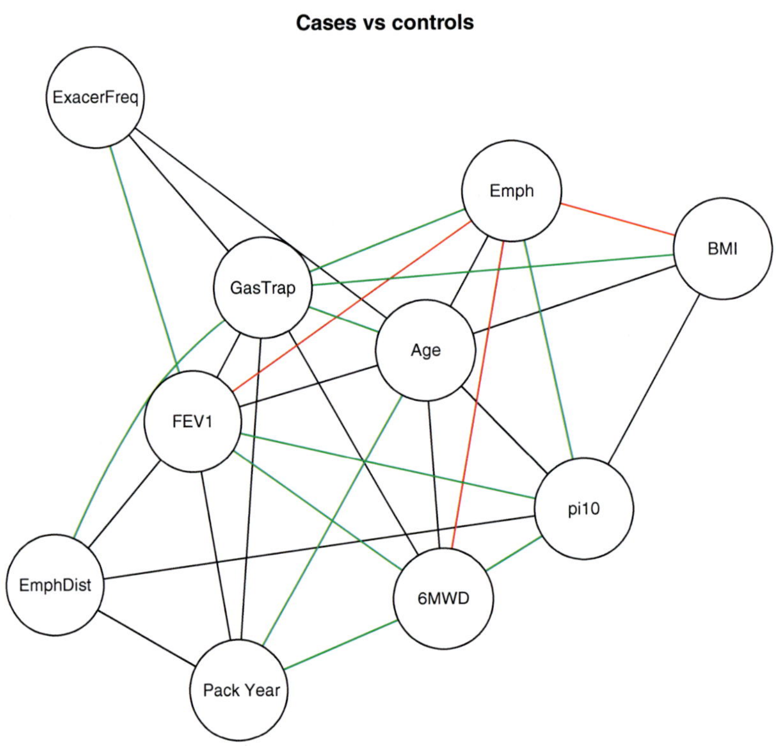

Fig. 22.5 *Comparing phenotypic networks in COPD cases and smoking controls* [36]. Partial correlation-based phenotypic networks were generated in 8141 COPDGene subjects. Differences in the network structure between COPD cases and controls were assessed by permutation analysis. Edges in *green* were seen in both COPD and control networks, with the same direction of correlation. Edges in *black* were seen in one group only. Edges in *red* were seen in both COPD cases and controls, but with opposite signs in those networks. Abbreviations include: *Emph* quantitative emphysema on chest CT at −950 HU, *BMI* body mass index, FEV_1 forced expiratory volume in 1 s, *Pack-year* smoking intensity in pack-years, *GasTrap* gas trapping at −856 HU on expiratory chest CT scan, *EmphDist* emphysema distribution in upper vs. lower thirds of the lung, *ExacerFreq* frequency of COPD exacerbations in the year before enrollment, *6MWD* 6-min walk distance, *pi10* square root of wall area of hypothetical 10 mm internal perimeter airway. (From Chu, BMC Systems Biology 2014; 8: 78, with permission)

relationships between COPD cases and control smokers in the COPDGene study are shown in a phenotypic network. A small number of edges, such as the relationship between emphysema and body mass index, are opposite in sign between COPD cases and smoking controls, pointing to potentially interesting biological differences. This inverse relationship makes biological sense, since increased emphysema is seen with lower BMI in severe COPD cases, while in subjects without substantial emphysema the increased radiation noise due to higher body mass could artifactually increase the amount of measured "emphysema" in subjects with high BMI.

The modeling approaches described above can be thought of as "top down" efforts to use Big Data to identify disease-related networks. However, "bottom up" approaches to build disease networks by identifying the biological mechanisms and pathway members for well-established COPD susceptibility genes like *SERPINA1*, *HHIP*, and *FAM13A* can also be used to create disease networks. Ideally, the top down and bottom up approaches can be used synergistically to identify the set of key molecules involved in COPD pathogenesis.

Potential of Integrative Research Approaches in COPD

As highlighted throughout this book, COPD is a heterogeneous syndrome rather than a single disease entity. Thus, it is not surprising that genome-wide association studies of the presence/absence of COPD, which we have described as First Generation Genetic Studies [37] (Fig. 22.6), have required large sample sizes and only accounted for a small percentage of the genetic contribution to COPD susceptibility. Second Generation Genetic Studies, which focus on identifying genetic determinants of an Omics data type like a gene expression level, require substantially smaller samples to find genetic associations to an Omics level, but subsequently still need to be linked to disease pathogenesis. With Network Medicine and

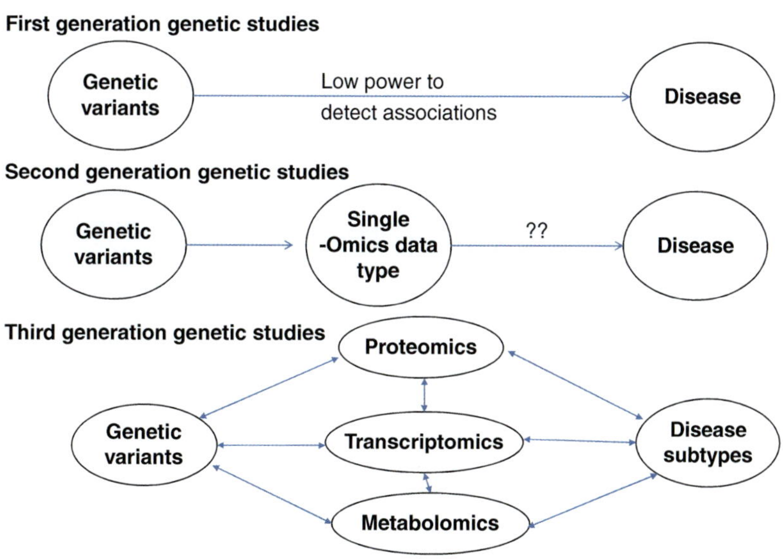

Fig. 22.6 *Evolution of complex disease genetic studies* [37]. First Generation Genetic Studies involve efforts to link genetic variants directly to disease. In Second Generation Genetic Studies, genetic association is assessed for an Omics data type, such as a gene expression, protein, or metabolite level. In Third Generation Genetic Studies, an integrated analysis of multiple Omics data types with genetic variants is performed in a network framework, with recognition of phenotypic heterogeneity (From Silverman/Loscalzo, Discovery Med 2012; 14: 143, with permission)

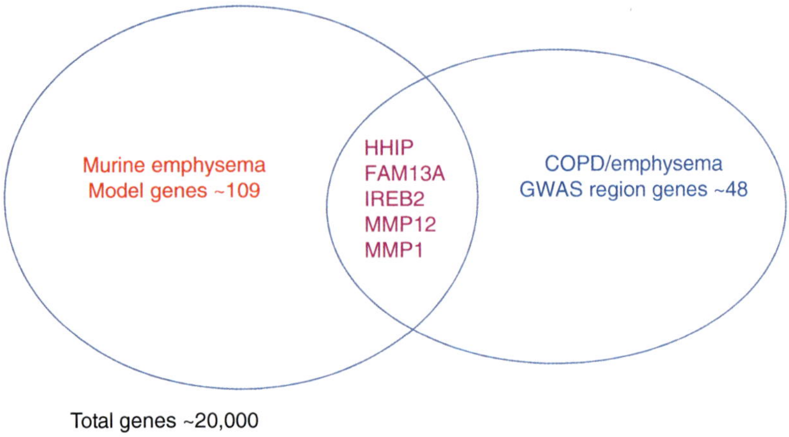

Fig. 22.7 *Overlap of murine emphysema model genes and COPD GWAS region genes*. Of approximately 20,000 mammalian genes, only five are located in both COPD genome-wide association regions and have been supported by a murine model of emphysema (e.g., transgenic, knockout)

Big Data, we can move toward Third Generation Genetic Studies, which will integrate multiple types of Omics data in a network framework, along with efforts to subtype COPD.

The identification of COPD subtypes—distinct groups of COPD subjects with different disease etiologies—will be essential to Third Generation Genetic Studies. Machine learning approaches [38] like unsupervised cluster analysis can be useful tools in this process. Based on four clinically relevant variables (FEV_1, % emphysema on CT, emphysema distribution in the upper vs. lower third of the lungs, and airway wall thickness), Castaldi and colleagues identified four clusters of subjects: resistant smokers, mild upper lobe predominant emphysema, airway-predominant disease, and severe destructive emphysema [39]. Of interest, the effect size for genetic association of several known COPD GWAS loci, such as *HHIP* and the chromosome 15q25 locus which includes *IREB2* and *CHRNA3/5*, was increased in specific clusters. Thus, identifying more phenotypically homogeneous groups of subjects may increase the magnitude of genetic effects observed. Future subtyping studies that integrate multiple Omics data have the potential to identify subjects with similar disease etiology more effectively.

Integration of multiple types of Big Data will be essential for Third Generation Genetic Studies. Leveraging both Omics and animal model experimental data can overcome the limitations of an individual method. A PubMed search identified about 109 genes that have been implicated in murine models of emphysema based on knock-outs or transgenics (Fig. 22.7). Thus, there are many ways to perturb the lungs that can lead to emphysema in a mouse. However, only a fraction of these potential perturbations are likely to be relevant for human COPD. In COPD GWAS studies, eight genomic regions have been significantly associated with COPD and/or emphysema. Some of these regions contain only a single gene while others contain multiple genes—approximately 48 genes are located within the eight COPD/emphysema GWAS loci; identifying the key gene within GWAS regions is a major challenge. Among the 109 murine emphysema genes and 48 COPD GWAS region genes, there are five overlapping genes: *HHIP* [35], *FAM13A* [40], *IREB2* [41], *MMP1* [42], and *MMP12* [43]. These five genes, supported by independent research approaches, have the greatest potential to play a key role in COPD pathogenesis. As more COPD GWAS and murine emphysema genes are detected, the number of such genes supporting by both approaches will increase.

The Future of COPD Research

How can we effectively manage and integrate the deluge of Big Data using Network Medicine and other advanced analytical approaches? We envision parallel efforts in Omics analysis of biological

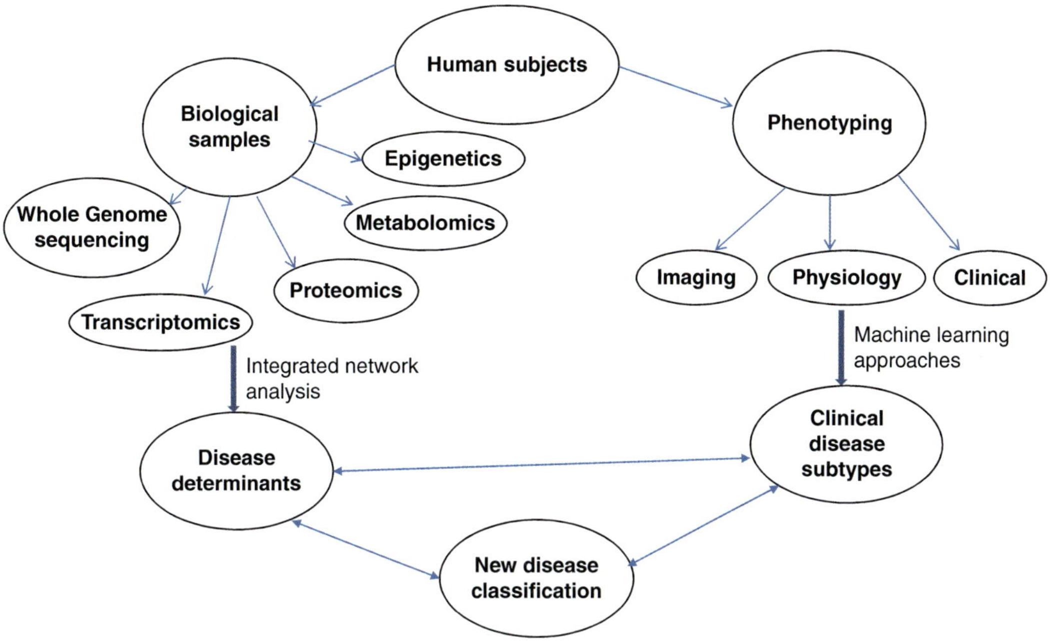

Fig. 22.8 *Reclassifying COPD using Network Medicine* [37]. Parallel efforts in phenotypic assessment using clinical, imaging, and physiological approaches and in genetics and other Omics approaches to identify disease determinants will be combined to reclassify COPD based on etiology. (Modified from Silverman/Loscalzo, Discovery Medicine 2012; 14: 143, with permission)

samples and clinical phenotyping data (Fig. 22.8). Clinical phenotyping will involve assessment of imaging, physiological, and other clinical information using machine learning and network analysis methods as well as standard epidemiological approaches. Omics analyses of biological samples will include genetics (ultimately with whole genome sequencing), transcriptomics, metabolomics, proteomics, and epigenetics in an integrated network framework to identify COPD molecular determinants. Using an iterative process that incorporates both molecular determinants and clinical subtypes, disease classification based on etiology could result, leading to more precise diagnosis, more accurate prognostic information, and more effective targeted therapies.

In order to make this vision come to reality, substantial changes in how we perform medical research will be required. Assessment of comprehensive Omics data is often viewed pejoratively as hypothesis-free "fishing expeditions" while focusing on a few selected genes, proteins, or metabolites is deemed to define a higher yield set of experiments that are testing focused hypotheses. I beg to differ with this perspective. Comprehensive Omics-based assessments still must test hypotheses, but they can test broad hypotheses: "Comprehensive metabolomic assessment will identify metabolites associated with COPD" instead of "Metabolite X is associated with COPD." Why is the broader approach better? We have experienced this dichotomy directly through the Candidate Gene Era of genetic association studies, which preceded the current era of genome-wide association studies. In the Candidate Gene Era for COPD (similar tales could be told for essentially every other complex disease), dozens of well-chosen biological candidates were associated with COPD case-control status in one study but not replicated in others, leading to a chaotic medical literature. In retrospect, the Candidate Gene Era studies suffered from small sample sizes and a variety of other problems [44], but a key challenge was that by only focusing on a small number of genetic variants in a specific manuscript, a genome-wide adjustment for multiple statistical testing was not performed (if any adjustment for multiple statistical testing was included)—resulting in many false-positive results. The realities were that our ability to select biologically important candidate genes was (and is) embarrassingly poor, and since the study population would typically be used for many different focused candidate gene studies, a genome-wide adjustment for multiple testing would have been much more appropriate. We do not need to relive this futile experience with the other Omics data types; we can leverage the technological advances that have made comprehensive Omics analysis feasible and use the appropriate analytical strategies for them.

There are a variety of other key research directions to explore that will involve Big Data and/or Network Medicine. Although COPD is often described as being caused by genetics and environmental exposures, we need to recognize that COPD is also potentially influenced by stochastic and dynamic effects—it develops in a developmental context within each patient. We also need to consider how to test for the effects of genetic, environmental, and developmental processes beyond differences in mean values; disease manifestations could also be influenced by factors that alter molecular variability. Genetic determinants of cell-to-cell variability in gene expression levels have been identified in yeast [45], and similar human genetic determinants could lead to differences in the "noise" levels of gene expression that could influence disease risk.

As we dissect COPD heterogeneity and understand the networks of interacting biological factors that are related to different COPD subtypes, new approaches to disease treatment will be required. Since COPD is a syndrome rather than a single disease, treatment for patients with different disease subtypes should reflect that heterogeneity. In addition, we will need to move away from efforts to identify single key molecular targets for disease treatment; multiple targets may need to be treated, potentially in a dynamic fashion. The intriguing results from Lee and colleagues [46] in triple negative breast cancer cell lines, in which only sequential treatment with an EGRF inhibitor followed by a DNA damaging chemotherapeutic agent caused effective killing of these breast cancer cells, could provide a key lesson for benign diseases like COPD as well. Restructuring the approaches for COPD drug development and testing would be required for this systems pharmacology-based approach [47], with Omics read-outs of potential drug efficacy [48].

In sum, Big Data and Network Medicine have the potential to transform the diagnosis and treatment of COPD. However, to realize the potential of these exciting opportunities, we will need to restructure the way we study the pathogenesis of COPD and the approaches that we utilize to develop new COPD treatments.

Acknowledgements The author thanks Dawn DeMeo, Craig Hersh, Peter Castaldi, and Michael Cho for helpful comments on this manuscript.

Conflict of Interest Statement In the past 3 years, Edwin K. Silverman received honoraria and consulting fees from Merck, grant support and consulting fees from GlaxoSmithKline, and honoraria from Novartis.

References

1. Agusti A, Anto JM, Auffray C, Barbe F, Barreiro E, Dorca J, et al. Personalized respiratory medicine: exploring the horizon, addressing the issues. Summary of a BRN-AJRCCM workshop held in Barcelona on June 12, 2014. Am J Respir Crit Care Med. 2015;191(4):391–401.
2. Marx V. Biology: the big challenges of big data. Nature. 2013;498(7453):255–60.
3. Stephens ZD, Lee SY, Faghri F, Campbell RH, Zhai C, Efron MJ, et al. Big data: Astronomical or Genomical? PLoS Biol. 2015;13(7):e1002195.
4. Silverman EK, Mosley JD, Palmer LJ, Barth M, Senter JM, Brown A, et al. Genome-wide linkage analysis of severe, early-onset chronic obstructive pulmonary disease: airflow obstruction and chronic bronchitis phenotypes. Hum Mol Genet. 2002;11(6):623–32.
5. Silverman EK, Palmer LJ, Mosley JD, Barth M, Senter JM, Brown A, et al. Genomewide linkage analysis of quantitative spirometric phenotypes in severe early-onset chronic obstructive pulmonary disease. Am J Hum Genet. 2002;70(5):1229–39.
6. Hardin M, Silverman EK. Chronic obstructive pulmonary disease genetics: a review of the past and a look into the future. J COPD Found. 2014;1(1):33–46.
7. Cho MH, McDonald ML, Zhou X, Mattheisen M, Castaldi PJ, Hersh CP, et al. Risk loci for chronic obstructive pulmonary disease: a genome-wide association study and meta-analysis. Lancet Respir Med. 2014;2(3):214–25.

8. Cho MH, Boutaoui N, Klanderman BJ, Sylvia JS, Ziniti JP, Hersh CP, et al. Variants in FAM13A are associated with chronic obstructive pulmonary disease. Nat Genet. 2010;42:200–2.
9. Cho MH, Castaldi PJ, Hersh CP, Hobbs BD, Barr RG, Tal-Singer R, et al. A genome-wide association study of emphysema and airway quantitative imaging phenotypes. Am J Respir Crit Care Med. 2015;192(5):559–69.
10. Pillai SG, Ge D, Zhu G, Kong X, Shianna KV, Need AC, et al. A genome-wide association study in chronic obstructive pulmonary disease (COPD): identification of two major susceptibility loci. PLoS Genet. 2009;5(3):e1000421.
11. Wilk JB, Chen TH, Gottlieb DJ, Walter RE, Nagle MW, Brandler BJ, et al. A genome-wide association study of pulmonary function measures in the Framingham Heart Study. PLoS Genet. 2009;5(3):e1000429.
12. Castaldi PJ, San Jose Estepar R, Mendoza CS, Hersh CP, Laird N, Crapo JD, et al. Distinct quantitative computed tomography emphysema patterns are associated with physiology and function in smokers. Am J Respir Crit Care Med. 2013;188(9):1083–90.
13. Castaldi PJ, Cho MH, San Jose Estepar R, McDonald ML, Laird N, Beaty TH, et al. Genome-wide association identifies regulatory loci associated with distinct local histogram emphysema patterns. Am J Respir Crit Care Med. 2014;190(4):399–409.
14. Ryan DM, Vincent TL, Salit J, Walters MS, Agosto-Perez F, Shaykhiev R, et al. Smoking dysregulates the human airway basal cell transcriptome at COPD risk locus 19q13.2. PLoS One. 2014;9(2):e88051.
15. Cho MH, Castaldi PJ, Wan ES, Siedlinski M, Hersh CP, Demeo DL, et al. A genome-wide association study of COPD identifies a susceptibility locus on chromosome 19q13. Hum Mol Genet. 2012;21(4):947–57.
16. Kim WJ, Lim JH, Lee JS, Lee SD, Kim JH, Oh YM. Comprehensive analysis of transcriptome sequencing data in the lung tissues of COPD subjects. Int J Genomics. 2015;2015:9.
17. Telenga ED, Hoffmann RF, Ruben TK, Hoonhorst SJ, Willemse BW, van Oosterhout AJ, et al. Untargeted lipidomic analysis in chronic obstructive pulmonary disease. Uncovering sphingolipids. Am J Respir Crit Care Med. 2014;190(2):155–64.
18. Bowler RP, Jacobson S, Cruickshank C, Hughes GJ, Siska C, Ory DS, et al. Plasma sphingolipids associated with chronic obstructive pulmonary disease phenotypes. Am J Respir Crit Care Med. 2015;191(3):275–84.
19. Lomas DA, Silverman EK, Edwards LD, Locantore NW, Miller BE, Horstman DH, et al. Serum surfactant protein D is steroid sensitive and associated with exacerbations of COPD. Eur Respir J. 2009;34(1):95–102.
20. Lomas DA, Silverman EK, Edwards LD, Miller BE, Coxson HO, Tal-Singer R. Evaluation of serum CC-16 as a biomarker for COPD in the ECLIPSE cohort. Thorax. 2008;63(12):1058–63.
21. Sin DD, Miller BE, Duvoix A, Man SF, Zhang X, Silverman EK, et al. Serum PARC/CCL-18 concentrations and health outcomes in chronic obstructive pulmonary disease. Am J Respir Crit Care Med. 2011;183(9):1187–92.
22. Duvoix A, Dickens J, Haq I, Mannino D, Miller B, Tal-Singer R, et al. Blood fibrinogen as a biomarker of chronic obstructive pulmonary disease. Thorax. 2013;68(7):670–6.
23. Yonchuk JG, Silverman EK, Bowler R, Agusti A, Lomas DA, Miller BE, et al. Circulating sRAGE as a biomarker of emphysema and the RAGE Axis in the lung. Am J Respir Crit Care Med. 2015;192(7):785–92.
24. Cheng DT, Kim DK, Cockayne DA, Belousov A, Bitter H, Cho MH, et al. Systemic soluble receptor for advanced glycation endproducts is a biomarker of emphysema and associated with AGER genetic variants in patients with chronic obstructive pulmonary disease. Am J Respir Crit Care Med. 2013;188(8):948–57.
25. Terracciano R, Pelaia G, Preiano M, Savino R. Asthma and COPD proteomics: current approaches and future directions. Proteomics Clin Appl. 2015;9(1–2):203–20.
26. Wan ES, Qiu W, Baccarelli A, Carey VJ, Bacherman H, Rennard SI, et al. Cigarette smoking behaviors and time since quitting are associated with differential DNA methylation across the human genome. Hum Mol Genet. 2012;21(13):3073–82.
27. Qiu W, Baccarelli A, Carey VJ, Boutaoui N, Bacherman H, Klanderman B, et al. Variable DNA methylation is associated with chronic obstructive pulmonary disease and lung function. Am J Respir Crit Care Med. 2012;185(4):373–81.
28. Barabasi AL. Network medicine--from obesity to the "diseasome". N Engl J Med. 2007;357(4):404–7.
29. Barabasi AL, Gulbahce N, Loscalzo J. Network medicine: a network-based approach to human disease. Nat Rev Genet. 2011;12(1):56–68.
30. Vidal M, Cusick ME, Barabasi AL. Interactome networks and human disease. Cell. 2011;144(6):986–98.
31. Jia P, Zheng S, Long J, Zheng W, Zhao Z. dmGWAS: dense module searching for genome-wide association studies in protein-protein interaction networks. Bioinformatics. 2011;27(1):95–102.
32. McDonald ML, Mattheisen M, Cho M, Liu Y-Y, Harshfield B, Hersh C, et al. Beyond GWAS in COPD: probing the landscape between gene-set associations, genome-wide associations and protein-protein interaction networks. Hum Hered. 2014;78:131–9.
33. Langfelder P, Horvath S. WGCNA: an R package for weighted correlation network analysis. BMC Bioinformatics. 2008;9:559.
34. Glass K, Huttenhower C, Quackenbush J, Yuan GC. Passing messages between biological networks to refine predicted interactions. PLoS One. 2013;8(5):e64832.
35. Lao T, Glass K, Qiu W, Polverino F, Gupta K, Morrow J, et al. Haploinsufficiency of hedgehog interacting protein causes increased emphysema induced by cigarette smoke through network rewiring. Genome Med. 2015;7(1):12.

36. Chu JH, Hersh CP, Castaldi PJ, Cho MH, Raby BA, Laird N, et al. Analyzing networks of phenotypes in complex diseases: methodology and applications in COPD. BMC Syst Biol. 2014;8:78.
37. Silverman EK, Loscalzo J. Network medicine approaches to the genetics of complex diseases. Discov Med. 2012;14(75):143–52.
38. Jordan MI, Mitchell TM. Machine learning: trends, perspectives, and prospects. Science. 2015;349(6245):255–60.
39. Castaldi PJ, Dy J, Ross J, Chang Y, Washko GR, Curran-Everett D, et al. Cluster analysis in the COPDGene study identifies subtypes of smokers with distinct patterns of airway disease and emphysema. Thorax. 2014;69(5):415–22.
40. Jiang Z, et al. A chronic obstructive pulmonary disease susceptibility gene, FAM13A, regulates protein stability of b-catenin. Am J Resp Crit Care Med 2016;194:185–97.
41. Cloonan SM, et al. Mitochondrial iron chelation ameliorates cigarette smoke-induced bronchitis and emphysema in mice. Nature Medicine 2016;22:163–74.
42. D'Armiento J, Dalal SS, Okada Y, Berg RA, Chada K. Collagenase expression in the lungs of transgenic mice causes pulmonary emphysema. Cell. 1992;71(6):955–61.
43. Hautamaki RD, Kobayashi DK, Senior RM, Shapiro SD. Requirement for macrophage elastase for cigarette smoke-induced emphysema in mice. Science. 1997;277:2002–4.
44. Hersh CP, Demeo DL, Lange C, Litonjua AA, Reilly JJ, Kwiatkowski D, et al. Attempted replication of reported chronic obstructive pulmonary disease candidate gene associations. Am J Respir Cell Mol Biol. 2005;33(1):71–8.
45. Ansel J, Bottin H, Rodriguez-Beltran C, Damon C, Nagarajan M, Fehrmann S, et al. Cell-to-cell stochastic variation in gene expression is a complex genetic trait. PLoS Genet. 2008;4(4):e1000049.
46. Lee MJ, Ye AS, Gardino AK, Heijink AM, Sorger PK, MacBeath G, et al. Sequential application of anticancer drugs enhances cell death by rewiring apoptotic signaling networks. Cell. 2012;149(4):780–94.
47. Sorger PK, Allerheiligen SRB, Abernethy DR, Altman RB, Brouwer KLR, Califano A, et al. Quantitative and systems pharmacology in the post-genomic era: new approaches to discovering drugs and understanding therapeutic mechanisms. October 2011. Report No.
48. Silverman EK, Loscalzo J. Developing new drug treatments in the era of network medicine. Clin Pharmacol Ther. 2013;93(1):26–8.

Index

S.-D. Lee (ed.), *COPD*, DOI 10.1007/978-3-662-47178-4

R

S